ESSENTIALS *of* RADIOLOGY

ESSENTIALS *of* RADIOLOGY

Second Edition

Fred A. Mettler, Jr., M.D., M.P.H
Department of Radiology
New Mexico Federal Regional Medical Center
and
Professor
University of New Mexico
School of Medicine
Health Sciences Center
Albuquerque, New Mexico

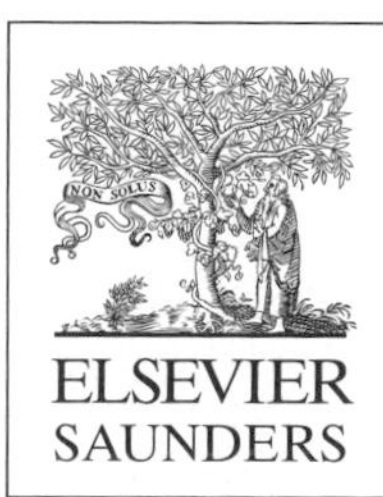

ELSEVIER
SAUNDERS

The Curtis Center
170 S. Independence Mall W. 300 E.
Philadelphia, Pennsylvania 19106-3399

ESSENTIALS OF RADIOLOGY ISBN 0–7216–0527–3

NOTICE

Radiology is an ever-changing field. Standard safety precautions must be followed, but as new research and clinical experience broaden our knowledge, changes in treatment and drug therapy may become necessary or appropriate. Readers are advised to check the most current product information provided by the manufacturer of each drug to be administered to verify the recommended dose, the method and duration of administration, and contraindications. It is the responsibility of the treating physician, relying on experience and knowledge of the patient, to determine dosages and the best treatment for each individual patient. Neither the Publisher nor the editor assumes any liability for any injury and/or damage to persons or property arising from this publication.

The Publisher

Library of Congress Cataloging-in-Publication Data
Mettler, Fred A.
Essentials of radiology / Fred A. Mettler, Jr.—2nd ed.
p.; cm.
Includes bibliographical references and index.
ISBN 0–7216–0527–3
1. Radiography, Medical. I. Title.
[DNLM: 1. Radiography—methods. WN 445 M595eb 2004]
RC78.M397 2005
616.07′57—dc22

2004041764

Printed in the United States of America

Last digit is the print number: 9 8 7 6 5 4 3 2 1

Preface (Second Edition)

Radiology receives little attention in most medical school curricula except perhaps as an elective. This is astonishing given that the physician most commonly encounters human internal anatomy and function through radiology. Physicians must be well grounded in the essentials of imaging to properly care for their patients. Some authors have argued the need for "imaging literacy." I hope this text can contribute to such a goal.

With a basic text containing fundamentals, one might wonder why a second edition would be needed. Even though many aspects of radiology have remained unchanged over the last decade, rapid and significant changes have occurred in both technology and applications. Radiology over the last century relied predominantly on film as the image receptor. Now images are commonly obtained, interpreted, transmitted, and stored in digital format. As with digital cameras, film is becoming a thing of the past. These changes will not be immediately apparent to the reader of this text. Access to digital images is much more convenient. Chest x-rays often appear on computers in intensive care units and, to the great relief of medical students, interns, and residents, little time will be lost in tracking down films. Indeed, there is much less reason for a physician to visit the radiology department. In-person consultations with radiologists are becoming less frequent. Greater expertise in radiology will be required as medical students, residents, and others will be interpreting digital images at sites remote from the radiology department.

Uses of computed tomography (CT) scanning have significantly expanded. CT scanners have evolved from single-slice, rather slow, machines to helical 16-slice scanners capable of imaging large portions of the body in a matter of a few seconds. Applications that previously could not be performed, because of patient or organ motion, now are no problem. In addition to procedures allowed by the new technology, much more clinical experience has been gained. CT scans have largely replaced intravenous pyelograms (IVPs) for evaluation of renal or ureteral stones, and CT has become a mainstay in the diagnosis of many abdominal, pelvic, and retroperitoneal pathologies (e.g., appendicitis). CT scans are rapidly replacing most plain films of the abdomen.

In nuclear medicine, rapid growth has been seen in positron emission tomography (PET) scanning. The most common applications are for evaluation and staging of neoplasms. Even the boundary between radiology and nuclear medicine has become blurred with the advent of hybrid CT/PET scanners.

The major changes to the second edition of *Essentials of Radiology* are an increased emphasis on CT scanning and PET imaging. Information has been added on the appropriate workup of common clinical problems such as headache, hypertension, and low back pain. I have endeavored to include this information without expanding the total volume of the text and yet retaining the essentials. Because readers often have questions about the cost and radiation dose associated with common examintations, this information has been retained in the appendix.

Fred A. Mettler, Jr.

Preface (First Edition)

Writing a basic textbook on medical imaging is a daunting task. There are, of course, many radiologists who have walked down this path before. Some have been much more successful than others.

The challenge comes from a basic question: "What should be included in such a book?" The answer depends on the intended audience. I have spent many hours interviewing medical students and entry-level residents in departments other than radiology about what they did and did not like about the many radiology textbooks currently available. The most common complaint was that most books written by radiologists address what radiologists think is important, rather than answering the questions faced by nonradiologists engaged in daily patient care.

After many hours of deliberation, three criteria were chosen to govern what should be included here. The first criterion was the inclusion of normal images and common variants. A clinician needs to be able to recognize and differentiate abnormal from normal on frequently done examinations. The second criterion was that clinicians be able to identify abnormalities that are common in day-to-day practice. The third criterion was that life-threatening abnormalities, even if somewhat rare, be included.

A large number of excellent images were collected and then put aside, because the pathology was quite rare, easily visible, or not immediately important to patient care. For such cases the clinician will seek out a radiologist for consultation. I have included selected examples of techniques (such as angioplasty, magnetic resonance imaging, and so on) to indicate what the radiologist's armamentarium has to offer clinicians.

Educators, medical students, and residents have encouraged me to include more images, tables, and differential diagnoses, and at the same time to make the text relatively brief. They also have asked that common terminology (such as *chest x-ray* instead of *chest radiograph*) be used. Whether all these aims have been met successfully, only time will tell.

Fred A. Mettler, Jr.

Acknowledgments (Second Edition)

I thank Ruth Ann Bump and Daniel Sandoval for their help in preparing the figures and Dr. Michael Hartshorne for allowing me the academic time to work on the book.

Contents

1 Introduction

AN APPROACH TO IMAGE INTERPRETATION

The first step in medical imaging is to examine the patient and determine the possible cause of his or her problem. Only after this is done can you decide which imaging study is the most appropriate. A vast number of algorithms or guidelines have been developed, but no consensus exists on the "right" one for a given symptom or disease because a number of imaging modalities have similar sensitivities and specificities. In this text, I have chosen to give you my opinion on the initial study to order in a specific clinical setting.

What should you expect from an imaging examination? Typically, one expects to find the exact location of a problem and hopes to make the diagnosis. Although some diseases present a very characteristic picture, most can appear in a variety of forms depending on the stage. As a result, image interpretation will yield a differential diagnosis that must be placed in the context of the clinical findings.

Examination of images requires a logical approach. First you must understand the type of image, the orientation, and the limitations of the technique used. For example, I begin by mentally stating, "I am looking at a coronal computed tomography (CT) scan of the head done with intravenous contrast." This is important, because intravenous contrast can be confused with fresh blood in the brain.

Next I look at the name and age on the film label to avoid mixing up patients, and it allows making a differential diagnosis that applies to a patient of that age and sex. You would not believe the number of times that this seemingly minor step will keep you from making very dumb mistakes.

The next step is to determine the abnormal findings on the image. This means that you need to know the normal anatomy and variants of that particular part of the body as well as their appearance on the imaging technique used. After this, you should describe the abnormal areas, because it will help you mentally to order a differential diagnosis. The most common mistake is to look at an abnormal image and immediately to name a disease. When you do this, you will find your mind locked on that diagnosis (often the wrong one). It is better to say to yourself something like, "I am going to give a differential diagnosis of generalized cardiac enlargement with normal pulmonary vasculature in a 40-year-old male," rather than to blurt out "viral cardiomyopathy" in a patient who really has a malignant pericardial effusion.

After practicing for 20 years or so, a radiologist knows the spots where pathology most commonly is visualized. Throughout this text, I point out the high-yield areas for the different examinations. Although no absolute rules exist, knowing the pathology and natural history of different diseases will help you. For example, if you are interested in hyperparathyroidism, a film of the hands may be all that is needed, because bone resorption is likely to occur there first. When you have the hand film, the optimal place to look is on the radial aspect of the middle phalanges.

After reviewing the common causes of the x-ray findings that you have observed, you should reorder the etiologies in light of the clinical findings. At this point, you probably think that you are finished. Not so. Often a plethora of information is contained in the patient's film jacket or in the hospital computer information system. This comes in the form of previous findings and histories supplied for the patient's other imaging examinations. Reviewing the old reports has directed me to areas of pathology on the current film that I would have missed if I had not looked into the medical information system. A simple example is a pneumonia that has almost but not completely resolved or a pulmonary nodule that, because of inspiratory difference, is hiding behind a rib on the current examination.

You probably think that you are finished now. Wrong again. A certain number of entities could cause the findings on the image, but you just have not thought of them all. After I have finished looking at a case, I try to go through a set sequence of categories in search of other differential possibilities. The categories I use are congenital, physical/chemical, infectious, neoplastic, metabolic, circulatory, and miscellaneous.

X-RAY

Regular x-rays (plain x-rays) account for about 80% of imaging examinations. X-ray examinations, or plain x-rays, are made by an x-ray beam passing through the patient. The x-rays are absorbed in different amounts by the various tissues or materials in the body. Most of the beam is absorbed or scattered. This represents deposition of energy in the tissue but does not cause the patient to become radioactive or to emit radiation. A small percentage of the incident radiation beam exits the patient and strikes a detector.

The classic imaging receptor is a film/screen combination. The x-ray beam strikes a fluorescent screen, which produces light that exposes the film, and then the film is developed. Newer systems are called *computed radiography* or *digital radiography*. In computed radiography, the x-rays strike a plate that absorbs the x-rays and stores the energy at a specific location. The plate is then scanned by a laser, which releases a point of light from the plate. The location is detected and stored in a computer. In digital radiography detector systems, the x-ray hits a detector and then is converted to light immediately. Once either type of image is stored in the computer, it can be displayed on a monitor for interpretation or transmitted to remote locations for viewing.

Four basic densities, or shades, are visible on plain films. These are air, fat, water (blood and soft tissue), and bone. Air is black or very dark. On x-rays, fat is generally gray and darker than muscle or blood (Fig. 1-1). Bone and calcium appear almost white. Items that contain metal (such as prosthetic hips) and contrast agents also appear white. The contrast agents generally used are barium for most gastrointestinal stud-

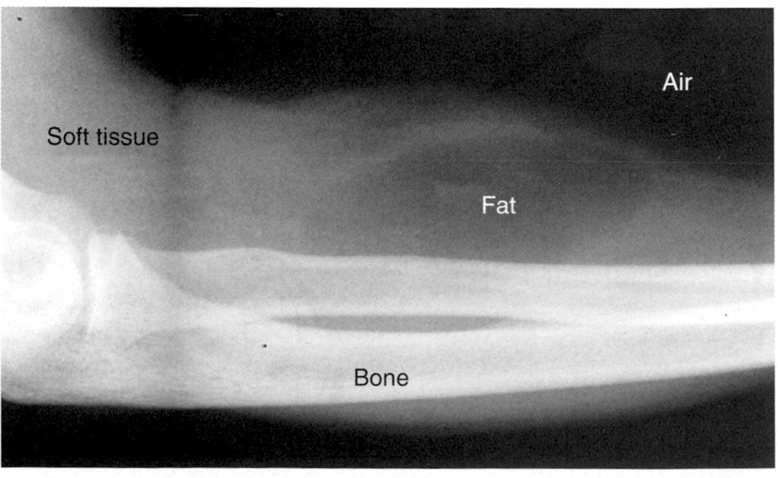

FIGURE 1-1 ■ The four basic densities on an x-ray. A lateral view of the forearm shows that the bones are the densest, or white; soft tissue is gray; fat is somewhat dark; and air is very dark. The abnormality in this case is the fat in the soft tissue of the forearm, which is due to a lipoma.

ies and iodine for most intravenously administered agents.

Remember that standard or plain x-rays are two-dimensional presentations of three-dimensional information. That is why frontal and lateral views are often needed. Without these, mistakes can easily be made. You must remember that an object visualized on a specific view is somewhere in the path of the x-ray beam (not necessarily in the patient). If an object projects outside the patient on any view, it is outside the patient. However, even if an object projects within the patient on two orthogonal views, it can still be located outside the patient. (Figs. 1-2 and 1-3). Each additional view needed to make a diagnosis requires an additional x-ray exposure and therefore adds to the patient's radiation dose.

The terminology used to describe images is usually quite straightforward. Chest and abdominal films are referred to as upright or supine, depending on the position of the patient. In addition, chest x-rays are usually described as posteroanterior (PA) or anteroposterior (AP) (Fig. 1-4). These terms indicate the direction in which the x-ray beam traversed the patient on its way to the detector. PA means that the x ray beam entered the *p*osterior aspect of the patient and exited *a*nteriorly. AP means that the beam direction through the patient was *a*nterior to *p*osterior. A left lateral decubitus view is one taken with the patient's left side down.

Position is important to note, because it can affect magnification, organ position, and blood flow and therefore significantly affect image interpretation. For example, the heart appears larger on AP than on PA images because on an AP projection, the heart is farther from the detector and is magnified more by the diverging x-ray beam. It also appears larger on supine than on upright images because the hemidiaphragms are pushed up, making the heart appear wider. Portable chest images are taken not only in the AP projection but also with the tube closer to the patient than on upright films. This magnifies the heart even more.

Use of contrast agents permits visualization of anatomic structures that are not normally seen. For example, intravenous or intra-arterially injected agents allow visualization of blood vessels (Fig. 1-5). If imaging is done with standard format, the blood vessels appear white. Digital imaging allows subtraction or removal of unwanted structures, such as the bones, from an image (Fig. 1-5B). Often the computer manipulation is done in such a way that the arteries may appear black instead of white, although this usually does not present a problem in interpretation.

Contrast agents are used to fill either a hollow viscus (such as the stomach) or anatomic tubular structures that can be accessed in some way (such as blood vessels, ureter, and common bile duct). When you see an abnormality on one of these studies, you must determine whether

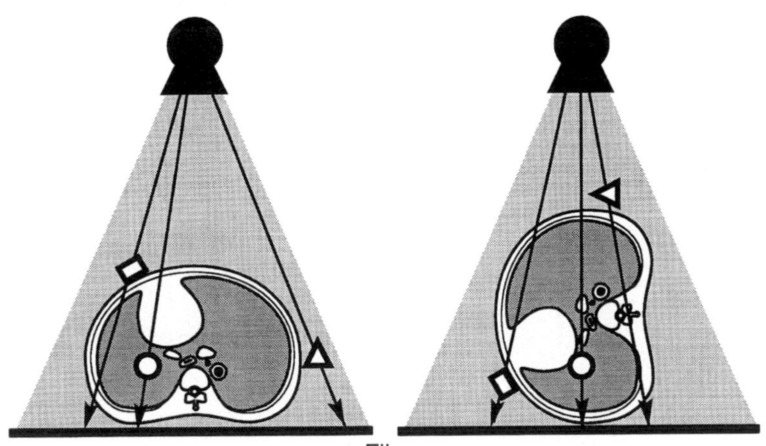

FIGURE 1-2 ■ Spatial localization on an x-ray. On both anteroposterior (AP) and lateral projections, the square and round objects will be seen projecting within the view of the chest, even though the square object is located outside the chest wall. If you can see an object projecting outside the chest wall on at least one view (the triangle), it is outside the chest. If, however, an object looks as though it is inside the chest on both views, it may be either inside or outside.

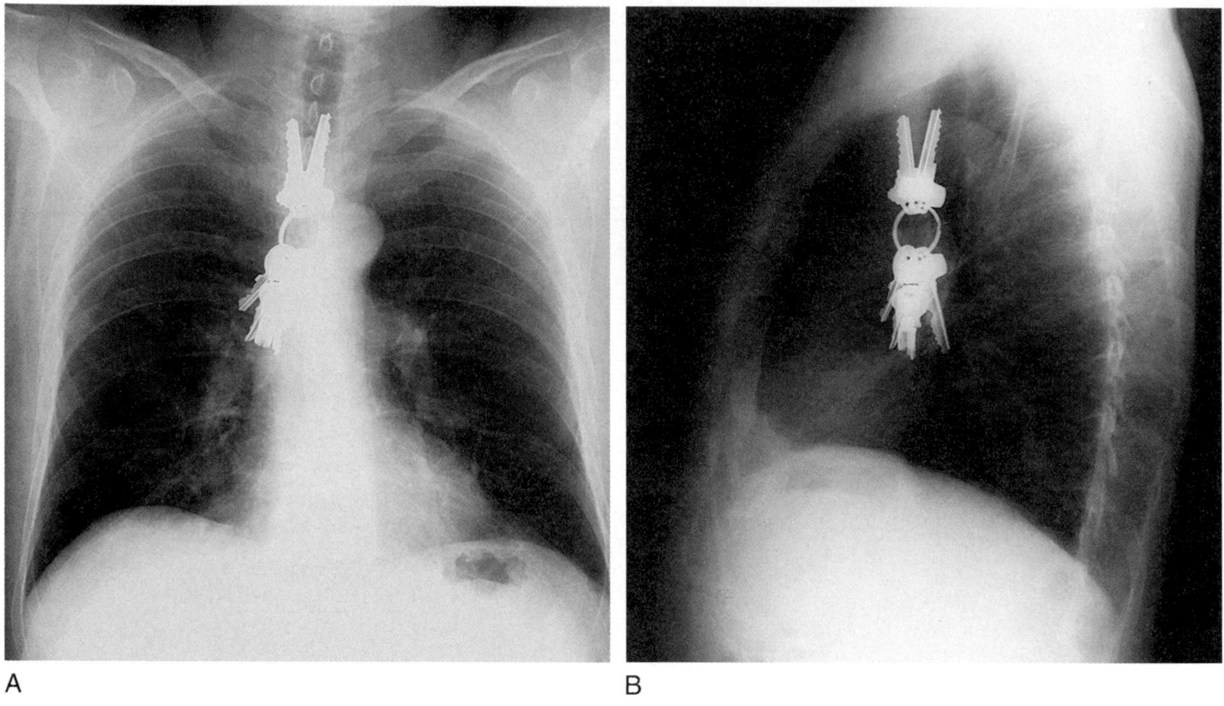

FIGURE 1-3 ■ **What is the location of the keys?** On both the posteroanterior (PA) view of the chest *(A)* and the lateral view *(B),* the keys seem to be within the center of the chest. Actually if you look carefully, you will notice that the keys do not change position at all, even though the patient has rotated 90 degrees. The keys are located on the receptor cassette and are not in the patient.

FIGURE 1-4 ■ **Typical x-ray projections.** X-ray projections are typically listed as AP or PA. This depends on whether the x-ray beam passed to the patient from anterior to posterior (AP) or the reverse. Lateral (LAT) and oblique (OBL) views also are commonly obtained.

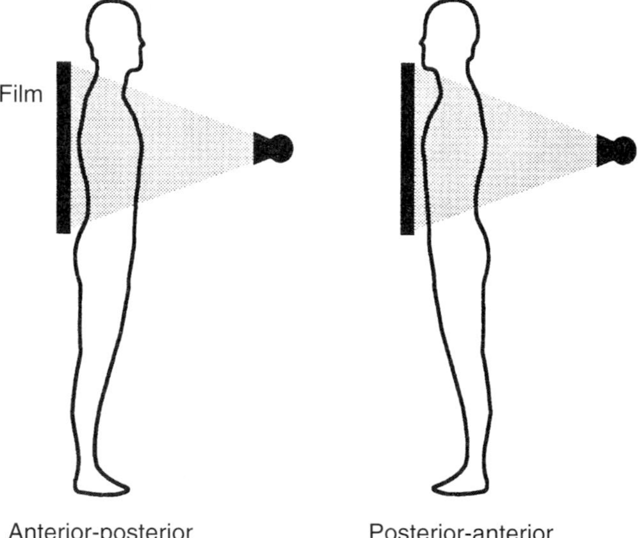

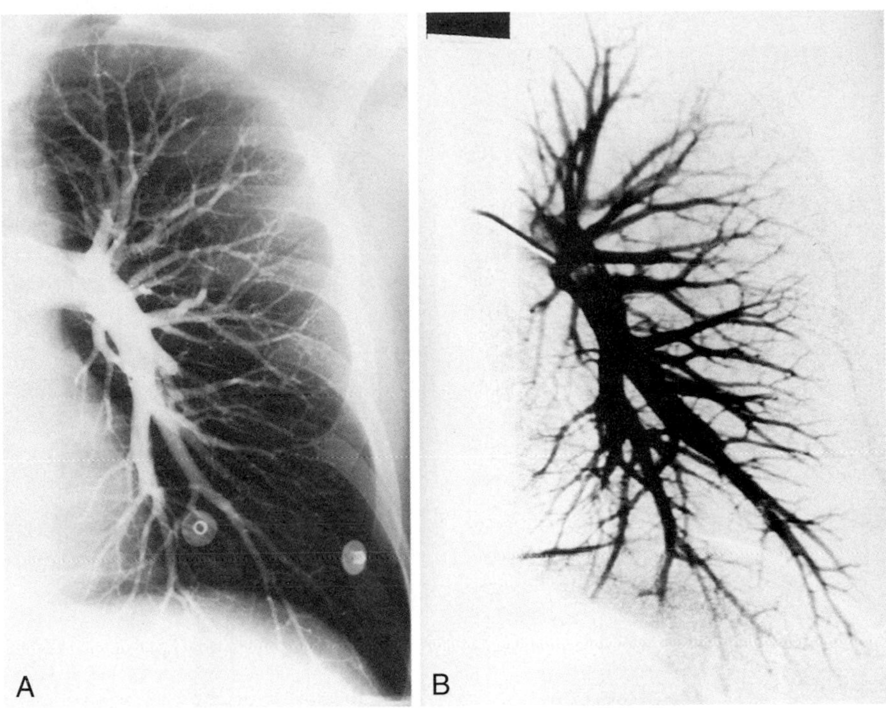

FIGURE 1-5 ■ **Pulmonary angiogram.** A conventional view of blood vessels can be obtained by injecting iodinated contrast material into the vessels *(A)*. On these images, the vessels will appear white, and the bones will be seen as you would normally expect (white). A digital subtraction technique with computers may show the vessels either as black *(B)* or as white, but the bones will have been subtracted from the image.

the location is intraluminal, mural, or extrinsic. This usually requires seeing the abnormality in perpendicular views (Fig. 1-6). Unless you are careful about this determination, you will make errors in diagnosis.

Contrast agents instilled orally, rectally, or retrograde into the ureter or bladder incur little or no risk unless aspiration or perforation occurs. With the intravenously or intra-arterially administered agents, a small but real risk of contrast reaction exists. This is something that you should consider before ordering an intravenous pyelogram or a contrast-enhanced CT scan. About 5% of patients will experience an immediate mild reaction, such as a metallic taste or a feeling of warmth; some experience nausea and vomiting, wheeze, or get hives as a result of these contrast agents. Some of these mild reactions can be treated with 50 mg of intramuscular diphenhydramine (Benadryl). Because contrast agents also can reduce renal function, they should not generally be used in patients with compromised renal function or multiple myeloma.

A small number (about 1 in 1000) patients have a severe reaction to intravascular contrast. This may be a vasovagal reaction, laryngeal edema, severe hypotension, an anaphylactic-type reaction, or cardiac arrest. A vasovagal reaction can be treated with 0.5 to 1.0 mg of intravenous atropine. The most important initial therapeutic measures in these severe reactions are to establish an airway, ensure breathing and circulation, and give intravenous fluids. Other drugs obviously also may be necessary. The risk of death from a study using intravenously administered contrast agents is between 1 in 40,000 and 1 in 100,000.

COMPUTED TOMOGRAPHY

Computed tomography (CT) is accomplished by passing a rotating fan beam of x-rays through the patient and measuring the transmission at thousands of points. The data are handled by a computer that calculates exactly what the x-ray absorption was at any given spot in the patient.

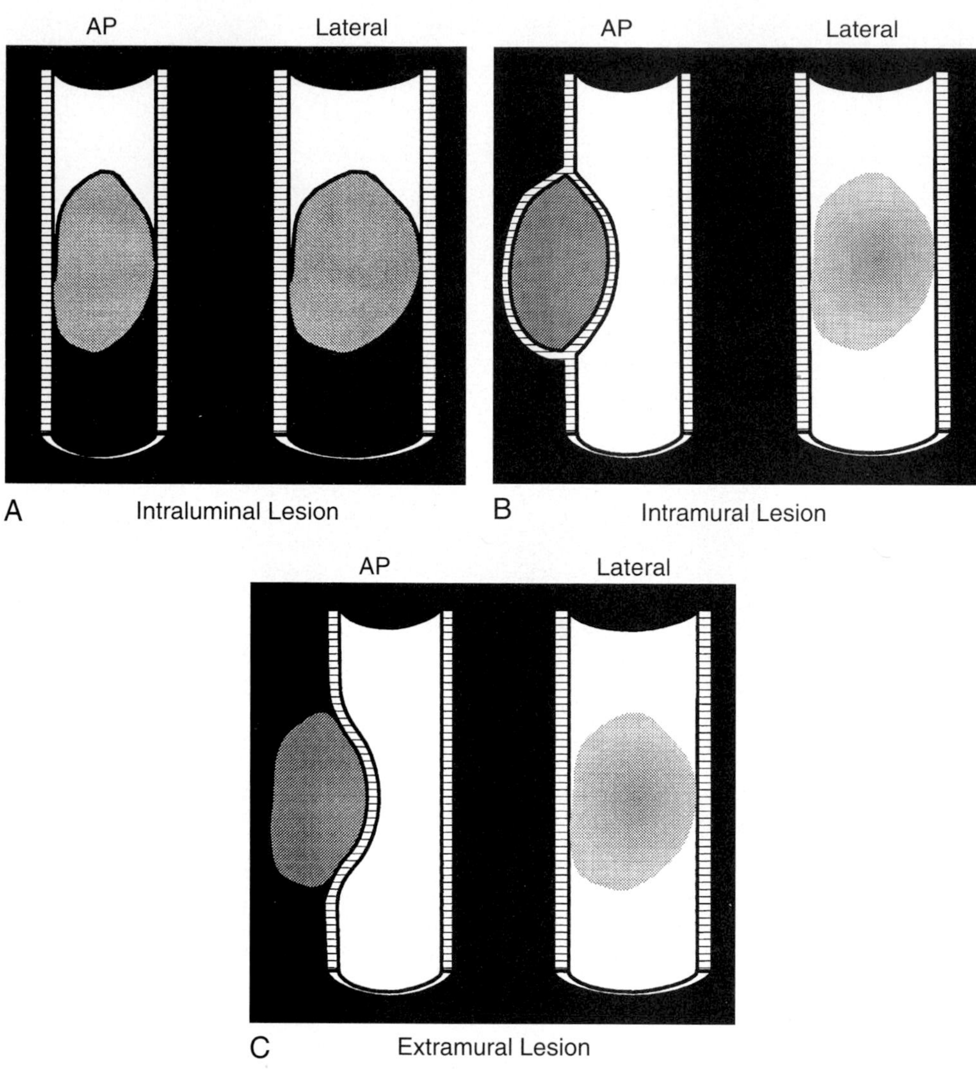

FIGURE 1-6 ■ Appearances of different lesions depending on their location when using contrast. Contrast medium is used to visualize tubular structures, including the spinal canal, blood vessels, gastrointestinal tract, ureters, and bladder. Intraluminal lesions *(A),* such as stones or blood clots within the lumen of the given structure, produce a central defect on both AP and lateral projections. On the AP and lateral views, the contrast will show acute angles on both sides and in both projections. Intramural lesions *(B)* will produce a defect that indents the column of contrast. When seen tangentially, an acute angle will appear between the normal wall and the beginning of the indentation. Extramural lesions *(C)* also can indent the wall, but at the point of indentation, the angle will be somewhat blunted as compared with the intramural lesion.

The data can be manipulated in a number of ways, displayed on a screen, or photographed. Because the data points are in the computer memory, it is possible to "window" the image and obtain a number of filmed pictures without additional radiation exposure (Fig. 1-7). The computers can even display the data as a three-dimensional rotating image, although this is rarely necessary for diagnosis. Compared with plain x-rays, CT uses about 10 to 100 times more radiation.

On early CT scanners, the x-ray tube rotated around the patient to obtain a single "slice," and then the table was incremented before another slice was obtained. Newer scanners allow the x-ray tube to stay on and rotate at the same time that the table is moving. This is called a spiral or helical scanner. The most modern scanners not only have the helical motion but also have multiple rows of detectors and can obtain up to 16 slices at once.

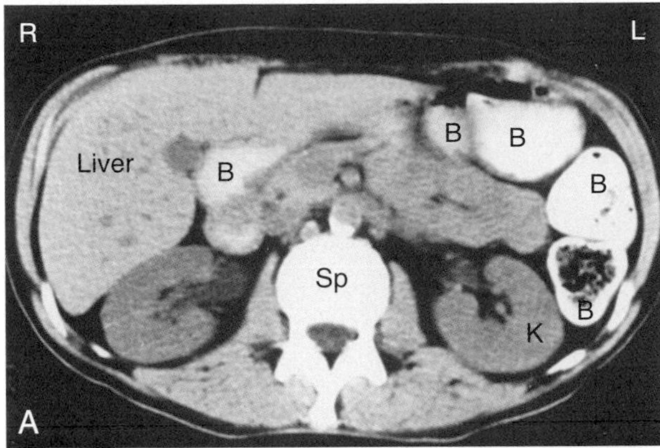

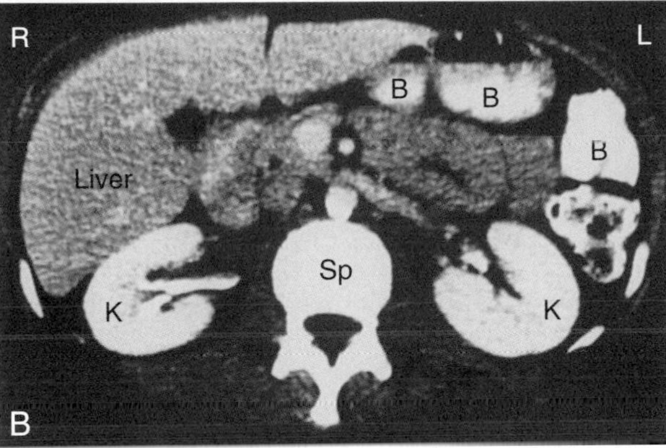

FIGURE 1-7 ■ **Computed tomography (CT).** Images of the abdomen are presented here. *A,* The image was made by using relatively wide windows during filming, and no intravenous contrast was used. *B,* The windows have been narrowed, producing a rather grainy image, and intravenous contrast has been administered so that you can see enhancement of the aorta, abdominal vessels, and both kidneys (K). In both images, contrast has been put in the bowel (B) to differentiate bowel from solid organs and structures.

The appearance of tissues on CT scan depends to some extent on the computer manipulation, but in general, the basic four densities on CT images are the same as those in plain x-rays: air is black, fat is dark gray, soft tissue is light gray, and bone or calcium and contrast agents are white. One advantage of CT is that actual x-ray absorption of a specific tissue can be displayed. The units used are Hounsfield units, and the density of water is zero. The greater sensitivity of CT compared with plain x-rays allows areas of tiny punctate calcification to be seen.

CT scans are presented as a series of slices of tissue. The method is similar in principle to slicing a loaf of bread and pulling up one slice at a time to examine it. Thus CT is a two-dimensional display of two-dimensional information, and objects appear where they really are in space. The scans or slices are shown as if you are viewing the patient from the foot of the patient's bed. Thus the individual's right side is on your left (Fig. 1-8). This also is the convention used for the transverse images of ultrasound and magnetic resonance imaging (MRI).

Contrast agents, frequently used in CT scans, are usually the same water-soluble oral, rectal, or intravenous iodinated agents used in other imaging studies. Intravenous contrast agents are common, being used in probably 75% of all CT studies, and obviously carry the risk of contrast reactions discussed previously.

The appeal of CT is that a large number of structures are visualized simultaneously. In a patient with abdominal pain, one CT examination shows the liver, adrenal glands, kidneys, spleen, aorta, pancreas, and other structures. This allows the clinician to identify macroscopic pathology quickly.

ULTRASOUND

Ultrasound examination uses high-frequency sound waves to make images. The technology is that of sonar or a glorified fish-finder used by fishermen. The image is made by sending high-frequency sound into the patient and assessing the magnitude and time of returning echoes. Echoes are the result of interfaces or changes in density. Typically, a cyst has few if any echoes, because it is mostly water. Tissues such as liver and spleen give a picture with rather homogeneous small echoes due to the fibrous interstitial tissue (Fig. 1-9). High-intensity echoes are caused by calcification, fat, and air.

The technology of ultrasound is attractive because it does not use ionizing radiation, and the machines are relatively inexpensive. For these reasons, ultrasound has found widespread use in obstetrics. The use of so-called real-time ultrasound allows the images to be seen in sequential frames just as in a movie. This capability has proved popular for imaging rapidly moving structures, such as the heart. Unfortunately, ultrasound images can be quite dependent on

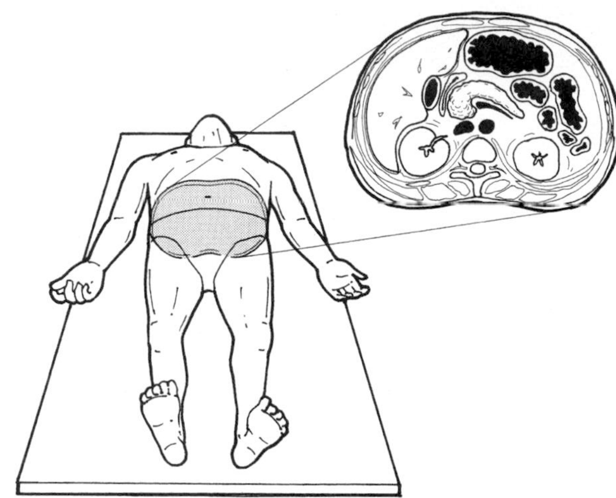

FIGURE 1-8 ■ Orientation of computed tomography (CT) and magnetic resonance (MR) images. CT and MR usually present images as transverse (axial) slices of the body. If, as you stand and look at the patient from the foot of the bed, you think of these images as slices lifted out of the body, you will have the orientation correct.

operator-set parameters, and the field of view within the patient is limited. Thus unless clear labels are placed relative to orientation, the images can be difficult or impossible for the novice to interpret. Ultrasound images are usually presented as white echoes on a black background but occasionally as black echoes on a white background.

FIGURE 1-9 ■ Ultrasound examination of the liver and kidney. This is a longitudinal image, and you are essentially looking at the patient from the right side. The patient's head is to your left. The liver has rather homogeneous echoes, and the kidney is easily seen as a bean-shaped object posterior to the right lobe of the liver.

In addition to using echoes to generate images, you can analyze the returning echo frequencies. This Doppler analysis allows identification of moving blood as well as its direction and magnitude. One example of its use is to identify and quantitate stenoses of the carotid arteries.

NUCLEAR MEDICINE

Nuclear medicine images are made by giving the patient a short-lived radioactive material. The most commonly used radionuclides decay rapidly and have half-lives of only hours. Most materials administered are not detectable within a day or so after administration. With the attachment of a radionuclide (such as technetium 99m) to specific carrier compounds, concentration of the radioactivity can be measured in a chosen organ or tissue, such as the thyroid, bone, lung, heart, abscess, or tumor. Few, if any, significant patient reactions are found to radiopharmaceuticals used for diagnosis.

Nuclear medicine images are made by a gamma camera or positron emission scanner that records radiation emanating from the patient and makes an image of the distribution of the radioactive material (Fig. 1-10). The radiation dose to the patient is determined by the amount of radioactive material initially injected into the body. Therefore once the radiopharmaceutical has been given, additional images can

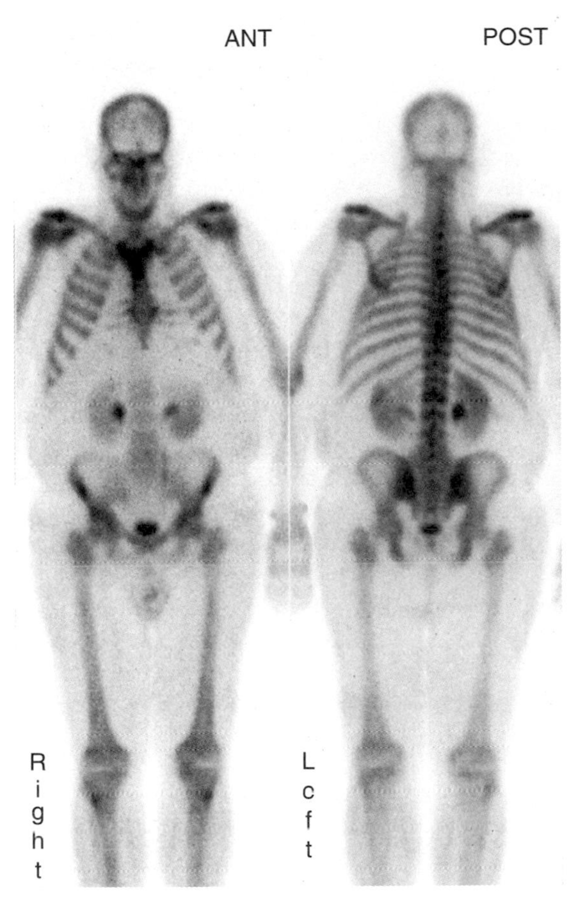

FIGURE 1-10 ■ **Nuclear medicine bone scan.** Radioactivity has been introduced intravenously and localizes in specific organs. In this case, a tracer makes the radioactivity localize in the bone and the kidneys. Nuclear medicine can obtain images of a number of organs, including lungs, heart, and liver.

be obtained without increasing the radiation dose. Images are usually obtained as planar images that, like plain x-rays, display three-dimensional data in two dimensions. These images are labeled as anterior, lateral, and so forth. Computer technology (similar to CT) has been applied to nuclear medicine and allows images to be displayed as slices of the tissue of interest. The major advantage of nuclear medicine is its ability to obtain an image of physiologic function. For example, virtually no other imaging technique can assess regional pulmonary ventilation or hepatobiliary function.

MAGNETIC RESONANCE IMAGING

Magnetic resonance imaging (MRI) generates images by applying a varying magnetic field to the body. The magnetic field aligns atoms. When the field is released, radio waves are generated. The frequency of the emitted radio waves is related to the chemical environment of the atoms as well as to their location. With computer analysis of these data, MR images (which are essentially hydrogen maps) can be generated.

Although many MRI techniques exist, the two basic types of images are T1 and T2. T1 images show fat as a white or bright signal, whereas water (or cerebrospinal fluid [CSF]) is dark. On a T2 image, fat is dark, and blood, edema, and CSF appear white (Fig. 1-11). Unfortunately, calcium and bone are difficult to

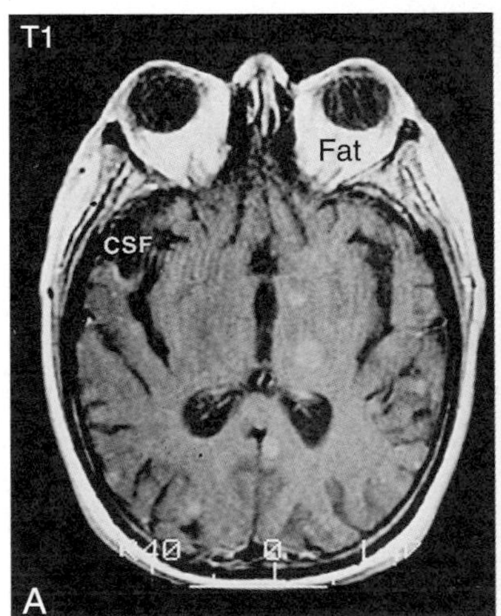

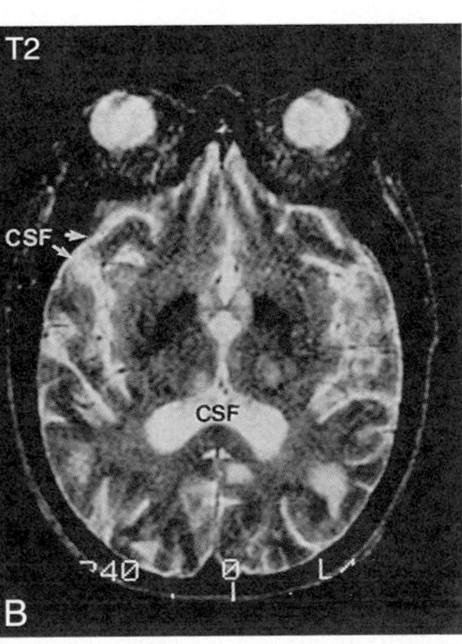

FIGURE 1-11 ■ **Magnetic resonance (MR) imaging of the brain.** A wide variety of imaging parameters can make tissues appear very different. The two most common presentations are T1 images *(A),* in which fat appears white, water or cerebrospinal fluid (CSF) appears black, and brain and muscle appear gray. In almost all MR images, bone gives off no signal and will appear black. With T2 imaging *(B),* fat is dark, and water and CSF have a high signal and will appear bright or white. The brain and soft tissues still appear gray.

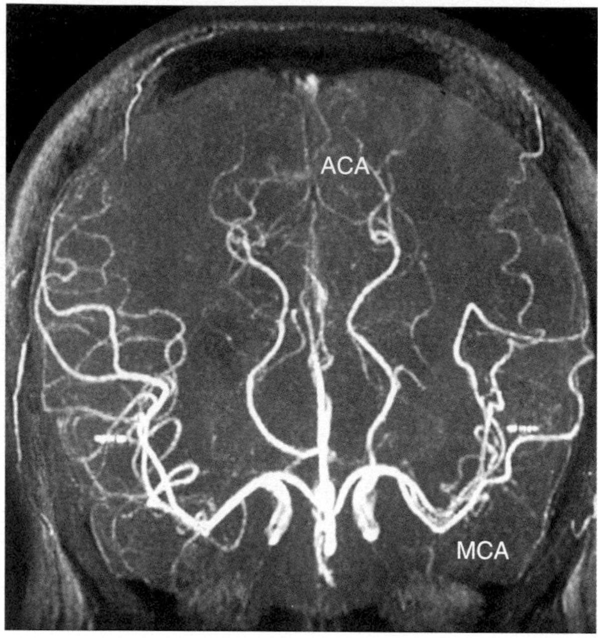

FIGURE 1-12 ■ **Magnetic resonance angiogram.** An anterior view of the head showing intracerebral vessels, including the anterior cerebral artery (ACA) and the middle cerebral artery (MCA). These images were obtained without injection of any contrast agent.

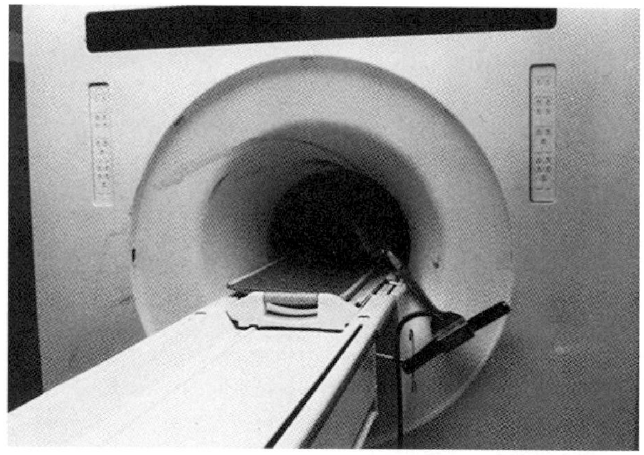

FIGURE 1-13 ■ **Floor polisher in a magnet.** The high magnetic field strength of a magnetic resonance machine is shown by a heavy floor polisher sucked into the scanner. The polisher was inadvertently brought into the room by cleaning personnel. (Courtesy of T. Haygood, M.D.)

see on MR images. What people think are the (white) bones is really visualization of fat in the marrow. Computer manipulation of MR images allows slices similar to those of CT orientation to be used. An intravenous contrast agent (gadolinium) is often used in conjunction with MRI. Not many significant patient reactions occur with this agent.

The primary advantages of MRI are that it obtains exquisite images of the central nervous system and stationary soft tissues (such as the knee joint). It also does not use ionizing radiation. Recent developments and shorter imaging times have allowed images of the heart and blood vessels to be generated without the need to inject anything into the patient (Fig. 1-12).

Disadvantages of MRI have been artifacts due to patient motion, the inability to bring ferrous objects near the magnet, and cost. The major safety problem with these magnets is that they are so strong that if you bring a ferromagnetic object (such as a wrench) into the room, it can accelerate to 150 miles per hour as it is ripped out of your hand and flies into the bore of the magnet. Large floor polishers have been sucked into magnets (Fig. 1-13). If a patient is in the machine at the time, lethal consequences will result. Be aware that some "sandbags" used for neck stabilization actually contain small BBs and can destroy magnets.

Suggested Basic Textbooks

GENERAL RADIOLOGY

Juhl J, Crummy A, Kuhl JE: Paul and Juhl's Essentials of Radiologic Imaging, 7th ed. Philadelphia, Lippincott Williams & Wilkins, 1998.

Harris JH, Harris WH: Radiology of Emergency Medicine, 4th ed. Philadelphia, Lippincott Williams & Wilkins, 1999.

Keats TE, Anderson MW: Atlas of Normal Roentgen Variants That May Simulate Disease, 7th ed. Philadelphia, WB Saunders, 2001.

NUCLEAR MEDICINE

Mettler F, Guiberteau M: Essentials of Nuclear Medicine Imaging, 4th ed. Philadelphia, WB Saunders, 1998.

Wahl RL, Buchanan JW: Principles and Practice of Positron Emission Tomography. Philadelphia, Lippincott Williams & Wilkins, 2002.

ULTRASOUND

Meire HB, Cosgrove D, Dewbury D, Farrant P: Clinical Ultrasound, 2nd ed. A Comprehensive Text. Philadelphia, WB Saunders, 2001.

COMPUTED TOMOGRAPHY AND MAGNETIC RESONANCE

Lee JT, Sagel SS, Stanley RJ, Heiken JP: Computed Body Tomography, 3rd ed. Philadelphia, Lippincott Williams & Wilkins, 1997.

Runge VM: Clinical MRI. Philadelphia, WB Saunders, 2002.

Stark D, Bradley WG, Bradley WG Jr: Magnetic Resonance Imaging. St. Louis, Mosby-Yearbook, 1998.

2 Head and Soft Tissues of Face and Neck

SKULL AND BRAIN

The appropriate initial imaging studies for various clinical problems are shown in Table 2-1.

The Normal Skull and Variants

Normal anatomy of the skull is shown in Figure 2-1. The most common differential problem on plain skull films is distinguishing cranial sutures from vascular grooves and fractures. The main sutures are coronal, sagittal, and lambdoid. A suture also runs in a rainbow shape over the ear. In the adult, sutures are symmetrical and very wiggly and have sclerotic (very white) edges. Vascular grooves are usually seen on the lateral view and extend posteriorly and superiorly from just in front of the ear. They do not have sclerotic edges and are not perfectly straight.

A few common variants are seen on skull films. Hyperostosis frontalis interna is a benign condition of female subjects in which sclerosis, or increased density, is seen in the frontal region and spares the midline (Fig. 2-2). Large, asymmetrical, or amorphous focal intracranial calcifications should always raise the suspicion of a benign or malignant neoplasm. Occasionally, areas of lucency (dark areas) are found where the bone is thinned. The most common normal variants that cause this are vascular lakes or biparietal foramen. Asymmetrically round or ill-defined "holes" should raise the suspicion of metastatic disease (Fig. 2-3).

Paget's disease can affect the bone of the skull. In the early stages, very large lytic, or destroyed, areas may be seen. In later stages, increased density (sclerosis) and marked overgrowth of the bone, causing a "cotton-wool" appearance of the skull, may be seen (Fig. 2-4). Always be aware that both prostate and breast cancer can cause multiple dense metastases in the skull and that both diseases are more common than Paget's disease.

BRAIN

Normal Anatomy

Table 2-2 gives a methodology to follow or checklist of items for use when examining a computed tomography (CT) scan. Both CT and magnetic resonance imaging (MRI) are capable of displaying anatomic "slices" in a number of different planes. Usually the study that you are looking at will show a "scout view," which is an image with numbered lines drawn across it (Fig. 2-5). This view can be helpful in orienting yourself with regard to a particular slice. The normal anatomy of the brain on CT and MR images is shown in Figures 2-6 and 2-7. You should be able to identify some anatomy on these images.

Intracranial Calcifications

Intracranial calcifications can be seen occasionally on a skull film, but they are seen much more

TABLE 2-1 ■ **Imaging Modalities for Cranial Problems**

Suspected Cranial Problem	Initial Imaging Study
Skull fracture (depressed)	CT brain scan including bone windows
Major head trauma	CT (neurologically unstable); MRI (neurologically stable)
Mild head trauma	Observe; CT (if persistent headache)
Acute hemorrhage	Noncontrasted CT
Suspected intracerebral aneurysm or arteriovenous malformations	MRI
Hydrocephalus	Noncontrasted CT
Transient ischemic attack	Noncontrasted CT, MRI if vertebrobasilar findings; consider carotid ultrasonography if bruit present
Acute transient or persistent CNS symptoms or findings	See Table 2-3
Acute stroke (suspected hemorrhagic)	Noncontrasted CT
Acute stroke (suspected nonhemorrhagic)	MRI
Multiple sclerosis	MRI of the brain
Tumor or metastases	MRI
Aneurysm (chronic history)	MR angiogram or contrasted CT
Abscess	Contrasted CT or MRI
Preoperative for cranial surgery	Contrast angiography
Meningitis	Lumbar tap; CT only to exclude complications
Seizure (new onset or poor therapeutic response)	MRI
Seizure (febrile or alcohol withdrawal without neurologic deficit)	Imaging not indicated
Neurologic deficit with known primary tumor elsewhere	MRI if associated sensorineural findings
Vertigo (if suspect acoustic neuroma or posterior fossa tumor)	MRI or contrasted CT
Headache	See Table 2-3
Dementia	Nothing, or MRI
Alzheimer's disease	Nuclear medicine SPECT scan
Sinusitis	See Table 2-6

CNS, central nervous system; CT, computed tomography; MRI, magnetic resonance imaging; SPECT, single-photon emission computed tomography.

often on CT. Intracranial calcifications may be due to a myriad of causes. Normal pineal as well as ependymal calcifications may occur. Scattered calcifications can occur from toxoplasmosis, cysticercosis, tuberous sclerosis (Fig. 2-8), and granulomatous disease. Unilateral calcifications are very worrisome, because they can occur in arteriovenous malformations, gliomas, and meningiomas.

Headache

Headaches can be due to a myriad of causes and should be characterized by location, duration, type of pain, provoking factors, and age and sex of the patient. In the primary care population, only fewer than 0.5% of acute headaches are the result of serious intracranial pathology. Simple headaches, tension headaches, migraine headaches, and cluster headaches do not warrant imaging studies. A good physical examination is essential, including evaluation of blood pressure, urine, eyes (for papilledema), temporal arteries, sinuses, ears, neurologic system, and neck. In a patient with a febrile illness, headache, and stiff neck, a lumbar puncture should be performed. In only a few circumstances is imaging indicated (Table 2-3).

In general, imaging is indicated when a headache is accompanied by neurologic findings, syncope, confusion, seizure, and mental status changes, or after major trauma. Sudden onset of the "worst headache of one's life" (thunderclap headache) should raise the question of subarachnoid hemorrhage. Sudden onset of a unilateral headache with a suspected carotid or vertebral dissection or ipsilateral Horner's syndrome should prompt an MRI and possible magnetic resonance angiogram.

Sinus headaches can usually be differentiated from other etiologies because they worsen when the patient is leaning forward or with

Text continued on page 22

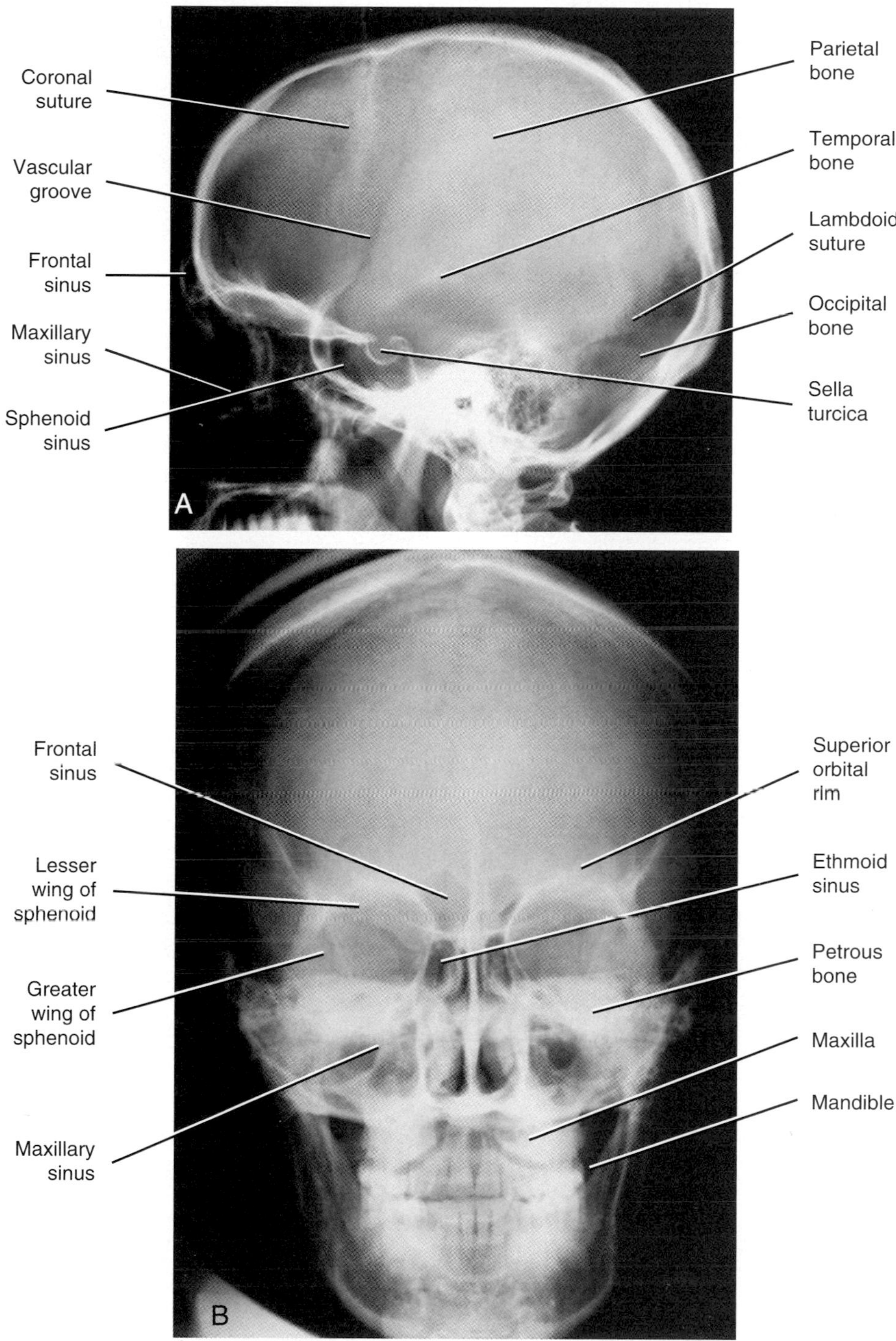

FIGURE 2-1 ■ **Normal skull.** Lateral *(A)*, anteroposterior (AP) *(B)*, AP Towne's projection *(C)*, and the AP Waters' view *(D)*.

Continued

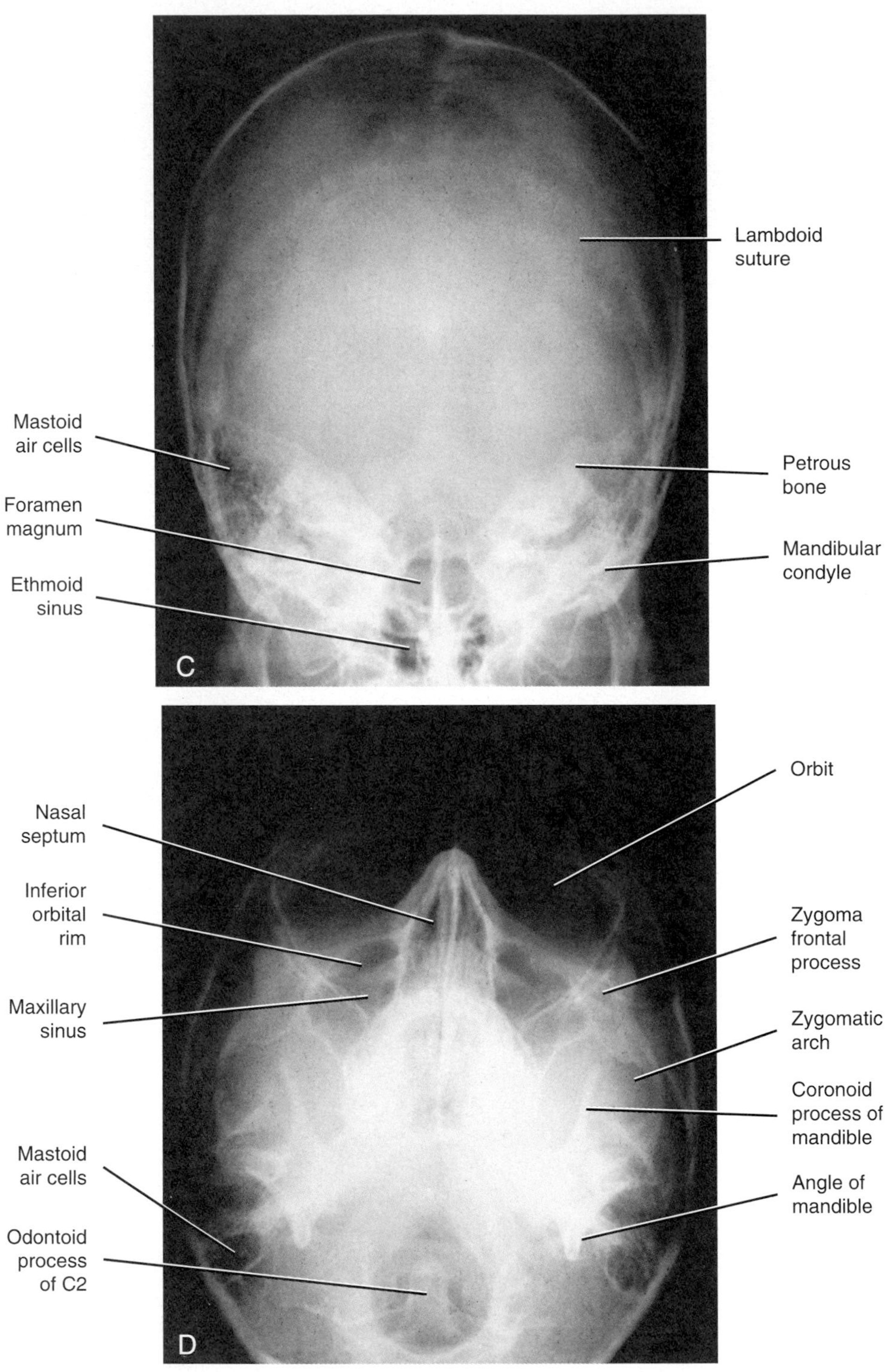

FIGURE 2-1 cont'd

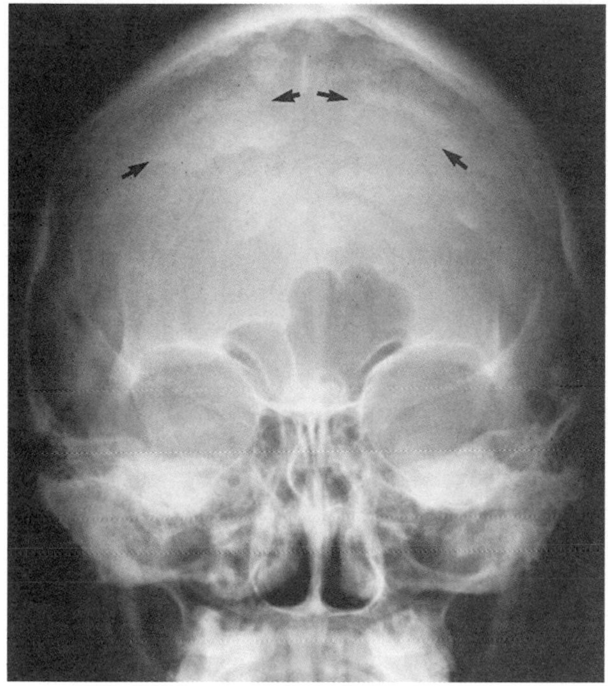

FIGURE 2-2 ■ Hyperostosis frontalis interna. A normal variant, most common in female patients, in which increased density of the skull occurs in the frontal regions. Notice that sparing of the midline is present.

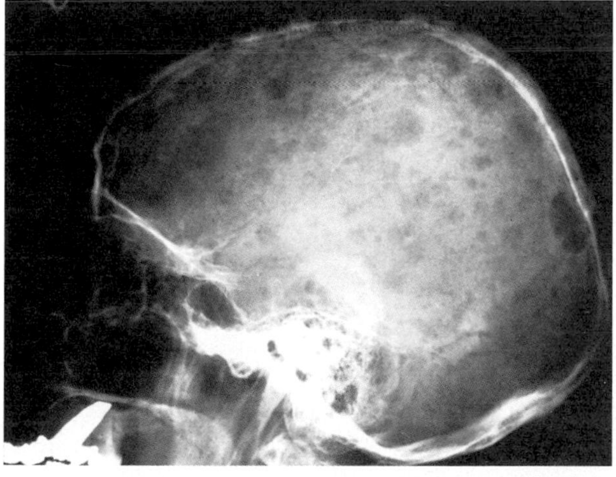

FIGURE 2-3 ■ Multiple myeloma. Multiple asymmetric holes in the skull are seen only with metastatic disease. Metastatic lung or breast carcinoma can look exactly the same as this case of multiple myeloma.

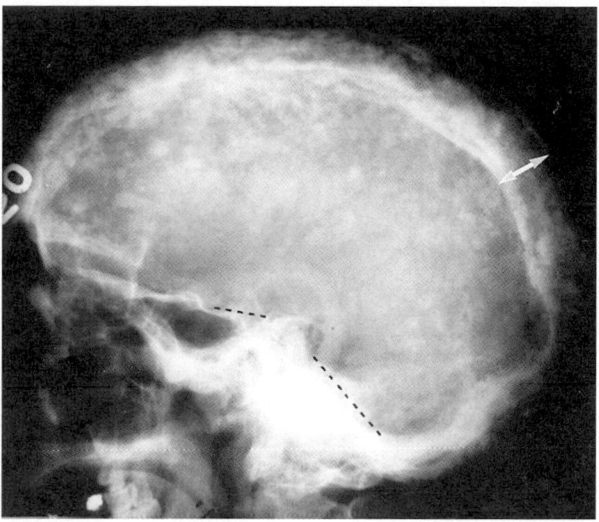

FIGURE 2-4 ■ Paget's disease. The fluffy cotton-wool densities overlying the skull are caused by bone expansion. Note also that the calvarium is very thick *(arrow)*. The base of the skull has become softened; the cervical spine and foramen magnum look as though they are pushed up, but in reality, the skull is sagging around them.

TABLE 2-2 ■ **Examination of a Computed Tomography (CT) Brain Scan**

Look for
- focally decreased density (darker than normal) due to stroke, edema, tumor, surgery, or radiation
- increased focal density (whiter than normal) on a noncontrasted scan
  - in ventricles (hemorrhage)
  - in parenchyma (hemorrhage, calcium, or metal)
  - in dural, subdural, or subarachnoid spaces (hemorrhage)
- increased focal density on contrasted scan
  - all items above
  - tumor
  - stroke
  - abscess or cerebritis
  - aneurysm or arteriovenous malformation (AVM)
- asymmetrical gyral pattern
  - mass or edema (causing effacement of sulci)
  - atrophy (seen as very prominent sulci)
- midline shift
- ventricular size and position (look at all ventricles)
- sella for masses or erosion
- sinuses for fluid or masses
- soft tissue swelling over skull
- bone windows for possible fracture

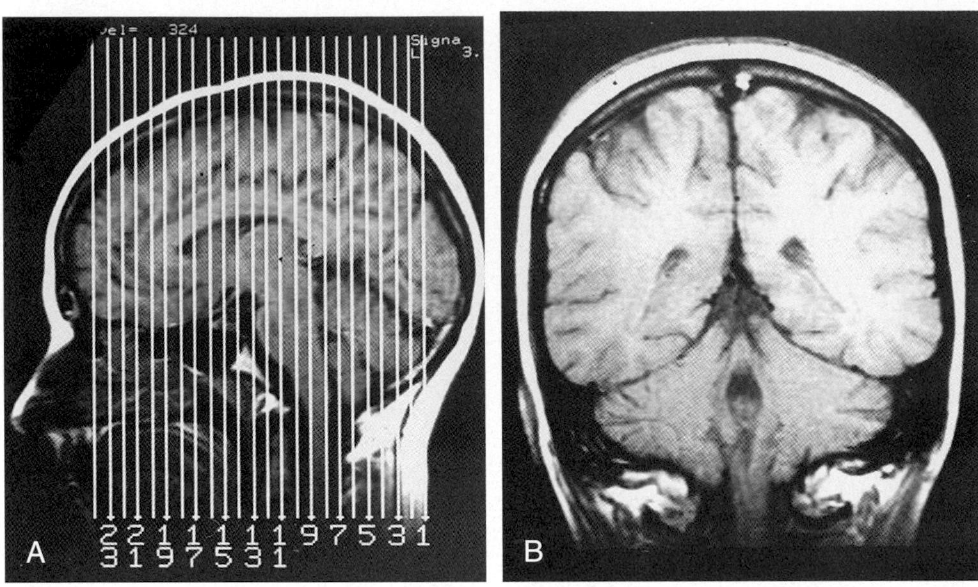

FIGURE 2-5 ■ Scout view image. Scout view images *(A)* are commonly obtained during computed tomography (CT) and magnetic resonance (MR) imaging. Lines are seen across the image; the numbers at one end help to localize the slice. In this case, slice 8 has been pulled out and turned sideways, showing a coronal view of the brain *(B)*.

FIGURE 2-6 ■ Normal anatomy of the brain in transverse (axial) CT and MR images. *A* to *H*, Noncontrasted computed tomography (CT) and T1–weighted magnetic resonance (MR) images are shown for the same levels.

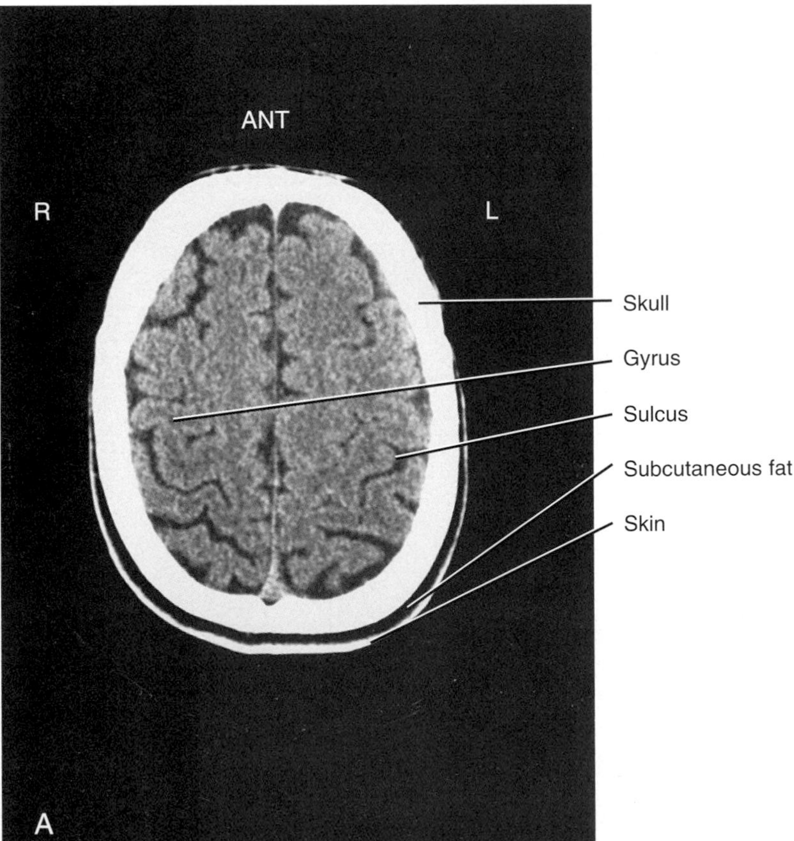

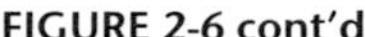

FIGURE 2-6 cont'd

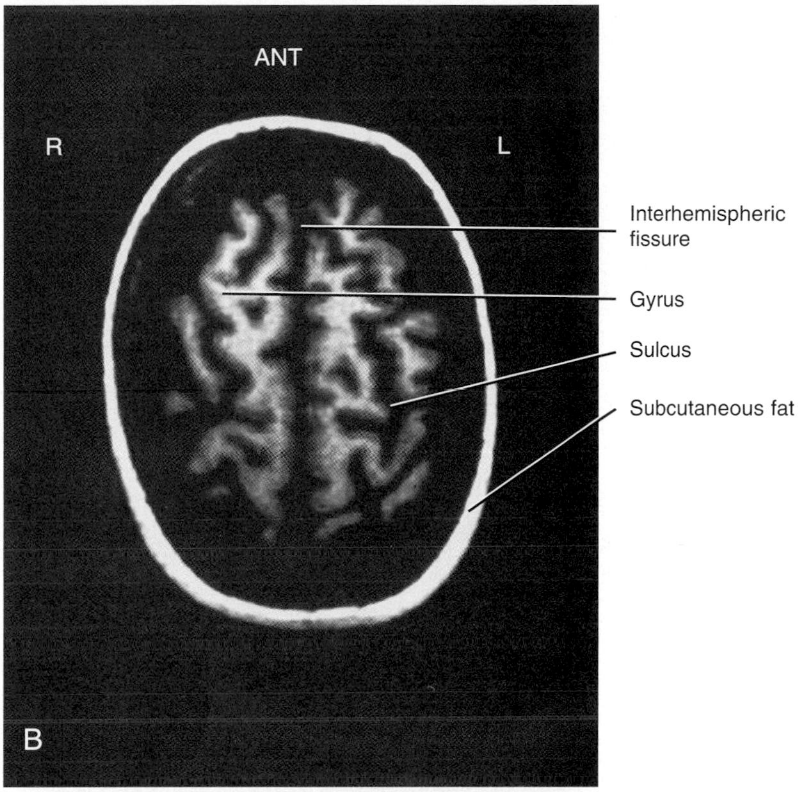

ANT
R
L
Interhemispheric fissure
Gyrus
Sulcus
Subcutaneous fat
B

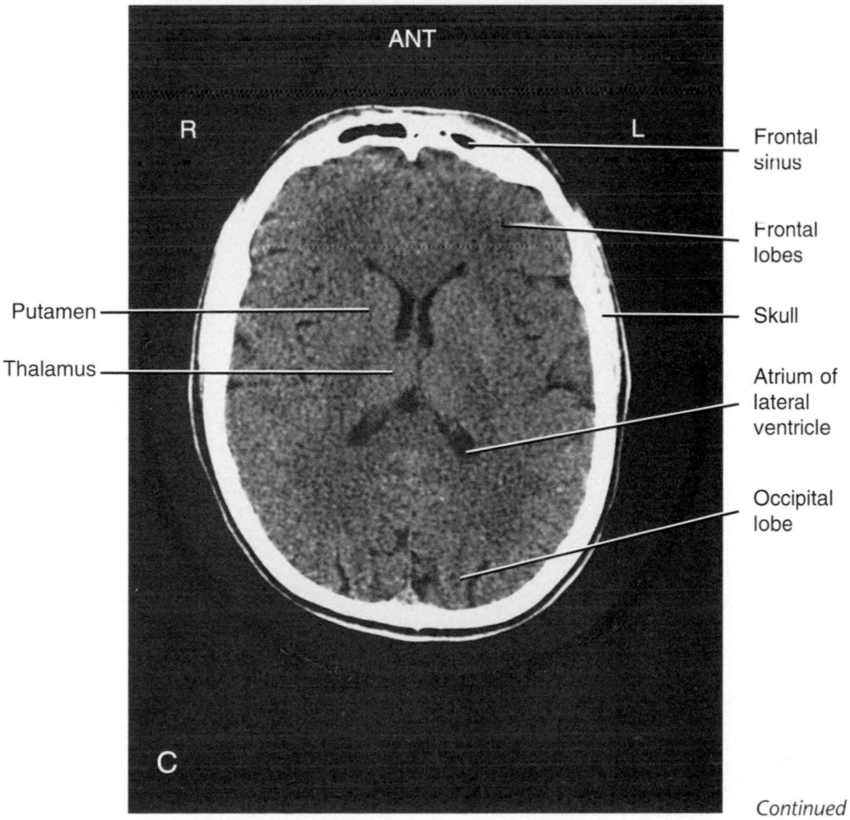

ANT
R
L
Frontal sinus
Frontal lobes
Putamen
Skull
Thalamus
Atrium of lateral ventricle
Occipital lobe
C

Continued

FIGURE 2-6 cont'd

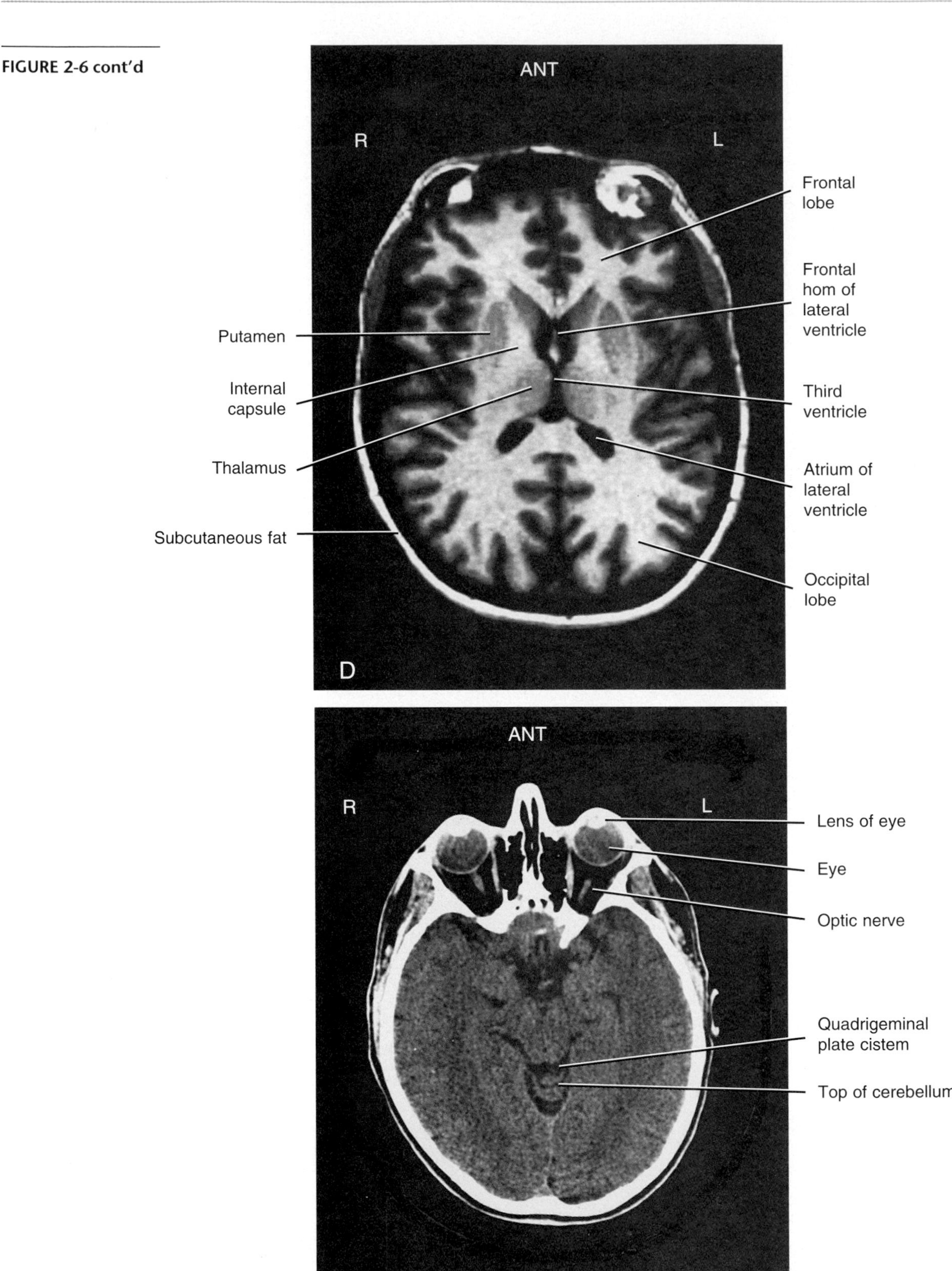

FIGURE 2-6 cont'd

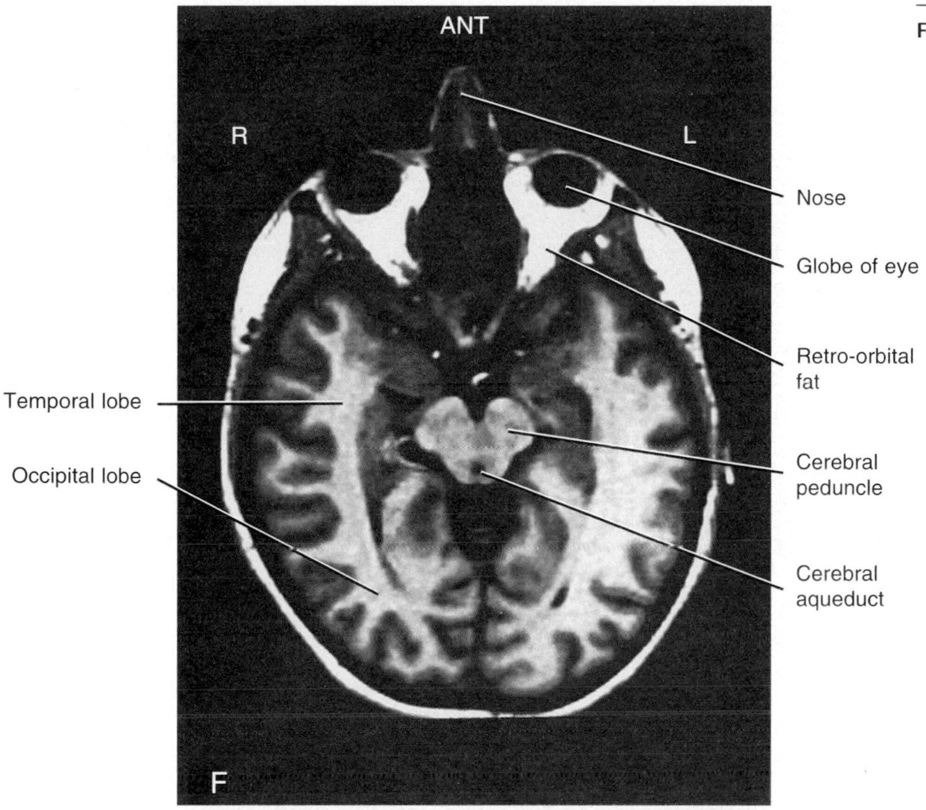

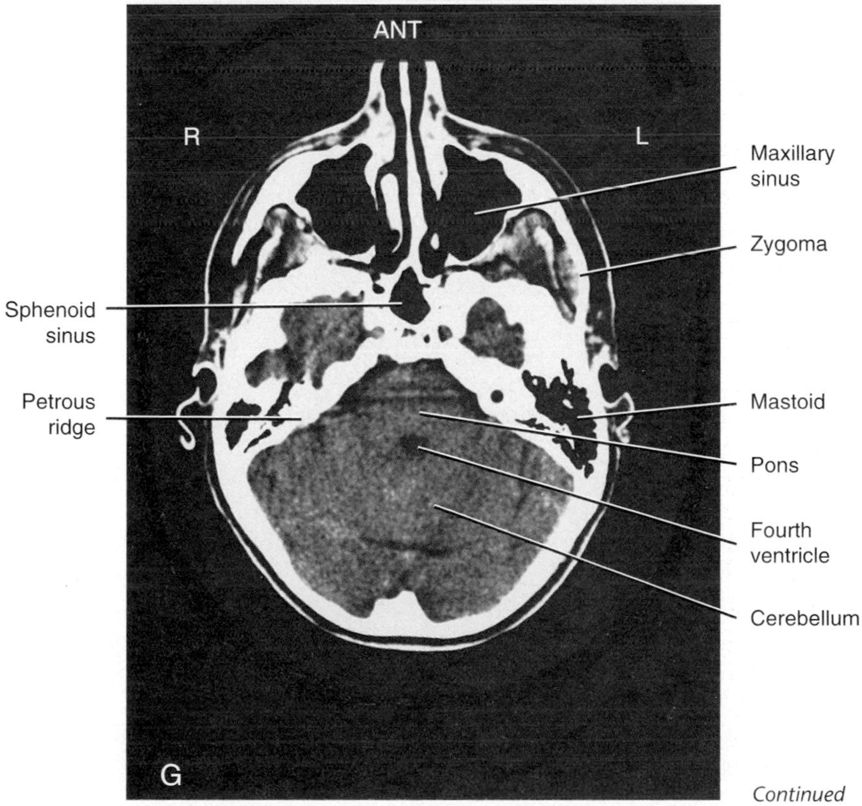

ANT
R
L
Nose
Globe of eye
Retro-orbital fat
Temporal lobe
Cerebral peduncle
Occipital lobe
Cerebral aqueduct
F

ANT
R
L
Maxillary sinus
Zygoma
Sphenoid sinus
Petrous ridge
Mastoid
Pons
Fourth ventricle
Cerebellum
G

Continued

FIGURE 2-6 cont'd

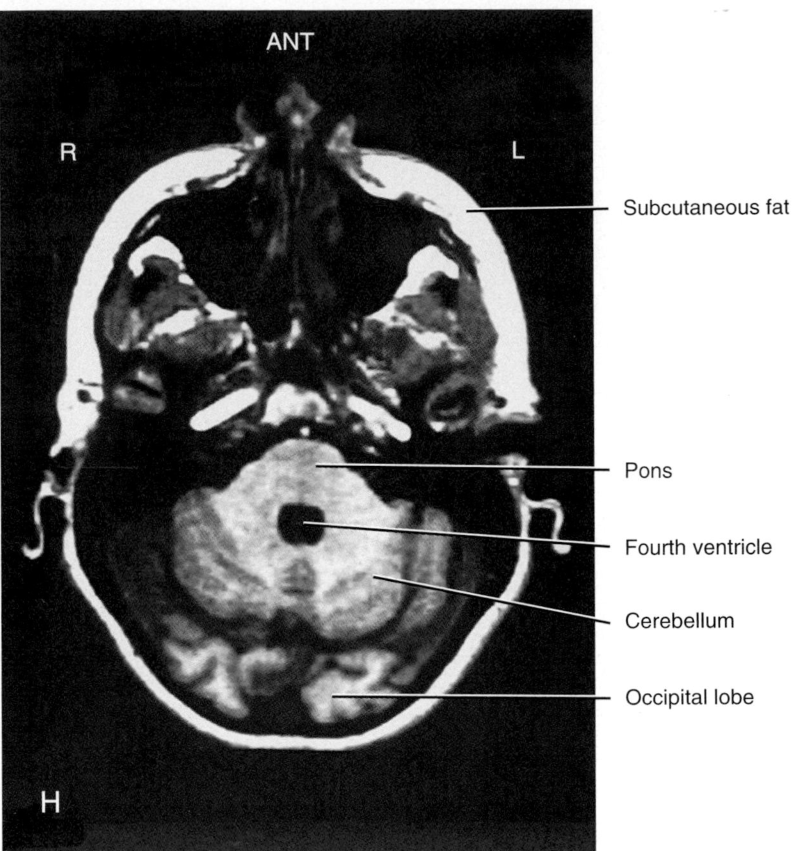

application of pressure over the affected sinus. Indications for CT use in sinus headaches are presented later in Table 2-6.

Head Trauma

On skull x-rays, fractures are dark lines that have very sharp edges and tend to be very straight (Fig. 2-9). If a fracture is present over the middle meningeal area, an associated epidural hematoma may be found. If a depressed fracture is present, the lucent fracture lines can be stellate or semicircular (Fig. 2-10). In either of these cases, substantial brain injury may be present, and a CT scan, including bone windows, is indicated.

Skull films are ordered much too frequently. A skull fracture without loss of consciousness is very rare. Significant brain injury may be found without a skull fracture. The patient should be examined clinically and a decision made as to whether physical findings and the history indicate moderate to severe head injury or mild head injury. CT, MRI, or skull radiography is not needed for low-risk patients. Low risk is defined as those who are asymptomatic or have only dizziness, mild headache, scalp laceration, or hematomas; are older than 2 years; and have no moderate- or high-risk findings.

Patients at moderate risk are those who have any of the following conditions: history of change in the level of consciousness at any time after the injury, progressive or severe headache, post-traumatic seizure, persistent vomiting, multiple trauma, serious facial injury, signs of basilar skull fracture (hemotympanum, "raccoon eyes," cerebrospinal fluid [CSF] rhinorrhea or otorrhea), suspected child abuse, bleeding disorder, or age younger than 2 years (unless the injury is trivial).

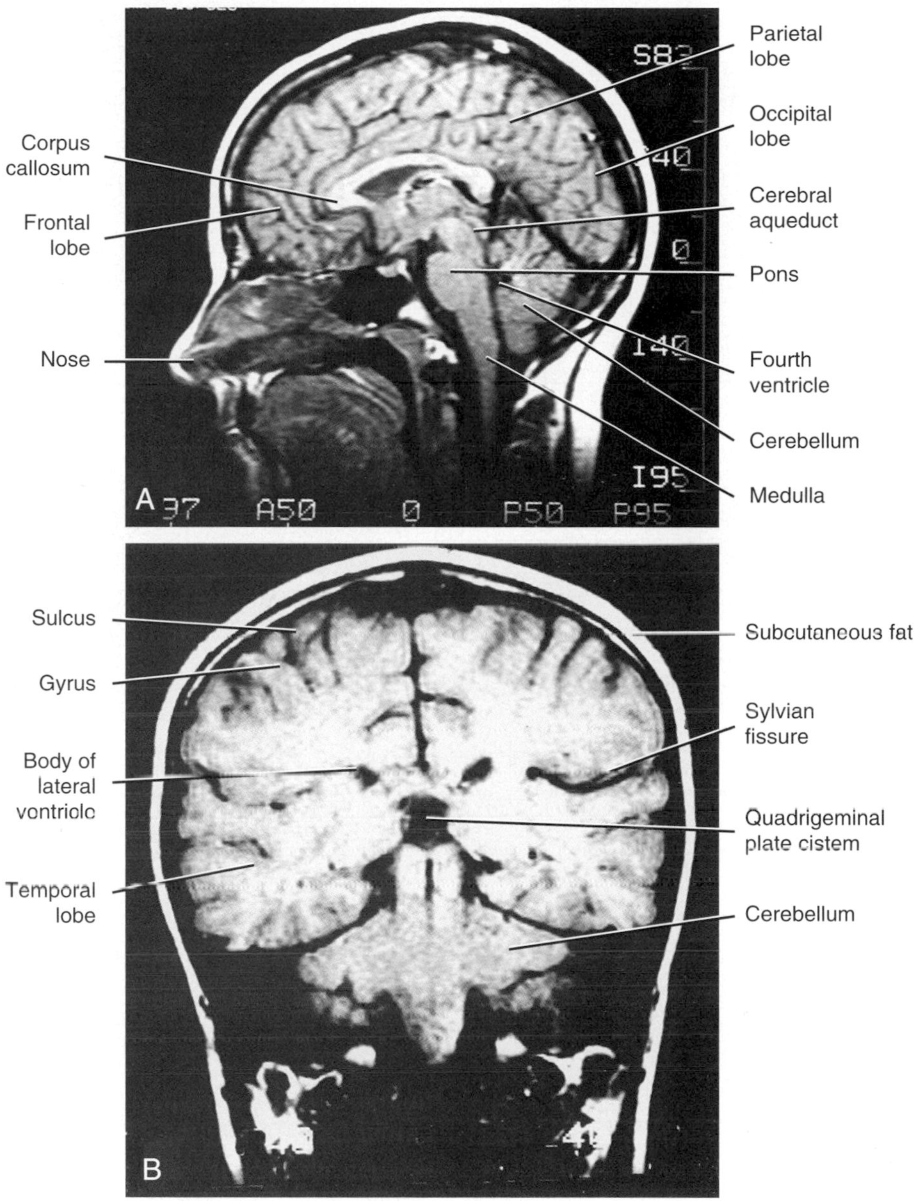

FIGURE 2-7 ■ *A* and *B*, Normal magnetic resonance imaging (MRI) anatomy of the brain in coronal and sagittal projections, respectively.

High-risk patients are those with any of the following conditions: focal neurologic findings, a Glasgow Coma Scale score of 8 or less, definite skull penetration, metabolic derangement, postictal state, or decreased or depressed level of consciousness (unrelated to drugs, alcohol, or other central nervous system [CNS] depressants). If a moderate or severe injury is present and the patient is neurologically unstable, a CT scan should be done to exclude a hematoma. If the patient is neurologically stable, an MR scan is preferable to look for parenchymal shearing

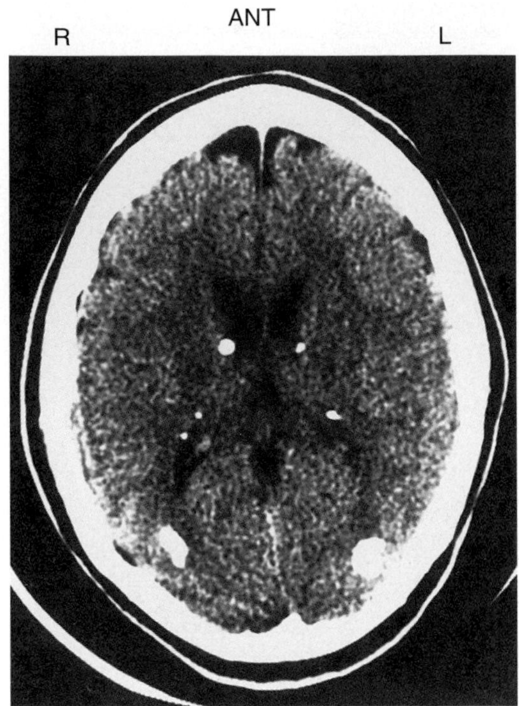

FIGURE 2-8 ■ Tuberous sclerosis. Scattered calcifications are seen about the ventricles in the posterior parietal regions. Other diseases that could show this appearance include intrauterine TORCH infections (*t*oxoplasmosis, *r*ubella, *c*ytomegalovirus (CMV), *h*erpes).

TABLE 2-3 ■ **Imaging Indications for Headaches**

MRI is indicated for the following:
- Sudden onset of the "worst headache of one's life" (thunderclap headache)
- A headache that
  - worsens with exertion
  - is associated with a decrease in alertness
  - is positionally related
  - awakens one from sleep
  - changes in pattern over time
- A new headache in an HIV-positive individual
- Associated with papilledema
- Associated with focal neurologic deficit
- Associated with mental status changes

For most of the above indications, CT is acceptable if an MRI is not feasible or available. MRI is usually not indicated for sinus headaches. See Table 2–6 for CT indications in sinus disease.

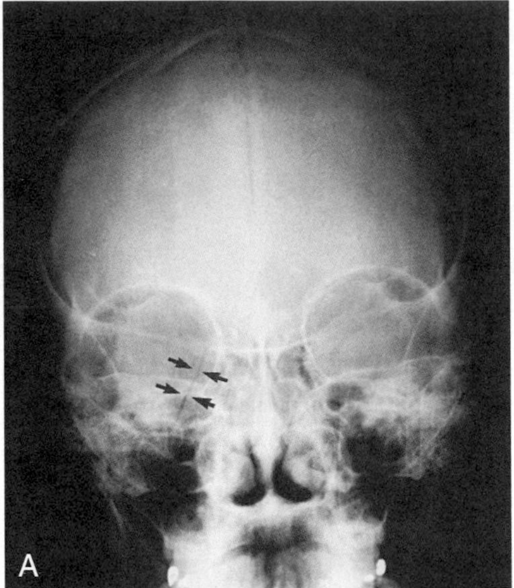

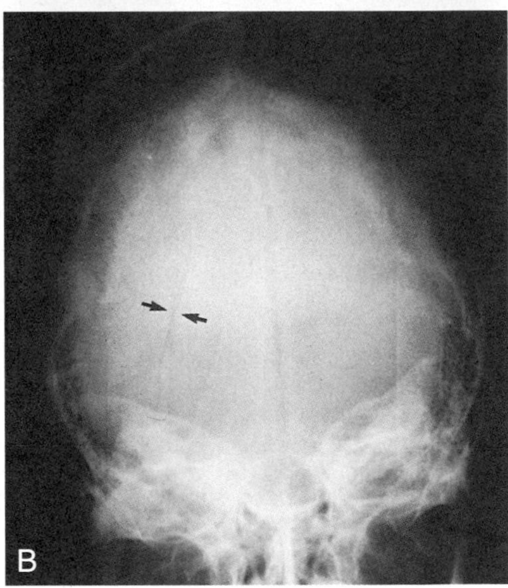

FIGURE 2-9 ■ Linear skull fracture. Skull fractures *(arrows)* are usually dark lines that are very sharply defined and do not have white margins. On the anteroposterior (AP) view *(A)*, it cannot be determined whether the fracture is in the front or the back of the skull. With a Towne's view, however, in which the neck is flexed and the occiput is raised *(B)*, this fracture can clearly be localized to the occipital bone.

injuries. In mild head injury (with no loss of consciousness or neurologic deficit), the patient may be observed. If a persistent headache occurs after trauma, CT scanning should be performed.

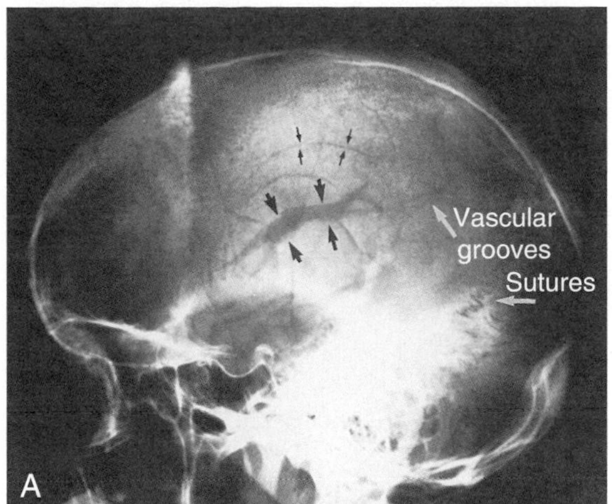

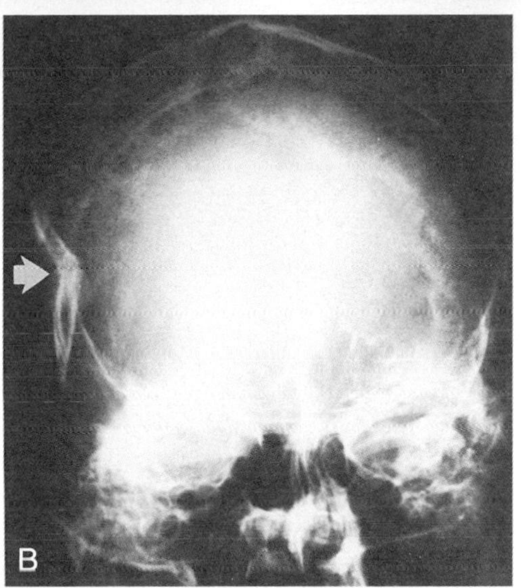

FIGURE 2-10 ■ Depressed skull fracture. This patient was hit in the head with a hammer. The lateral view *(A)* shows the central portion of the fracture, which is stellate *(large arrows)*, and the surrounding concentric fracture line *(small arrows)*. Note the very wiggly posterior suture lines and the normally radiating vascular grooves. The anteroposterior (AP) view *(B)* shows the amount of depression of the fracture, although this is usually much better seen on a computed tomography (CT) scan.

Suspected Intracranial Hemorrhage

If the presence of acute intracranial hemorrhage is suspected, the study of choice is a CT scan done without intravenous contrast. The scan is done without contrast because acute hemorrhage appears to be white on a CT scan (Fig. 2-11), and so does intravenously administered contrast. Hemorrhage into the ventricles is usually seen in the posterior horns of the lateral ventricles. Blood is denser than CSF and therefore settles dependently. This settling process is not seen with subarachnoid or intraparenchymal blood. The presence of hemorrhage is a contraindication to anticoagulation.

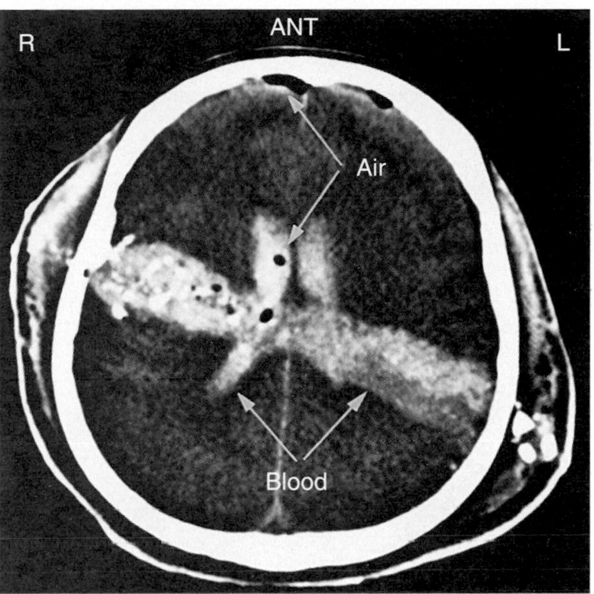

FIGURE 2-11 ■ Gunshot wound of the head. A noncontrasted computed tomography (CT) scan shows bilateral soft tissue swelling and a hemorrhagic track across the brain. Blood appears white, and it also is seen within the lateral ventricles. Several small air bubbles are seen in the lateral ventricles along the track and along the anterior surface of the brain.

Intraparenchymal bleeding can result from a ruptured aneurysm, stroke, trauma, or tumor, which are common complications of hypertension. Grave prognostic factors are large size or brainstem location. Most (80%) hypertensive bleeds occur in the basal ganglia. Ten percent occur in the pons, and 10%, in the cerebellum. An associated mass effect may be present with compression of the ventricles or midline shift. The findings of acute hemorrhage on a noncontrasted CT scan indicate increased density in the parenchyma (Fig. 2-12). Differentiation from calcification usually is easily made by clinical history and, if necessary, by having the area of interest measured on the scan in terms of density (Hounsfield units).

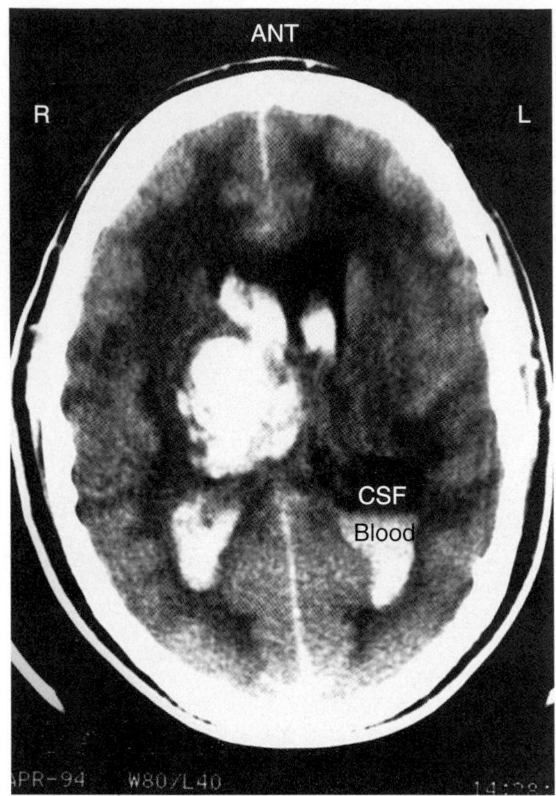

FIGURE 2-12 ■ Intracerebral hemorrhage. In this hypertensive patient with an acute severe headache, the noncontrasted computed tomography (CT) scan shows a large area of fresh blood in the region of the right thalamus. Blood also is seen in the anterior and posterior horns of the lateral ventricles. Because blood is denser than cerebrospinal fluid (CSF), it is layered dependently.

Subdural hematomas are seen as crescent-shaped abnormalities between the brain and the skull. They can cross suture lines, but they do not cross the tentorium or falx. In some cases, subdural hematomas can be quite difficult to see, because new blood appears denser or whiter than brain tissue. (Fig. 2-13*A*). As the blood ages (over a period of several weeks), it becomes less dense than brain (Fig. 2-13*B*). Obviously, it follows that a subacute phase occurs during which the blood is the same density as the brain (isodense). In this stage, sometimes the only clue that a subdural hematoma is present is effacement of the gyral pattern on the affected side, a midline shift away from the affected side, or ventricular compression on the affected side.

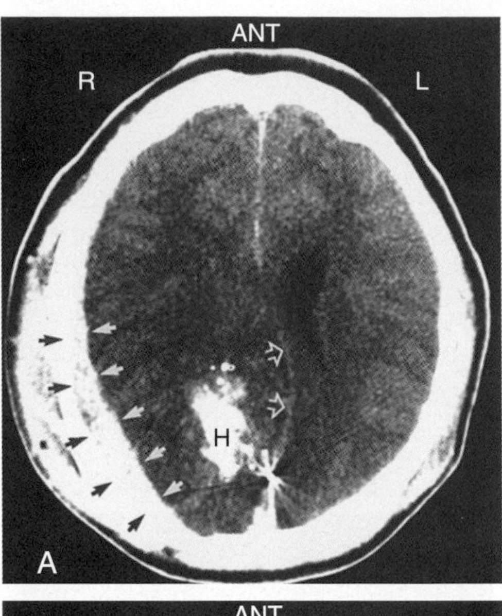

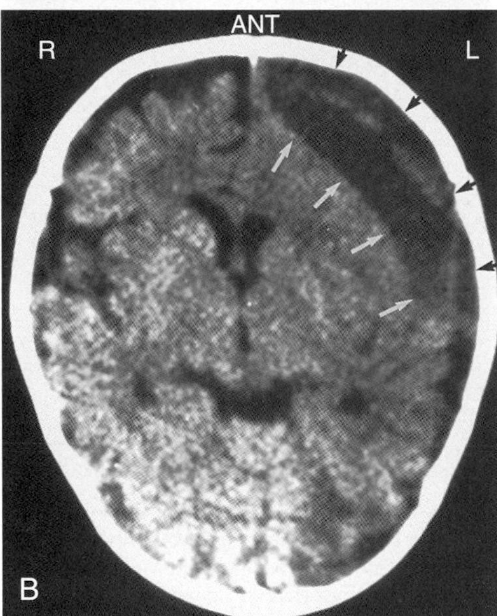

FIGURE 2-13 ■ Subdural hematomas. A noncontrasted computed tomography (CT) scan of an acute subdural hematoma *(A)* shows a crescentic area of increased density *(arrows)* in the right posterior parietal region between the brain and the skull. An area of intraparenchymal hemorrhage (H) also is seen; in addition, mass effect causes a midline shift to the left *(open arrows)*. A chronic subdural hematoma is seen in a different patient *(B)*. An area of decreased density appears in the left frontoparietal region effacing the sulci, compressing the anterior horn of the left lateral ventricle, and shifting the midline somewhat to the right.

Epidural hematomas follow the same changing pattern of density as do subdural hematomas. The major differential point from an imaging viewpoint is that they are lenticular rather than crescentic (Fig. 2-14) and tend not to cross suture lines of the skull. Epidural hematomas are associated with temporal bone fractures that have resulted in a tear of the middle meningeal artery.

Subarachnoid hemorrhage is usually the result of trauma or a ruptured aneurysm. It is most often accompanied by a very severe sudden-onset headache. Subarachnoid hemorrhage can really be visualized only in the acute stage, when the blood is radiographically denser (whiter) than the CSF. The most common appearance is increased density in the region around the brainstem in a pattern sometimes referred to as a "Texaco star" (Fig. 2-15). Increased density due to the presence of blood also can be seen as a white line in the sylvian fissures, in the anterior interhemispheric fissure, or in the region of the tentorium. In the absence of trauma, a ruptured aneurysm should be suspected. As is discussed in Chapter 9, in infants, both intraventricular and intra-

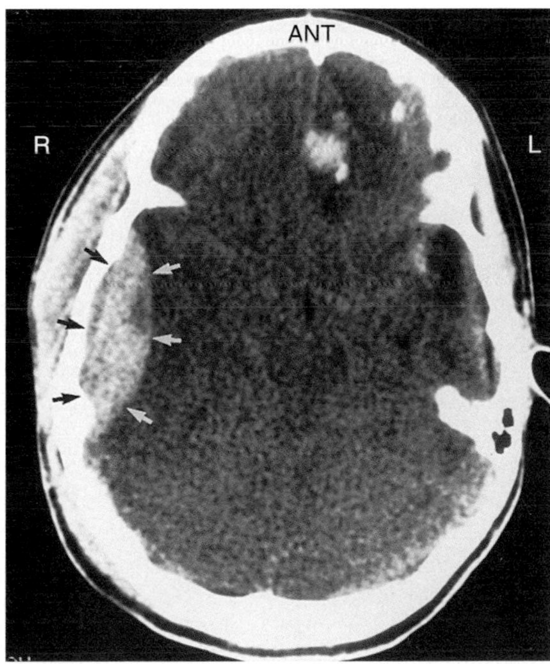

FIGURE 2-14 ■ Epidural hematoma. In this patient, who was in a motor vehicle accident, a lenticular area of increased density is seen on a noncontrasted axial computed tomography (CT) scan in the right parietal region. These typically occur over the groove of the middle meningeal artery. Areas of hemorrhage also are seen in the left frontal lobe.

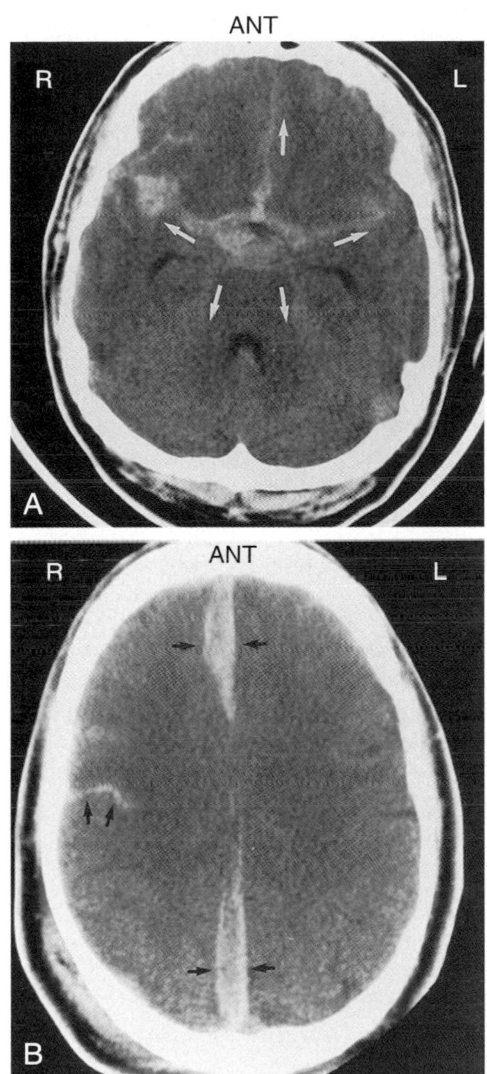

FIGURE 2-15 ■ Acute subarachnoid hemorrhage. A noncontrasted axial computed tomography (CT) scan shows the blood as areas of increased density. A transverse view *(A)* near the base of the brain shows blood in the "Texaco star" pattern, formed by blood radiating from the suprasellar cistern into the sylvian fissures and the anterior interhemispheric fissure. A higher cut *(B)* shows blood as an area of increased density in the anterior and posterior interhemispheric fissures, as well as in the sulci on the right.

parenchymal hemorrhage can be visualized and monitored by using ultrasound. This can be done only if the fontanelles have not closed.

Pneumocephalus

Air within the cranial vault is almost always the result of trauma. Even tiny amounts of air are easily seen on CT as decreased density (blackness) (see Fig. 2-11). It is preferable to do a CT scan instead of an MRI examination because of the superior ability of CT to localize skull fractures and fresh hemorrhage. It also is easier to manage an unstable patient in a CT scanner than in an MRI machine.

TABLE 2-4 ■ **Imaging Indications with a New Neurologic Deficit**

Acute onset or persistence of the following neurologic deficits is an indication for computed tomography or magnetic resonance imaging:
- New vision loss
- Aphasia
- Mental status change (memory loss, confusion, impaired level of consciousness)
- Sensory abnormalities (hemianesthesia/hypesthesia including single limb)
- Motor paralysis (hemiparesis or single limb)
- Vertigo with headache, diplopia, motor or sensory deficit, ataxia, dysarthria, or dysmetria

Hydrocephalus

Dilatation of the ventricles can be either obstructive or nonobstructive. The ventricles are easily seen on a noncontrasted CT or MRI study. If the cause is obstructive, both modalities have a good chance of finding the site of obstruction.

Transient Ischemic Attack

A transient ischemic attack (TIA) is defined as a neurologic deficit that has an abrupt onset and from which rapid recovery occurs, often within minutes, but always within 24 hours. The imaging indications for patients with a new neurologic deficit are shown in Table 2-4. A TIA indicates that the patient may be at high risk for stroke. In the acute setting, the initial test of choice is a CT scan to differentiate an ischemic event from a hemorrhagic one. A second CT scan can be obtained in 24 to 72 hours if the diagnosis is in doubt, but an MRI is more sensitive in identifying early ischemic damage and may establish the cause of the TIA. If initial vertebrobasilar findings are seen, an MRI provides better evaluation of the posterior fossa than does a CT scan. Regardless of whether a carotid bruit is present in this setting, a duplex Doppler ultrasound examination of the carotid arteries is indicated if the patient would be a surgical candidate for endarterectomy. Magnetic resonance angiography can be used to visualize carotid stenosis, but many vascular surgeons want a true contrast angiogram (because of better spatial resolution) before surgery.

Stroke

A stroke may be ischemic or associated with hemorrhage. An acute hemorrhagic stroke is most easily visualized on a noncontrasted CT scan, because fresh blood is quite dense (white). A diagnosis of stroke cannot be excluded even with normal results on a CT scan taken within 12 hours of a suspected stroke. A purely ischemic acute stroke is difficult to visualize on a CT scan unless mass effect is present. This is noted as compression of the lateral ventricle, possible midline shift, and effacement of the sulci on the affected side. One key to identification of most strokes is that they are usually confined to one vascular territory (such as the middle cerebral artery). An acute ischemic stroke is very easy to see on an MRI study, because the edema (increased water) can be identified as a bright area on T2 images. In spite of this, an MRI scan is not needed in a patient with an acute stroke. Because anticoagulant therapy is often being contemplated, a noncontrasted CT scan can be obtained to exclude hemorrhage (which would be a contraindication to such therapy).

After about 24 hours, the edema associated with a stroke can be seen on a CT scan as an area of low density (darker than normal brain). If a contrasted CT scan is done 1 day to several days after a stroke, enhancement (increased density or whiteness) may be seen at the edges of the area (so-called *luxury perfusion*). During the months after a stroke, atrophy of the brain occurs, which can be seen as widened sulci and a focally dilated lateral ventricle on the affected side (Figs. 2-16 and 2-17).

Intracranial Aneurysm

Intracranial aneurysms occur in approximately 2% to 4% of the population and are a cause of intracranial hemorrhage. Most aneurysms occur in the anterior communicating artery or near the base of the brain. The best initial way to visualize intracranial aneurysms is with CT or MRI. In a setting of acute headache and suspected acute intracranial bleeding, a noncontrasted CT study should be done. If the noncontrasted CT is negative, it is followed by a contrasted CT. The noncontrasted study will show extravascular acute hemorrhage as denser (whiter) than normal brain. If this is seen, an angiogram is done, and the contrasted CT scan is skipped (Fig. 2-18). A completely thrombosed aneurysm is frequently seen as a hypodense region with a surrounding thin ring of calcium. On the contrasted study, a large nonthrombosed aneurysm will fill with contrast, although only partial filling may be seen because of a thrombus. With MRI, the aneurysm may be seen as an area signal void (black) on the T1 images. If gadolinium contrast is used, the aneurysm may fill and have an increased signal (white) (Fig. 2-19).

In the acute setting, CT or MRI is usually followed by a conventional contrast arteriogram before surgery. This is done because of the very high spatial resolution of the conventional arteriogram. Some CT and MR machines can give excellent angiographic images, but many surgeons still demand a regular angiogram. Patients who have an acute bleeding episode as the result of a ruptured aneurysm may have associated spasm (occurring after a day or so and lasting up to a week). This can make the aneurysm hard or impossible to see on an arteriogram. For this reason, if subarachnoid hemorrhage is present and an aneurysm is not seen, the angiogram is often repeated a week or so later. For patients who have a long history of headache, or a familial history of aneurysms, a noninvasive MR arteriogram is probably the procedure of choice.

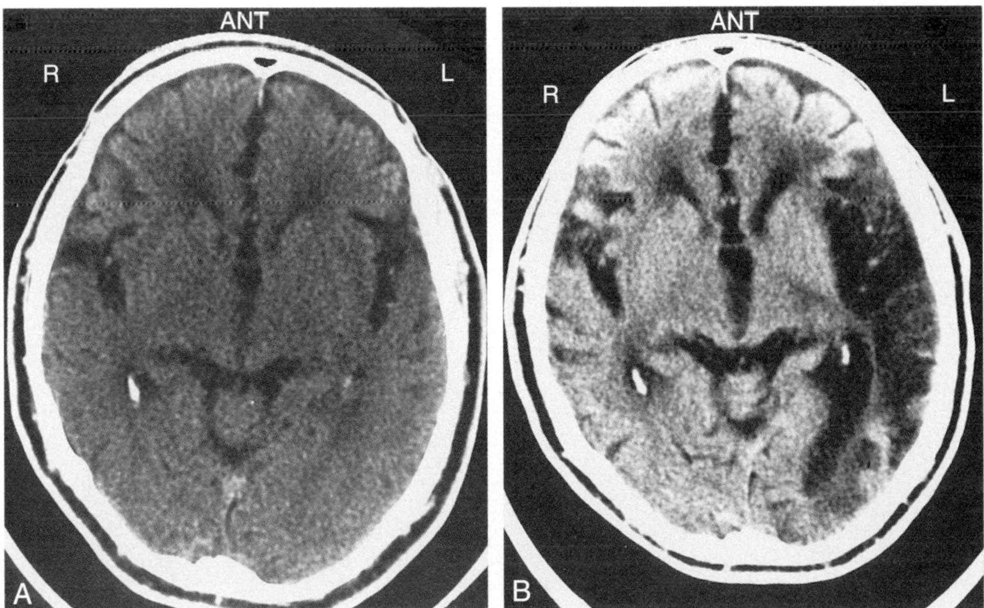

FIGURE 2-16 ■ Acute and chronic stroke on CT. An axial computed tomography (CT) scan performed on a patient with an acute stroke *(A)* has little, if any, definable abnormality within the first several hours. Later, some low density and mass effect may appear as a result of edema. Another scan, approximately 2 years later *(B)*, shows an area of atrophy and scarring as low density in the region of the distribution of the left middle cerebral artery.

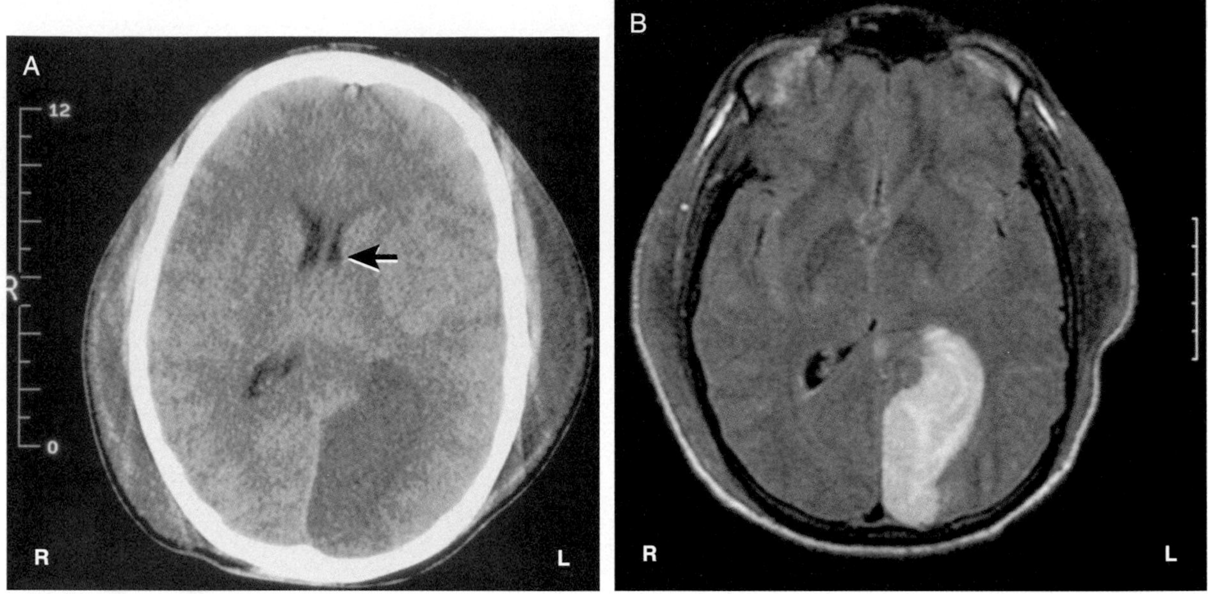

FIGURE 2-17 ■ Stroke on computed tomography (CT) and magnetic resonance imaging (MRI) scans. In this man 3 days after stroke, the CT scan *(A)* shows a low-density area posteriorly on the left with mass effect and clear midline shift *(arrows)*. The MRI scan *(B)* done on the same day shows the infarcted area much more clearly.

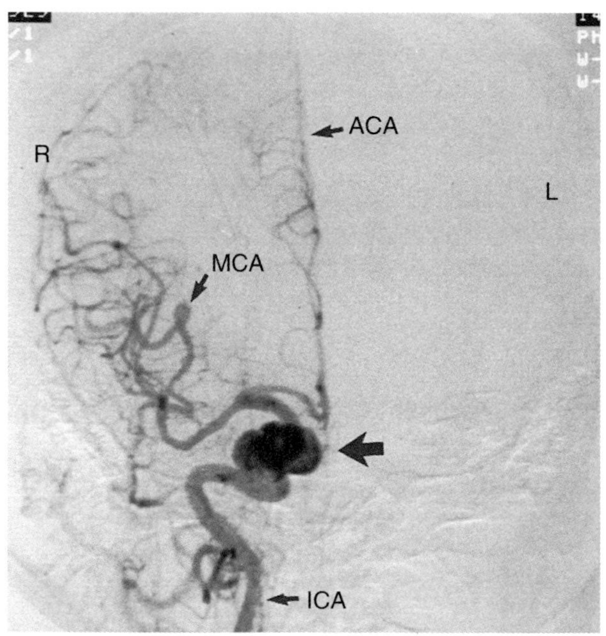

FIGURE 2-18 ■ Intracerebral aneurysm. An anteroposterior projection from a digital angiogram shows the right internal carotid artery (ICA), the anterior cerebral artery (ACA), and the middle cerebral artery (MCA). A large rounded density seen in the region of the circle of Willis is an aneurysm *(large arrow)*.

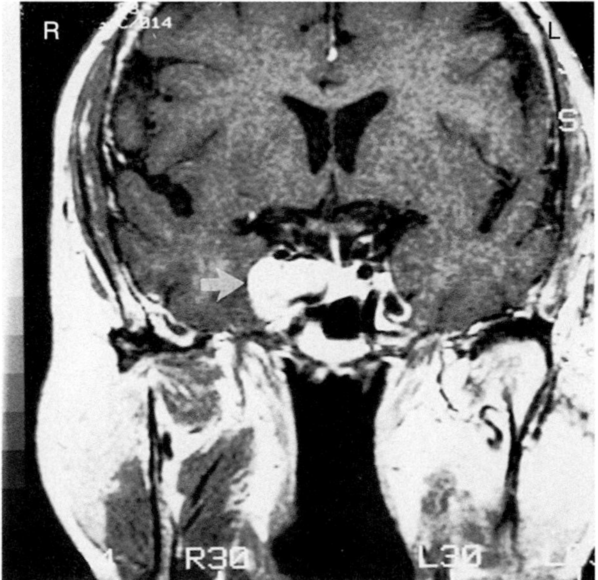

FIGURE 2-19 ■ Magnetic resonance image of intracranial aneurysm. A gadolinium contrast–enhanced scan in the coronal projection shows a large area of enhancement *(arrow)* representing an aneurysm.

Primary Brain Tumors and Metastases

A variety of brain tumors is found. Meningiomas occur along the surface of the brain. They grow quite slowly and often contain calcium. The study of choice is a CT scan with and without intravenous contrast. The noncontrasted scan may show the calcification, whereas the contrasted scan will show the extent of this typically vascular tumor (Fig. 2-20). Astrocytomas can be high or low grade and typically occur within the brain substance. Low-grade tumors may contain some calcium, but they are low density (dark) on a noncontrasted CT scan and have minimal surrounding low-density edema. The more edema and the more enhancement after administration of intravenous contrast, the more malignant the lesion is likely to be. On MR scans, these tumors are usually low signal (dark) in T1 images and high signal (bright) on T2 images. They also can show enhancement when intravenously administered gadolinium is used as a contrast agent (Fig. 2-21).

Other intracranial tumors, such as pinealomas, papillomas, lipomas, epidermoids, and others, have variable appearances and are not considered here. A reasonable differential diagnosis can be made from the appearance and location of the lesions on either CT or MR scans.

The wide variety of pituitary tumors range from benign microadenomas to malignant craniopharyngiomas. The examination with the best resolution for the pituitary region is MRI, although relatively large lesions can be imaged with thin-cut (1 to 1.5 mm) CT scans of the sellar region. In either case, the studies are usually done with and without intravenous contrast, because differential enhancement of the tumor and the pituitary allows the margins to be delineated (Fig. 2-22).

Metastatic disease is best identified using MRI with intravenous gadolinium (Fig. 2-23). A contrasted CT scan can be used, but it is not as sensitive as MRI. Most metastases enhance with contrast agents. The reason for ordering any study should be carefully considered to determine that the findings would affect the treatment. Usually little reason is found to do a cranial MR or CT scan on a patient who has known metastases elsewhere. Almost all metastases to the brain are quite resistant to all forms of therapy.

Vertigo and Dizziness

Sometimes vertigo and dizziness are confused. Symptoms of vertigo are quite specific and occur in only a small subset of patients who complain of dizziness. Nystagmus almost always accompanies true vertigo but is usually absent between episodes. The workup of most patients with vertigo rarely involves the use of imaging procedures. If the patient does not

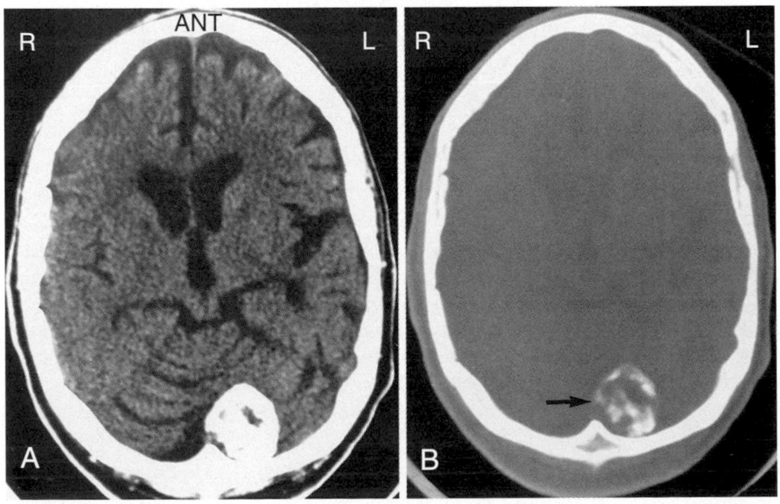

FIGURE 2-20 ■ **Meningioma.** A noncontrasted computed tomography (CT) scan *(A)* shows a very dense, peripherally based lesion in the left cerebellar area. A bone-window image *(B)* obtained at the same level shows that the density is due to calcification within this lesion.

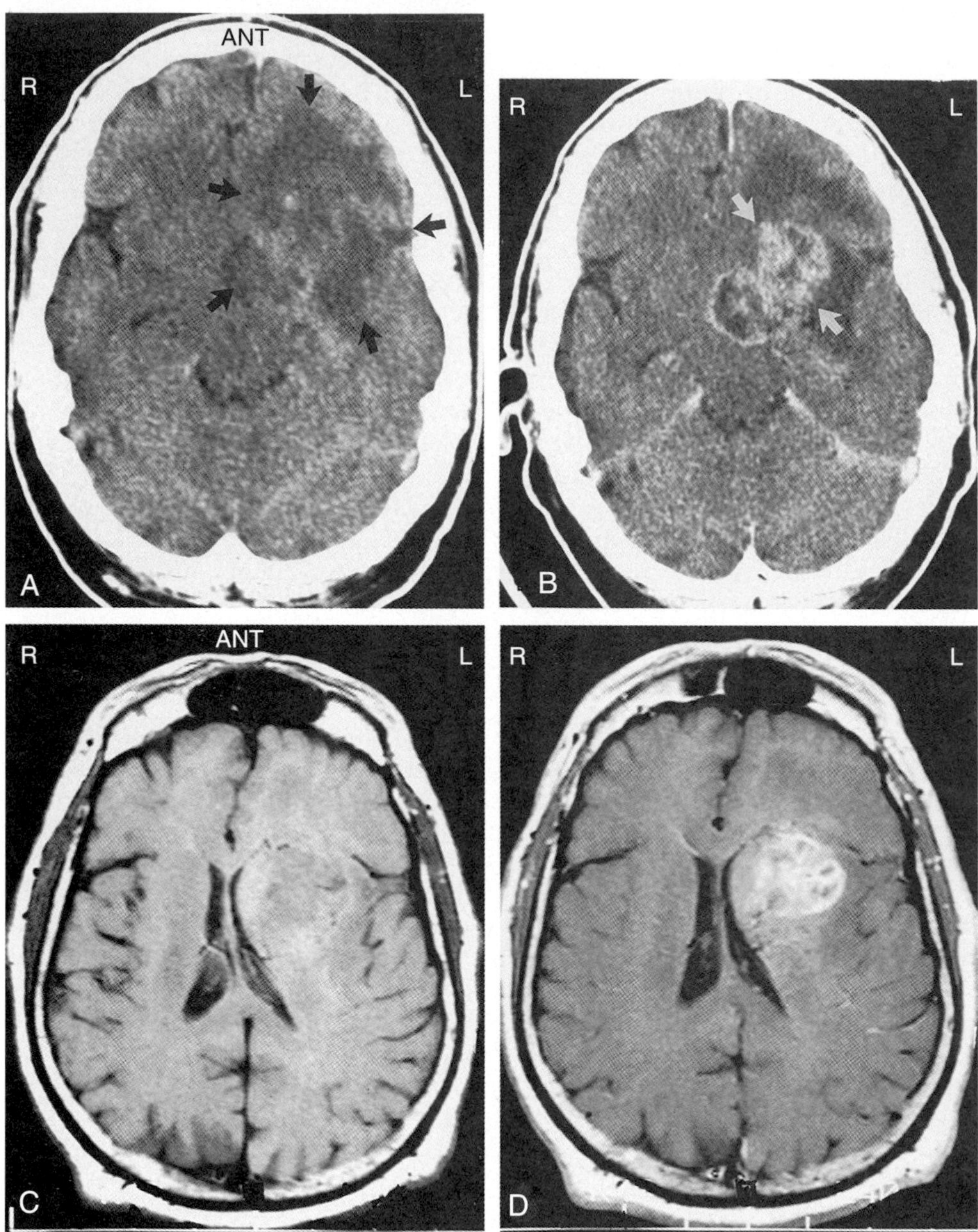

FIGURE 2-21 ■ **Astrocytoma.** These contrasted and noncontrasted computed tomography (CT) and magnetic resonance (MR) images were obtained of the same patient and demonstrate a left astrocytoma with a large amount of surrounding edema. The noncontrasted CT scan *(A)* shows only a large area of low density that represents the tumor and edema *(arrows)*. A contrasted CT scan *(B)* shows enhancement of the tumor (arrows) surrounded by the dark or low-density area of edema. A noncontrasted T1–weighted MR image *(C)* clearly shows a mass effect due to impression of the tumor on the left lateral ventricle and some midline shift. A gadolinium-enhanced T1–weighted MR image *(D)* clearly outlines the tumor, but the edema is difficult to see.

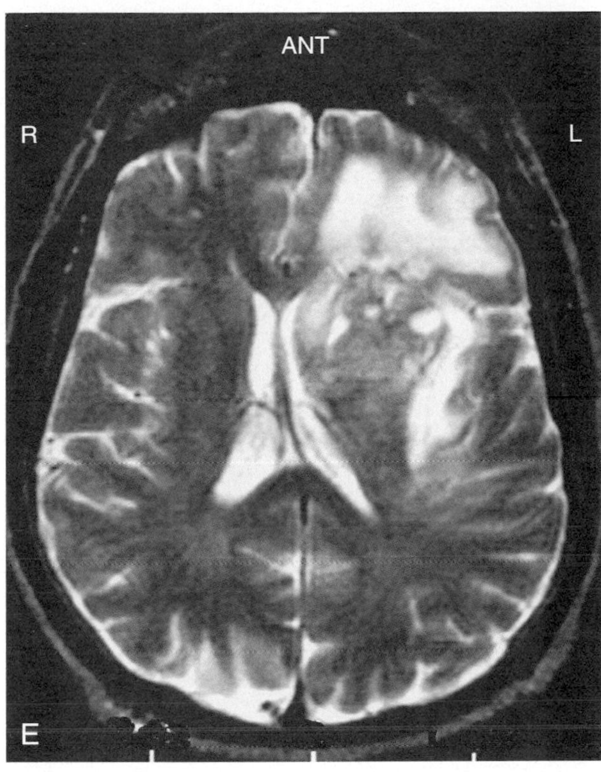

FIGURE 2-21 cont'd ■ *(E)* A T2-weighted magnetic resonance (MR) image *(E)* shows the tumor rather poorly, but the surrounding edema is easily seen as an area of increased signal (white).

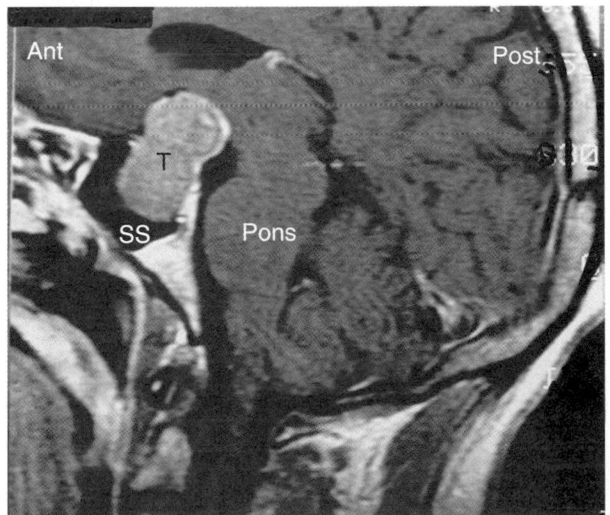

FIGURE 2-22 ■ **Pituitary adenoma.** A sagittal view of the base of the brain on a T1-weighted magnetic resonance imaging (MRI) scan shows the pituitary tumor (T) and its extension down into the sphenoid sinus (SS).

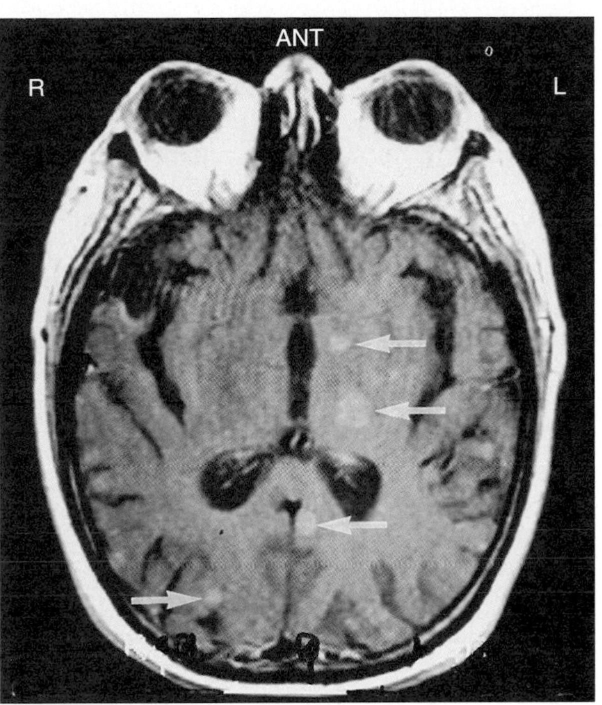

FIGURE 2-23 ■ **Metastatic disease to the brain.** A gadolinium-enhanced T1-weighted image shows multiple metastases as areas of increased signal *(arrows)*.

respond to conservative measures, imaging studies should be considered in consultation with an ear, nose, and throat specialist. If the patient has vertigo with sensorineural hearing loss or suspected acoustic neuroma or posterior fossa tumor, an MRI is indicated. If conductive hearing loss and vertigo are present, a noncontrasted CT scan of the petrous bone may be indicated. Other types of dizziness may have a wide range of etiologies ranging from postural hypotension to TIAs. Few, if any, imaging tests are indicated for dizziness until the underlying etiology becomes clear.

Suspected Intracranial Infection

Most, if not all, suspected intracranial infections are best imaged by MRI. Probably the only exception to this is when a sinus infection is suspected, and then a CT should be ordered. It should be remembered that the primary method for diagnosis of meningitis is lumbar puncture. In patients who have acquired immunodeficiency syndrome (AIDS) or are human immunodeficiency virus (HIV) positive, CNS complications such as toxoplasmosis, *Cryptococcus*, and lymphoma may develop. These complications are being seen less because of better treatment; however, patients who have neurologic finding or a headache often have a contrasted MRI scan for evaluation. A CT scan also may be used but it is not as sensitive.

Multiple Sclerosis

Multiple sclerosis is effectively imaged only by MRI. Often small high-signal (bright) lesions are seen on either T1 or T2 images (Fig. 2-24). These plaques can have contrast enhancement to varying degrees in the same patient. Whether the enhancement is related to activity of disease remains a matter of debate.

Dementia and Slow-onset Mental Changes

Imaging of the brain in most patients with dementia is usually an unrewarding exercise. Most of the time, a CT scan shows atrophy compatible with age and nothing else. As mentioned, an MR scan can effectively exclude multiple sclerosis, tumor, metastases, and hydrocephalus. Often it is ordered to exclude these rather than to find the true cause of most dementias. It is possible to do a nuclear medicine tomographic brain scan (brain single-photon emission CT [SPECT] or positron emission tomography [PET]) by using radioactive substances that are extracted on the first pass through the cerebral circulation. It appears that these scans show bilateral reduced blood flow to the temporoparietal areas in Alzheimer's disease and scattered areas of reduced perfusion in multi-infarct dementias. Such studies may not be cost effective unless you have effective therapy for these entities.

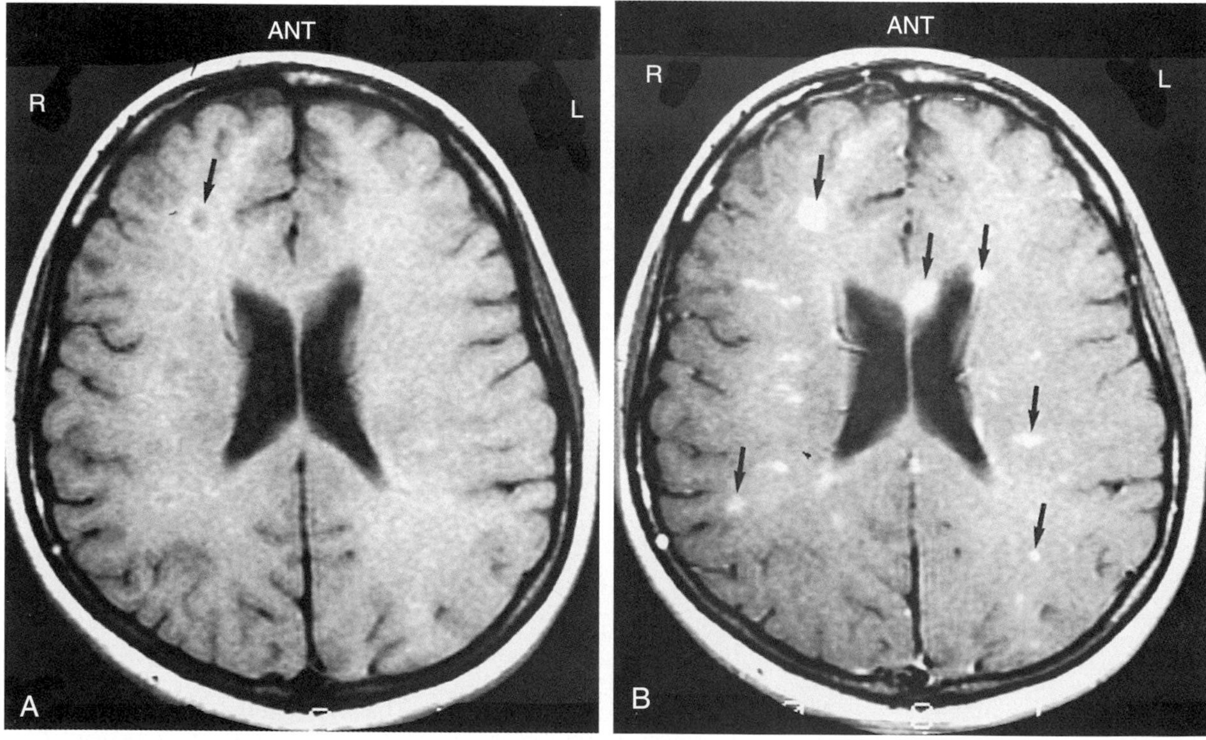

FIGURE 2-24 ■ **Multiple sclerosis.** The noncontrasted T1–weighted magnetic resonance imaging (MRI) scan *(A)* is generally unremarkable, with the exception of one lesion in the right frontal lobe (*arrow*). A gadolinium-enhanced scan *(B)* is much better and shows many enhancing lesions, only some of which are indicated by the *arrows*.

Seizures

Examination of a patient with a seizure should include a thorough medical history, physical examination, and blood and urine evaluation. Particularly pertinent history includes information regarding seizures (personally or in the family), drug abuse, and trauma. Noncontrasted MRI is the imaging procedure of choice, although contrasted CT scanning may be used. Imaging is usually done for persons who are otherwise healthy with a new onset of seizures, those who have epilepsy with a poor therapeutic response, alcoholics with a new onset of seizures, or seizure patients with a neurologic deficit or abnormal EEG. Noncontrasted CT scanning is usually used in patients with seizures and acute head trauma or other emergency pathology. Imaging is not usually needed in children who have a suspected febrile seizure and in adults without neurologic deficits who are in chemical withdrawal or who have metabolic abnormalities.

Psychiatric Disorders

Imaging studies of most psychiatric patients usually have a low yield for diagnostic information. One must remember that a number of CNS abnormalities may first be seen with apparent psychiatric symptoms, particularly in the elderly. For example, common conditions that may be mistaken for a depressive disorder include infections, malignancies, and stroke. Patients treated for chronic alcoholism may have unrecognized subdural hematomas. Obtaining a thorough history and performing a careful physical examination are essential. If associated neurologic findings or disparities are noted between the psychiatric findings and common diagnoses, imaging may be in order. In such circumstances, an MRI is the initial study of choice.

Some authors have suggested that neuroimaging studies are unnecessary if the mental status examination, neurologic examination, and EEG are normal. If the patient is younger than 40 years, has no history of head injury, and has normal mental status and neurologic examinations but abnormal EEG, the imaging examination is not likely to give additional diagnostic information.

FACE

Indicated imaging for face and neck problems is shown in Table 2-5.

TABLE 2-5 ■ **Indicated Imaging for Face and Neck Problems**

Suspected Face and Neck Problem	Initial Imaging Study
Unilateral proptosis, periorbital swelling or mass	CT or MRI
Facial fracture	Plain x-ray, CT for complicated cases
Mandibular fracture	Panorex
Carotid bruit	Duplex ultrasound
Epiglottitis	Lateral soft tissue x-ray of neck
Foreign body	Plain x-ray if calcified or metallic (fish bones not visible)
Retropharyngeal abscess	Lateral soft tissue x-ray film; if positive, CT to determine extent
Lymphadenopathy fixed, nontender (or no decrease in size over 4 wk)	CT (preferred) or MRI
Hyperthyroidism	Serum TSH and free T_4 (no imaging needed)
Suspected goiter or ectopic thyroid	Nuclear medicine thyroid scan
Thyroid nodule (palpable)	Fine needle aspiration (no imaging needed)
Known thyroid cancer (postoperative)	Nuclear medicine whole body radioiodine scan
Exclude recurrent thyroid tumor	Serum thyroglobulin
Suspected hyperparathyroidism	CT or nuclear medicine scan

CT, computed tomography; MRI, magnetic resonance imaging; TSH, thyroid-stimulating hormone; T_4, thyroxine.

Sinuses and Sinusitis

The frontal skull film is best uses to evaluate the frontal and ethmoid sinuses. The frontal Waters' view (done with the head tipped back), is used to evaluate the maxillary sinuses. The lateral view is used for evaluation of the sphenoid sinus (Fig. 2-25). Sinus series are often inappropriately ordered to rule out sinusitis in children. Sinuses are not developed or well pneumatized until children are about 5 to 6 years old (Fig. 2-26). In adults, often hypoplasia of the frontal sinuses is seen.

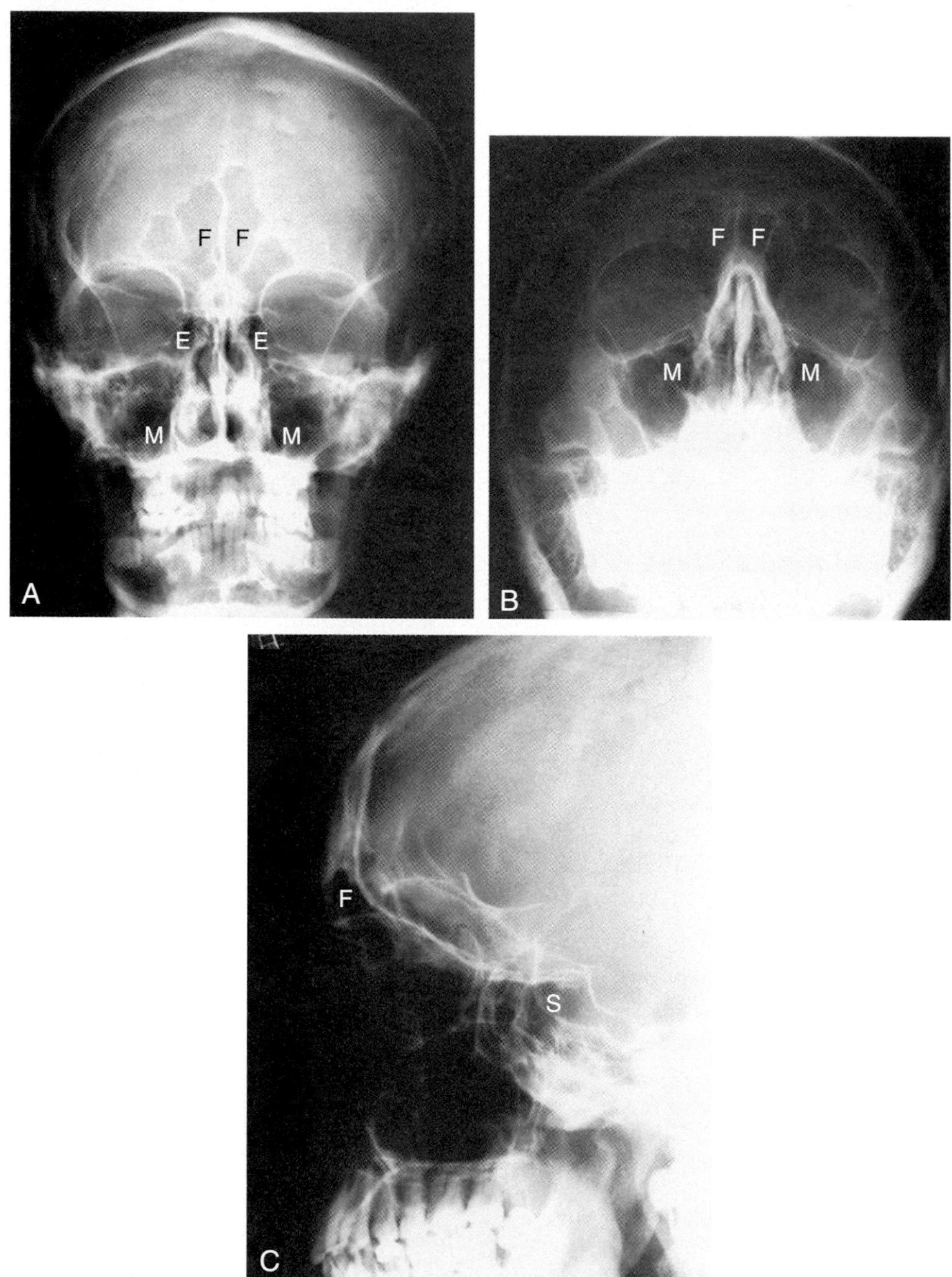

FIGURE 2-25 ■ Normal radiographic anatomy of the sinuses. Typical radiographic projections are anteroposterior (AP) *(A)*, Waters' view *(B)*, and lateral view of the face *(C)*.

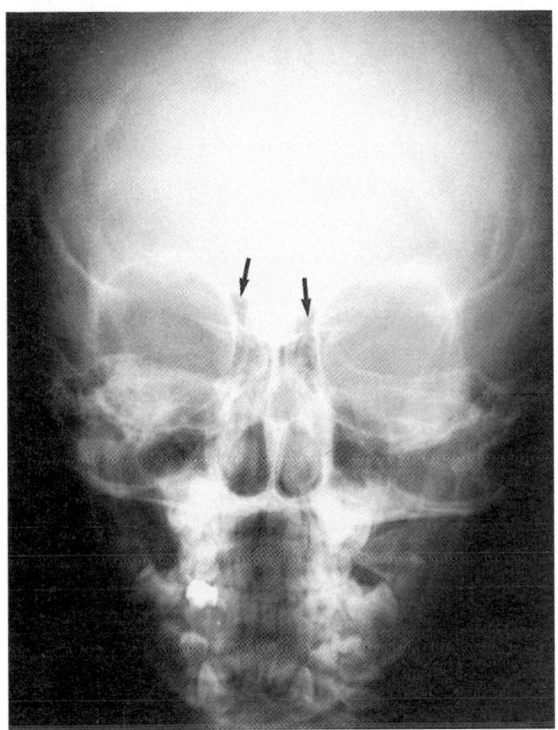

FIGURE 2-26 ■ Hypoplastic frontal sinuses. This adult has had only minimal development of both frontal sinuses (arrows). This is a common normal variant.

TABLE 2-6 ■ Indications for Computed Tomography (CT) in Sinus Disease

CT scanning is indicated in acute complicated sinusitis if the patient has
- Sinus pain/discharge and
- Fever and
- A complicating factor such as
  - mental status change
  - facial or orbital cellulitis
  - meningitis by lumbar puncture
  - focal neurologic findings
  - intractable pain after 48 hr of intravenous antibiotic therapy
  - immunocompromised host
- Three or more episodes of acute sinusitis within 1 yr in which the patient has signs of infection

CT scanning is indicated in chronic sinusitis if
no improvement is seen after 4 wk of antibiotic therapy based on culture or
no improvement or seen after 4 wk of intranasal steroid spray
CT scanning also is indicated in cases of suspected sinus malignancy

Most patients with suspected sinusitis do not need sinus films for clinical management (Table 2-6). Sinusitis is most common in the maxillary sinuses. Acute sinusitis is diagnosed radiographically if an air/fluid level in the sinus (Fig. 2-27) or complete opacification is found. After trauma, hemorrhage also can

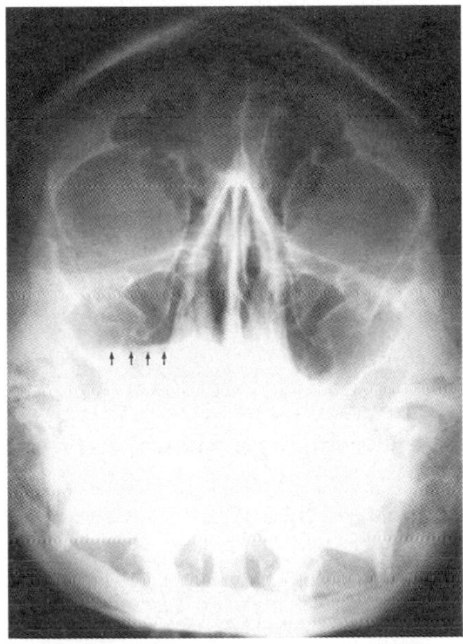

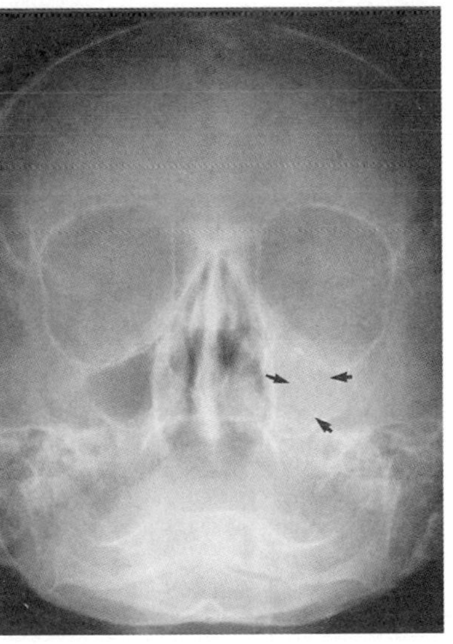

FIGURE 2-27 ■ Sinusitis. A Waters' view taken in the upright position *(A)* may show an air/fluid interface *(arrows)* in acute sinusitis. In another patient who is a child *(B)*, opacification of the left maxillary antrum *(arrows)* is seen, and this may represent either acute or chronic sinusitis.

cause an air/fluid level. With chronic sinusitis, thickening and indistinctness of the sinus walls appear. CT is vastly superior to radiography and MRI for evaluation of the paranasal sinuses, mastoid sinuses, and adjacent bone. Malignancy should be suspected if recurrent episodes occur of unilateral epistaxis with no visible bleeding site, constant facial pain, anosmia, recurrent unilateral otitis media, a soft tissue mass, or bone destruction on a sinus or dental x-ray.

Facial Fractures

Zygoma. Fractures of the zygoma usually result from a direct blow to the arch or to the zygomatic process. The arch and the skull form a rigid bony ring. Just like a pretzel, it cannot be broken in only one place. The view that should be ordered if an arch fracture is suspected is the "jug handle" view (Fig. 2-28). If only one fracture is seen in the arch, then films of the facial bones should be obtained to exclude a so-called tripod fracture. The tripod fracture results from a direct blow to the zygomatic process. It actually consists of four fractures, not three, as the name suggests. The fractures are of the zygomatic arch, lateral orbital rim, inferior orbital rim, and lateral wall of the maxillary sinus (Fig. 2-29).

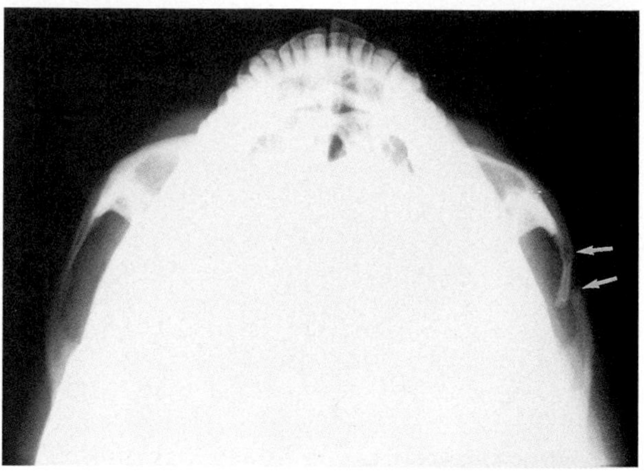

FIGURE 2-28 ■ Depressed zygomatic fracture. A view of the skull from the bottom (jug-handle view) shows the zygomatic arches very well. In this patient, a direct blow to the zygoma has caused a depressed fracture *(arrows).*

Nasal. Nasal films are really useful only to look for depressed fractures or lateral deviation. The latter is often clinically obvious. On the lateral view, the nasal bone has normal lucent lines that are often mistaken for fractures. If the lucent

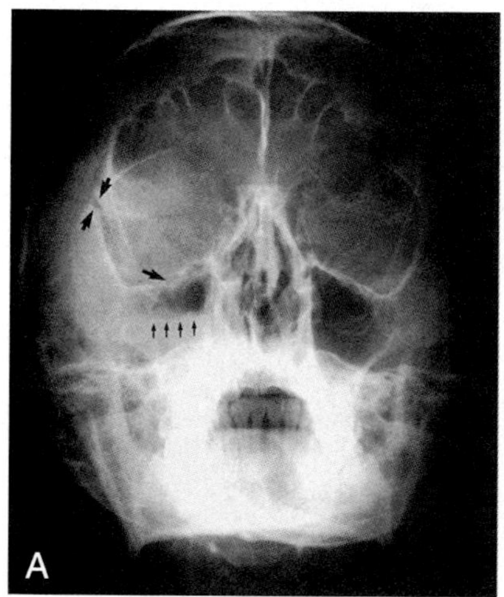

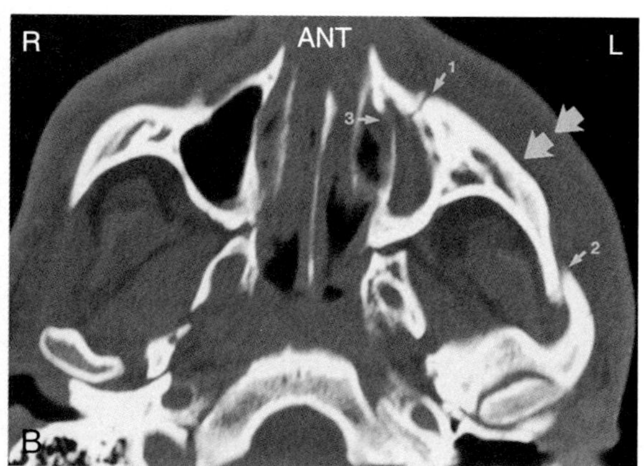

FIGURE 2-29 ■ Tripod (zygomatic) fracture. In this patient who had a direct blow to the zygomatic process, the anteroposterior (AP) Waters' view of the skull obtained in the upright position *(A)* shows an air/fluid level (as a result of hemorrhage) in the right maxillary antrum. Discontinuity of the inferior and right lateral orbital walls represents a fracture. A transverse computed tomography (CT) view in a different patient *(B)* shows a tripod fracture on the left caused by a direct blow in the direction indicated by the *large arrows.* Fractures of the anterior (1) and posterior (2) zygoma, as well as the medial wall of the left maxillary sinus (3), are seen.

lines follow along the length of the nose, however, they are not fractures. Fractures are seen as dark lines that are perpendicular or sharply oblique to the length of the nose (Fig. 2-30).

Orbital. Blowout fractures occur from a direct blow to the globe of the eye. The pressure on the eyeball fractures the weak medial or inferior walls of the orbit. The usual blowout fracture is down through the orbital floor. The Waters view affords the best image to look for this. The findings that may be present are discontinuity of the orbital floor, a soft tissue mass hanging down into the maxillary antrum (Fig. 2-31), fluid in the maxillary antrum, and, rarely, air in the orbit (coming up from the sinus). Blowout fractures also can occur medially into the ethmoid sinus (Fig. 2-32). You will see this on the frontal skull view only as opacification (whiteness) in the affected ethmoid sinus.

Le Fort Fractures of the Face. These rare injuries are produced by massive facial trauma. They are associated with many other smaller fractures. A Le Fort 1 fracture is a fracture through the maxilla, usually caused by being hit in the upper mouth with something like a baseball bat. A Le Fort 2 fracture involves the maxilla, nose, and inferior and medial orbital walls. A Le Fort 3 fracture is a facial/cranial dissociation or a separation between the face and the skull. Owing to the massive trauma required for the type 3 fracture, a high fatality rate occurs from the associated brain injury.

Mandible. Mandibular fractures should be suspected especially if malocclusion after trauma is present. Occasionally temporomandibular joint dislocation is found. The easiest way to visualize these entities is to order a panorex view of the mandible. This displays the mandible as if it were flattened out (Fig. 2-33). If a panorex machine is not available, standard oblique views of the mandible are satisfactory but harder to interpret.

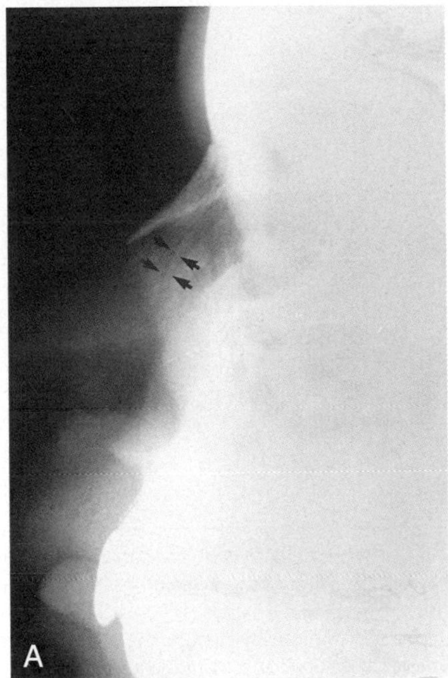

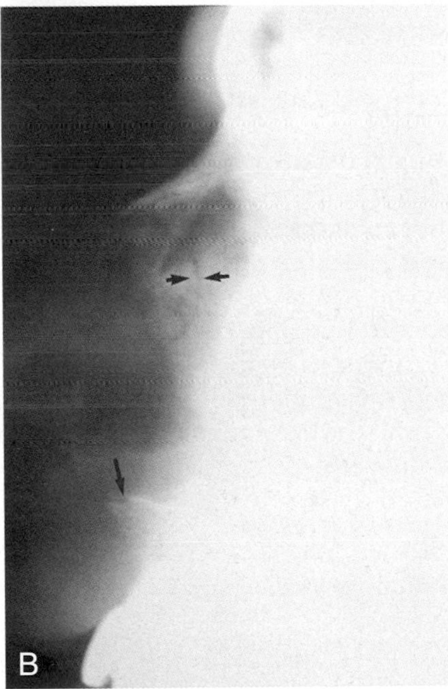

FIGURE 2-30 ■ Normal and fractured nasal bones. A normal lateral view *(A)* of the nose shows normal dark longitudinal lines in the nasal bone. A nasal fracture *(B)* is seen as a lucent line that is not in the long axis of the nose *(arrows)*. A fracture of the anterior maxillary spine also is seen in this patient.

SOFT TISSUES OF THE NECK

For a discussion of cervical fractures and dislocation, refer to Chapter 8.

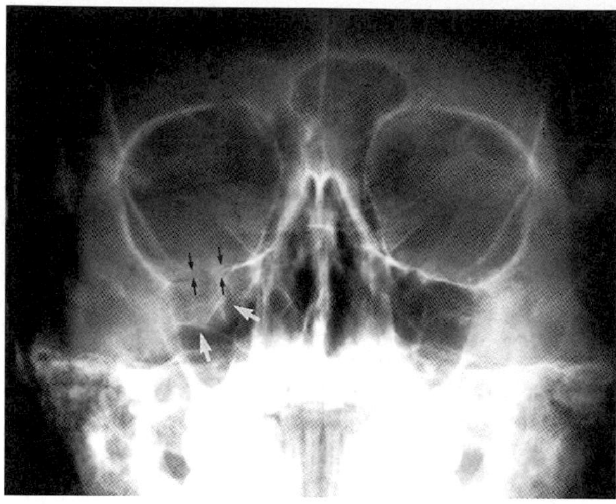

FIGURE 2-31 ■ Inferior blowout fracture of the orbit. An anteroposterior (AP) view of the face shows air in the orbit, discontinuity of the floor of the right orbit *(black arrows)*, as well as a soft tissue mass hanging down from the orbit into the maxillary antrum *(white arrows)* and blood in the dependent part of the sinus.

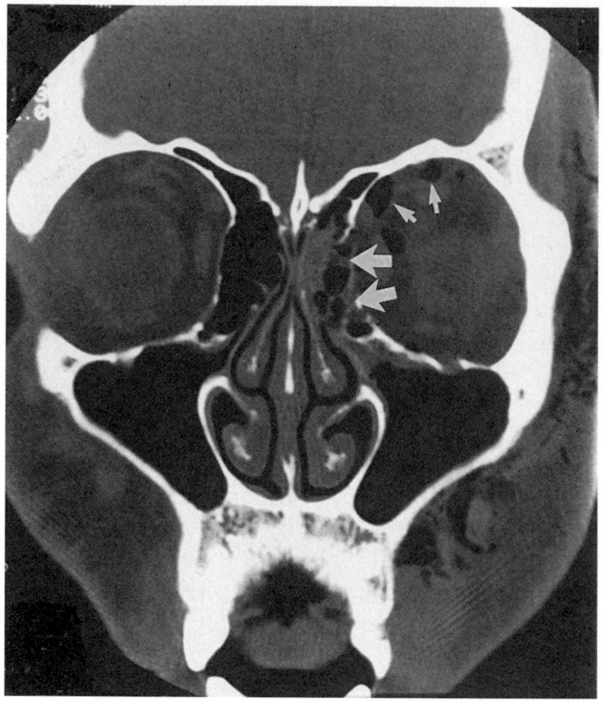

FIGURE 2-32 ■ Medial blowout fracture. A coronal computed tomography (CT) scan shows a fracture of the medial orbital wall with hemorrhage into the left ethmoid sinus *(large arrows)*. Air within the orbit *(small white arrows)* is seen in this case.

Epiglottitis

Epiglottitis is usually thought of as a childhood disease, but it can occur in adults as well. The best initial imaging modality for upper airway obstruction or suspected foreign body is a lateral soft tissue view of the neck. This is essentially an underexposed lateral cervical spine view, and the airway is usually well seen. With epiglottitis, swelling of the epiglottis is seen easily on the lateral view, and the epiglottis looks somewhat like a thumbprint rather than a thin delicate curved structure (Fig. 2-34). For a discussion of croup and pediatric epiglottitis, refer to Chapter 9.

Retropharyngeal Abscess

Retropharyngeal abscess is another cause of upper airway obstruction as well as a cause of

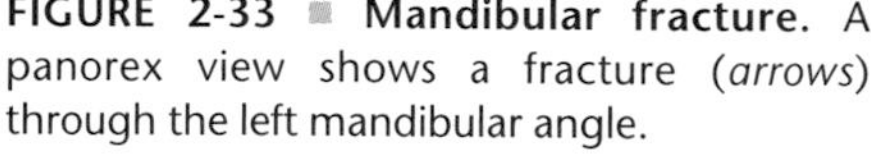

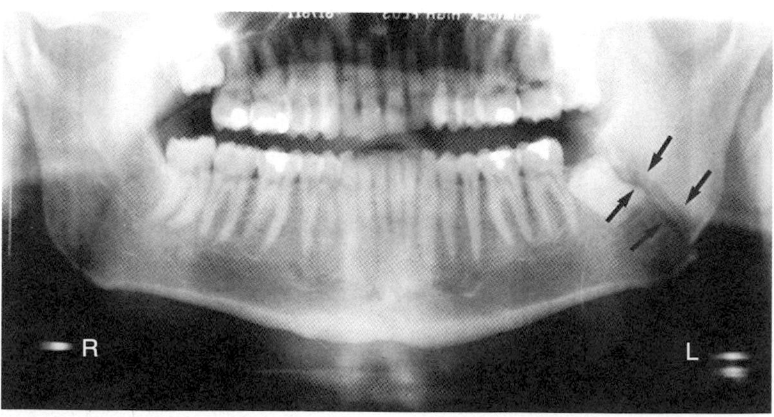

FIGURE 2-33 ■ Mandibular fracture. A panorex view shows a fracture (*arrows*) through the left mandibular angle.

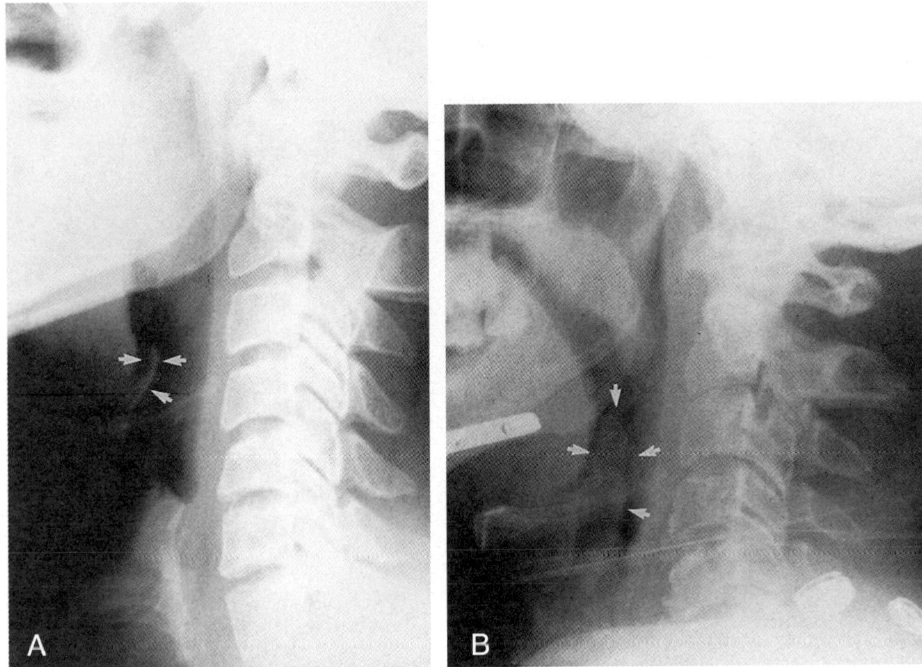

FIGURE 2-34 ■ Normal epiglottis and epiglottitis. The normal epiglottis is well seen on the lateral soft tissue view of the neck *(A)* as a delicate curved structure. In a patient with epiglottitis *(B)*, the epiglottis is swollen and significantly reduces the diameter of the airway.

dysphagia. The soft tissue lateral x-ray is the initial imaging procedure of choice, usually showing prevertebral soft tissue swelling. Air may or may not be within these swollen soft tissues (Fig. 2-35). An intravenously contrasted CT scan is often of great value to help discern the lateral and inferior margins of the abscess and the location of the great vessels of the neck. Retropharyngeal abscesses can extend interiorly into the mediastinum or laterally into the region of the carotid artery and jugular vein.

Subcutaneous Emphysema

In addition to air within the soft tissues of the retropharynx, you should also be aware of dark vertical lines of air within the anterior and lateral soft tissues of the neck. If you see these, you should look at the concurrent chest x-ray, or order one, to exclude either a pneumothorax or mediastinal emphysema. These are both potentially life-threatening abnormalities, and the air from these commonly dissects up into the neck. (See Chapter 3 for a full description of these entities.)

Thyroid

The thyroid is a symmetrical gland that lies lateral and anterior to the trachea just above the thoracic inlet. Large goiters can compress the trachea in a symmetrical fashion, although this is unusual. More commonly, asymmetrical enlargement occurs, and the trachea is deviated to one side or the other. Before diagnosing tracheal deviation, you must be sure that the patient is not rotated. On a well-positioned posteroanterior (PA) or anteroposterior (AP) film, the medial aspect of the clavicles is equidistant from the posterior spinous processes (Fig. 2-36).

A number of patients will present with hyperthyroidism and a smoothly enlarged gland (Graves' disease) (Fig. 2-37) or a lumpy enlarged

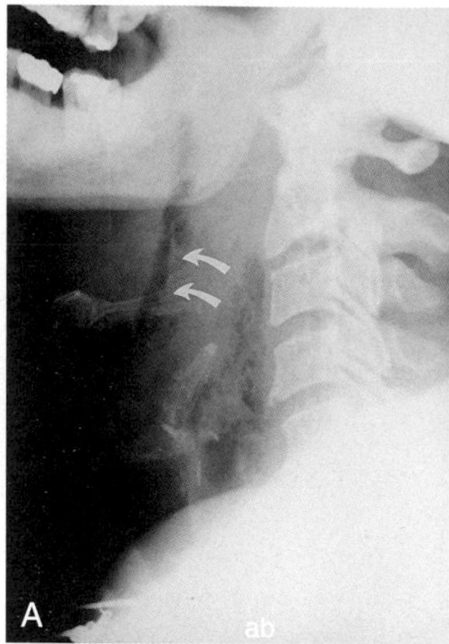

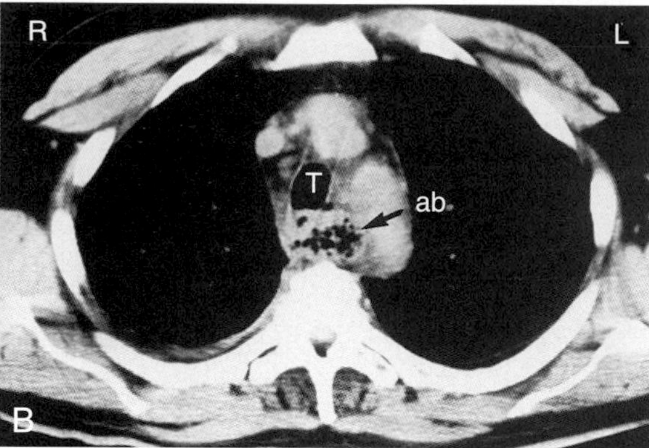

FIGURE 2-35 ■ Retropharyngeal abscess. On a lateral soft tissue view of the neck *(A)*, the normal air column is displaced forward *(curved arrows)*. A large amount of soft tissue swelling occurs in front of the cervical spine; gas, which represents an abscess (ab), is seen in the lower portion. A computed tomography (CT) scan through the upper thorax in the same patient *(B)* shows extension of the abscess (ab) down into the mediastinum between the trachea (T) and the spine.

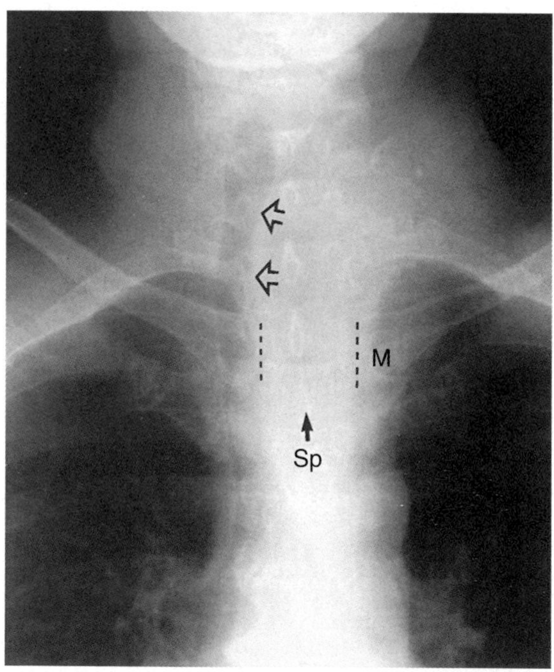

FIGURE 2-36 ■ Thyroid mass. A large thyroid adenoma has displaced the trachea to the right *(open arrows)*. This pattern can be simulated if the patient is rotated slightly when the radiograph is taken. In this case, however, the medial aspects of the clavicles *(dotted lines)* can be seen to be centered over the posterior spinous processes, indicating that, in this case, the patient was not rotated, and a mass is truly present.

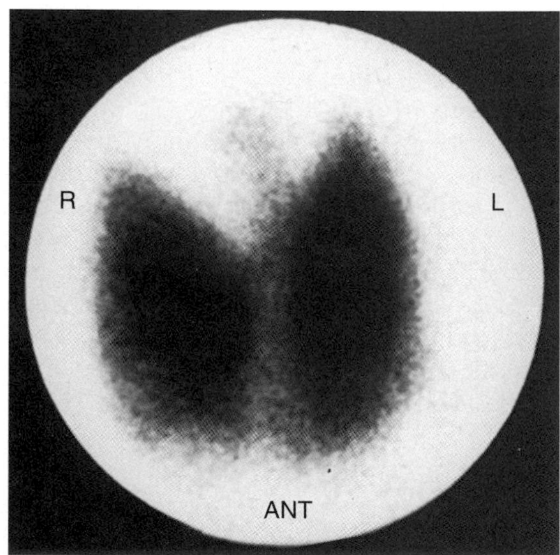

FIGURE 2-37 ■ Graves' disease. An iodine 123 nuclear medicine scan shows a very enlarged right and left lobe of the thyroid. Activity projecting from the upper portion of the left lobe represents a pyramidal lobe commonly seen in Graves' disease patients.

gland (multinodular goiter). The most appropriate imaging study for these patients is a nuclear medicine thyroid scan done after administration of a radioactive material that concentrates in the thyroid gland (such as technetium 99m pertechnetate or iodine 123). Radioactive iodine 131 is often given orally to treat both hyperthyroidism and thyroid cancer.

A nuclear medicine scan is a common imaging study for patients who have a palpable thyroid nodule to ascertain whether the nodule has function similar to that of the normal tissue. If it does, it is not likely to be a cancer. If the nodule has less than normal accumulation of radioactivity, it may be a cancer (Fig. 2-38), a necrotic adenoma, or a colloid cyst. Although ultrasound can be performed, it usually does not add much diagnostic information. Ultrasound is commonly used to direct fine-needle aspiration of cells for pathologic examination.

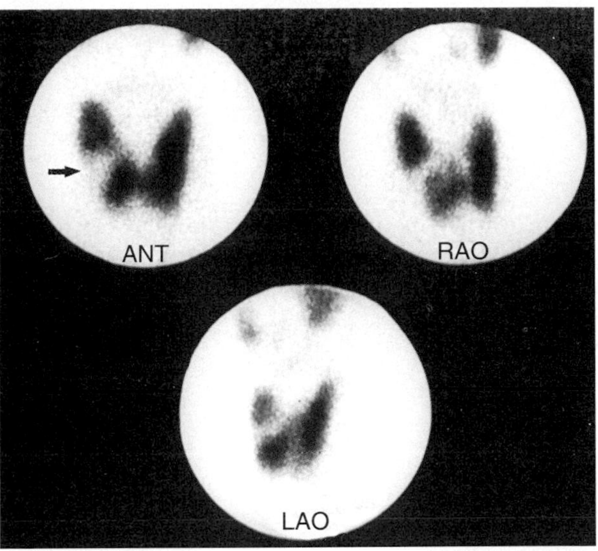

FIGURE 2-38 ■ Thyroid carcinoma. The right and left lobes of the thyroid are well seen; however, a "cold" lesion appears in the middle of the right lobe *(arrow)*. Lack of uptake of the radioactive tracer can be due to a number of entities, including a cyst or an adenoma, but in this case, it was due to thyroid carcinoma.

Parathyroid

The most common parathyroid problem requiring imaging is hypercalcemia secondary to a parathyroid adenoma (80%) or to hyperplasia (20%). Because adenomas can be very difficult to locate at surgery, a nuclear medicine scan using radioactive compounds that accumulate in the thyroid or parathyroid or both should be done. The resulting images are very accurate in localizing the adenomas (Fig. 2-39). Parathyroid adenomas can be imaged by CT, MRI, or ultrasound, but the interpretation is more difficult.

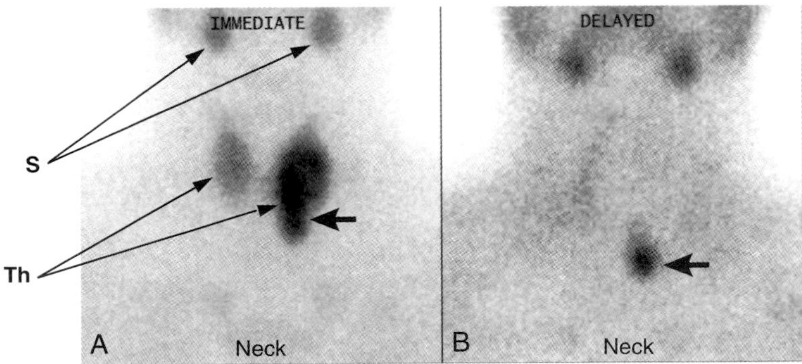

FIGURE 2-39 ■ Parathyroid adenoma. A nuclear medicine scan done with technetium 99 sestamibi. The initial image *(A)* shows the thyroid (Th), submandibular glands (S), and a parathyroid adenoma *(arrow)*. On a delayed 2-hour image *(B)*, the radioactivity has faded in the thyroid and submandibular glands.

Suggested Textbooks on the Topic

Brant-Zawadzki M, Bradley WG Jr, Cambray-Forker J, Lufkin RB: MRI of the Brain II, 2nd ed. Philadelphia, Lippincott Williams & Wilkins, 2001.

Orrison WW: Neuroimaging. Philadelphia, WB Saunders, 2000.

Osborne A: Diagnostic Neuroradiology. St. Louis, CV Mosby, 1994.

Som PH, Curtin HD: Head and Neck Imaging, 4th ed. Philadelphia, WB Saunders, 2003.

3 Chest

THE NORMAL CHEST IMAGE

Technical Considerations

Exposure. Making a properly exposed chest x-ray is much more difficult than making x-rays of other parts of the body because the chest contains tissues with a great range of contrast. The range stretches from small vessels in air-filled lungs to dense bony structures located behind the heart. A correctly exposed film should allow visualization of vessels to at least the peripheral one third of the lung and at the same time allow visualization of the paraspinous margins and the left hemidiaphragm behind the heart.

Overexposure causes the image to be dark. Under these circumstances, the thoracic spine, mediastinal structures, retrocardiac areas, and nasogastric and endotracheal tubes are well seen, but small nodules and the fine structures in the lung cannot be seen (Fig. 3-1*A*). If the image was obtained by using either digital or computed radiography, the image can be "windowed" lower on the computer, resulting in an interpretable image.

Underexposure causes the image to be quite white. This is a major problem for adequate interpretation. It will make the small pulmonary blood vessels appear prominent and may lead to thinking that there are generalized infiltrates when none are really present. Underexposure also makes it impossible to see the detail of the mediastinal, retrocardiac, or spinal anatomy (Fig. 3-1*B*). Even with digital or computed radiography, nothing can be done to an underexposed image to improve the image.

Male versus Female Chest. The major difference between male and female chest x-rays is caused by differences in the amount of breast tissue. This is generally relevant only in interpretation of a posteroanterior (PA) or an anteroposterior (AP) projection and not of the lateral projection. Breast tissue absorbs some of the x-ray beam, essentially causing underexposure of the tissues in the path. This results in the lung behind the breasts appearing whiter and the pulmonary vascular pattern in the same area appearing more prominent. If the breasts are pendulous, on the PA or AP projection, bilateral basilar lung infiltrates may appear to be present.

One common problem is encountered in the woman who has had a unilateral mastectomy. In this circumstance, the lung density will be asymmetrical. The lung on the side of the mastectomy will appear darker than the lung on the normal side. In these circumstances, recognition of the mastectomy will prevent you from making an erroneous diagnosis of an infiltrate or effusion based on the relatively increased density on the side with the remaining breast (Fig. 3-2).

Visualization on a PA or an AP chest x-ray of a single well-defined "nodule" in the lower lung zone should raise the suspicion that you are seeing a nipple shadow and not a real pulmonary nodule. Nipple shadows are common in both men and women. First, look at the opposite lung to see if a comparable nodule appears there. If one does, usually you can stop worrying (Fig. 3-3), but before you completely stop worrying, also look at the lateral film and make sure that the "nodule" is not seen projecting within the lung. If only one "nodule" is found projecting

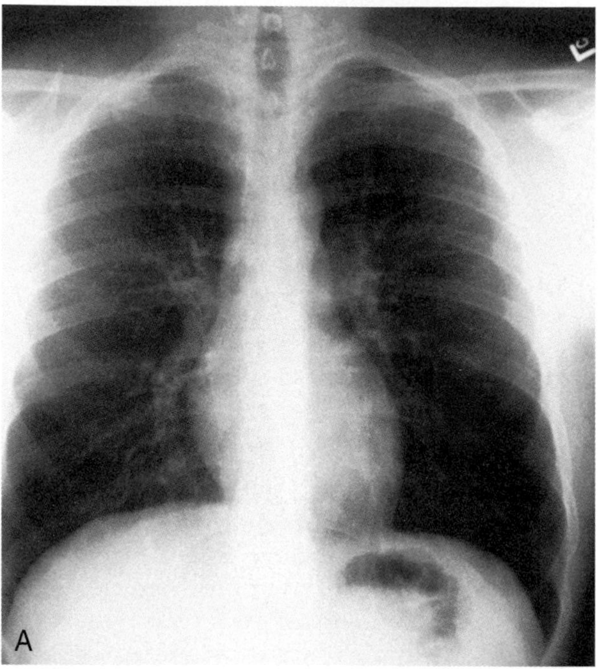

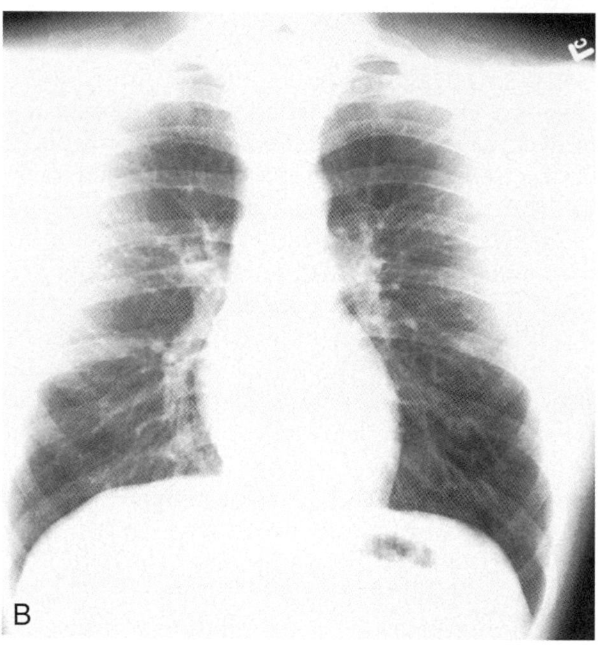

FIGURE 3-1 ■ Effect of over- and underexposure on a chest x-ray. Overexposure *(A)* makes it very easy to see behind the heart and the regions of the clavicles and thoracic spine, but the pulmonary vessels peripherally are impossible to see. Underexposure *(B)* accentuates the pulmonary vascularity, but you cannot see behind the heart or behind the hemidiaphragms.

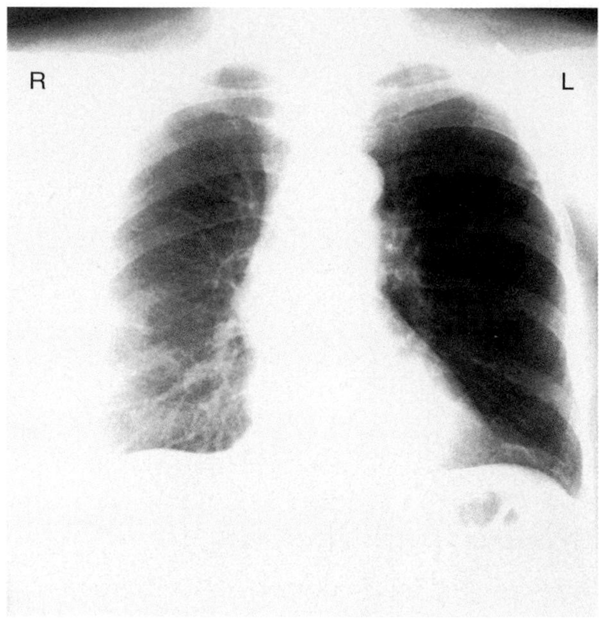

FIGURE 3-2 ■ Left mastectomy. The right breast, which remains, causes the pulmonary vessels at the base of the right lung to be accentuated, and this can be mistaken for a right lower lobe infiltrate. In contrast, the left lung appears darker than the right, and you might mistakenly think there is hyperinflation of the left lung.

over a lung in the PA projection, and no nodule is seen on the lateral view, a small metallic BB can be taped over the nipples and the single PA view repeated to see whether the nipple was being visualized.

Posteroanterior versus Anteroposterior Chest X-rays. Chest x-rays on ambulatory patients are usually done with the subject's chest up against the film holder or detector plate. The x-ray tube is behind the patient, and the x-ray beam passes in from the back and exits the front of the chest. This is referred to as a PA (posterior to anterior) projection. If the patient is lying down, it is standard practice to take the image with the x-ray beam entering the front of the chest and to have the film cassette or detector plate behind the patient. This is called an AP (or anterior to posterior) chest x-ray.

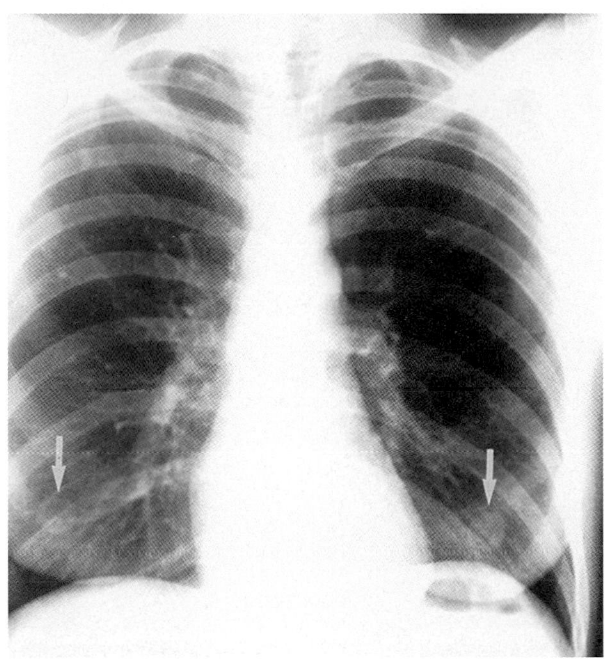

FIGURE 3-3 ■ **Nipple shadows.** Prominent nipple shadows can be seen in both men and women and are seen in the midclavicular line over the lower half of both the right and the left lung *(arrows).* These should be bilateral and sometimes can be seen on the anterior soft tissue of the chest on the lateral view.

For interpretive purposes, the main difference is that the heart will be more magnified on the AP projection (Fig. 3-4). This is because in the AP projection, the heart is farther from the film or detector plate, and the x-ray beam diverges as it goes farther from the tube. Thus the shadow of the heart appears larger on an AP chest x-ray than on a PA view. Simply remember to make sure that you are looking at a PA view before you interpret an image as showing mild or moderate cardiomegaly. Usually the technician will have written the projection on the x-ray requisition, and occasionally it may be marked on the image.

Upright versus Supine Chest X-rays. As you can imagine, patients who are able to stand or sit up usually have their chest x-rays done in that position for a number of reasons. The amount of inspiration is greater in these positions, spreading the pulmonary vessels and allowing clearer visualization. It is obviously easier to see a bird

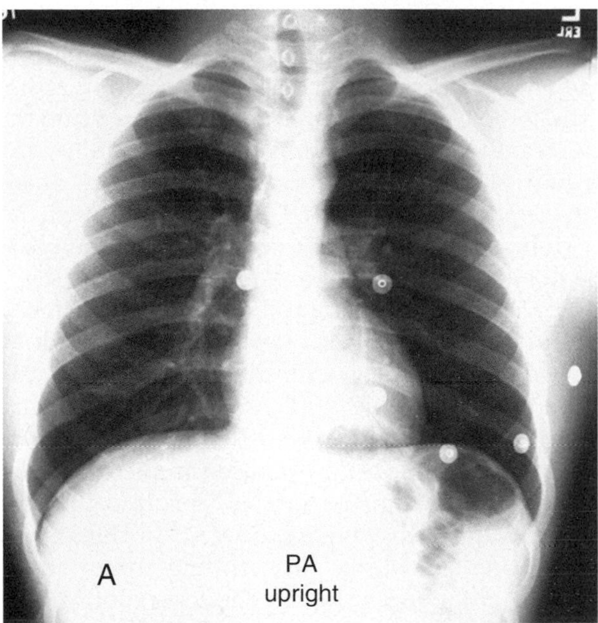

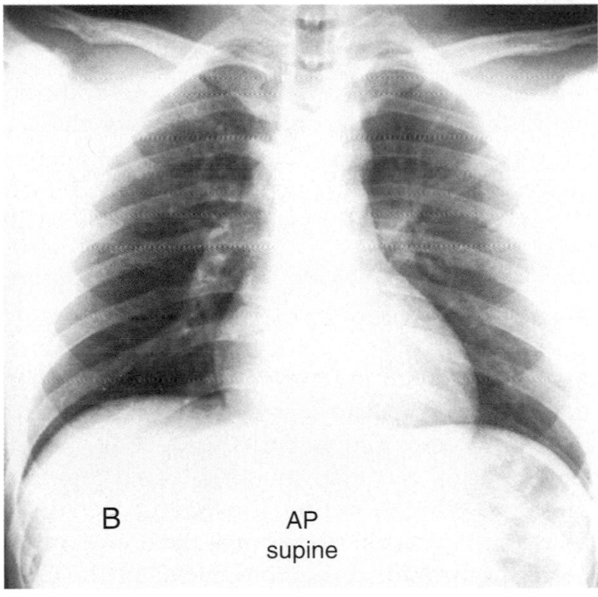

FIGURE 3-4 ■ **Effect of position on the chest x-ray.** A posteroanterior (PA) upright view *(A)* allows fuller inspiration than does a supine view. The small round objects over the left lower chest are snaps on the patient's clothing. In an anteroposterior supine view *(B),* the abdominal contents are pushing the hemidiaphragms up, and the chest appears hypoinflated. This projection also magnifies the heart relative to a PA view.

in a tree if the branches can be spread out instead of being squashed together. Another reason for preferring an upright examination is that small pleural effusions tend to run down into the normally sharp costophrenic angles, allowing relatively small effusions to be identified. Small pneumothoraces tend to go to the lung apex and can be relatively easy to see on an upright chest x-ray.

Now let us think about a patient lying in bed (supine). The typical chest x-ray will be done with a detector cassette under the patient. No lateral view is done. Under these circumstances, the patient cannot take a full inspiration; the liver and abdominal contents push up on the lungs and heart, and the result is that the pulmonary vessels are crowded. In the supine position, the blood flow to the upper lungs essentially equals that in the lower lobes, and this will mimic congestive failure. On a supine image, the standard AP projection combined with the cephalic push of the abdominal contents will make a normal heart appear large. In addition, with the patient in a supine position, small pleural effusions will layer in the posterior pleural space, whereas small pneumothoraces will go to the anterior pleural surface, and both will easily be missed. As a result you must be much more conservative and careful when interpreting the image of a supine, portable examination.

Inspiration and Expiration Chest X-rays. The degree of inspiration is important not only for assessing the quality and limitations of the examination but also for diagnosing different diseases. When standing, most adults can easily take an inspiration that brings the domes of the hemidiaphragms down to the level of the tenth posterior ribs. When the patient is sitting or lying down, often the level is between the eighth and tenth ribs. If the image has the domes of the diaphragms at the seventh posterior ribs, the chest should be considered hypoinflated, and you must be very careful before diagnosing basilar pneumonia or cardiomegaly (Fig. 3-5). You should be cognizant of the major differences in the appearance of a chest x-ray as a result of combining all the factors mentioned earlier. Unless you are aware of these issues, you will diagnose cardiomegaly, lung infiltrates, and con-

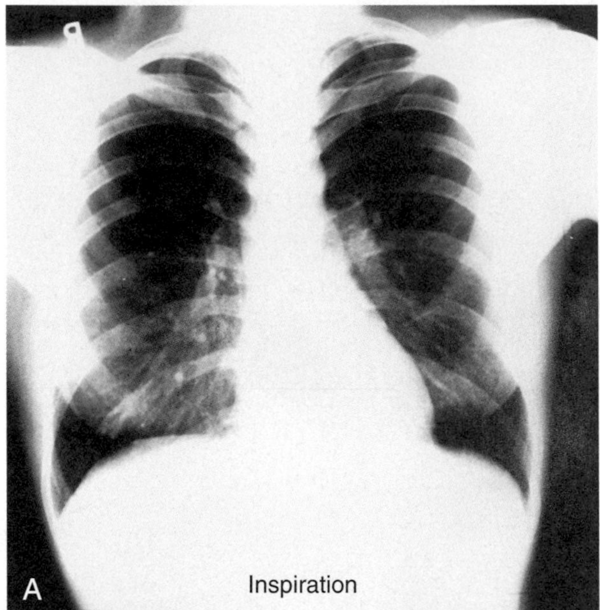

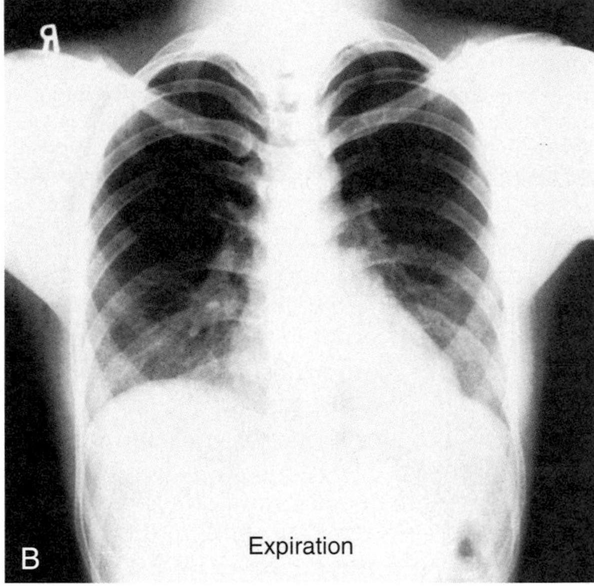

FIGURE 3-5 ■ Effect of respiration. Good inspiration on a chest x-ray *(A)* makes the hemidiaphragms come down to about the level of the posterior tenth or eleventh ribs. The breast shadows are clearly seen on both sides, and this overlying soft tissue accentuates the pulmonary markings behind them. On an expiration view *(B)*, the hemidiaphragms are higher, making the heart appear larger and crowding the basilar pulmonary vessels. The breast shadows overlap the hemidiaphragms, and these findings together may make you think that bilateral basilar lung infiltrates are present, when this is a normal chest.

gestive heart failure (CHF) in a patient who is, in fact, normal (Fig. 3-6).

Expiration films do have occasional constructive uses. If a small pneumothorax is present, an expiration view makes the lung smaller and denser, and at the same time, it makes the pneumothorax relatively larger and easier to see.

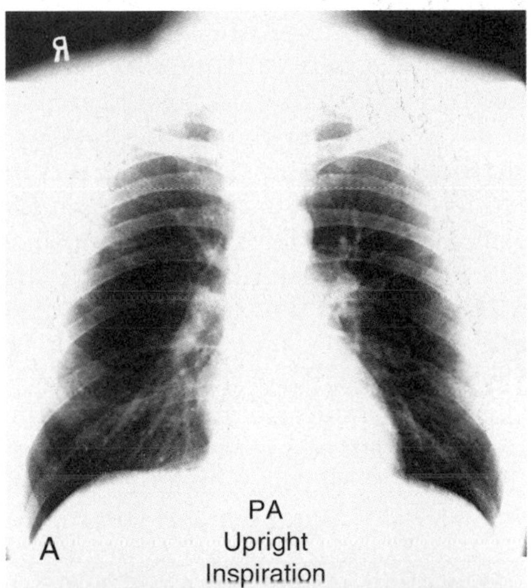

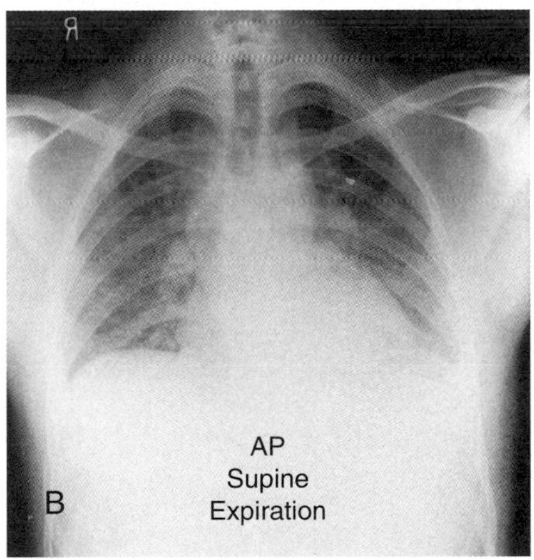

FIGURE 3-6 ■ Summation of the effect of position, projection, and respiration. A normal posteroanterior upright chest x-ray with full inspiration *(A)*. Another x-ray was taken of this perfectly healthy college student 1 minute later; it was done in an anteroposterior projection while he was lying supine and during expiration *(B)*. The wide cardiac shadow and prominent pulmonary vascularity could easily trick you into thinking that this individual was in congestive heart failure.

Thus if your prime interest is in identification of a small pneumothorax, order an upright expiration image. In the case of a foreign body (such as a peanut) lodged in a major bronchus, both inspiration and expiration examinations should be ordered. Either postobstructive atelectasis or a ball-valve phenomenon may be seen. In the latter case, the air can get in past the object during inspiration, but during expiration (as the bronchus gets smaller), the air cannot get out around the object. As a result, on the expiration film, air trapping will occur in the affected lung with shift of the mediastinum toward the normal side.

Before hyperinflation is diagnosed on a chest x-ray, the lateral image should be examined. With hyperinflation, the diaphragms should be flattened on the lateral view. Many young adults can normally take a very deep inspiration, but on the lateral view, they will not have an increased AP diameter or truly flattened hemidiaphragms. In long-standing chronic obstructive pulmonary disease (COPD), additional findings may appear, such as an increased AP diameter and an increase in the clear space between the sternum and the ascending aorta.

Chest X-ray versus Rib Technique. A typical chest x-ray is done by using an energy of the x-rays that is a compromise for visualizing lung markings, soft tissues, and bones at the same time. Bones can be well seen by using relatively low voltage x-rays, but then the pulmonary markings are hard to see (Fig. 3-7). If you are interested in rib or spine fractures or other abnormalities of bone, order either a "rib" or a "spine" examination rather than a chest x-ray. This will accentuate the detail of the bones.

Normal Anatomy and Variants

Normal anatomy as visualized on a chest x-ray is important to understand, and major structures are shown in Figure 3-8. A method for examining a chest x-ray is given in Table 3-1. The appropriate imaging study to order in various clinical circumstances is shown in Table 3-2. Some circumstances in which a chest x-ray is not indicated are shown in Table 3-3.

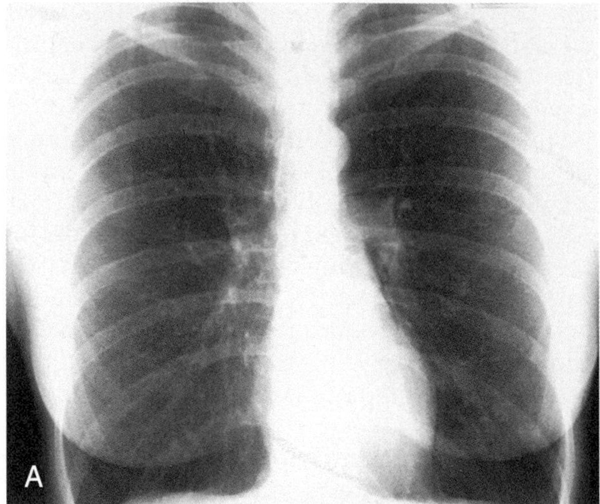

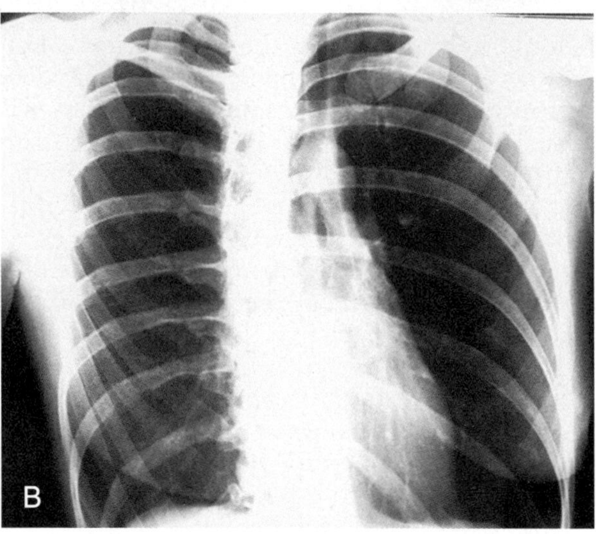

FIGURE 3-7 ■ Chest versus rib technique. A normal chest x-ray *(A)* is taken at a relatively high voltage, allowing you to see heart, pulmonary vessels, and skeletal structures. By lowering the voltage of the x-ray beam, the pulmonary vessels become much harder to see, and the bones become easier to see *(B)*.

The heart is the easiest thing to see, so we begin there. On the PA view of the heart, the left border is much more prominent than the right. It would be nice and simple to say that the left ventricle is on the left and the right ventricle is on the right. Unfortunately, the heart chambers are somewhat twisted in the chest, and on the PA and lateral views, the cardiac chambers mostly overlie each other. As a general rule, if the right side of the heart is enlarged more than the left, a right chamber lesion is present. The same holds true for the left side.

On an upright PA chest x-ray, the greatest width of the heart should be less than half the width of the thoracic cavity at its widest point (Fig. 3-9). This is determined by finding the farthest right and left portions of the cardiac silhouette. These will not be at the same horizontal level, but that is all right. Find the horizontal distance between the two most lateral cardiac margins. Sometimes patients have either dextrocardia or situs inversus (Fig. 3-10). Before the latter diagnosis is made, it is important to make sure that the technician did not misplace the right or left marker on the image.

The upper mediastinal structures that are visualized on the right are the brachiocephalic vessels, azygos vein, and ascending aorta. The right border of the ascending aorta can be seen beginning below the right hilum. The aortic arch is most commonly seen to the left of the trachea. The descending thoracic aorta can usually be visualized only along its left lateral border, where it abuts the left lung. The trachea should be midline and can be followed down to the carina. The right and left major bronchi are easily seen. The esophagus is not normally seen on a standard chest x-ray.

Hila and Lungs. The hila are made up of the main pulmonary arteries and major bronchi. The right hilum is usually somewhat lower than the left; it should not be at the same level or higher. The pulmonary veins usually are more difficult to see than the arteries. They converge on the atria at a level 1 to 3 inches below the pulmonary arteries. Lymph nodes are not normally seen on a chest x-ray, either in the hilar regions or in the mediastinum.

The lungs are composed mostly of air, and therefore, normally not much is seen other than blood vessels. These should be distinct and remain that way as they are traced back to the hila. If you cannot see blood vessels clearly near the hila, a perihilar infiltrate or fluid may be present (such as from CHF). Normal hila are sometimes indistinct on portable x-rays because the exposure takes longer, and the vessels are blurred by motion.

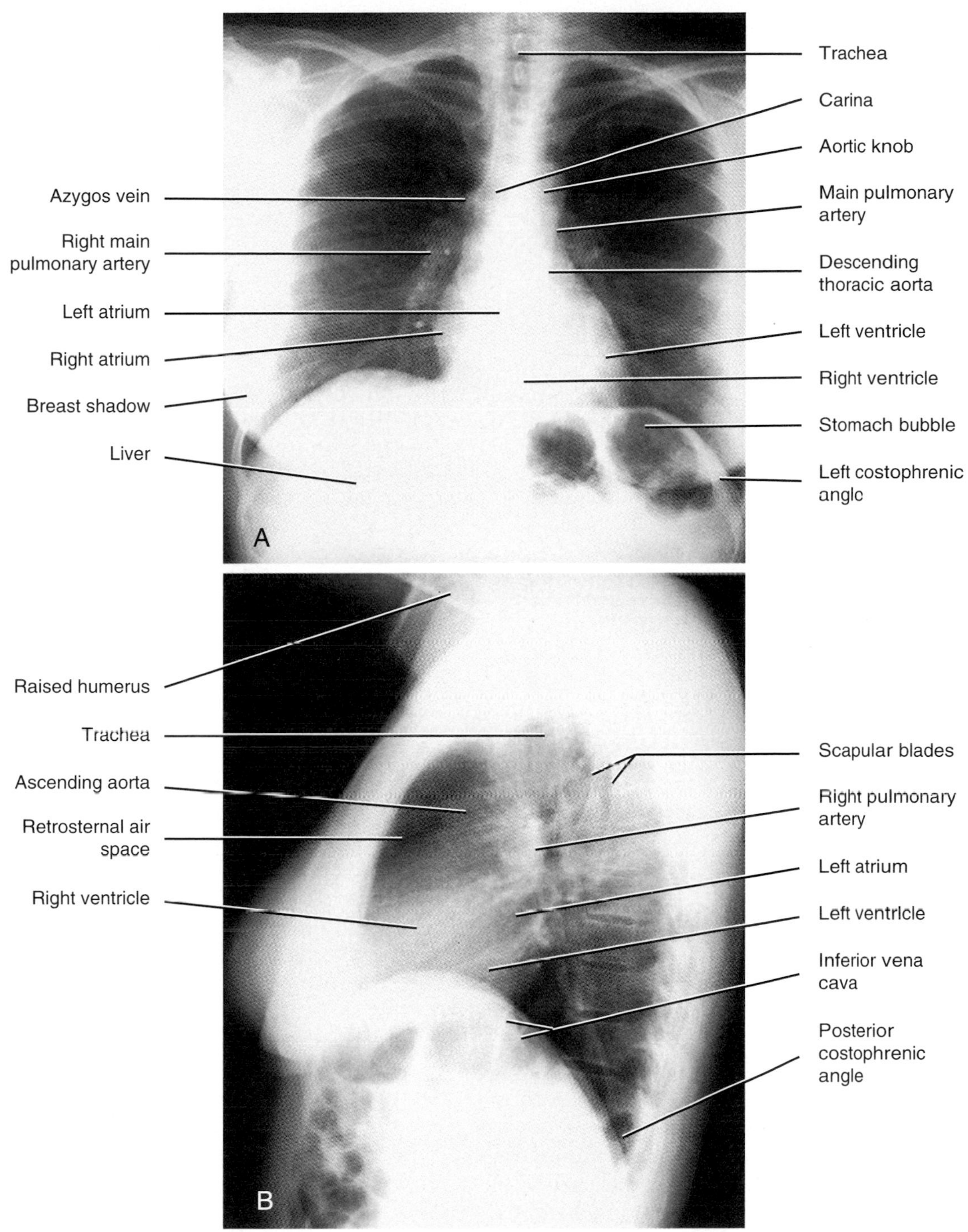

FIGURE 3-8 ■ Normal anatomy on the female chest x-ray in the upright posteroanterior projection *(A)* and the lateral *(B)* projection.

TABLE 3-1 ■ **How to Look at a Chest X-ray**

Determine the age, sex, and history of the patient
Identify the projection and technique used:
  AP, PA, lateral, portable, or standard distance
Identify the position of the patient:
  Upright, supine, decubitus, lordotic
Look at the inspiratory effort:
  Adequate, hypoinflated, hyperinflated
Identify the obvious and common abnormalities:
  Heart size, large or normal
  Heart shape, specific chamber enlargement
  Upper mediastinal contours
  Examine airway, tracheal deviation
  Lung symmetry
    Any mediastinal shift?
    Hilar position
  Lung infiltrates, masses, or nodules
  Pulmonary vascularity
    Increased, decreased, or normal
    Lower greater than upper
  Pleural effusions, blunting of costophrenic angles
  Rib, clavicle, and spine fractures or other lesions
  Check tube placement
Recheck what you thought was normal anatomy and look at typical blind spots
  Behind the heart
  Behind the hemidiaphragms
  In the lung apices
  Pneumothorax present?
  Costophrenic angles
  Chest wall
  Lytic rib lesions
  Shoulders
Look for old films, not just the last one
Decide what the findings are and their location
Give a common differential diagnosis correlated with the clinical history

AP, anteroposterior; PA, posteroanterior.

The blood vessels in the lung are usually clearly seen out to within 2 to 3 cm of the chest wall. Some people say that visualization of vessels in the outer third of the lung is abnormal, but this is not true. It depends on the quality of the film and on how hard you look. Lines located within 2 cm of the chest wall are abnormal and probably represent edema, fibrosis, or metastatic disease. Secondary bronchi are not normally visualized except near the hilum, where they can sometimes be seen end-on. The walls of the visualized bronchi normally should not be thicker than a fine pencil point.

A normal variant called an azygos lobe can occasionally be seen in the right upper lung. This is seen on the PA view as a fine, curved line extending from the right lung apex down toward the mediastinum (Fig. 3-11). It has a teardrop shape at its lower edge. This is caused embryologically by the azygos vein migrating inferiorly from the lung apex while trapping some of the lung medially.

Remember that on a PA or an AP chest x-ray, the lungs go behind the heart, behind and below the dome of the hemidiaphragms, and behind and in front of mediastinal structures. Forty percent of the lung area and 25% of the lung volume will be obscured by these other structures. If you do not look carefully at these regions, you will miss a significant amount of pulmonary pathology.

Diaphragms. The diaphragms are typically dome-shaped, although many persons have polyarcuate diaphragms that look like several domes rather than one. This is an important normal variant and should not be mistaken for a pleural or diaphragmatic tumor; it should not be called an eventration (Fig. 3-12). The right hemidiaphragm is usually higher than the left, and most people believe that this is because the liver is pushing up the right hemidiaphragm. This is nonsense, because the liver, which weighs many pounds, cannot push up into the lungs while the person is standing. The diaphragms are at different levels because the heart is pushing the left hemidiaphragm down. The edges of both hemidiaphragms form acute angles with the chest wall, and blunting of these angles should raise the suspicion of pleural fluid.

Most people have trouble telling the right from the left hemidiaphragm on the lateral view, but several ways exist to tell them apart. The right hemidiaphragm is usually higher than the left and can be seen extending from the anterior chest wall to the posterior ribs. The left side usually can be seen only from the posterior aspect of the heart to the posterior ribs. It also is the hemidiaphragm most likely to have a gas bubble (stomach or colon) immediately beneath it.

Bony Structures. Skeletal structures of interest on a chest x-ray include the ribs, sternum, spine,

TABLE 3-2 ■ **Suggested Imaging Procedures for Various Chest Problems**

Clinical Problem	Imaging Study
Pneumonia (diagnosed clinically)	Chest x-ray (confirmatory)
COPD (with acute exacerbation)	Chest x-ray
CHF (new or worsening)	Chest x-ray, echocardiogram
Trauma	Chest x-ray, CT
Chest pain (in adults older than 40 yr or positive physical examination)	Chest x-ray (additional studies depend on suspected cause)
Shortness of breath (severe or long duration or in adults age 40 yr or older)	Chest x-ray
Asthma (suspected superimposed disease or resistant to therapy)	Chest x-ray
Interstitial lung disease	Chest x-ray, pulmonary function studies
Immunosuppressed patient (with fever, cough, or dyspnea)	Chest x-ray
Foreign body	Inspiration/expiration chest x-ray
Aspiration pneumonia	Chest x-ray
Mediastinal mass	Contrasted CT
Solitary pulmonary nodule	PA and lateral chest x-ray (possibly with nipple markers), high-resolution CT of nodule, regular CT of chest, CT of chest to include adrenals
Lung tumor	Chest x-ray and CT or bronchoscopy
Pleural mass or fluid	CT
Localization of pleural effusion for thoracentesis	Stethoscope, ultrasound
Suspected pneumothorax	Chest x-ray (possibly expiration view as well)
Hemoptysis	Chest x-ray/bronchoscopy
Pericardial effusion	Cardiac ultrasound
Myocardial thickness	Cardiac ultrasound
Cardiac wall motion	Cardiac ultrasound
Cardiac ejection fraction	Nuclear medicine (gated blood pool study) or ultrasound
Pulmonary embolism	Chest x-ray, CT scan or nuclear medicine (ventilation/perfusion scan)
Coronary ischemia	Stress ECG, stress nuclear medicine (myocardial perfusion scan) or stress echocardiogram, coronary angiogram
Aortic aneurysm	Contrasted CT or transesophageal ultrasound
Aortic tear	CT or angiogram
Aortic dissection	Contrasted CT or transesophageal ultrasound

COPD, chronic obstructive pulmonary disease; CHF, congestive heart failure; CT, computed tomography; ECG, electrocardiogram; PA, posteroanterior.

and shoulder girdle. Twelve ribs should appear, but only the upper ones are completely seen on a PA chest x-ray. Ribs are very difficult to evaluate on the lateral view owing to superimposition of the right and left ribs and the many soft tissue structures. Evaluation should include searches for cervical ribs (Fig. 3-13), fractures, deformity, missing ribs (from surgery), and lytic (destructive) lesions. The upper margin of the ribs is usually well seen, because the rib is rounded here. The lower edge of the ribs is usually very thin, and the inferior cortical margin can be difficult to appreciate. Look for symmetry between the right and left ribs at the same level. If they are symmetrical, they are usually normal. At the anterior ends of the ribs, cartilage connects to the sternum. In older individuals, significant calcification of this cartilage may occur; this is a normal finding (Fig. 3-14).

The sternum is well seen only on the lateral view of the chest. On this view, look for pectus deformity, fractures, and lytic lesions. A pectus deformity can cause apparent cardiomegaly, because the sternum is depressed and squashes the heart against the spine, making the heart look wider than normal on the PA chest view (Fig. 3-15). Occasionally overexposed oblique views of the chest can show the sternum well. If this does

TABLE 3-3 ■ **Circumstances in Which a Chest X-ray Is Not Indicated**

Prenatal chest x-ray
Routine admission or preoperative (no cardiac or chest problem) in a patient younger than 65 yr
Routine pre-employment
Screening for occult lung cancer
Screening for tuberculosis
Uncomplicated asthmatic attack
Chronic obstructive pulmonary disease without acute exacerbation
Dyspnea of short duration and intensity in an adult younger than 40 yr
Chest pain in an adult younger than 40 yr with a normal physical examination and no history of trauma
Uncomplicated hypertension
Chronic bronchitis
Acute respiratory illness in an adult younger than 40 yr with a negative physical examination and no other symptoms or risk factors

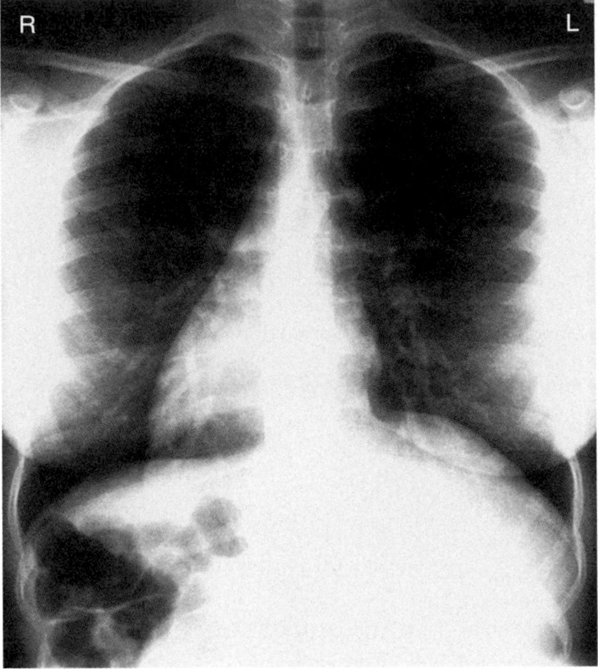

FIGURE 3-10 ■ **Situs inversus.** The heart, stomach, and liver are all in reversed positions. Before you make this diagnosis, make sure that the technician has placed the right and left markers correctly.

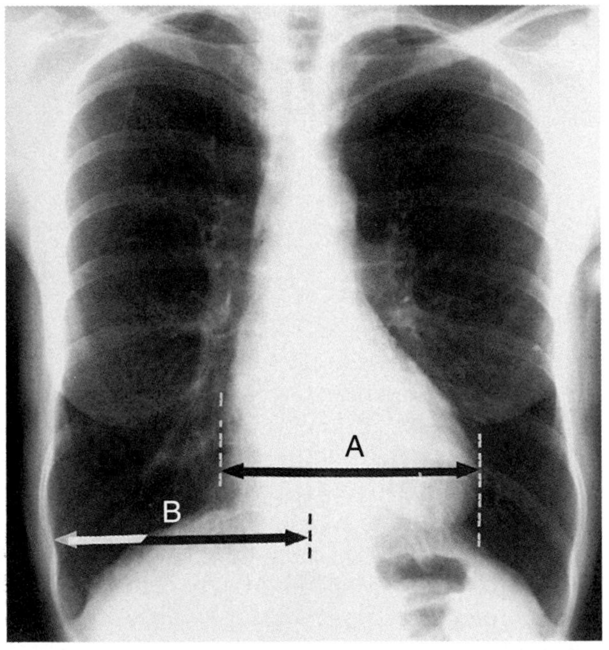

FIGURE 3-9 ■ **Measurement of cardiomegaly.** The width of the normal heart from its most lateral borders *(A)* should not exceed the width of half of the hemithorax measured from the middle of the spine to the widest portion of the inner ribs *(B)*.

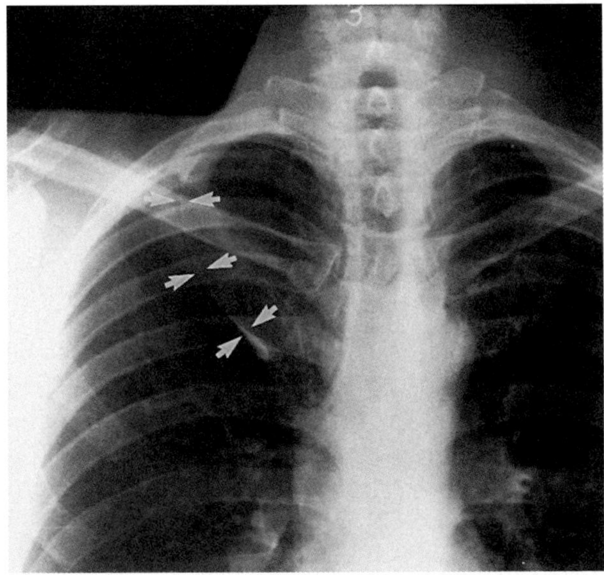

FIGURE 3-11 ■ **Azygos pseudolobe.** A thin curvilinear line extends from the right lung apex down and medially toward the azygos vein *(arrows)*. The line has a teardrop bottom end. This normal variant is seen only on the right side.

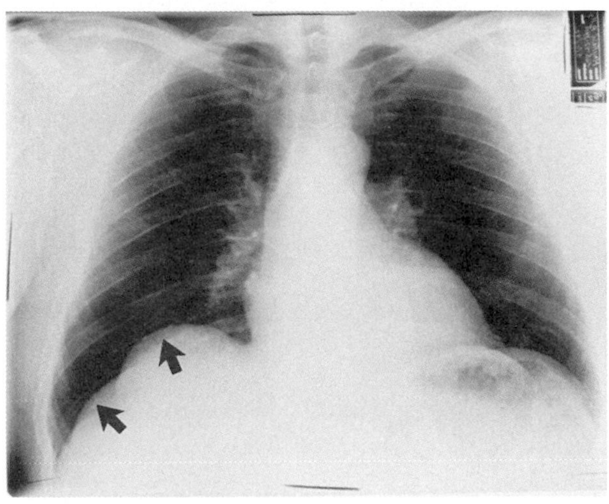

FIGURE 3-12 ■ Polyarcuate diaphragm. This is a common normal variant in which the diaphragm has several small domes instead of one large one.

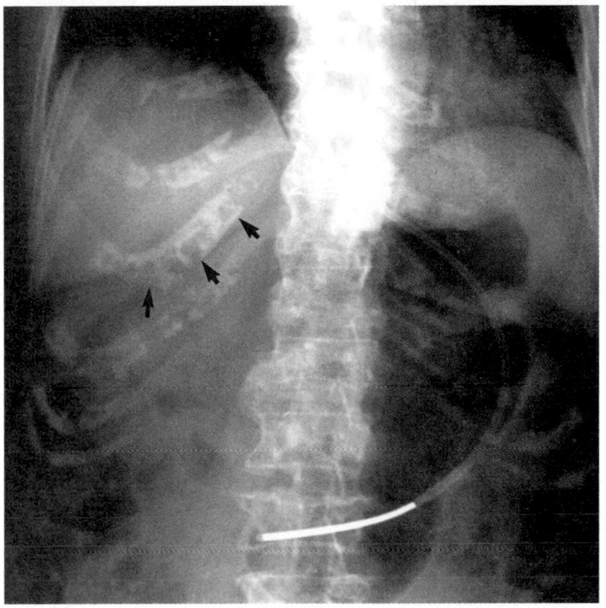

FIGURE 3-14 ■ Costochondral calcification. Calcification between the anterior ends of the ribs and the sternum is quite common, particularly in older persons, and can be quite striking *(arrows)*. A Dobbhoff feeding tube is noted in this patient as well.

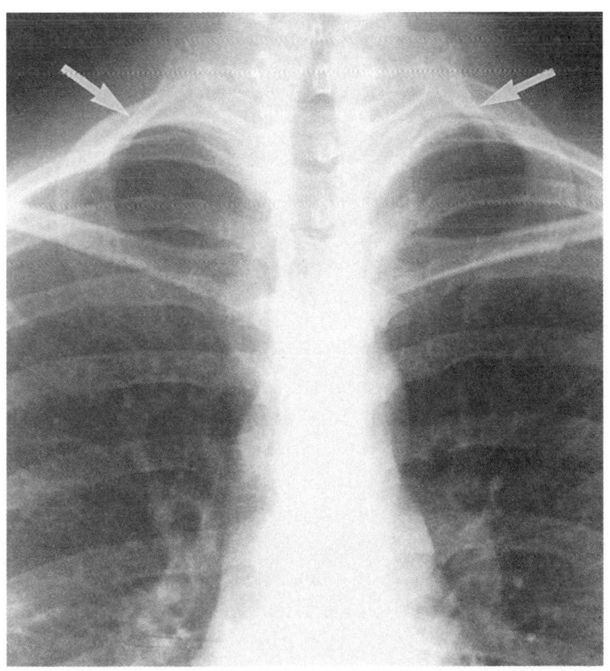

FIGURE 3-13 ■ Cervical ribs. A congenital abnormality in which small ribs project off the lateral aspect of C7 *(arrows)*. Occasionally these can be symptomatic.

not work, you may need to resort to a computed tomography (CT) scan with bone windows.

The clavicles and shoulders also should be routinely examined. Often a scalloped appearance is seen of the inferior and medial portions of the clavicle. This is called a rhomboid fossa, and it is bilateral. It should not be mistaken for a pathologic bone lesion (Fig. 3-16). The medial aspect of the scapula projects over the upper lateral aspect of the lungs and sometimes can be mistaken for a pathologic line, such as a pneumothorax. When you think that you see a pneumothorax, make sure that it is not the scapular border. Note that the medial scapular border is usually straight rather than curved, and trace the outline of the scapula.

The thoracic spine is seen only incompletely on a standard chest x-ray because, on the frontal view, it is obscured by the heart and mediastinal structures. In older people, substantial degenerative changes or bone spurs may extend laterally from the vertebral bodies. These can often be seen on the PA view

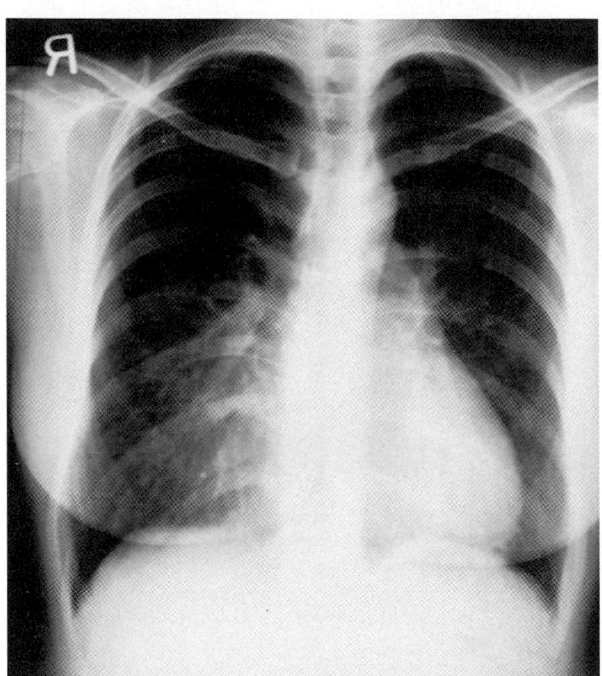

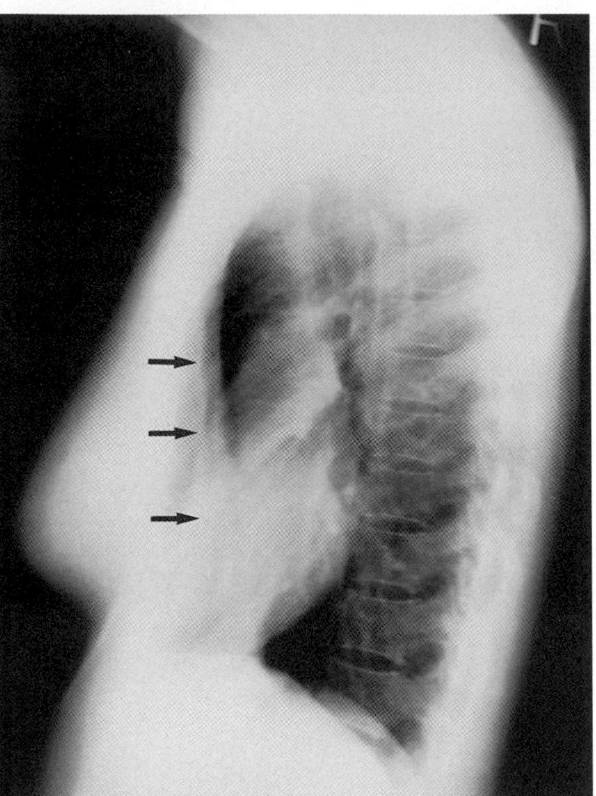

FIGURE 3-15 ■ **Pectus excavatum.** A congenital abnormality in which the sternum is depressed. Because the heart is squashed between the sternum and spine, it appears big in the frontal view *(A)* of the chest, and the right heart border is indistinct, suggesting a right middle lobe infiltrate. A lateral view *(B)* clearly shows the depressed position of the sternum *(arrows)*.

(Fig. 3-17), and on the lateral view, the spurs can look like pulmonary nodules. A key to differentiating bony spurs from nodules is that spurs project over the vertebral disks on the lateral view and do not look like round nodules on the frontal chest x-ray.

Soft Tissues. The soft tissues also should be examined. We have already seen the problems in interpretation that can arise as a result of a mastectomy or nipple shadows, but other soft tissues also are important. It is important to look for asymmetry of soft tissues or for air or calcium within them. Calcification may be seen in the carotid arteries or great vessels in older persons (Fig. 3-18). A common confusing artifact can be caused by hair (especially braids). If the hair is greasy and braided, very strange artifacts (Fig. 3-19) that may be mistaken for apical lung infiltrates can be seen.

Normally, not much soft tissue or water density should exist between the peripheral aerated lung and the ribs. The pleura are not normally seen at the lung margins. In some adults, a collection of fat appears along the chest wall between the lung and the ribs. This is extrapleural fat, which is usually seen only on the PA view of the chest and almost always in the upper outer portion of the thoracic cavity (Fig. 3-20). The biggest pitfall is mistaking this for bilateral pleural effusions. If no other sign of effusion (such as costophrenic angle blunting) is noted and if the finding is bilateral, is seen near the upper lateral lung zones, and does not exceed 3 to 4 mm in thickness, it is almost certainly extrapleural fat rather than pleural fluid.

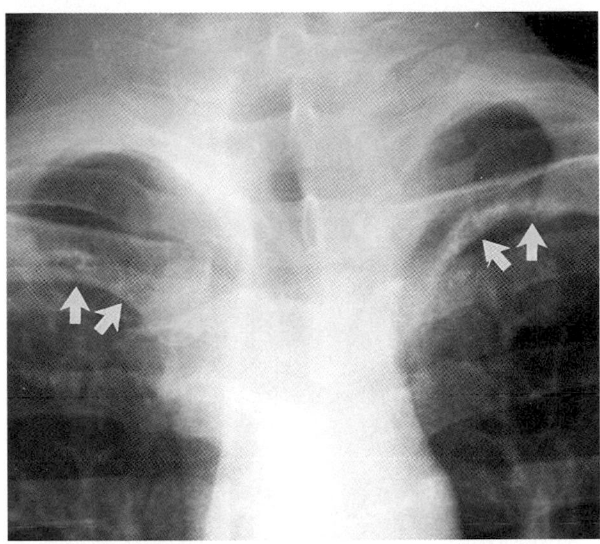

FIGURE 3-16 ■ Rhomboid fossa. A normal finding in which an indentation appears along the medial and inferior aspects of the clavicles *(arrows)*. This should be bilateral and is of no clinical significance.

Computed Tomography (CT) Anatomy. The cross-sectional anatomy of the chest is very important to understand, because CT is very commonly used for evaluation of thoracic pathology. CT scanning of the chest may be done with or without intravenous contrast. Most standard CT scanning techniques provide CT "slice" images that are 0.8 cm thick. To evaluate a lung nodule, use thinner cuts, and intravenous contrast is not needed. For evaluation of a potential dissecting aortic aneurysm, a bolus of intravenous contrast is essential. Consult a radiologist if you are in doubt about what to order. The radiologist usually will use the correct technique, provided you have supplied complete clinical information. If available, spiral, or multidetector, CT is often done because the entire chest can be scanned in several seconds while the patient holds his or her breath. After the scan is done, the technologist will film the computer data by using both mediastinal windows and pulmonary parenchymal windows. This affords

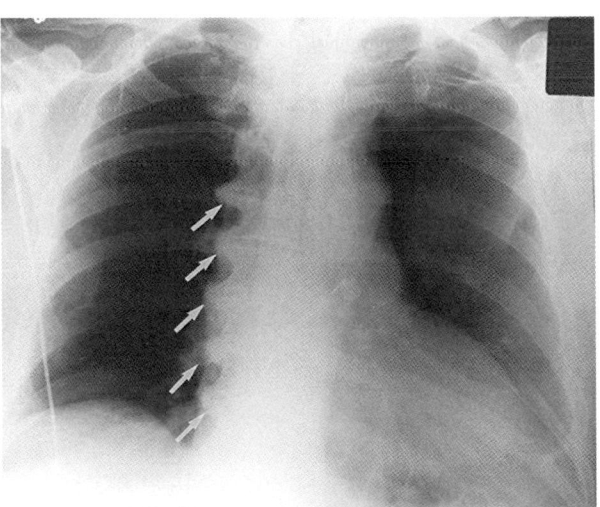

FIGURE 3-17 ■ Degenerative spurs or osteophytes. These projections occur at the level of the disks and can cause an unusual appearance along the lateral aspect of the thoracic spine. On the lateral chest x-ray, these bony spurs can simulate nodules projecting near or over the thoracic spine.

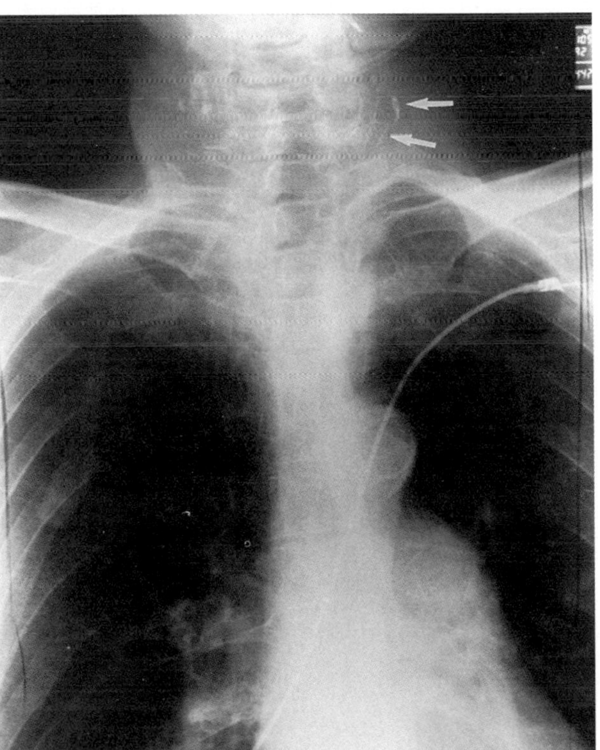

FIGURE 3-18 ■ Carotid calcification. In older patients, as a result of atherosclerosis, calcification of the aortic arch and great vessels often is seen. In this case, calcification is seen in the carotid arteries *(arrows)*.

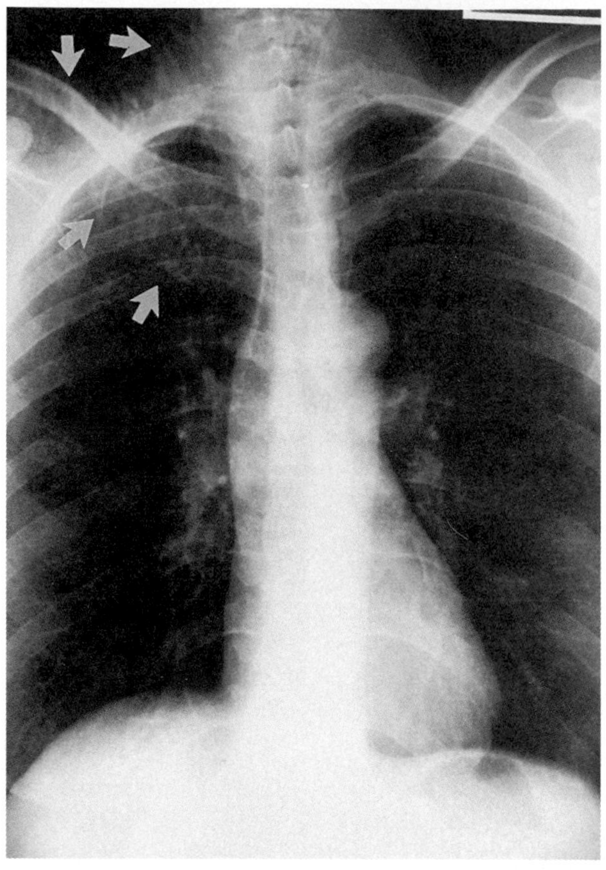

FIGURE 3-19 ■ Braid artifacts. Tightly woven or greasy hair can cause streaky artifacts that may resemble an upper lobe infiltrate. A key finding is that these artifacts can be seen extending above the apex of the lung and projecting over the cervical soft tissue region.

a good look at the pulmonary parenchyma and still allows differentiation of mediastinal structures (Fig. 3-21).

In some special circumstances, you will want to look at the fine detail of the lung. In these circumstances, high-resolution CT (HRCT) can be done. The "slices" that are obtained are 1 to 2 mm thick. This usually is not done for the whole lung, because it would involve too many images and it is not necessary to make most diagnoses. For this reason, a regular CT scan is often done with thin cuts at selected levels (Fig. 3-22).

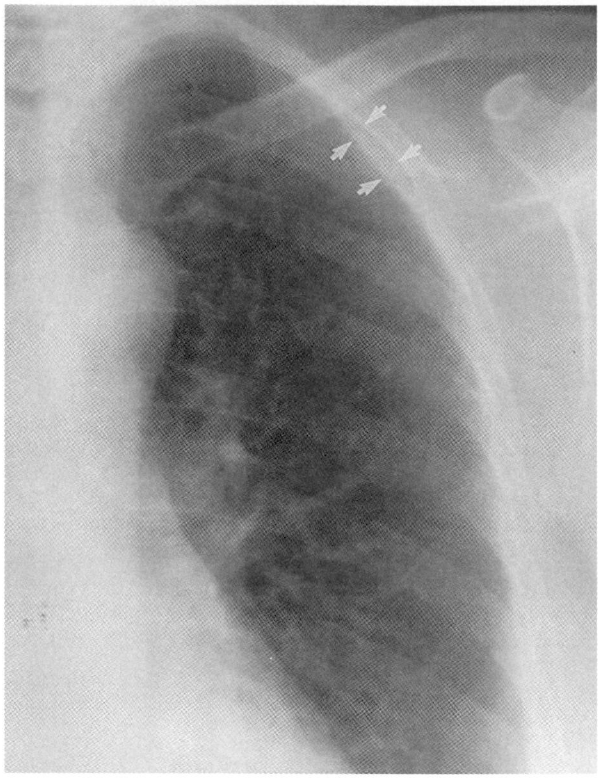

FIGURE 3-20 ■ Extrapleural fat. This normal finding in the upper and lateral hemithorax is symmetrical between right and left and should not be mistaken for a pleural effusion.

THE ABNORMAL CHEST IMAGE

Admission, Preoperative, and Prenatal Chest X-rays

Routine admission chest x-rays have a low yield and are not indicated. If a patient is being admitted with a cardiothoracic problem, cancer, or a febrile illness, a chest x-ray is appropriate. In a similar fashion, routine preoperative chest x-rays are not indicated (e.g., before foot or knee surgery). Preoperative chest x-rays are indicated in patients undergoing neck or chest surgery, in those who have a history of respiratory or cardiac problems, who are febrile, immunocompromised, have altered mental status, an acute abdomen, a known or suspected cancer, or are older than 65 years. A chest x-ray also is appropriate for children who are admitted to an intensive care unit for any reason.

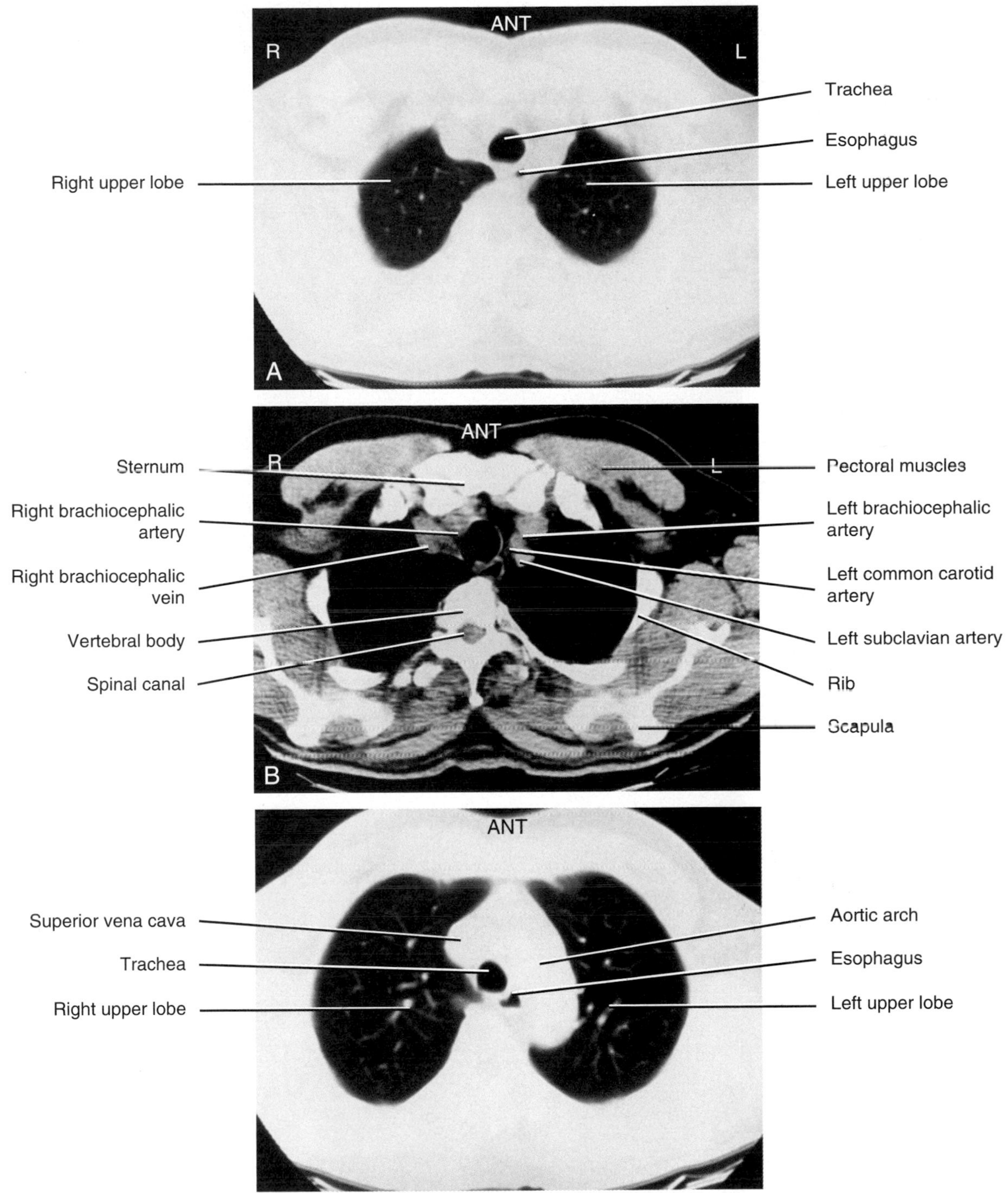

FIGURE 3-21 ■ Normal anatomy of the chest on transverse (axial) computed tomography scans. Identical levels have been filmed by using pulmonary parenchymal windows and soft tissue windows (*A* through *L*).

Continued

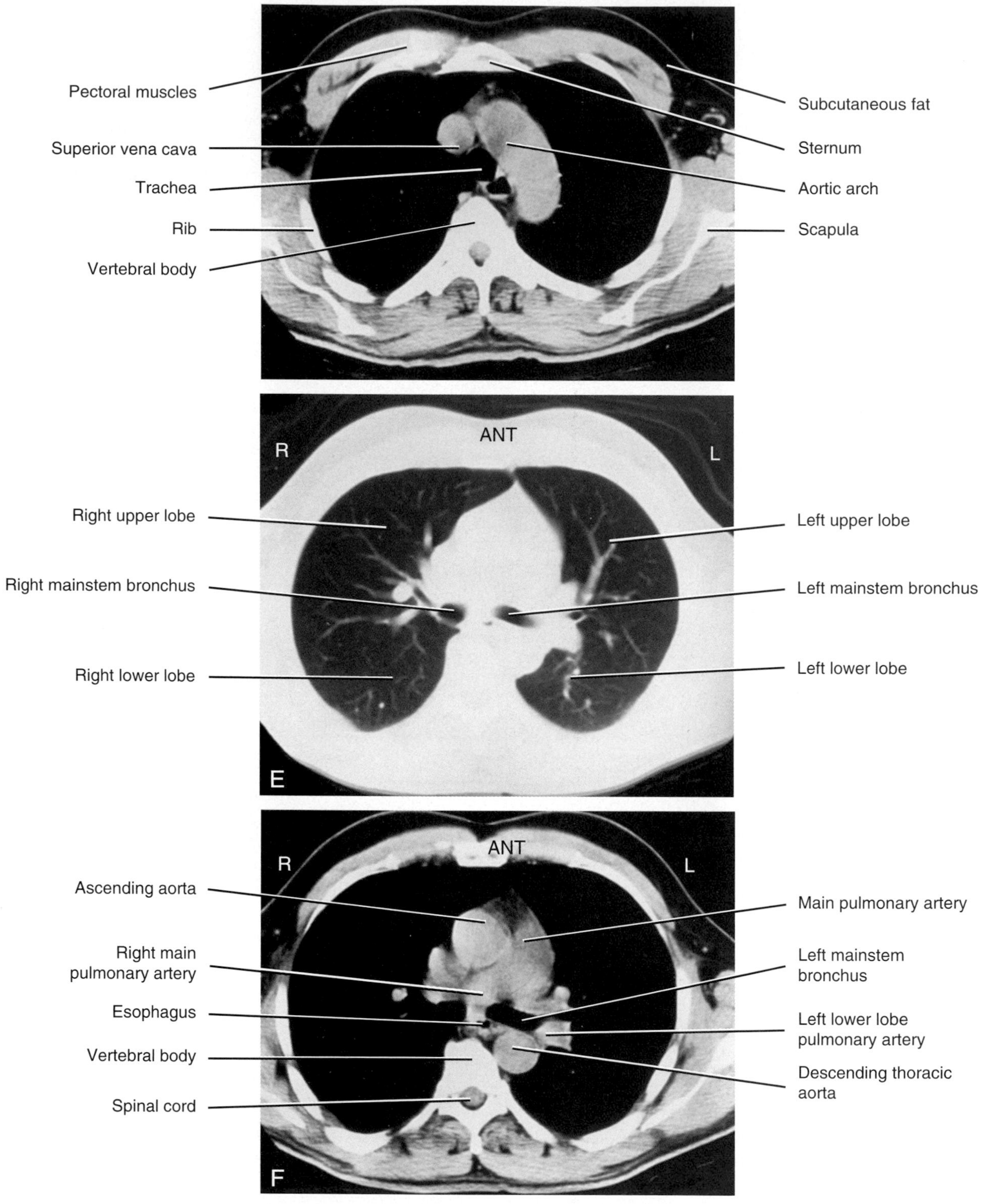

FIGURE 3-21 cont'd

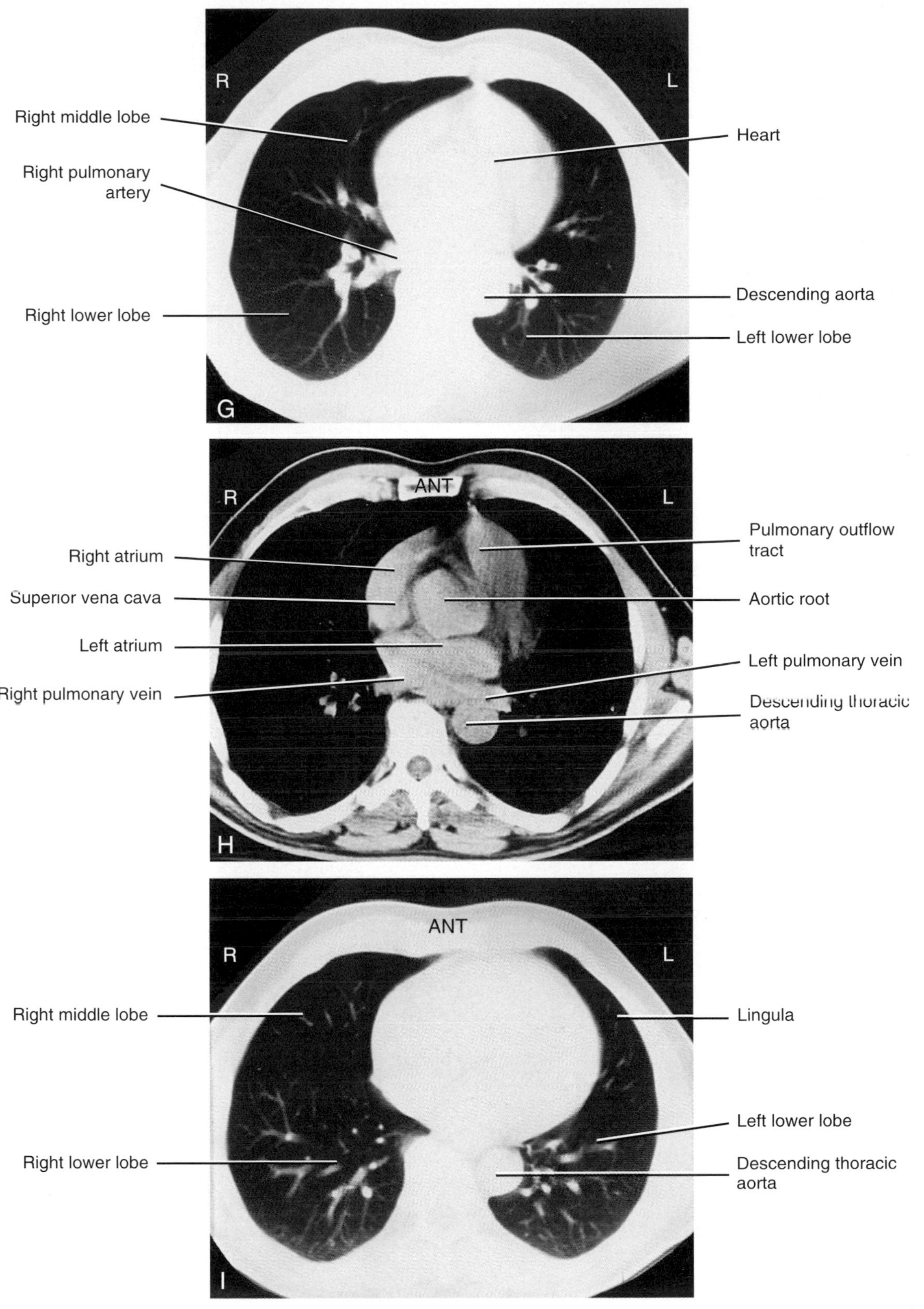

FIGURE 3-21 cont'd

Continued

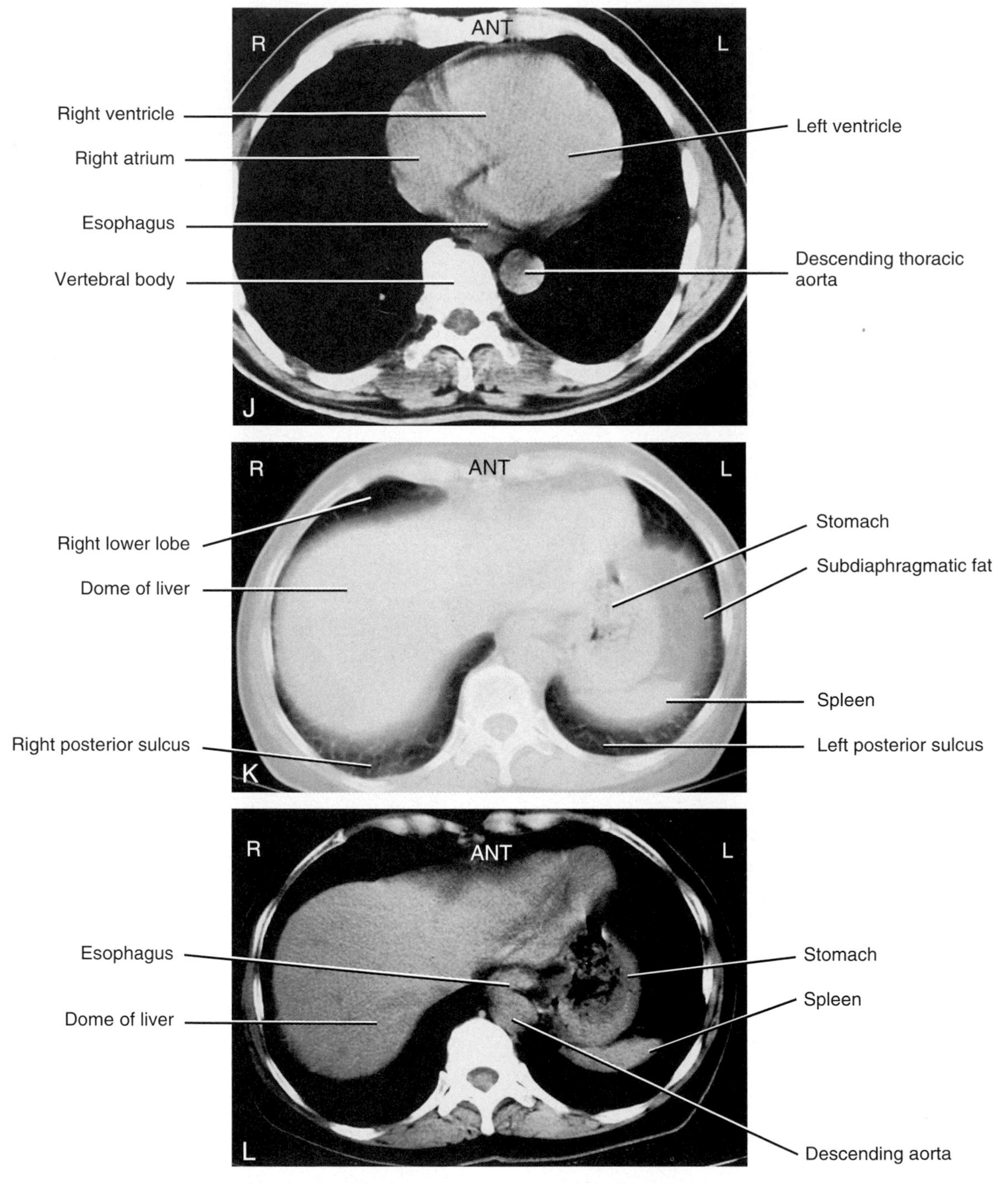

FIGURE 3-21 cont'd

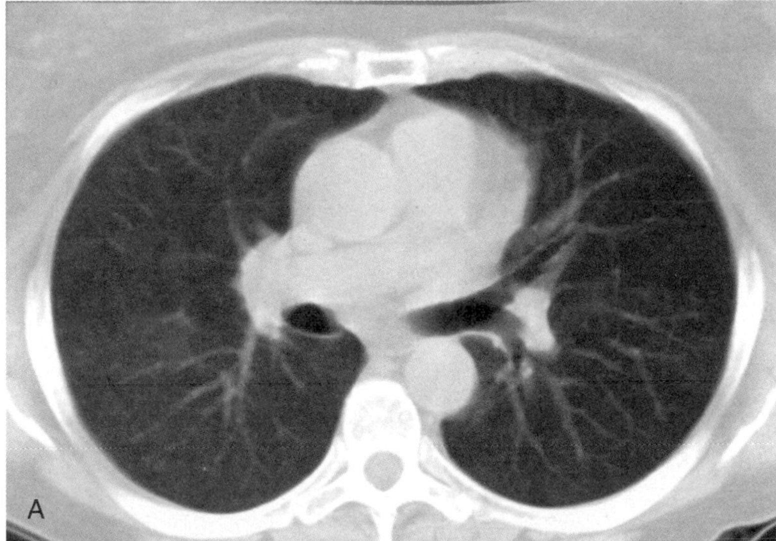

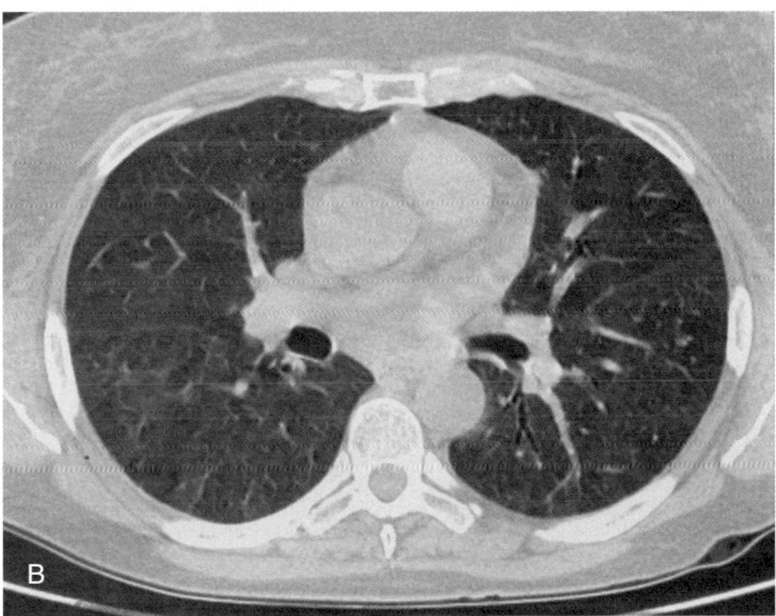

FIGURE 3-22 ■ **Normal and high-resolution computed tomography (CT) of the lungs.** The normal slice thickness *(A)* of a CT scan of the chest is 0.8 cm. A high-resolution slice *(B)* taken at exactly the same level is 1.5 mm in thickness and shows much greater detail of the vessels and bronchi.

Chest X-ray Examinations in Occupational Medicine

Pre-employment and preplacement chest x-rays should be done selectively based on pertinent factors in the medical history, clinical examination, and proposed work assignment. Surveillance of persons who work with or may be exposed to substances that adversely affect pulmonary function or cause pulmonary disease should be done if this is the diagnostic procedure with the greatest accuracy and earliest detection. The periodicity of such testing would vary with the particular circumstance.

Silhouette Sign

The silhouette sign is one of the most useful signs in interpreting a chest x-ray. It helps determine the location of an abnormality in relation to normal structures. Loss of a normal border occurs if an abnormality is contiguous with that structure. For example, if an infiltrate is identified on the PA or AP image in the lower right lung zone, it could be in either the right middle or the right lower lobe. If a loss of the normally distinct right heart border is found, then the infiltrate must abut the heart and can be only in the medial segment of the right middle lobe. If, however, loss of the outline of the right hemidiaphragm is found, the infiltrate is almost certainly in the right lower lobe. The silhouette sign also can be used in the reverse fashion. If, on a PA chest x-ray, a mass projects over the aortic knob and the aortic knob is clearly defined, then the mass must be either in front of, or behind, the aortic knob.

Portable Chest Radiography in the Intensive Care Unit

Much has been written about the utility or overuse of chest x-rays in intensive care units. In general, standing or routine orders for chest x-ray should be avoided. However, by definition, patients in intensive care units are very sick, are usually lying supine all day, and are not ventilating normally. Almost all these patients have supporting tubes or lines that are changed or repositioned frequently. Daily chest x-rays are indicated on patients with endotracheal tubes or a recently placed tracheostomy tube. In such patients, about 60% of daily chest x-rays do not disclose either new major or minor findings, and about 20% have new minor findings. However, about 20% of the time, new major findings are clinically unsuspected and are seen only on the x-ray. Chest x-rays also are indicated after a chest tube or central venous line has been placed, to assess the position and potential presence of a pneumothorax. Abnormalities to look for on a postsurgical or post-trauma chest x-ray are shown in Table 3-4.

TABLE 3-4 ■ **Abnormalities to Look for on a Postsurgical or Post-traumatic Chest X-ray Examination**

Position of the endotracheal tube, pleural tubes, venous catheters
Upper mediastinal widening
Left apical pleural cap
Ill-defined aortic knob or anteroposterior window (signs of aortic tear)
Pneumothorax
Apical
Loculated or basilar
Mediastinal emphysema
Subcutaneous emphysema
Infiltrates (? changing)
Mediastinal shift
Atelectasis
Lobar
Focal
Pleural fluid collection
Rib or sternal fractures
Spine fractures (including paraspinous soft tissue widening)
Shoulder fractures and dislocations
Free air under the diaphragms

TUBES, WIRES, AND LINES

Evaluation of the placement and associated complications of various tubes, wires, and lines is a very common reason for ordering a chest x-ray. On patients who are very sick and in intensive care units, the portable chest x-ray often resembles a plate of spaghetti with tubes, lines, and wires all over the place. Your job is to figure out which parts of the tubes and wires are inside the patient and which are simply lying on the patient. In addition, you need to know if the lines and tubes that are inside the patient are going to the right place or are at the correct level.

Endotracheal (ET) Tube

An endotracheal tube (ET) is probably the easiest item to identify, because it is within the air shadow of the trachea. In an adult or child, the ET tip should be at least 1 cm above the carina, and preferably slightly more. A tube in a lower position can obstruct air flow to one side and cause atelectasis (collapse) of a lung or a portion of a lung. An ET tube in low position usually will go into the right main-stem bronchus because it is more vertically oriented than the left main-stem bronchus (Fig. 3-23). The highest that an ET tube tip should be is at the level of the suprasternal notch (which is midway between the proximal clavicles).

Nasogastric (NG) Tube

A nasogastric (NG) tube should follow the course of the esophagus on the frontal chest

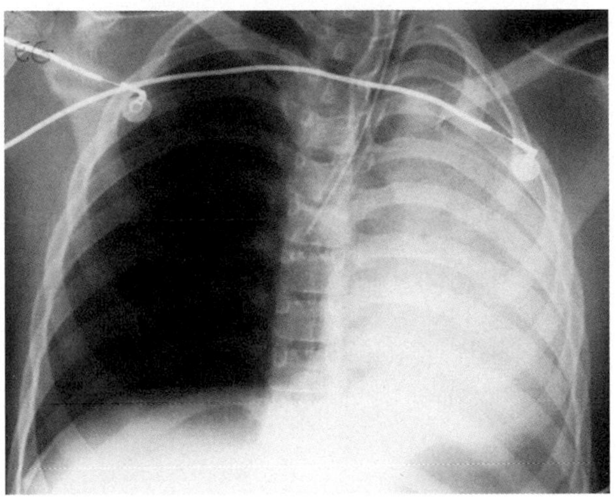

FIGURE 3-23 ■ Left lung atelectasis. The endotracheal tube is down too far, and the tip is located in the right main-stem bronchus. The left main-stem bronchus has become totally obstructed, the air in the left lung has been resorbed, and volume loss is seen in the left lung with shift of the mediastinum to the left.

x-ray, and on the lateral view, it should pass behind the trachea and then along the posterior aspect of the heart (Fig. 3-24). You must ascertain the position of the tip of an NG tube before putting any liquid through the tube. The position often can be determined by clinical means without resorting to a chest x-ray. The most common method is to put air into the tube and listen over the stomach with a stethoscope.

NG tubes have two favorite abnormal positions. The most common is with the NG tube only partway down the esophagus or coiled in the esophagus. Fluid placed down the tube can reflux and be aspirated into the lungs. Less commonly during insertion, the NG tubes can pass into the trachea instead of going into the esophagus. When this happens, they tend to go

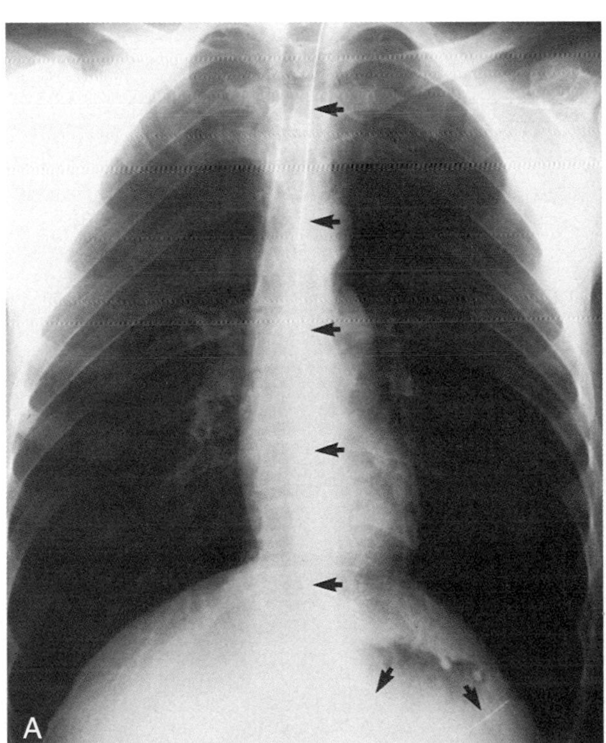

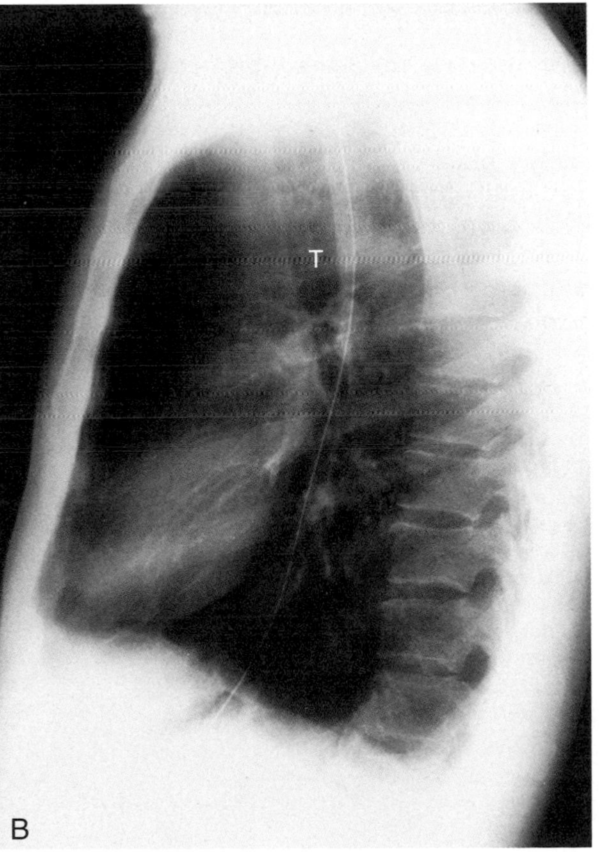

FIGURE 3-24 ■ Normal course of a nasogastric (NG) tube. In the posteroanterior projection of the chest *(A)*, the NG tube passes directly behind the trachea until it gets past the carina and then curves slightly to the left at the gastroesophageal junction. On the lateral view *(B)*, the NG tube can be seen behind the trachea (T) and going down behind the heart.

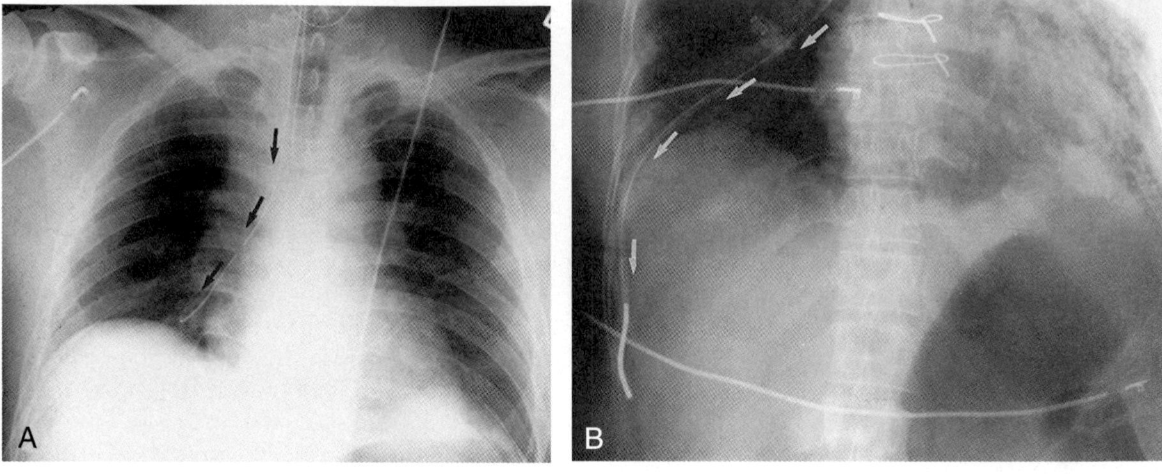

FIGURE 3-25 ■ Nasogastric (NG) tube in right main-stem bronchus. If the NG tube gets into the trachea, it will usually go down the right main-stem bronchus *(A)*. These tubes are quite rigid and, if pushed, can perforate the lung and go out into the pleural space *(B)*.

down the right main-stem bronchus (just as do ET tubes that are advanced too far). Because NG tubes can be stiff and have a rigid end, if pushed hard enough, they can perforate the lung and go out into the pleural space (Fig. 3-25). Many patients require alimentation via NG tube; this works best if the tube tip is in the distal aspect of the duodenal loop near the ligament of Treitz.

Jugular or Subclavian Venous Line

This is a very common route of venous access. The tip of the catheter should optimally be placed in the superior vena cava (SVC). On the frontal chest x-ray, the catheter tip should be about 1 to 4 cm below the medial aspect of the right clavicle (Fig. 3-26). The favorite abnormal positions of subclavian catheter tips are

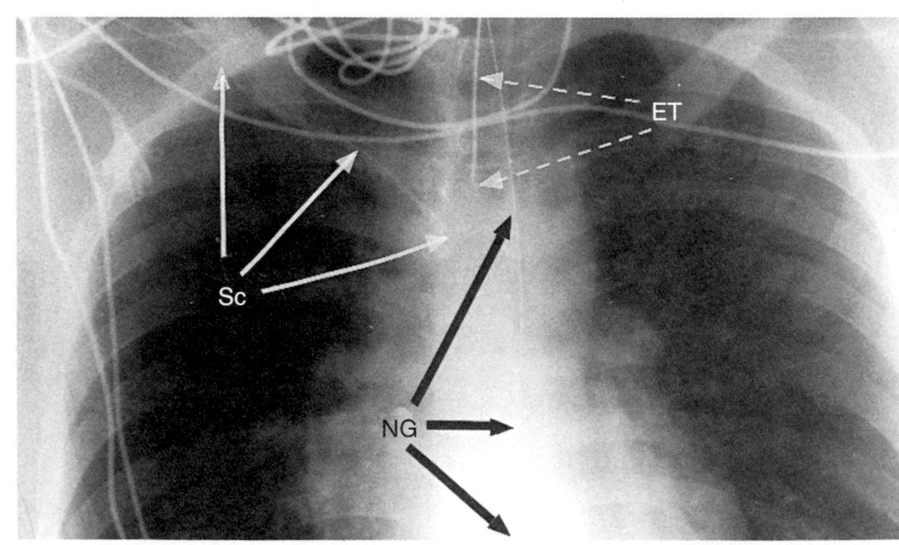

FIGURE 3-26 ■ Normal subclavian catheter course. The subclavian catheter (Sc) should progress medially and then inferiorly to the medial clavicle, with the tip located in the superior vena cava. An endotracheal tube (ET) and nasogastric tube also are present. The remainder of overlying and coiled wires are electrocardiogram leads.

those that have turned up into the jugular vein rather than down into the SVC (Fig. 3-27*A*), and those that have crossed the midline and extended into the opposite subclavian vein (Fig. 3-27*B*).

Swan-Ganz or Pulmonary Artery Catheter

Central lines are usually placed to monitor cardiac or pulmonary arterial pressures. The normal course is almost circular: down the SVC, through the right atrium and right ventricle, and out into the main pulmonary and peripheral pulmonary arteries. The most common natural course that the catheter follows leads it into the right rather than the left main pulmonary artery (Fig. 3-28). Some venous catheters are placed from the inguinal region. In this case, the catheter usually follows a gentle "S" curve from the inferior vena cava (IVC) into the right atrium and right ventricle and into the pulmonary artery (Fig. 3-29). A central venous catheter placed too far out into a pulmonary artery will obstruct blood flow and can result in pulmonary infarction (Fig. 3-30). The tip of a central venous pressure (CVP) line should not extend more than halfway between the hilum and the lung periphery, or lung infarction can occur. Another problem encountered can be the passage of such a catheter from the SVC into the IVC instead of into the right heart (Fig. 3-31).

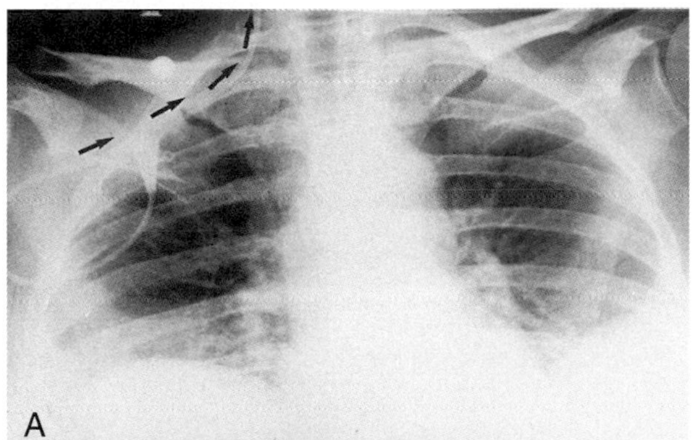

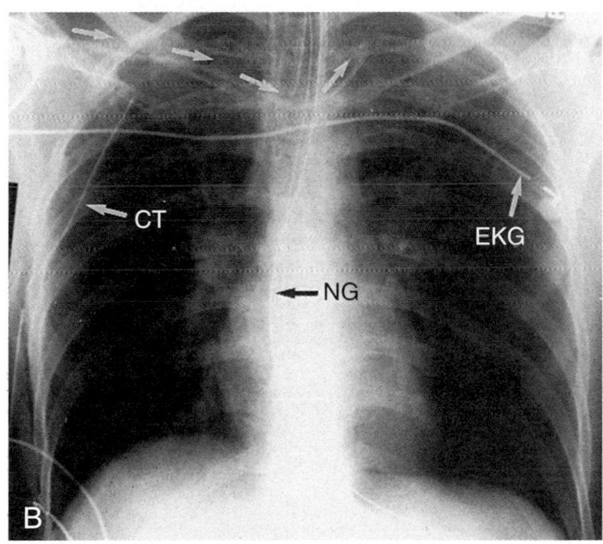

FIGURE 3-27 ■ Abnormal courses of subclavian catheter. Common abnormal courses include the tip of the catheter going up the jugular vein *(A)* or across the brachiocephalic vein into the opposite subclavian vein *(B)*. Nasogastric (NG) tube and electrocardiogram leads (EKG) also are seen. A chest tube (CT) is seen on the right. Note the discontinuity in the radiodense line of the pleural tube just outside the ribs. This discontinuity represents a tube port, indicating that the chest tube has not been inserted far enough.

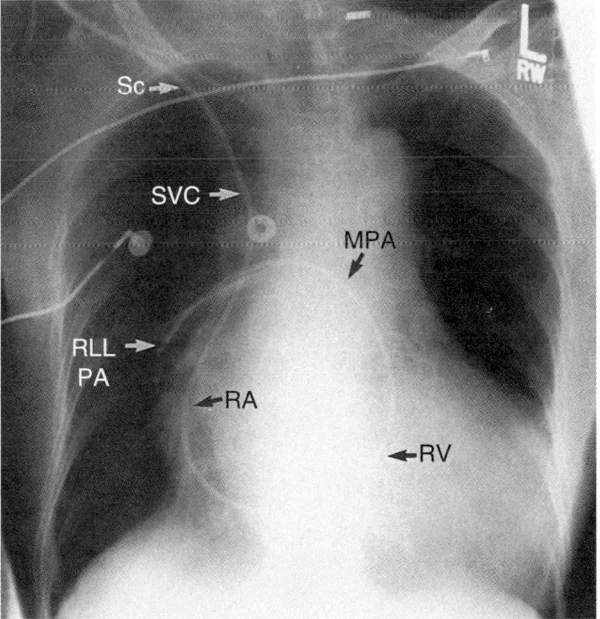

FIGURE 3-28 ■ Normal course of a Swan-Ganz catheter. A Swan-Ganz catheter inserted on the right goes into the subclavian vein (Sc), into the superior vena cava (SVC), right atrium (RA), right ventricle (RV), main pulmonary artery (MPA), and in this case, the right lower lobe pulmonary artery (RLL PA).

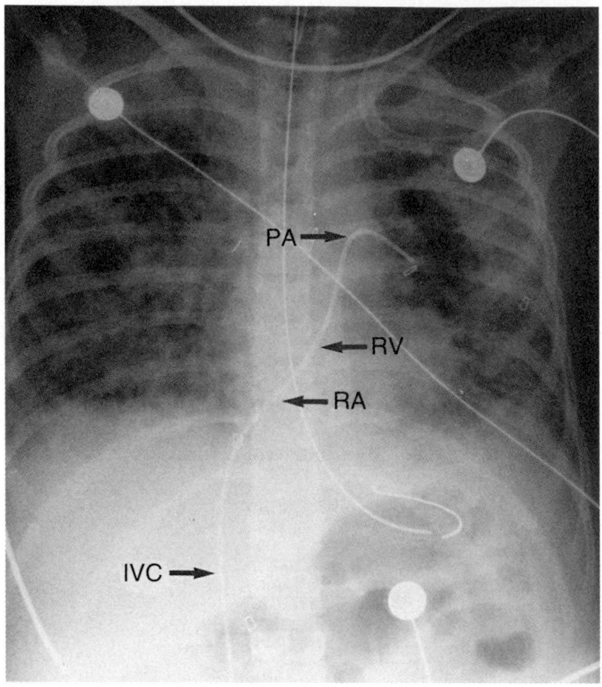

FIGURE 3-29 ■ Swan-Ganz catheter inserted via a femoral approach. This catheter proceeds up the inferior vena cava (IVC) and follows a gentle S curve through the right atrium (RA), right ventricle (RV), and, in this case, the left main pulmonary artery (PA). The patient also has a nasogastric tube, a left subclavian catheter, and multiple electrocardiogram leads.

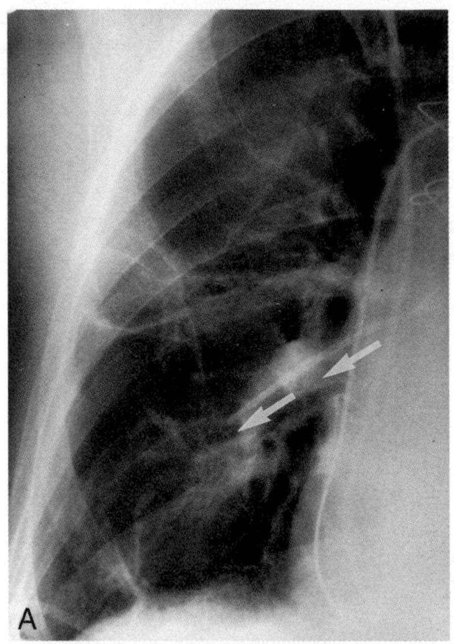

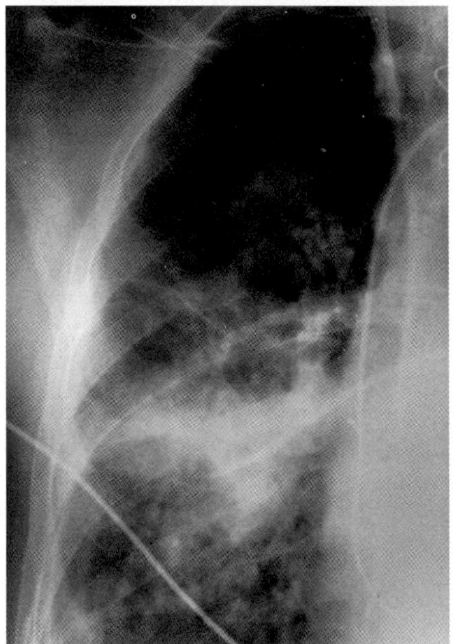

FIGURE 3-30 ■ A Swan-Ganz catheter causing infarction. A Swan-Ganz catheter has been inserted too far into the right lower lobe pulmonary artery *(A)*. Several hours later, an infiltrate is present in this region *(B)* as a result of lung infarction, because the catheter obstructed blood flow.

Pleural Tubes

Pleural tubes are typically placed to evacuate a pneumothorax or drain a pleural fluid collection. They are relatively large bore and are inserted between the ribs in the mid- or lower-lateral chest. One common question about these tubes concerns the location of the tip and side port. The tip should not abut the mediastinum. The side port can be seen as a discontinuity in the radiodense marker line, and it should be inside the chest cavity and not out in the soft tissues of the chest (see Fig. 3-27*B*). Another question relates to whether the tube has kinked and whether it is working to reduce the pneumothorax or fluid collection. Remember, a posteriorly placed tube will have a hard time removing a pneumothorax if the patient is supine and the air collection is located anteriorly.

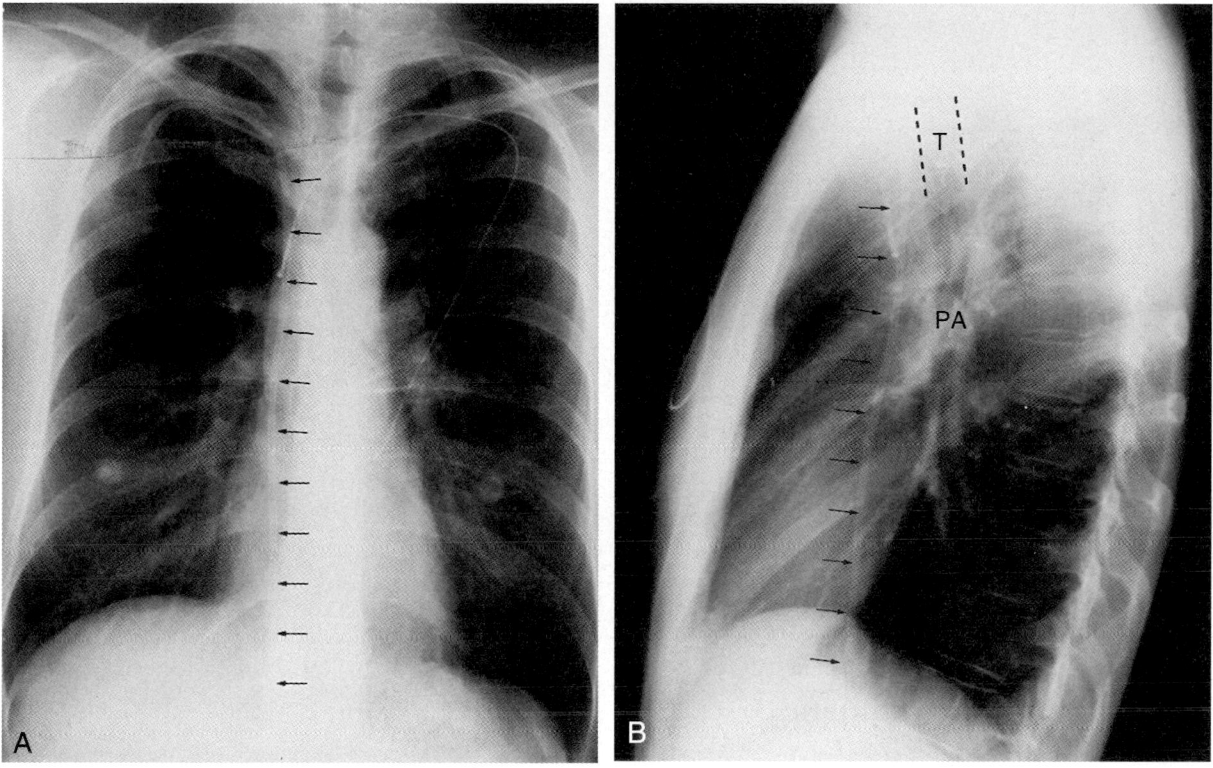

FIGURE 3-31 ■ **Abnormal course of Swan-Ganz catheter.** This catheter was inserted from a right subclavian approach, and on the posteroanterior view of the chest, it is seen extending down along the right side of the spine to below the level of the hemidiaphragms *(A)*. On the lateral view *(B)*, it can be seen extending down the inferior vena cava through the heart and down into the inferior vena cava *(arrows)*. The patient also has a left subclavian catheter with tip in the superior vena cava.

Cardiac Pacers

Cardiac pacers are wires that extend from a pacing source, down the SVC, through the right atrium, and to the right ventricular apex (Fig. 3-32). Not much that can go wrong with these can be identified on a conventional chest x-ray; however, in the case of pacer failure, look for a broken wire.

Overlying Electrocardiogram (ECG) Wires and Tubes

Electrocardiogram (ECG) leads are metallic wires and therefore are denser than most tubes and catheters. They also can be recognized because they usually have a button or snap on the end, usually are over the upper chest, and do not follow any reasonable internal anatomic pathway (such as venous structures) (see Fig. 3-27*B*). Other overlying objects that are often confusing are oxygen supply lines to nasal cannulas and masks. These can look like catheters, but they too do not follow normal vascular or anatomic pathways and are seen mostly over the upper chest and neck. If an unsolved issue appears, perform a visual examination of the patient rather than ordering another radiographic study.

Trauma

A chest x-ray is often obtained in the emergency department in patients with major trauma. This allows rapid identification of moderate to large pneumothoraces and pleural fluid collections. Because the patients are usually supine, a small anterior pneumothorax or posterior fluid collection can easily be missed. These are often incidentally noted on a chest CT obtained later

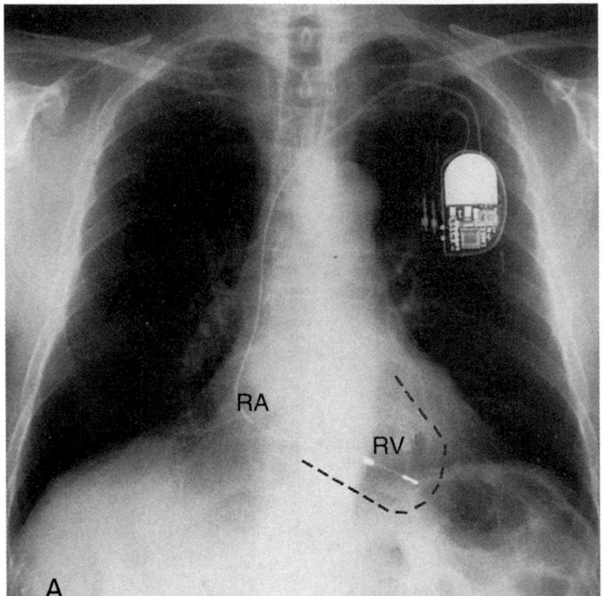

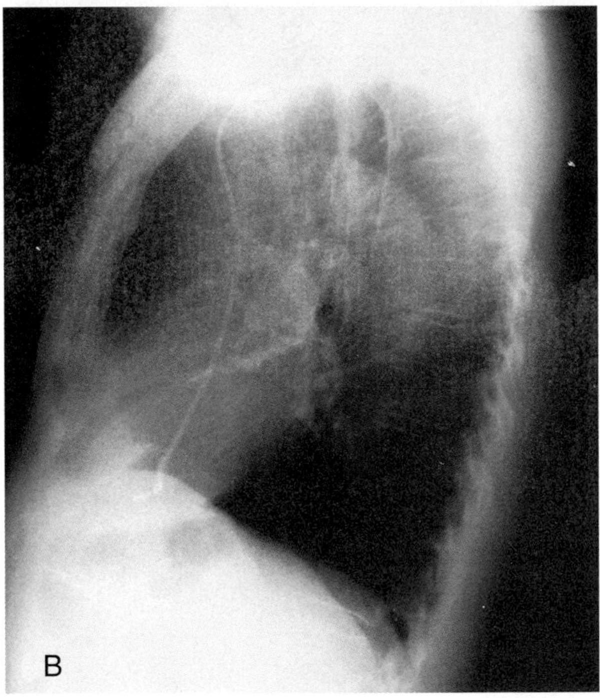

FIGURE 3-32 ■ Cardiac pacer. On the posteroanterior view *(A)*, the control portion is underneath the skin and is seen projecting over the right lung apex. It extends into the brachiocephalic vein and down into the right atrium (RA) and has the tip in the right ventricle (RV). On the lateral view *(B)*, the course can be clearly identified.

(see Fig. 3-75). With major chest trauma, consideration of spine and sternal injuries may require additional x-rays. Dedicated rib films are usually not needed because no change in treatment would occur as the result of an uncomplicated rib fracture. A widened mediastinum on a chest x-ray raises the question of vascular injury, and a contrasted CT scan is indicated. Plain x-ray examinations often underestimate the extent of soft tissue injuries, and as a result, it is common for trauma surgeons to order a CT scan of the chest, abdomen, and pelvis. This is being done much more commonly to identify life-threatening injuries that require prompt surgical intervention.

Pulmonary infiltrates are common after lung trauma. Pulmonary contusions can occur without rib fractures and are seen within hours of an accident. About 50% of such patients will have hemoptysis. Contusions are seen radiographically as ill-defined pulmonary parenchymal infiltrates caused by hemorrhage and edema. If uncomplicated, they normally resolve over a period of 4 to 5 days. Pulmonary hematomas are caused by bleeding as a result of shearing injuries of the lung parenchyma. These can appear as nodules or masses, and they may cavitate. They take weeks to resolve completely. Pneumomediastinum or subcutaneous emphysema also should be identified. The latter indicates a high probability of rib fracture, pneumothorax, or penetrating injury. The various entities related to trauma are discussed and shown with examples later in this chapter.

A post-traumatic abnormality that can produce bilateral, ill-defined infiltrates is fat embolism. This is not seen except with fracture of a large bone (such as the femur) that has undergone surgical manipulation. These patients usually initially have a clear chest film and have a sudden onset of dyspnea some time afterward. The diagnosis is made by looking for fat globules in the urine.

The Airways

Issues related to epiglottitis and retropharyngeal abscesses were discussed in Chapter 2. You should be able to recognize several major problems related to airways.

Occlusion. Lung cancer can narrow or totally occlude a bronchus. If the airway is only partially occluded, difficulty will occur in clearing mucus, and a postobstructive pneumonia may be found. In any older adult who has a focal pneumonia, you should look carefully at the nearby bronchi. In an adult with recurrence of pneumonia in a particular location, you should suspect a lung tumor, and bronchoscopy may be indicated.

If a tumor or mucous plug totally obstructs an airway, resorption of air distally will be accompanied by volume loss. If the obstruction is of a major bronchus, rapid opacification (whiteness) of the lung may be found, accompanied by shift of the trachea and mediastinal structures toward the affected side as a result of volume loss. A major bronchus obstruction can often be identified on the frontal chest x-ray. Additional studies, such as CT, can be useful to determine the extent of tumor, the presence of enlarged lymph nodes, and so forth (Fig. 3-33). If the patient is young or very sick, a mucous plug is a more likely cause of obstruction and volume loss than is a tumor. Bronchoscopy or pulmonary therapy should be suggested rather than a CT scan of the chest.

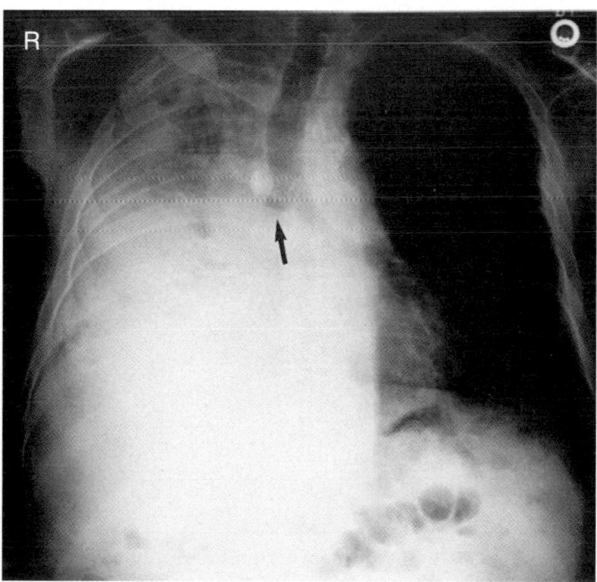

FIGURE 3-33 ■ Tumor obstructing right main-stem bronchus. A sharp cutoff of the air column is clearly identified *(arrow)*. The obstruction has caused a postobstructive infiltrate, with resorption of the air from the right lung, volume loss, and resultant shift of the mediastinum to the right.

Foreign bodies are usually the result of aspiration or swallowing an object that was in the mouth. In the case of aspiration, depending on the density of the offending object, it may or may not be seen on a chest x-ray. Metal objects are easily seen (Fig. 3-34), whereas items such as plastic toys and peanuts do not differ in density from soft tissues. The typical location of aspirated foreign bodies is in the right main-stem or right lower lobe bronchus because of the more vertical direction compared with the left side. As mentioned earlier, in cases in which a nonmetallic obstructing foreign body is suspected, you should order inspiration and expiration PA chest views. In uncooperative children, right and left decubitus chest views are sometimes used. The side that does not decrease in volume during expiration or when placed dependently is abnormal.

Chronic Obstructive Pulmonary Disease (COPD). A chest x-ray can detect only moderate or advanced chronic obstructive pulmonary disease (COPD). In early stages, the chest x-ray is normal, and you must rely on pulmonary function tests to make this diagnosis. In advanced stages, obvious signs of hyperinflation are noted. On the PA x-ray, the superior portions of the hemidiaphragms may be down to the level of the posterior twelfth ribs, and often blunting of the costophrenic angles is seen. With COPD, an increase in the AP diameter of the chest on the lateral view, a large anterior clear space between the sternum and ascending aorta, and marked flattening or even inversion of the hemidiaphragms are seen (Fig. 3-35). An associated finding may be the presence of bullae or large air cavities within the lungs as a result of destruction of alveoli. In very advanced COPD, what is known as a *saber sheath trachea* may be seen. This refers to a trachea that is compressed from the sides by the lungs, with the trachea appearing narrow on the PA x-ray and wide on the lateral film. I do not see this very often. Because most COPD is associated with smoking, also look for an occult lung cancer.

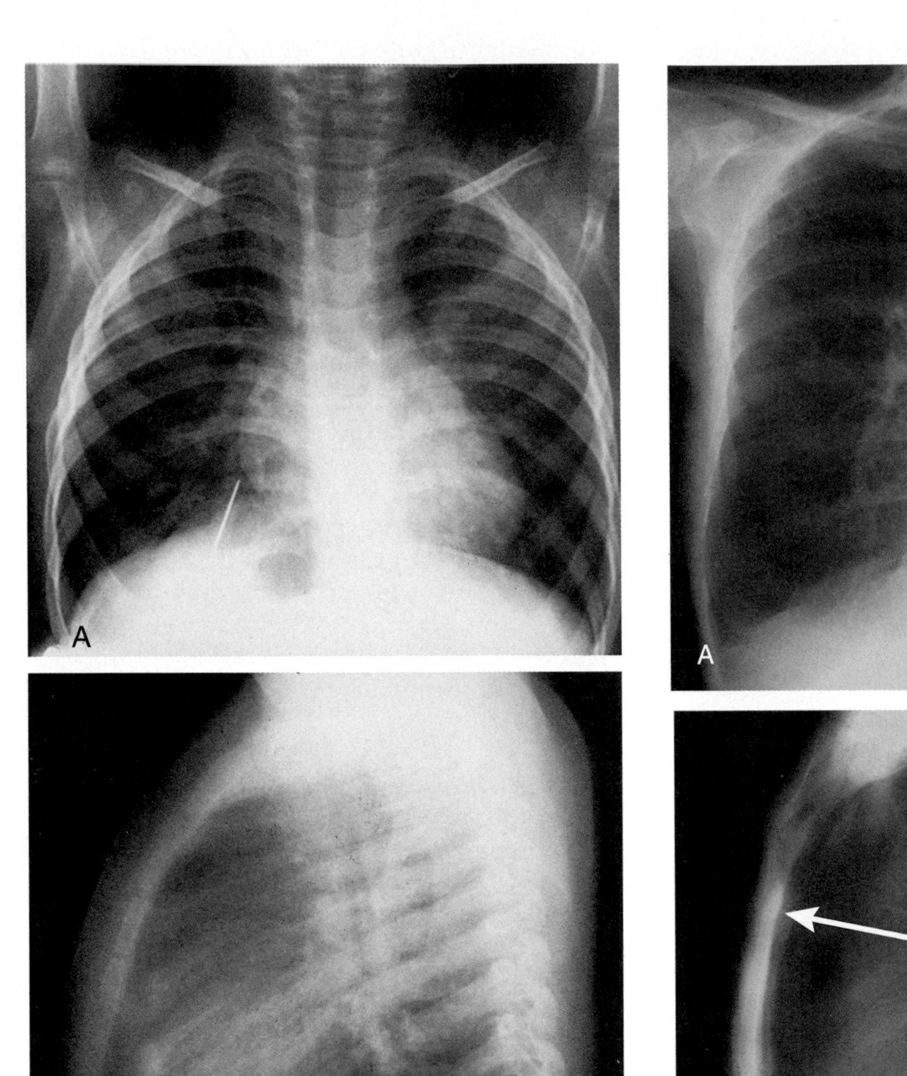

FIGURE 3-34 ■ Aspiration of a nonobstructing foreign body. A metallic straight pin can be seen in the right lower lobe on both the posteroanterior *(A)* and the lateral *(B)* chest x-rays.

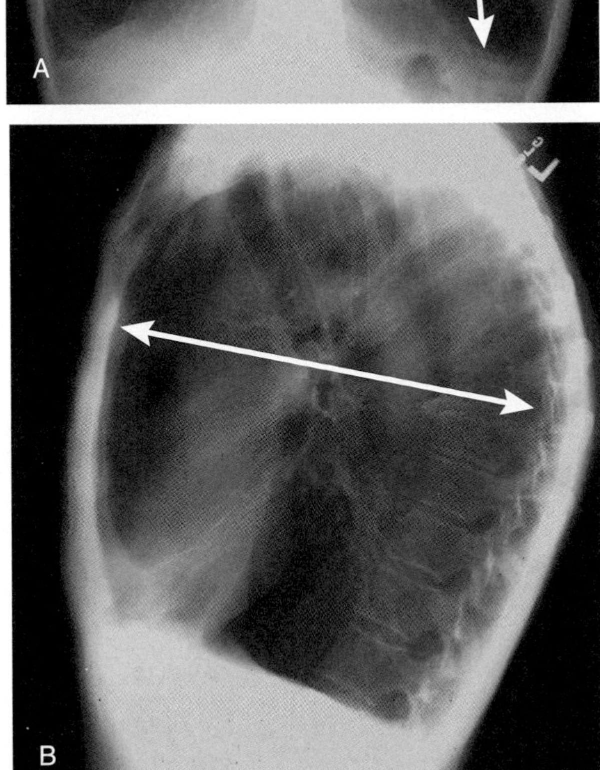

FIGURE 3-35 ■ Chronic obstructive pulmonary disease (COPD). The posteroanterior view *(A)* shows that the superior aspect of the hemidiaphragms is at the same level as the posterior aspect of the twelfth ribs. Hyperinflation also is seen on the lateral view *(B)* as an increase in the anteroposterior diameter and flattening of the hemidiaphragms.

Asthma. Imaging studies are usually not necessary in an uncomplicated asthma attack. A chest x-ray is ordered only with the suspicion of superimposed disease or if the attack is resistant to therapy. The findings of asthma on chest x-ray range from a normal appearance (about three fourths of the time) to signs of mild hyperinflation, such as slightly increased AP diameter or hemidiaphragms with the superior aspect level with the posterior tenth to eleventh ribs (Fig. 3-36). With asthma, it is very unusual to have enough hyperinflation either to drive the diaphragms lower than this or to significantly flatten them (as seen on the lateral view). An acute asthma attack can result in a pneumomediastinum but rarely in a pneumothorax. Patients with recurrent asthmatic attacks may have a prominent interstitial pattern due to scarring, and they may have slightly thickened bronchial walls. Also look for a focal infiltrate or pneumonia as the precipitating cause of the asthmatic attack.

Bronchiectasis. *Bronchiectasis* refers to diffuse or focal dilatation of the bronchi. This is usually the result of chronic or childhood infection and subsequent cartilage damage. It also is seen in patients with rare entities such as cystic fibrosis and allergic bronchopulmonary aspergillosis. Symptoms are chronic cough, purulent sputum, and sometimes hemoptysis. Bronchiectasis typically involves the medial aspects of both right and left lower lobes. This is visualized on a plain chest x-ray by the associated bronchial wall thickening, which is the result of infection.

Early bronchiectasis may be associated with a normal chest x-ray, although in later stages, the bronchial wall thickening causes the appearance of a stringy or honeycomb (coarse mesh) infiltrate at both lung bases. In addition, sometimes "tram-tracking" can be seen. This refers to two parallel linear densities seen as white lines that represent the thickened bronchial walls. Usually this is seen for only 2 or 3 cm before it disappears (Fig. 3-37*A* and *B*). Late bronchiectasis is seen as cavities or a honeycomb appearance at the lung bases. Although it is difficult to see bronchiectasis on a plain chest x-ray, it is quite easy to identify by using thin-slice or high-resolution CT scanning (Fig. 3-37*C*). You should

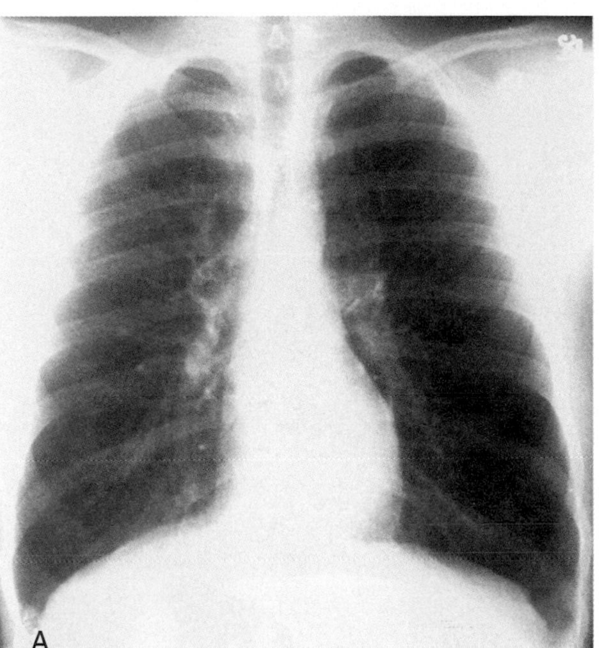

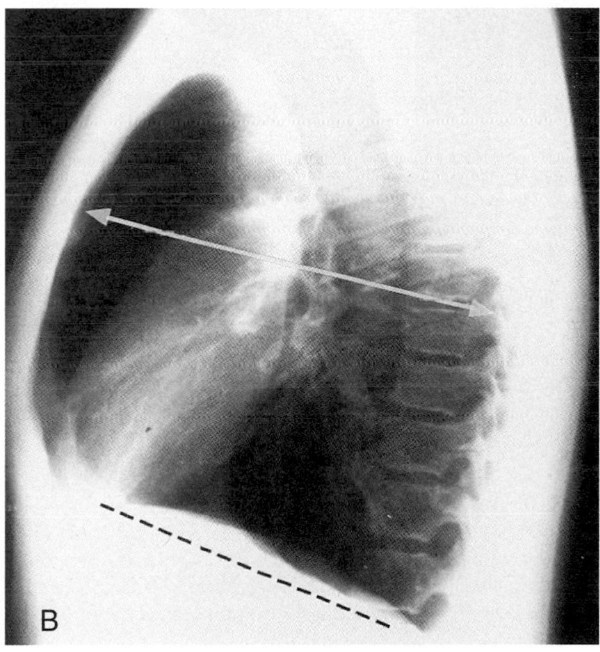

FIGURE 3-36 ■ Asthma. During a severe asthma attack, hyperinflation, similar to that seen in chronic obstructive pulmonary disease (COPD), can be seen. In this case, hyperinflation is seen, with the superior aspect of the hemidiaphragms located at the level of the posterior eleventh ribs *(A)*; a slight increase in the anteroposterior diameter and some flattening of the hemidiaphragm appear *(B)*. The patient does not have the barrel-shaped chest seen in COPD (Fig. 3-35*B*). Most patients with asthma have normal chest x-rays.

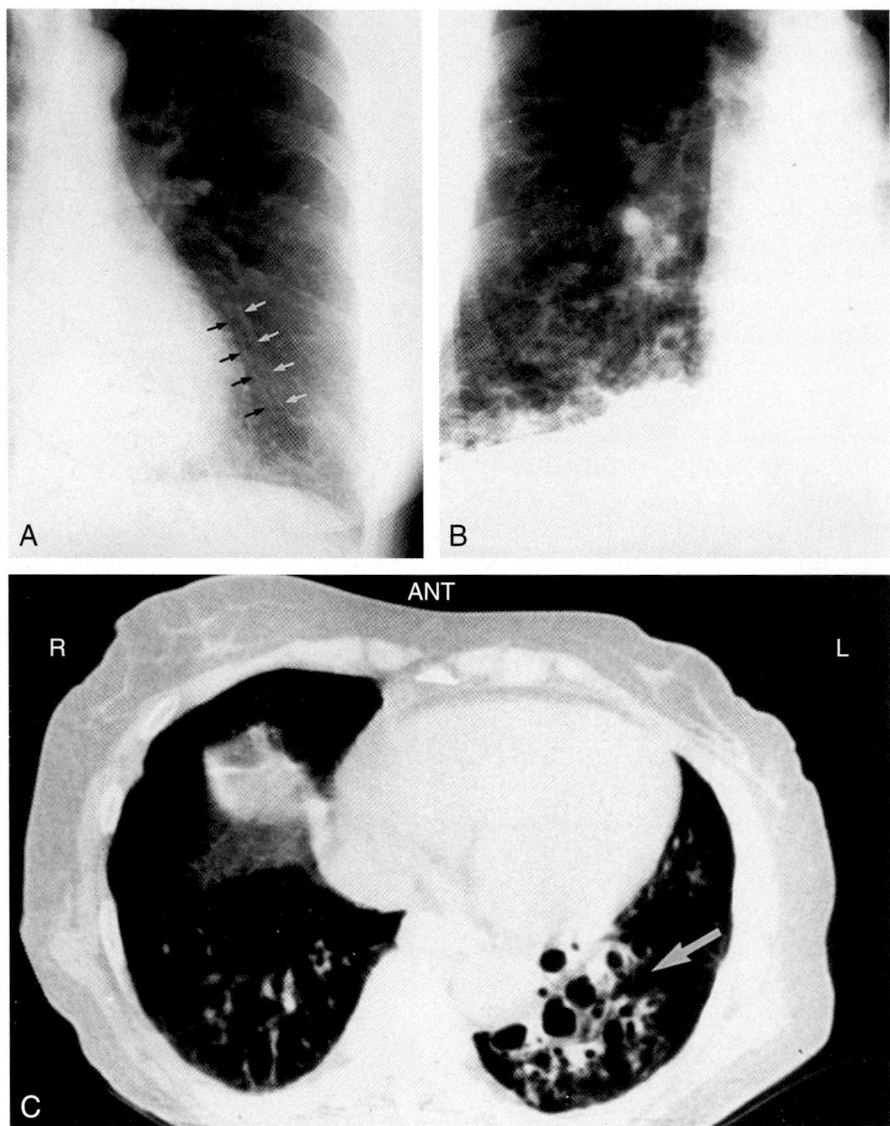

FIGURE 3-37 ■ Bronchiectasis. A posteroanterior chest x-ray in a patient with bronchiectasis demonstrates bronchial wall thickening, most pronounced at the lung bases *(A)*. This is often referred to as "tram tracking" or linear parallel lines that represent thickened bronchial walls *(arrows)*. In advanced bronchiectasis *(B)*, coarse basilar lung infiltrates may appear cavitary. Bronchiectasis is much better seen on a computed tomography scan *(C)* than on a chest x-ray. The findings are of dilated bronchi with thickened bronchial walls *(arrow)*.

not order a CT study unless it will make a difference in therapy or outcome.

Atelectasis. Atelectasis refers to collapse of a lung or portion of the lung with resorption of air from the alveoli. This can result from an obstructing bronchial lesion, extrinsic compression (from pleural effusions or bullae), fibrosis, or a loss of surface tension in the alveoli (as in hyaline membrane disease). Atelectasis can involve a small subsegmental region of a lung or the entire lung. Because atelectasis is a very common finding and has clinical implications, you should be familiar with the various appearances and progressions that are associated with focal or generalized volume loss in a lung.

Linear (discoid or platelike) atelectasis is almost always seen in the middle or lower lung zones as a horizontal or near-horizontal line of increased density (whiteness). This minimal form of subsegmental collapse is most commonly seen in patients who have difficulty breathing, such as after recent surgery or rib fractures. The atelectasis may appear very quickly (within hours) and can disappear just as quickly after the patient has been encouraged to breathe deeply or after respiratory therapy (Fig. 3-38).

Atelectasis, or collapse of entire lung segments, occurs typically as a result of a mucous plug, tumor, or malplacement of ET tubes. Early right upper lobe atelectasis is seen on the AP or PA x-ray as a hazy white density in the right upper lung zone. As air is resorbed from the right upper lobe, increasing density but decreasing right upper lobe volume may be seen. During this process, the right minor fissure moves from its normal horizontal position and becomes bowed upward. This looks like an upside-down white triangle at the right lung apex. With complete collapse of the right upper lobe, only a whitish density may appear, beginning at the right hilum and extending up along the right lateral aspect of the superior mediastinum and then curving out over the apex. In this late stage (complete right upper lobe collapse), the diagnosis can be difficult to make. Usually, however, other signs of volume loss point toward the right upper lobe. These include shift or pulling of the trachea to the right and elevation of the right hilum. Remember that the right hilum should normally be slightly lower than the left; if both right and left hila appear at the same level, think about right upper lobe volume loss as one possible cause for this finding.

Atelectasis of the right middle lobe is often difficult to appreciate on an AP x-ray, but it appears as a slightly increased density (whiteness) over the lower portion of the right lung, and loss of the normally distinct right cardiac margin is seen. On the lateral chest x-ray, a narrow white triangle will project over the heart, formed by the approximation of the minor fissure and the lower half of the major fissure.

With right lower lobe collapse, there is increasing density at the right lung base, loss of the right hemidiaphragm margin, and pulling down of the right hilum. On the lateral chest x-ray, posterior and inferior displacement of the major fissure and increasing density (or whiteness) over the lower thoracic spine appear (Fig. 3-39).

Lobar atelectasis, or collapse of left lung lobes, can be more difficult to appreciate than

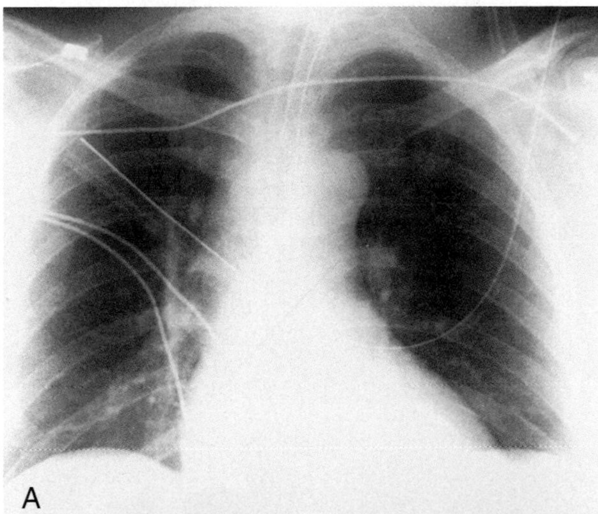

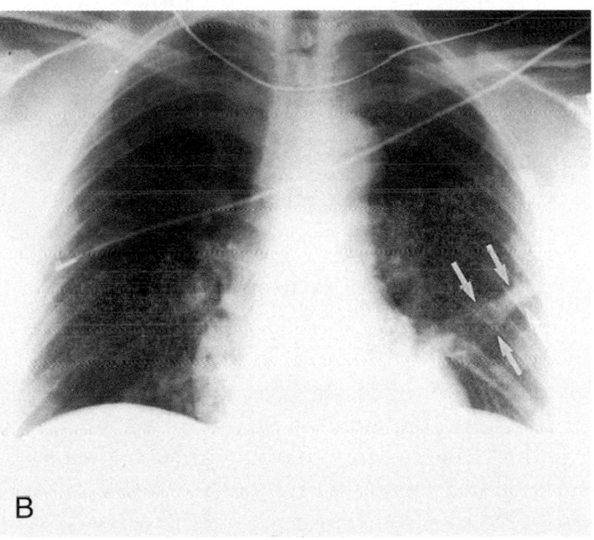

FIGURE 3-38 ■ Linear atelectasis. An immediate postoperative anteroposterior chest x-ray *(A)* is unremarkable with the exception of an endotracheal tube being present and overlying tubes and electrocardiogram leads. A chest x-ray obtained several hours after the patient had been extubated *(B)* shows an area of linear atelectasis *(arrows)*. This can clear up very quickly if the patient is given appropriate respiratory therapy.

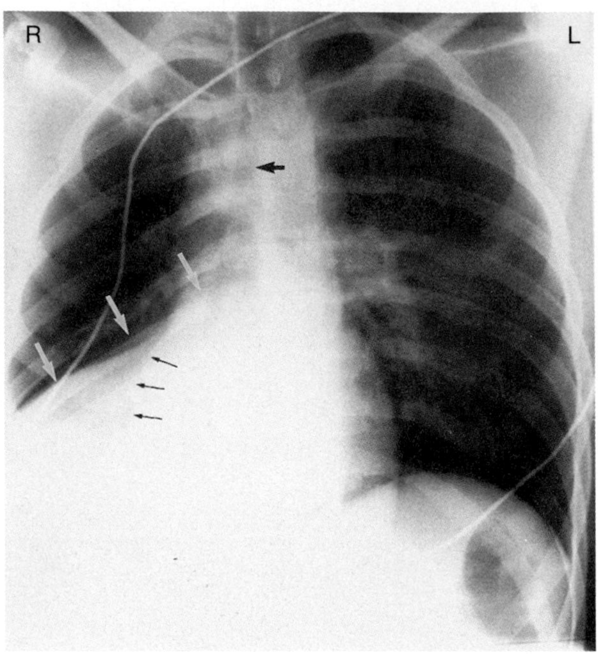

FIGURE 3-39 ■ Right lower lobe atelectasis. Complete collapse of the right lower lobe with volume loss evidenced by shift of the trachea and cardiac border to the right side *(black arrows)*. Air in the right lower lobe has been resorbed, resulting in a diffuse infiltrate *(white arrows)*.

you might suspect. On an AP or a PA chest x-ray, left lower lobe collapse appears as a haziness or increasing density at the left lung base and retrocardiac region. A retrocardiac density is more likely to be atelectasis than a pneumonia, particularly immediately after thoracic surgery. With left lower lobe atelectasis, the left hilum may be pulled down and level with the right one, and the left hemidiaphragm will be hard to see. On the lateral view, posterior and some inferior displacement of the major fissure are noted. As in right lower lobe collapse, increasing density over the lower thoracic spine is seen.

Both right and left lower lobe collapse can mimic or be mimicked by pleural effusions. The way to differentiate the two is to exclude the presence of a pleural effusion. This can be done by looking at the cardiophrenic angles on an upright frontal view of the chest to see if blunting or pleural fluid tracking up along the sides of the chest wall is present. If volume loss is seen (indicated by pulling down of the hilum or mediastinal shift toward the affected side), collapse should be suspected. With a large pleural effusion, often associated underlying lung atelectasis occurs as a result of direct compression, so do not be fooled into assuming that only one entity can exist at a given time.

Left upper lobe atelectasis is seen on the frontal chest x-ray as a generalized density in the left upper lung. In the early stages, increased density occurs anterior to the major fissure on the lateral chest x-ray. As atelectasis of the left upper lobe progresses and becomes complete, the collapsed left upper lobe becomes pancaked along the anterior chest wall and may be visualized only as a dense white line 1 or 2 cm thick in the retrosternal region (Fig. 3-40).

The most severe form of volume loss occurs after surgical removal of one lung. After a pneumonectomy, empty space fills with fluid over several weeks. As this progresses, the hemidiaphragm will elevate, the mediastinum will move toward the affected side, and the remaining lung will hyperinflate and often will herniate across the midline. If the mediastinal structures are displaced away from the resected lung, you should be suspicious of a postoperative malignant effusion or an empyema.

Blebs and Bullae. Both *blebs* and *bullae* refer to a portion of lung in which an air space is found without alveoli. Although I have never known a clear distinction to be made between these two entities, most people consider a bleb to be a relatively small air cavity, usually on the order of 1 cm or less. A bulla is greater than 1 cm and often significantly larger, measuring several inches in diameter. Both a bleb and a bulla should have walls that are very thin and well defined (if they can be seen at all) (Fig. 3-41). If a thick wall is present, think in terms of an inflammatory or cavitary neoplastic lesion. Because the walls of blebs and bullae are so thin, the sensitivity of a chest x-ray for detection of these lesions is quite poor, although they are easily seen on a CT scan. The presence of a bulla can sometimes be inferred on a chest x-ray by noting a region of lung that does not seem to have pulmonary vessels.

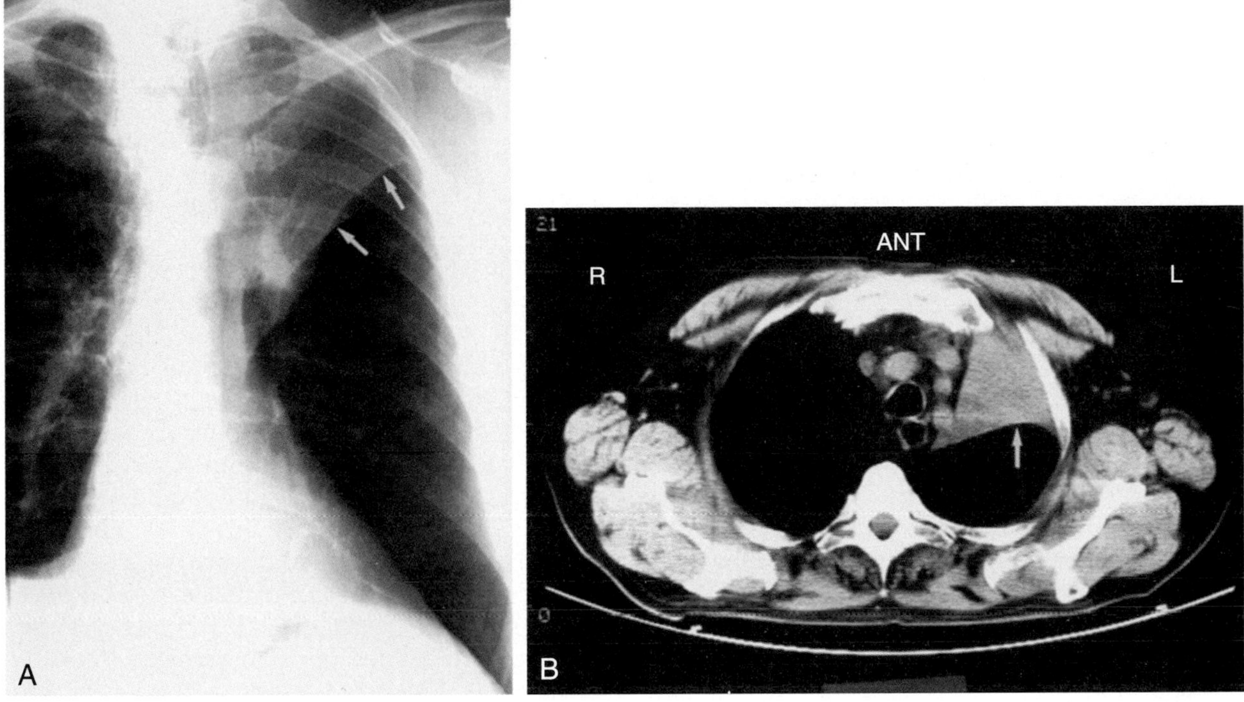

FIGURE 3-40 ■ Left upper lobe atelectasis. Right or left upper lobe atelectasis is often seen as a diffuse increase in density with upward bowing of the minor fissure. The volume loss also elevates the hilum on the affected side *(A)*. A computed tomography scan *(B)* also shows the atelectasis as a diffuse increase in density of the affected segment or lobe *(arrow)*.

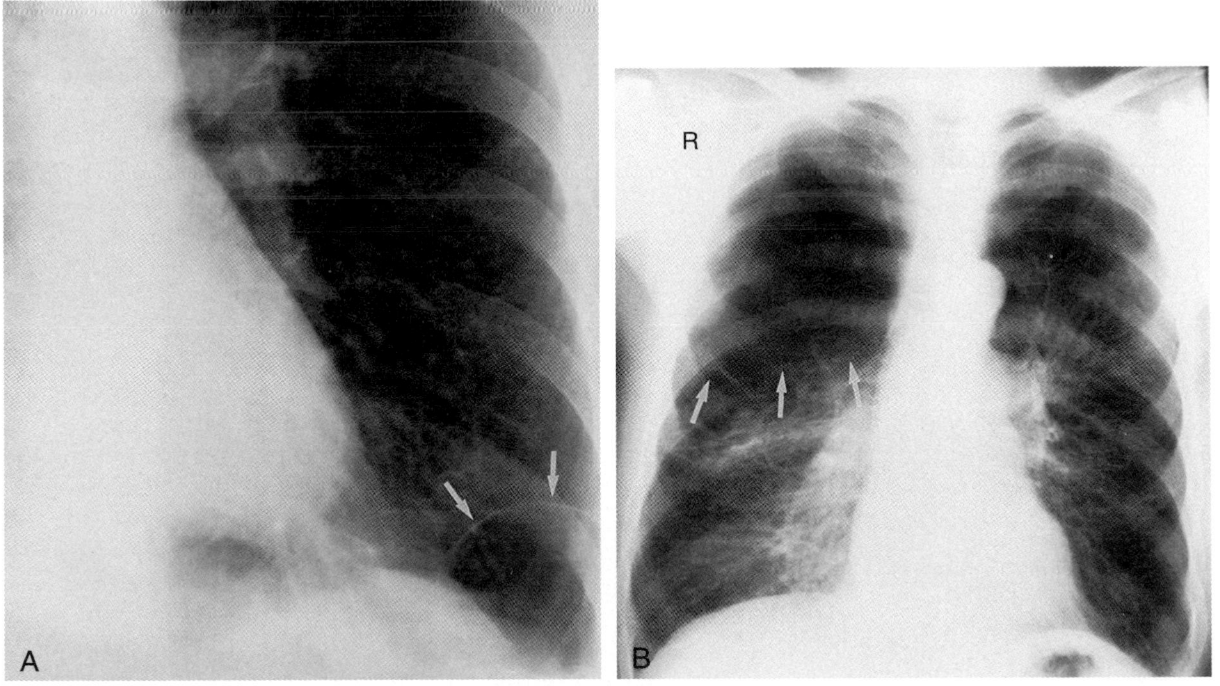

FIGURE 3-41 ■ Bullae. Sometimes small bullae can be seen on a chest x-ray *(A)* because their thin wall can be visualized. Larger bullae *(B)* are sometimes identified only by the fact that an area on the chest x-ray does not appear to have any pulmonary vessels *(arrows)*, and at the periphery, crowding of the normal lung and vessels may appear.

Air-Space Pathology

Infiltrates and Pneumonias. For appropriate diagnosis of a patchy or diffusely increased density in the lungs, characterize the x-ray appearance and correlate this with the clinical history. Most radiologists will report an infiltrate as alveolar, interstitial, nodular, or mixed, and they will tell you whether it is focal (e.g., in the right upper lobe) or diffuse. The terms *alveolar* and *interstitial* are often difficult for the novice and the expert radiologist to differentiate and agree on.

Alveolar simply means that the alveolar spaces are filled with some material. In simple terms, this means that the alveoli are filled with pus, blood, fluid, or cells. Given this, it is not possible radiographically to tell whether an alveolar infiltrate is due to a pneumonia (pus), pulmonary hemorrhage (blood), pulmonary edema (fluid), or alveolar tumor (cells) (Fig. 3-42). Most alveolar infiltrates either are somewhat fluffy or represent areas of complete consolidation. As filling of the alveoli progresses, the only things left with air in them are the bronchi, and thus "air bronchograms" can be seen (Fig. 3-43*A*). If you see a bronchus filled with air and outlined by increased density, you can be certain that you are dealing with an alveolar process.

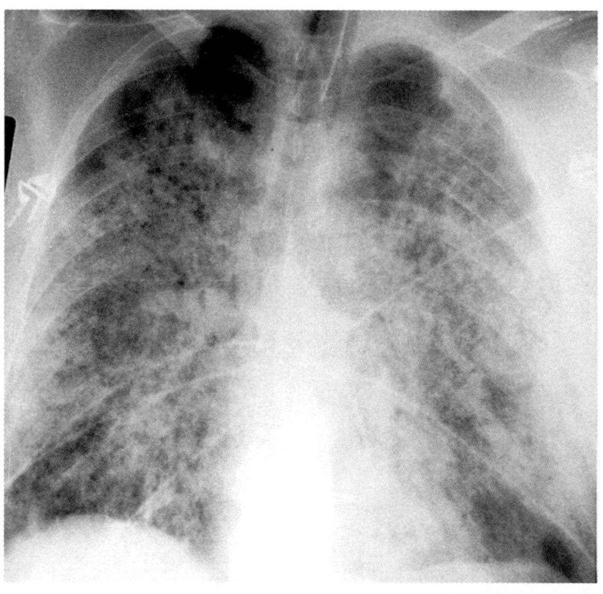

FIGURE 3-42 ■ Pulmonary hemorrhage. The fluffy alveolar pattern is produced by fluid filling the alveoli.

Interstitial infiltrates are caused by disease processes that affect tissues outside the alveoli. Interstitial processes are usually diffuse and are seen as thin white lines (Fig. 3-43*B*). Occasionally they may be somewhat honeycombed in appearance, and the differential diagnosis of these processes often depends on whether the interstitial infiltrate is acute or chronic. Again, the finding of an interstitial infiltrate is nonspecific. Increased fluid in the interstitium and interlobular septa can be seen in CHF. Interstitial changes also can be seen with what is commonly referred to as lymphangitic spread of tumor as well as idiopathic pulmonary fibrosis, collagen vascular diseases, and other entities. Do not be surprised if you think you see both interstitial and alveolar signs on the same chest x-ray. Many processes, such as CHF, can cause both findings (i.e., interstitial edema and pulmonary edema with alveolar filling).

Community-acquired Pneumonia in Adults. The diagnosis of pneumonia should be made clinically, based on fever, cough, dyspnea, pleuritic chest pain, rales, localized diminished breath sounds, percussion dullness, or egophony on auscultation. A chest x-ray is confirmatory and helps differentiate pneumonia from other conditions that may have similar symptoms (e.g., bronchial obstruction) and may demonstrate findings that suggest a complicated course or prolonged recovery, such as multilobar distribution and pleural effusions.

Most bacterial pneumonias produce lobar, segmental, or patchy infiltrates. Although this is an alveolar infiltrate, the alveolar filling and consolidation are usually not enough to be able to see distinct air bronchograms. Accurate localization of a pneumonia to a segment of the lung usually requires both PA and lateral chest x-rays. When the consolidation is fairly dense, the infiltrate is quite easy to localize. A right or left upper lobe infiltrate is usually seen as increased density in the upper portions of the lung on the AP or PA view. The lateral film generally is unnecessary for this diagnosis (Fig. 3-44).

A right middle lobe infiltrate or pneumonia can be in the medial or lateral segment, or both. An

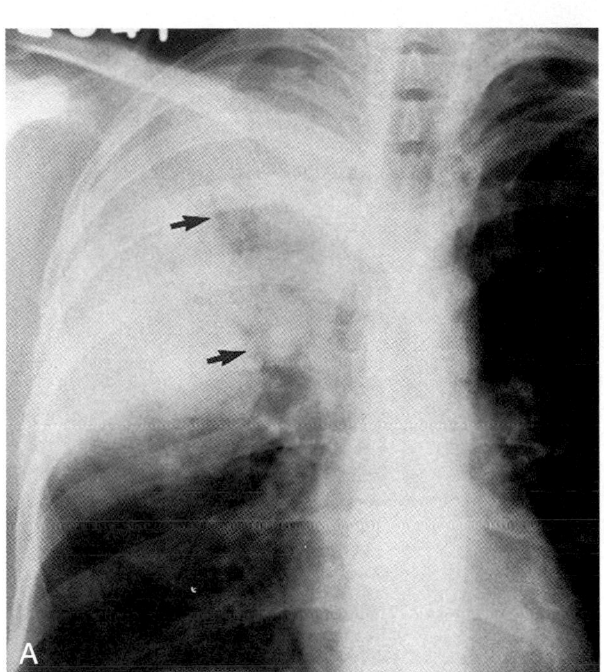

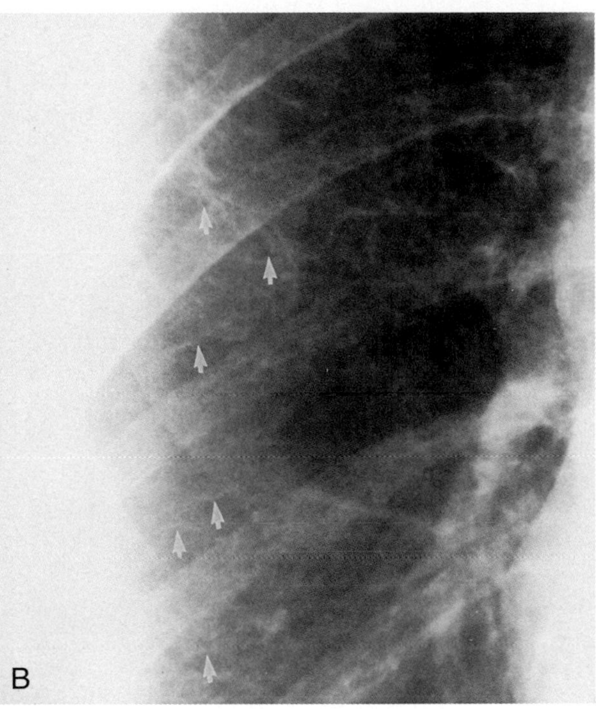

FIGURE 3-43 ■ Alveolar and interstitial pulmonary infiltrates. Alveolar lung infiltrates are seen initially as patchy densities, but as they become more confluent and the process fills the alveolar spaces *(A)*, the only air that remains is in the bronchi. This results in what is termed an air bronchogram *(arrows)*. An interstitial infiltrate is seen on the chest x-ray of a different patient as multiple, very white, thin lines *(B)*. Pulmonary vessels are not normally seen at the very periphery of the lung, and therefore the lines shown here by the *white arrows* represent an interstitial process.

infiltrate in the medial segment of the right middle lobe will obscure the right heart border on the frontal view, and on the lateral view, is seen as a triangular density radiating from the hilum toward the anterior and lower part of the chest (Fig. 3-45).

Right and left lower lobe infiltrates can be visualized by one of three methods. They may obscure the right or left hemidiaphragm on the frontal view. Remember, on an AP or a PA chest x-ray, you should normally be able to see the hemidiaphragms from the lateral costophrenic angles almost all the way to the spine (even behind the heart) (Fig. 3-46*A*). On the lateral view, lower lobe infiltrates can be identified as being behind the location of the major fissure (Fig. 3-46*B*); alternatively, they can be identified by utilizing the "spine sign." The vertebral bodies of the thoracic spine usually are darker as you proceed lower in the chest. If the vertebral bodies are darker down to about the midportion of the thoracic spine and then become whiter or lighter inferiorly, you should suspect a lower lobe infiltrate (Fig. 3-46*C*). Determining whether this is on the right or left will require correlation with the frontal chest x-ray.

Pneumonias need not always be segmental or lobar; they can be round or diffuse. Round pneumonias can simulate mass lesions, such as a neoplasm, although the clinical presentation is very different, and round pneumonias occur more commonly in children than in adults. These are usually due to *Streptococcus*.

Some characteristics of pneumonias can be used to guess the organism of origin, although none of these is specific. Lobar pneumonias are associated with streptococcal, staphylococcal, and gram-negative organisms. Lobar enlargement with an infiltrate is characteristically associated with *Klebsiella*. Cavitation in an acute pneumonia is associated with staphylococci and

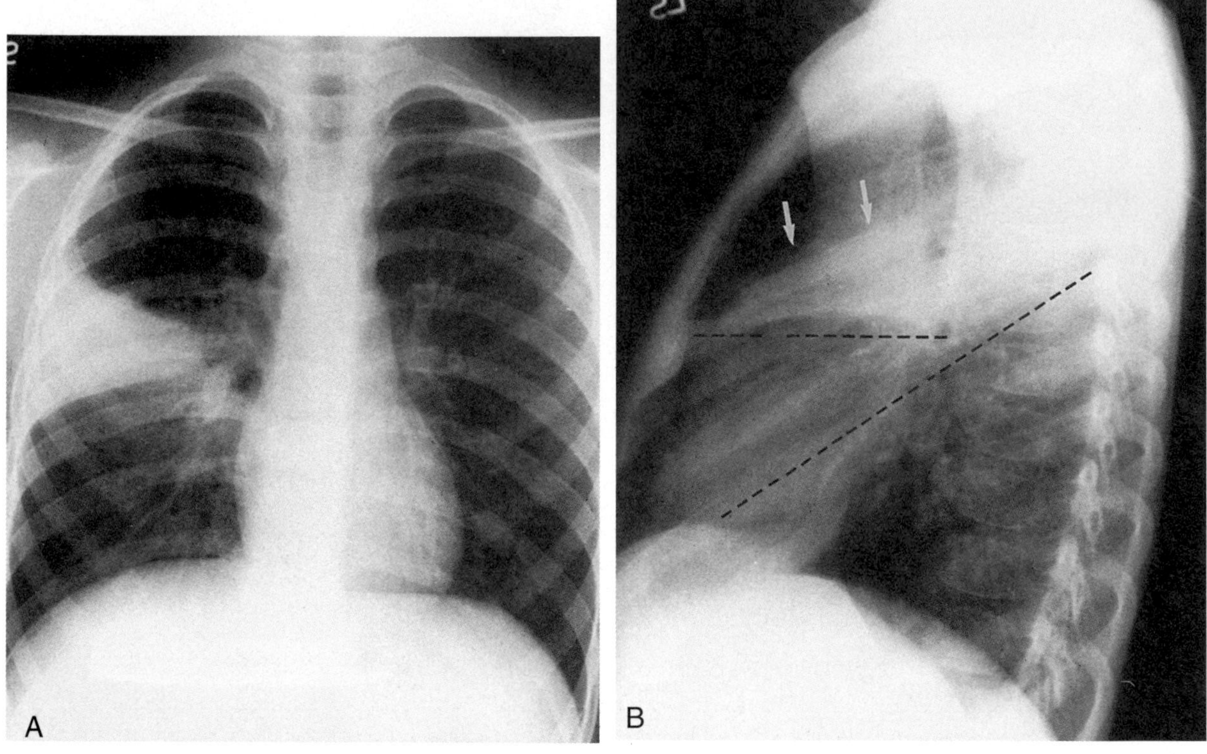

FIGURE 3-44 ■ Right upper lobe pneumonia. On the posteroanterior chest x-ray *(A)*, note that the right cardiac border is well seen. The alveolar infiltrate is seen in the right midlung. Localization is quite easy on the lateral view *(B)* by noting where the major and minor fissures should be. The infiltrate *(arrows)* can be seen above the minor fissure, indicating that it is in the upper lobe.

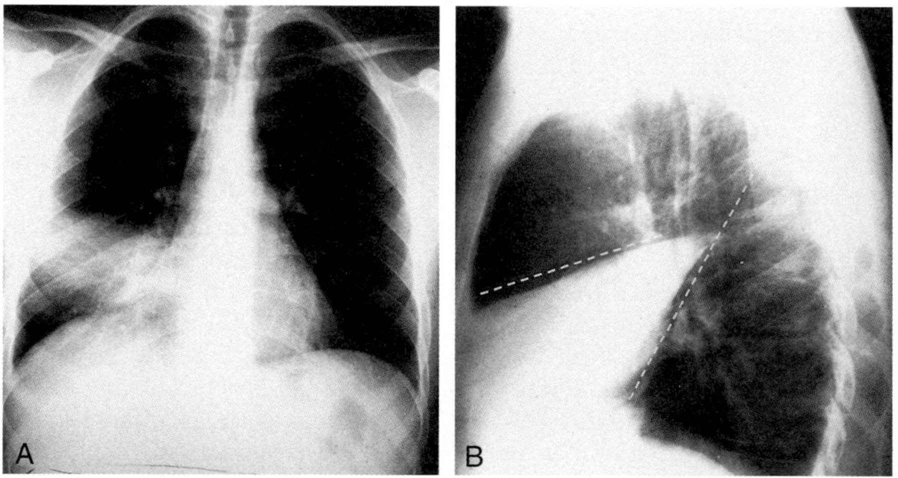

FIGURE 3-45 ■ Right middle lobe pneumonia. On the posteroanterior chest x-ray *(A)*, the alveolar infiltrate obscures the right cardiac border. This silhouette sign means that the pathologic process is up against the right cardiac border and therefore must be in the middle lobe. This is confirmed on the lateral view *(B)* by noting that the consolidation is anterior to the major fissure but below the minor fissure.

virulent streptococci. Chronic cavitation is associated with tuberculosis (TB), histoplasmosis, and fungal lesions.

Pneumonias that are interstitial and symmetrically diffuse throughout both lungs often are atypical pneumonias. These include pneumonias due to *Mycoplasma*, viruses, and *Pneumocystis*. Viral pneumonias and *Pneumocystis carinii* pneumonia (PCP) are rare in nonimmunocompromised adults; the most likely cause of an interstitial pneumonia in a nonimmunocompromised adult is mycoplasmal infection. Severe acute respiratory syndrome (SARS) is an atypical pneumonia. The imaging findings in SARS are nonspecific and include focal and patchy interstitial opacities as well as unilateral or bilateral areas of consolidation.

CT is not indicated for pneumonias unless a repeated chest x-ray after 2 weeks of therapy does not show improvement, or no improvement is found after two separate trials of antibiotic therapy based on Gram stain sputum and blood cultures. CT is indicated in a patient with recurrent pneumonia at the same site within 6 months.

Pneumonia in Immunocompromised Patients. In immunocompromised patients with a fever, a chest x-ray is indicated. If the x-ray is positive, the patient is treated and followed up clinically.

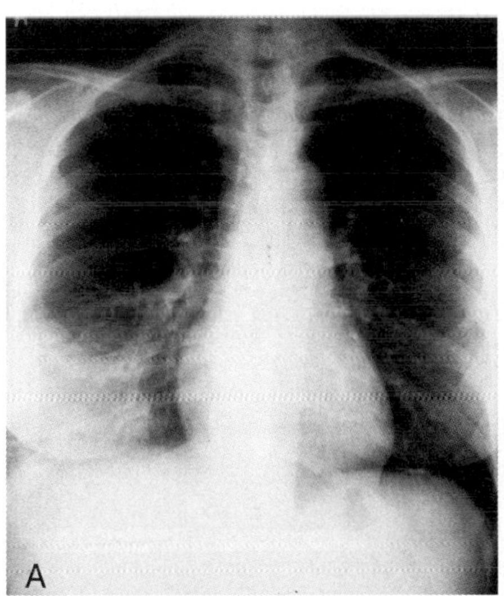

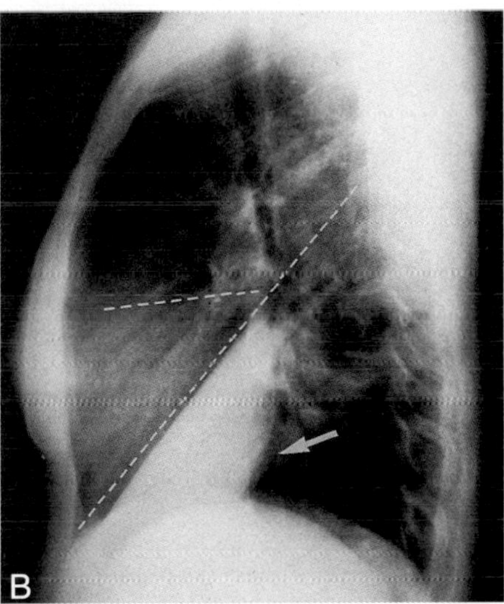

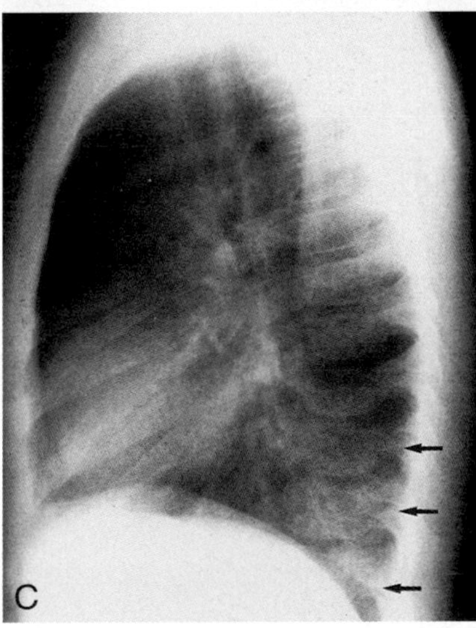

FIGURE 3-46 ■ Right lower lobe pneumonia. On the posteroanterior chest x-ray *(A)*, an alveolar infiltrate can easily be seen at the right lung base. The fact that the right heart border is clearly identified suggests that this is not in the right middle lobe but is probably in the lower lobe. The lateral view *(B)* shows that the infiltrate is behind the major fissure and is in the anterior segment of the right lower lobe. The lateral view in a different patient *(C)* also shows a right lower lobe infiltrate. In this case, the "spine sign" is used to detect an early infiltrate. The vertebral bodies of the spine should become darker as one goes from upper to lower thoracic spine, but those marked with *black arrows* are getting whiter rather than darker, indicating that an overlying infiltrate is present.

If the chest x-ray is negative and the patient is symptomatic or hypoxic, and the rest of the examination is negative, a CT scan may be indicated, but bronchoscopy usually provides sufficient information for diagnosis and management. In patients with acquired immunodeficiency syndrome (AIDS), it is best to characterize the air-space disease as diffuse, localized, or multiple nodules.

Lobar or segmental infiltrates in immunocompromised adults are most likely bacterial or fungal in origin. A chest x-ray in such a patient may reveal infiltrates (Fig. 3-47*A*), although a patient who has PCP can have a relatively normal chest x-ray. In these circumstances, a nuclear medicine gallium scan may show increased activity (Fig. 3-47*B*). Diffuse air-space disease in immunocompromised patients is due to *Pneumocystis* with or without cytomegalovirus infection. Early *Pneumocystis* infection can be seen as an interstitial infiltrate, although a more advanced condition may cause diffuse alveolar disease with air bronchograms. This can progress to consolidation within several days.

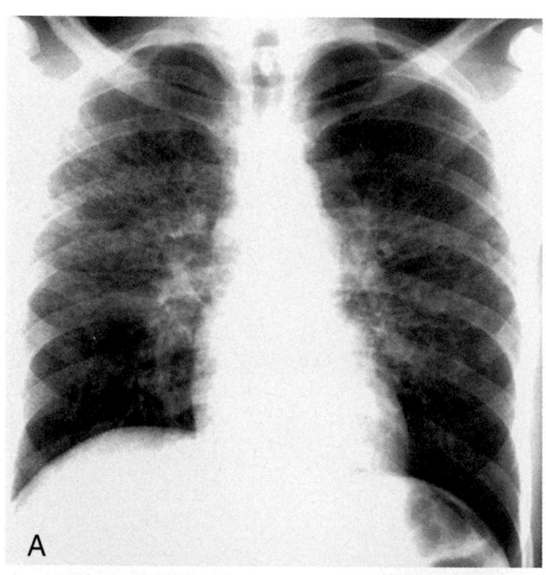

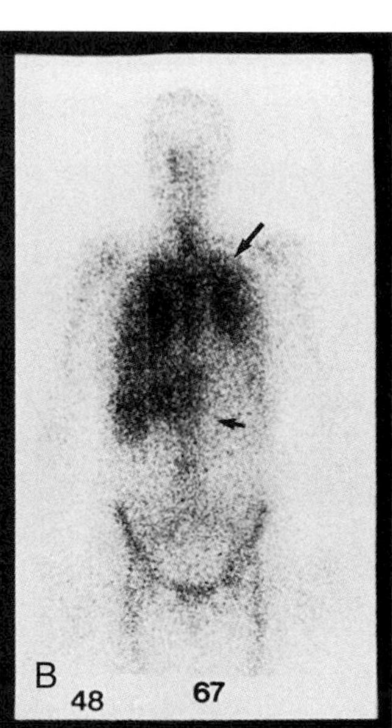

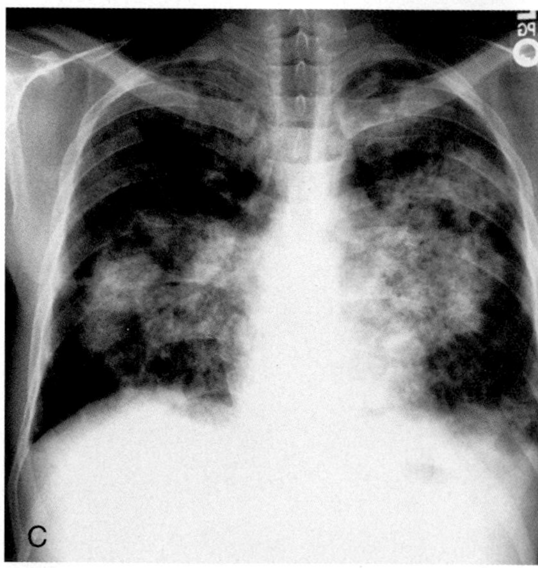

FIGURE 3-47 ■ Acquired immunodeficiency syndrome (AIDS) complications. A posteroanterior chest x-ray in a human immunodeficiency virus–positive patient shows a diffuse bilateral perihilar infiltrate due to *Pneumocystis* pneumonia *(A)*. In many patients with AIDS, the chest x-ray may be negative when *Pneumocystis* is present. A nuclear medicine gallium scan *(B)* can often show increased activity in the lungs of such patients. A chest x-ray in a different patient with AIDS *(C)* shows bilateral dense patchy alveolar infiltrates, in this case representing Kaposi's sarcoma.

Occasionally upper lobe air-filled cysts progress to pneumothorax or bronchopleural fistula. These latter findings mimic tuberculosis, but with PCP, adenopathy and pleural effusions are rare. Fungal infections in AIDS patients are uncommon.

In patients with AIDS, diffuse or nodular pulmonary involvement may be found with lymphoma or Kaposi's sarcoma (Fig. 3-47*C*). A nuclear medicine gallium scan will not be positive in patients with Kaposi's sarcoma but will be positive in PCP, most other infections, and lymphoma. Isolated hilar adenopathy in AIDS patients is more likely due to lymphoma than to mycobacterial infections.

Aspiration Pneumonia. A common indication for ordering a chest x-ray is to exclude aspiration pneumonia. The question of aspirated gastric contents may occur as the result of a seizure, cardiac resuscitation attempt, or alcoholic binge. In the case of aspiration, the chest x-ray is often normal within the first hour or so. If you get a normal chest x-ray interpretation after a recent suspected aspiration, a follow-up film should be obtained in approximately 12 hours. It often takes several hours for the gastric contents to react with the lung to cause fluid exudate and an alveolar infiltrate (Fig. 3-48). A number of other toxic agents, such as water (drowning), hydrocarbons, chlorine, smoke, heroin, and aspirin, as well as radiation therapy, can produce alveolar infiltrates. Some drugs, such as busulfan, bleomycin, and cyclophosphamide, produce toxic interstitial disease. Amiodarone can cause a wide variety of pulmonary abnormalities, but the characteristic finding seen on CT scan is increased lung density due to the iodine content of the drug.

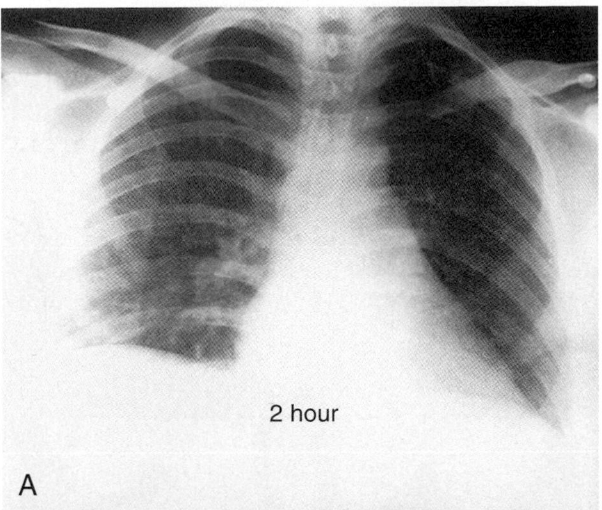

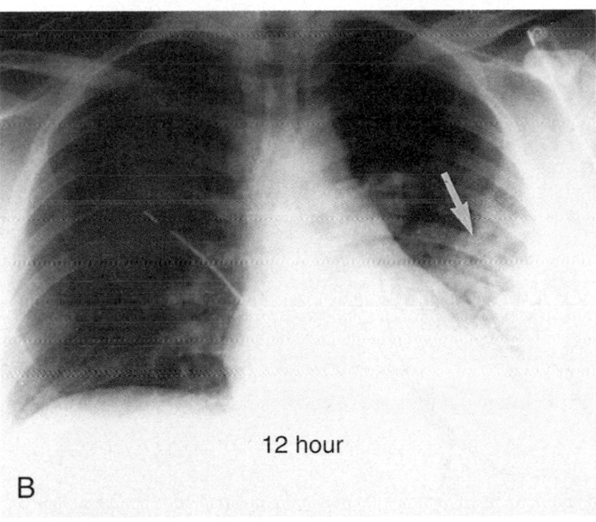

FIGURE 3-48 ■ **Aspiration pneumonia.** A chest x-ray obtained immediately after aspiration may be quite normal *(A)*. The chemical pneumonia takes 6 or 12 hours *(B)* to cause an alveolar infiltrate *(arrow)*.

Tuberculosis. Routine screening chest x-rays to detect TB are not indicated. Chest x-rays are often done on persons who have had a positive purified protein derivative (PPD) skin test, and 99% or more are normal. Guidelines exist for the use of chest x-rays in TB detection in asymptomatic patients. One should ascertain the results of a recent chest x-ray on elderly persons being admitted to nursing homes (and who may not react to skin tests). A chest x-ray also is indicated in a person with a first-time positive PPD skin test or a converter to determine if prophylaxis or multiple drug therapy should be initiated. It should be pointed out that a normal chest x-ray does not exclude active TB, because the TB that results in a positive skin test need not be in the lungs but can be in the kidneys or even in the spine.

When TB is visualized on a chest x-ray, the usual sequence of events is as follows. Primary TB is most commonly seen as a focal middle or lower lobe consolidation with lymphadenopathy and sometimes a pleural effusion. Cavitation is rare. Hilar adenopathy is present about 95% of the time and is more commonly seen in children than in adults. A pleural effusion is present about 10% of the time. Reactivation of a primary focus causes infiltrates in the posterior segments of the upper lobes and the superior segment of the lower lobes. Sequelae are miliary tuberculosis, cavitation (40%) (Fig. 3-49), and empyema.

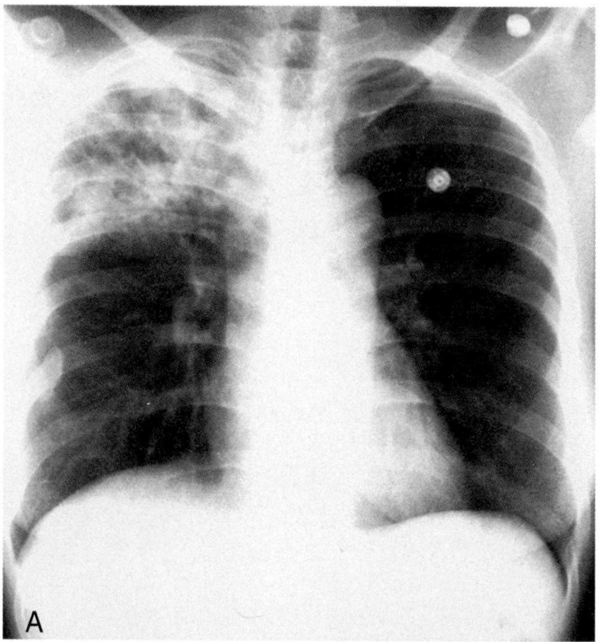

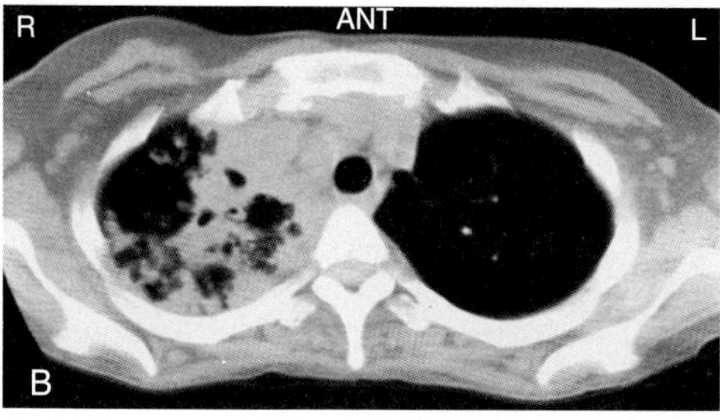

FIGURE 3-49 ■ Tuberculosis. The classic appearance of reactivation tuberculosis is that of an upper lobe infiltrate with cavities *(A)*. Over time, healing and fibrosis will occur, which will pull the hilum up on the affected side. If any question remains about whether the infiltrate is cavitated, a computed tomography scan *(B)* may be useful.

Adenopathy is rare compared with primary infectious TB. Healed TB may initially appear as fibrous changes in the apices or as areas of calcification, either within the lung parenchyma or in the region of the hilar or mediastinal lymph nodes. Most commonly, however, such focal calcifications are due to old histoplasmosis rather than to TB.

Miliary TB is seen as a diffuse bilateral process with very small nodules scattered throughout both lungs. The nodules are supposed to be the size of a millet seed. Because millet seeds are not very common, it is easier to remember that they are just slightly smaller than sesame seeds. Patients who initially have chest radiographic findings of miliary TB usually are extremely ill. Numerous very small lung nodules also can be seen with histoplasmosis, varicella pneumonia, and metastatic thyroid cancer.

Fungal Lesions. A wide variety of fungal lesions can affect the lung. These may be seen as focal infiltrates or as discrete lesions. Occasionally, a fungus ball or a mycetoma can be seen within a pulmonary cavitary lesion (Fig. 3-50). *Cryptococcus* sp. can be seen as a small cavitary lesion within the lung, and small satellite nodules are sometimes nearby.

Lung Abscess. Inhaled particulate matter or necrotic pneumonias can result in a lung abscess. A typical appearance is that of a lesion several centimeters in diameter that either looks solid (Fig. 3-51) or has a lucent (dark) air-filled center and a shaggy, thick wall. The wall typically is about 5 mm in thickness. The major differential diagnosis of a thick-walled cavitary lesion in the lung is a lung abscess or a cavitating neoplasm (usually squamous cell carcinoma). Lung abscesses may have an air/fluid level in the central portion, but so may infected cavitary neoplasms. CT scanning is commonly used to direct a needle biopsy of such lesions to obtain cultures and cytologic studies. Sometimes a lung abscess can be confused with an empyema, but abscesses are typically round, with the lung and blood vessels in normal position; if there is an air/fluid level, it is the same length on PA and lateral films. An empyema is

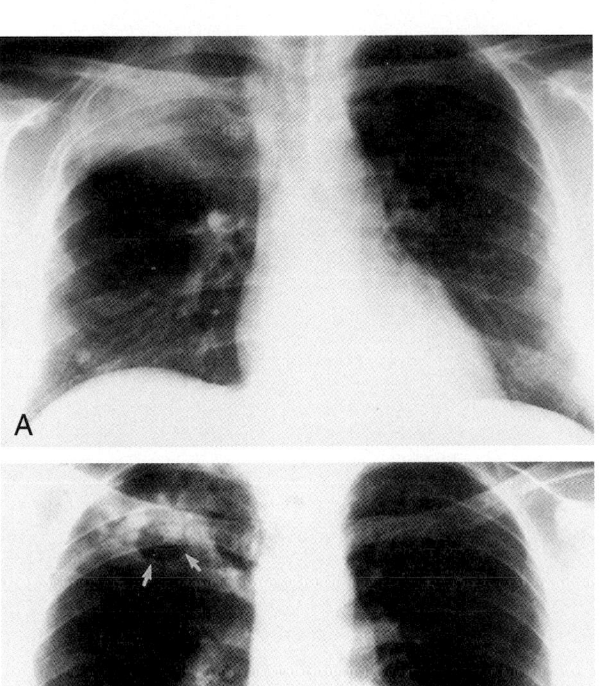

FIGURE 3-50 ■ **Fungal infection.** Fungal infections of the lung may initially be seen as an alveolar infiltrate *(A)*, but several days later *(B)*, they may show cavitation *(arrows)*, with a central loose mass representing a fungus ball.

usually elliptical, and the lung and blood vessels are displaced or compressed; if there is an air/fluid level, it often is of a different length on frontal and lateral films.

Adult Respiratory Distress Syndrome. Adult respiratory distress syndrome (ARDS) is of uncertain etiology, but the damage results from leakage of fluid from the alveolar capillary bed. It is typically seen in patients who have been in an intensive care unit for several days and who have been intubated. ARDS may occur in postoperative patients who have normal pulmonary function in the immediate postoperative period but in whom then tachypnea, anxiety, and breathing fatigue develop. Systemic nonpulmonary infections also can damage the pulmonary parenchyma and produce ARDS.

The usual pattern is that of diffuse or patchy alveolar infiltrates throughout both lungs (Fig. 3-52). The major difficulty in evaluating these patients is the exclusion of a concurrent bacterial pneumonia or congestive heart failure (CHF). The differential diagnosis is probably best made on clinical grounds, although if an alveolar infiltrate changes rapidly (within several hours or within 1 day), the infiltrates most likely represent CHF or fluid overload. In patients with CHF, usually Kerley B lines, pleural effusions, increased heart size, and perihilar or basilar infiltrates occur. With ARDS, Kerley B lines should not be present, pleural effusions occur only late, heart size is often normal, and alveolar infiltrates often extend to the lung periphery.

Bacterial pneumonias often take a day or more to change appearance, and patients with ARDS often have a relatively stable appearance over many days. The diagnosis of pneumonias is often made on the basis of bacterial cultures. Be aware that changes in the x ray technique or in the amount of positive-pressure respiratory therapy may cause significant changes in the appearance of the infiltrates in patients with ARDS.

Chronic Interstitial Lung Diseases

A wide variety of chronic lung abnormalities can occur. Bronchiectasis and COPD have already been described. Given the nonspecificity of the radiographic findings and the varied appearance of interstitial lung diseases, the diagnosis is best made by medical history and clinical findings. If the patient is not acutely ill, often no imaging needs to be done. If symptoms or decreased diffusing capacity, restrictive lung disease by pulmonary function tests, and interstitial prominence are seen on the chest x-ray, then an HRCT scan of the chest can be done to look for early infiltrative lung disease (such as unusual interstitial pneumonitis [UIP]). If the patient is acutely ill, and atypical pneumonia or heart disease is suspected, a CT scan is not needed.

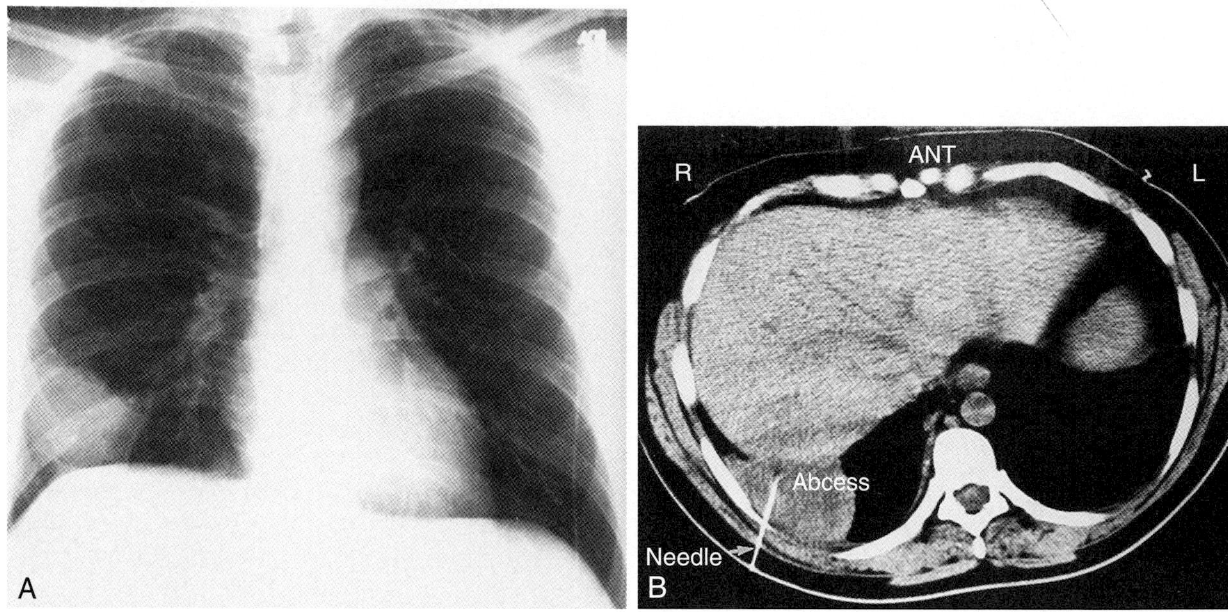

FIGURE 3-51 ■ **Lung abscess.** On a chest x-ray, a lung abscess may look to be a solid rounded lesion (*A*), or, if it has a connection with the bronchus, an air/fluid level may exist in a thick-walled cavitary lesion. Computed tomography scanning (*B*) can be used to localize the lesion and to place a needle for drainage and aspiration of contents for culture.

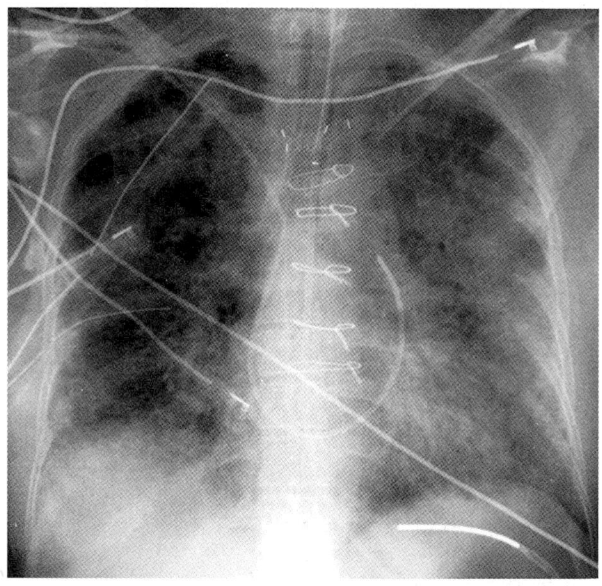

FIGURE 3-52 ■ **Adult respiratory distress syndrome (ARDS).** The findings of ARDS in this patient who has had a coronary artery bypass graft are diffuse bilateral alveolar infiltrates. Similar findings may be due to diffuse pneumonia or even pulmonary edema, and the differential diagnosis is ranked on clinical findings.

Diseases that preferentially affect the upper lobes are silicosis, sarcoidosis, and eosinophilic granuloma. Silicosis may have "eggshell" calcifications in the hilar nodes in addition to uniformly distributed small (1- to 10-mm) nodules (Fig. 3-53). These small nodules can coalesce to form upper lobe parenchymal masses (progressive massive fibrosis, Fig. 3-54).

Sarcoidosis is a disease of unknown etiology that most commonly occurs in African Americans. The manifestations on chest x-ray are hilar and mediastinal adenopathy and pulmonary parenchymal disease. About one third of patients will demonstrate symmetrical hilar lymph node enlargement and, occasionally, azygous adenopathy. About one third will have pulmonary parenchymal disease manifested as either interstitial or alveolar infiltrates, and one third will demonstrate both adenopathy and pulmonary parenchymal disease (Fig. 3-55). In late stages, a linear interstitial fibrotic pattern develops.

Conditions that preferentially affect the lower lobes are collagen vascular diseases, drug toxicity, asbestosis, interstitial fibrosis, and unusual interstitial pneumonias. My students like mnemonics

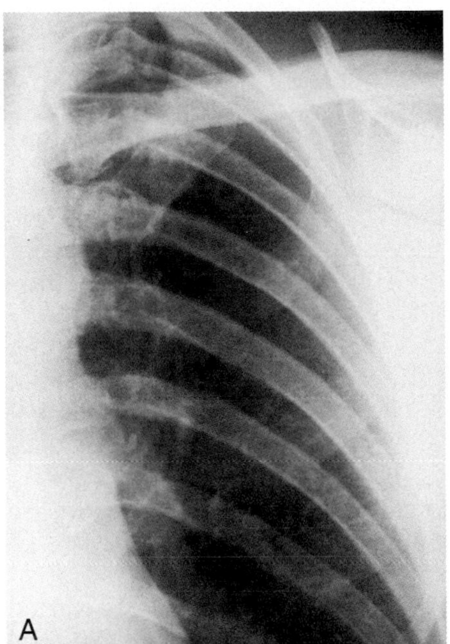

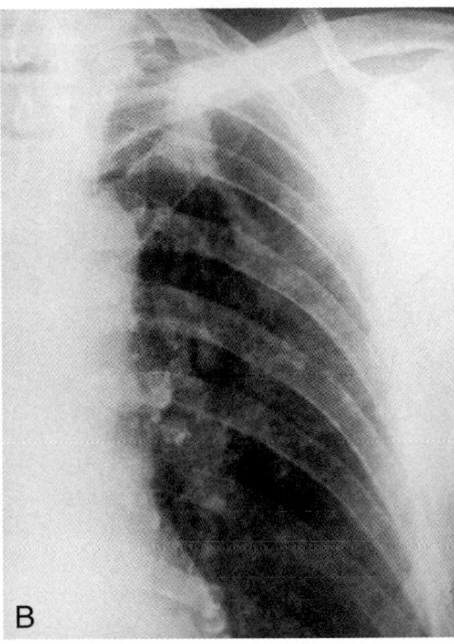

FIGURE 3-53 ■ Silicosis. Chest x-rays on the same person 20 years apart. The initial chest x-ray *(A)* shows an unremarkable left upper lobe. After many years of hard-rock mining, rounded calcifications are seen about the left hilum; a nodular appearance is seen in the lung parenchyma; and fibrosis is seen at the left apex *(B)*.

to help them remember, and they use BADAS for lower lobe diseases. This refers to *b*ronchiectasis, *a*spiration, *d*rugs, *a*sbestosis, and *s*cleroderma (or other collagen vascular diseases). For upper lobe diseases, they use CASSET P, which stands for *c*ystic fibrosis, *a*nkylosing spondylitis, *s*ilicosis, *s*arcoid, *e*osinophilic granuloma, *t*uberculosis, and *P*neumocystis carinii. For diffuse chronic interstitial disease, they use LIFE, which refers to *l*ymphangitic spread of tumor, *i*nflammation

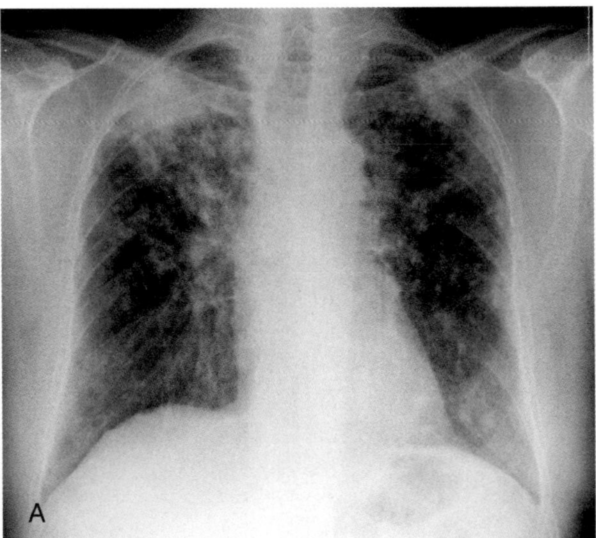

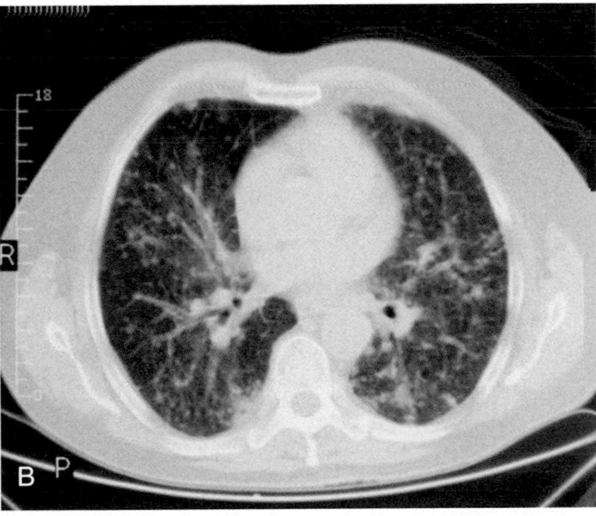

FIGURE 3-54 ■ Late stage of silicosis. The chest x-ray *(A)* shows significant parenchymal disease, predominant in the upper lobes, as a result of progressive massive fibrosis. The regular *(B)* and high-resolution *(C)* computed tomography scans show both coarse interstitial and nodular changes.

Continued

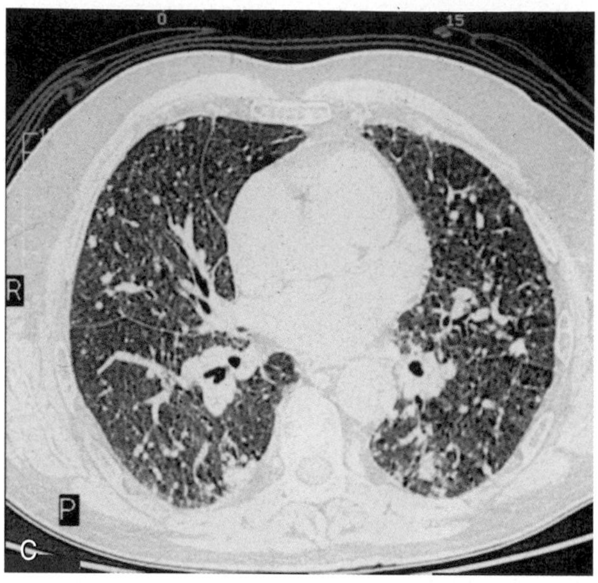

FIGURE 3-54 cont'd

(infection), *f*ibrosis, and *e*dema. For acute interstitial infiltrates, they use HEP, referring to *h*ypersensitivity (allergic alveolitis), *e*dema, and *p*neumonia (viral).

Lymphangitic carcinoma and sarcoid can have very small nodules that are concentrated about the bronchi and blood vessels, whereas most of the other entities have nodules that extend to the periphery of the lung. Most collagen vascular diseases can cause interstitial (fine lines), reticular (mesh-like), or honeycombing (coarse mesh-like) pulmonary parenchymal abnormalities. These can be seen with rheumatoid arthritis and systemic lupus erythematosus as well as with a number of other entities.

Some chronic lung disease can cause diffuse interstitial changes, honeycombing, or focal patchy infiltrates. Sarcoid already was mentioned. Other diseases that produce these varied findings include extrinsic allergic alveolitis (caused by a number of antigens such as mold or

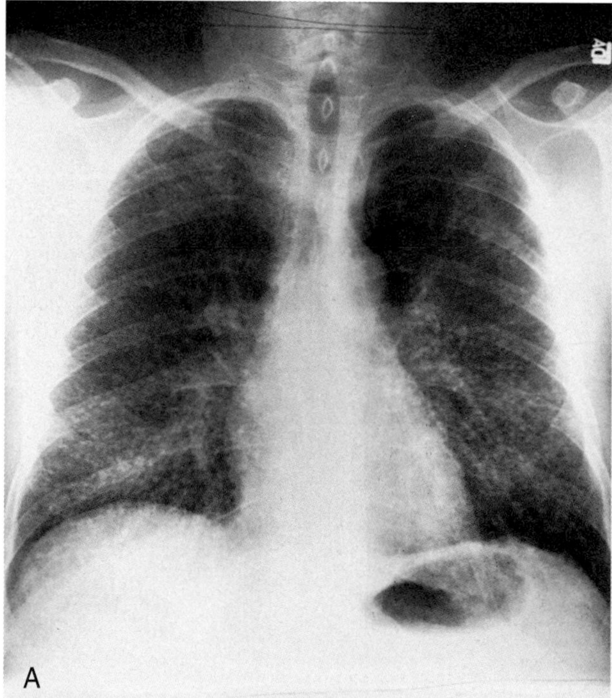

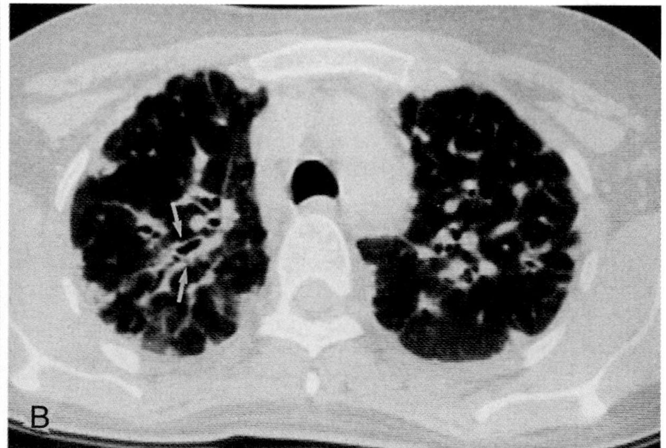

FIGURE 3-55 ■ Sarcoidosis. In the pulmonary parenchymal form, diffuse infiltrates are seen throughout both lungs *(A)*. Many of these patients also have associated lymphadenopathy about the hilum or in the paratracheal region. A high-resolution computed tomography scan *(B)* shows marked thickening of the bronchial walls *(arrows)*.

avian proteins), eosinophilic granuloma, bronchiolitis obliterans, and eosinophilic lung disease. Given the nonspecificity of the radiographic findings and the varied appearance of these diseases, the diagnosis is best made by history and clinical findings. The chest x-ray or high resolution CT can provide supporting information and be used to monitor progress of a given disease.

Bioterrorist Agents

Bioterrorist agents do not fit neatly into any specific imaging category. They are included here because they are infectious and many cause lung abnormalities, particularly air-space findings. A few of the agents (such as inhalational anthrax) have characteristic radiologic findings. Other agents, such as smallpox or viral hemorrhagic fevers, have striking clinical presentations. Regarding the imaging findings, anthrax has mediastinal adenopathy but not interstitial edema, focal consolidation, or diffuse air-space disease. Smallpox can have segmental or lobar consolidation after the skin lesions appear, and it occasionally exhibits pulmonary nodules in immunized hosts, but interstitial edema and adenopathy do not occur, and diffuse air-space disease is uncommon. Plague commonly has segmental or lobar consolidation and sometimes has adenopathy and diffuse air-space disease. Cavitation is rare. Tularemia commonly has segmental or lobar consolidation, occasional adenopathy, and cavitation. Interstitial edema and diffuse air-space disease is rare. Q fever commonly has segmental or lobar consolidation but not other thoracic imaging manifestations. American hantavirus commonly has interstitial edema and diffuse air-space disease but not adenopathy or segmental or lobar consolidation. Viral hemorrhagic fevers may have mild interstitial edema but no other thoracic imaging manifestations.

Hemoptysis

Bleeding from the gastrointestinal tract and nasopharynx is more common than is true hemoptysis, and these sites should be excluded as a cause of the patient's complaints. The initial imaging studies for hemoptysis are standard PA and lateral chest x-rays. The most common cause is bronchitis, although an endobronchial lesion or pulmonary embolism also should be considered. If the chest x-ray is normal and the patient is at low risk for bronchogenic carcinoma, a CT scan with high-resolution cuts to exclude bronchiectasis is the most useful imaging study. If the chest x-ray is normal and the patient is at high risk for lung cancer (>10 pack-years of smoking) or has a malignancy elsewhere, bronchoscopy is usually performed, although a CT also may be used. If an abnormality is seen on the chest x-ray, whether CT or bronchoscopy is used often depends on the nature of the abnormality. If it is peripheral, CT may be more helpful than bronchoscopy. If hemoptysis is present in a traumatized patient, a transected bronchus requiring surgery should be considered. In these latter cases, a chest x-ray usually reveals an associated pneumomediastinum.

Lung Cancer and Nodules

Solitary Pulmonary Nodule. A pulmonary nodule is really a small mass. I think of a nodule as being smaller than 3 cm in diameter, and when something in the lung is larger than 3 cm, I call it a mass. To me, anything approaching the size of a golf ball is very suggestive of a neoplasm; anything that is only 0.5 cm in diameter that you can see easily on a chest x-ray and is probably very dense is most likely a granuloma. Age also is a useful discriminating factor. In a patient younger than 40 years, a lung cancer may occur, but it is very, very rare.

A solitary pulmonary nodule can represent practically anything. As already mentioned, it may be due to a granuloma or lung cancer, but other etiologies include a single metastatic lesion, septic embolus, arteriovenous malformation, hamartoma, or even a small area of rounded atelectasis (Table 3-5). Several challenges appear when you have identified what you think is a solitary pulmonary nodule. The first is to determine that the nodule is within the lung and that you are not looking at a nipple shadow or wart that is on the skin surface. A nipple shadow is seen projecting within the

TABLE 3-5 ■ **Common Differential Diagnosis of Pulmonary Nodule(s)**

Solitary
Less than 3 cm
- Granuloma (especially if calcified)
- Lung cancer
- Single nipple shadow
- Wart on the skin
- Benign lung tumors
- Metastasis
- Rounded atelectasis
- Septic embolism

Large
- Lung cancer
- Round pneumonia
- Large solitary metastases
- Lung abscess

Multiple
- Granulomas
- Metastases
- Septic emboli

Cavitary
- Septic emboli
- Tuberculosis
- Fungal
- Squamous cell cancer

Benign Characteristics
- Small (<3 cm)
- Round
- Well-defined edges
- Slow growing (no appreciable change in 2 yr)
- Central calcification
- Solid (not cavitated)

Malignant Characteristics
- Large (>3 cm)
- Irregular shape
- Poorly defined edges
- Obvious growth in <2 yr
- Asymmetrical or no calcification
- Cavitated
- Active accumulation of fluorine-8-FDG on a PET scan

FDG, fluorodeoxyglucose; PET, positron emission tomography.

lung only on the frontal chest x-ray, is usually in the midclavicular line, and projects over the lower half of the lung. Small nipple markers (BBs) with a repeated chest x-ray may be of some use.

Locate the "nodule" in a horizontal plane on the frontal chest x-ray (for example, at the level of the aortic arch), and then look at the lateral chest x-ray (again at the horizontal plane of the aortic arch) and see whether you can find the nodule at the same level projecting within the chest on both views. If there is any doubt, you can obtain shallow oblique views; if the nodule is truly within the thoracic cavity, it should rotate less than the anterior and posterior ribs.

The second step is to characterize the nodule. If it is well defined and round, it is much more likely to be benign than if it is irregular or indistinct in its margins. Calcification that is very dense (Fig. 3-56) or within a nodule suggests that it is most likely a granuloma (Fig. 3-57). The calcification, however, should be centrally located in the nodule. If calcification is eccentrically located in a nodule, consider a neoplasm.

The third step of importance is to determine whether the nodule is new or old. A careful review of all available chest x-rays should be performed and phone calls to pertinent hospitals should be made before expensive or invasive studies are ordered. A nodule that has remained unchanged in size for 2 years can be considered benign. Stability for a period of 1 year is not enough, because slow-growing tumors may not change appreciably in a 12-month interval. If a 1-cm nodule doubles the number of cells that it contains, its diameter will grow only to 1.2 cm. A difference this small is hard to appreciate on a chest x-ray.

Further evaluation of a nodule can be obtained by doing a CT scan. In this case, ask for thin cuts at the level of the nodule of interest and include the entire lungs on the CT scan. Because CT scanning is more sensitive than a chest x-ray for detection of nodules, you may find that what you really have is the presence of multiple nodules; if this is the case, your differential diagnosis changes very quickly.

Positron emission tomography (PET) scans are used to help determine whether a nodule or mass is benign or malignant. This test is usually performed when a fine-needle aspiration is impractical or the patient has a known cancer and a new lung or mediastinal mass. The radioactive tracer used is fluorine-18 fluorodeoxyglucose (FDG). Malignant lesions have a high metabolism, and most will actively accumulate the tracer (Fig. 3-58). Malignant lesions must be about 8 mm in diameter to be visible on PET scan.

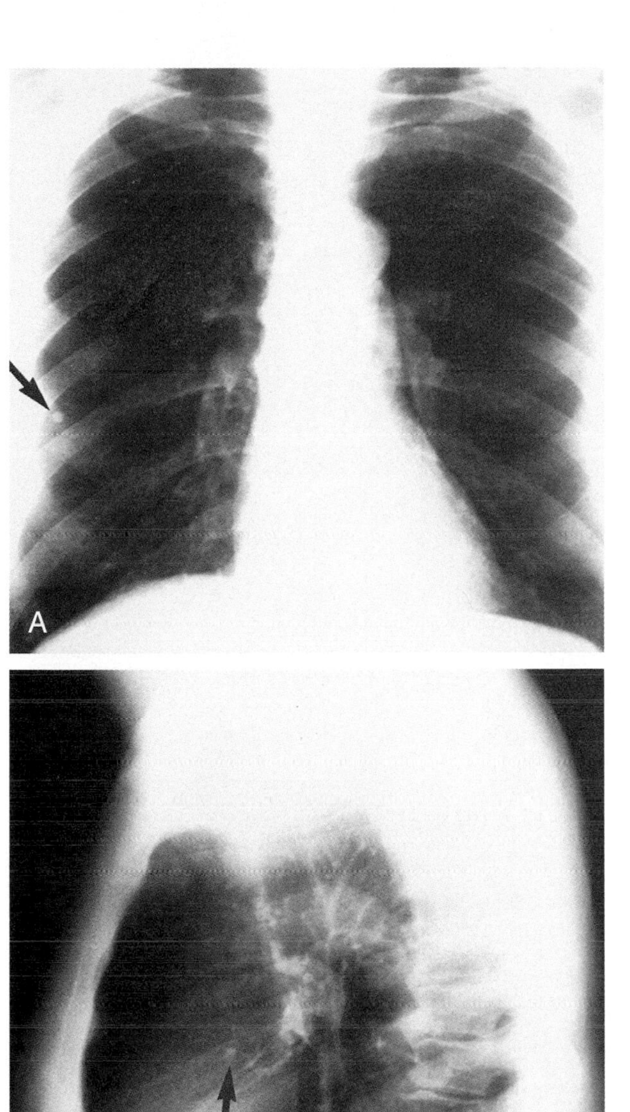

FIGURE 3-56 ■ Solitary calcified granuloma. A very dense pulmonary nodule is seen on both posteroanterior *(A)* and lateral *(B)* chest x-rays. This can be confidently called a granuloma; it needs no further workup, because it is much denser than even the surrounding ribs and therefore is clearly densely calcified.

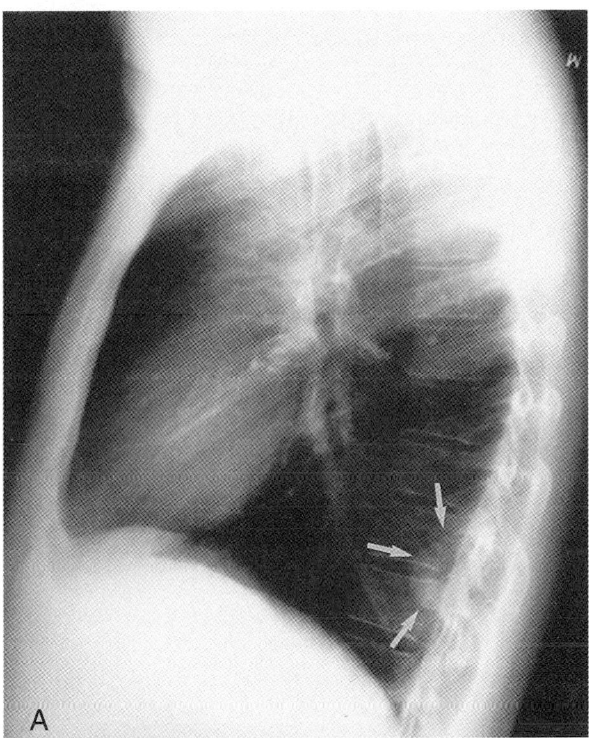

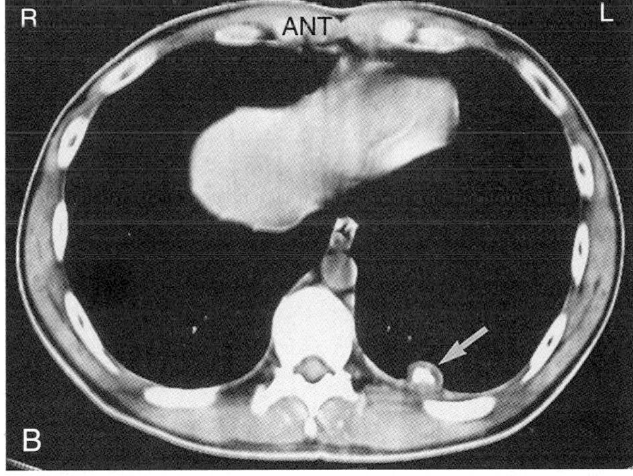

FIGURE 3-57 ■ Granuloma with central calcification. A lateral chest x-ray *(A)* showed what was thought to be a posterior pleural mass *(arrows)*. No definite calcification is seen on the chest x-ray; however, evaluation with computed tomography scan *(B)* clearly shows the lesion with dense central calcification *(arrow)*. If the calcification were not central in the mass, a neoplasm would have to be excluded.

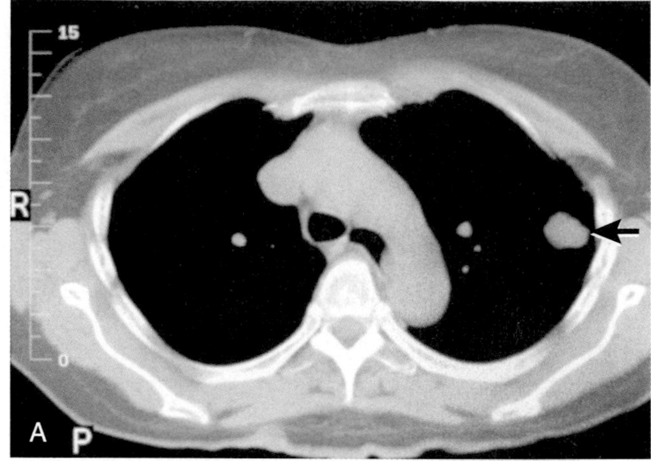

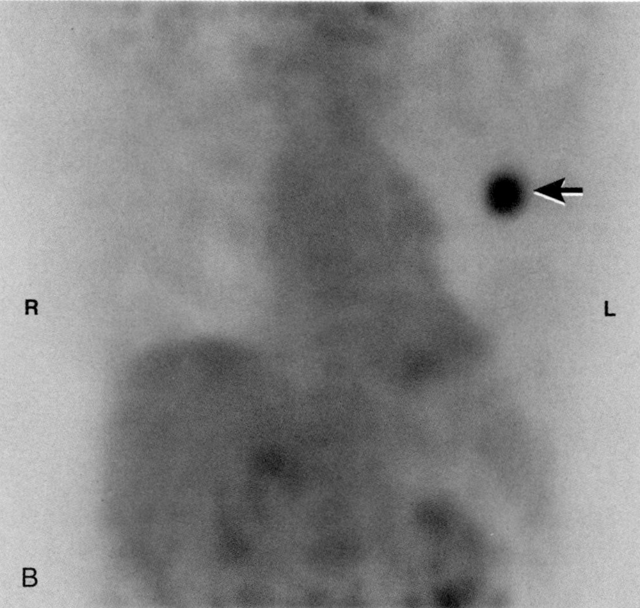

FIGURE 3-58 ■ **Lung cancer.** *A,* The computed tomography scan shows a 2-cm soft tissue mass in the middle portion of the left lung *(arrow)*. *B,* A whole-body positron emission tomography scan of the anterior chest and upper abdomen done with radioactively labeled glucose shows markedly increased activity at the same area, indicative of very high metabolic activity and a high probability of malignancy.

Screening for Lung Cancer. Many years ago, it was clear that annual chest x-rays did little or nothing to reduce mortality from lung cancer, even in smokers. By the time lesions were clearly identified, they were advanced enough that many had metastasized. Recently, much publicity and advertising, as well as some research projects, have been undertaken on the efficacy of annual screening CT chest examinations to detect lung cancer. It is clear that smaller lesions can be detected with CT; however, the experience to date has shown that, if smokers are screened, about 70% will have one or more visible "nodules." In some of the better-designed longitudinal studies, about 99% of these abnormalities are not cancer. This leaves the perplexing question of how to manage these patients. Many of the lesions are too small to perform an accurate percutaneous biopsy with a fine needle, and segmental resection carries at least a percentage or so mortality (Fig. 3-59). Usually the abnormalities are followed up with a 3-month CT

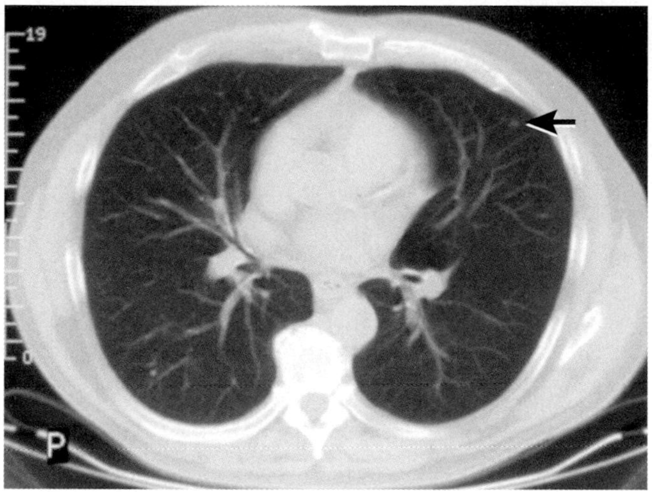

FIGURE 3-59 ■ Indeterminate tiny nodule. On a chest computed tomography (CT) scan done for other reasons, a 2-mm nodule was found in the anterior portion of the left lung *(arrow)*. The nodule is too small for a needle biopsy and usually will be followed up with serial CT scans. More than 99% of such incidental lesions are benign.

scan to assess for change. If there is none, the scan is repeated at 6 months, and if no change, then again at 12 months and 24 months. Now screening CT scans for detection of lung cancer are not recommended by the National Cancer Institute, the American Cancer Society, or the American College of Radiology.

Lung Cancer. The pathology of lung cancers is a bit confusing. Some confusion arises because a number of tumors exhibit more than one type of pathology; a number are undifferentiated; and the incidence of cell types varies depending on the type of series (surgical vs. autopsy) quoted. About 40% of lung cancers are adenocarcinomas, and 30% or so are squamous. Most of the remainder are small cell carcinomas (which includes oat cell types).

You may erroneously think that a 1-cm lung nodule, which turns out to be a lung cancer, is an early lesion. Nothing could be further from the truth. A 1-cm-diameter nodule has about 10 billion cells in it. In terms of doubling times, it is already two thirds of the way toward filling the entire hemithorax.

Primary lung cancers have a number of appearances. Adenocarcinoma occurs peripherally, whereas squamous cell types are central or peripheral. Squamous cell tumors of any origin tend to cavitate. Small cell carcinomas often initially appear as an indistinct hilar or perihilar mass. A unilateral hilar mass or persistent infiltrate in an adult older than 40 years should always raise the suspicion of a lung cancer.

A CT scan is the most valuable imaging method for initially and locally staging lung cancers. Intravenous contrast often is used with the CT scan, so that the tumor, adenopathy, and pulmonary vessels can be differentiated. However, if you have a good knowledge of anatomy, it is not necessary to use intravenous contrast. Analysis of a CT scan should include not only location and size of the pulmonary lesion but also whether it has a pleural or chest wall involvement and whether hilar or mediastinal lymphadenopathy is present (Fig. 3-60). The accuracy of CT in determining chest wall invasion is only about 50%, but invasion is suggested by pleural thickening, more than 3 cm of contact between pleura and tumor, obtuse angles between tumor and pleura, or an increased density of the extrapleural fat. A pleural effusion usually indicates a poor prognosis; however, only aspiration and cytologic confirmation of malignant cells in the effusion make the tumor unresectable. Staging of lung cancers with regard to mediastinal and distant spread is best

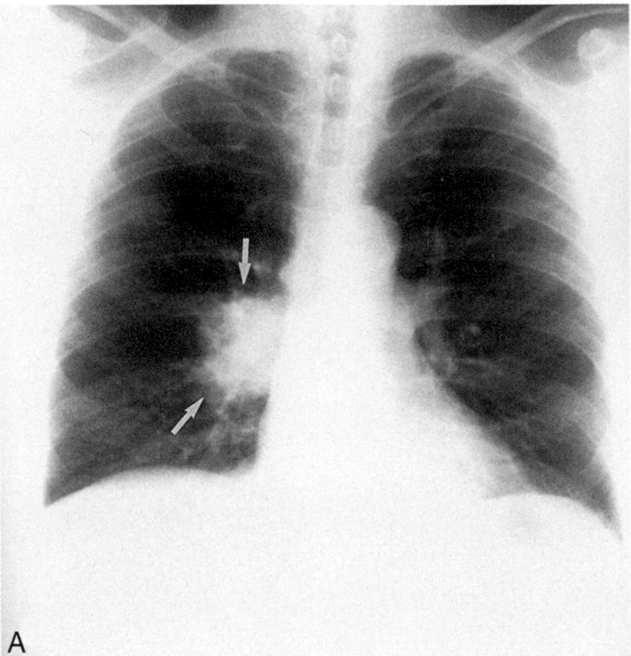

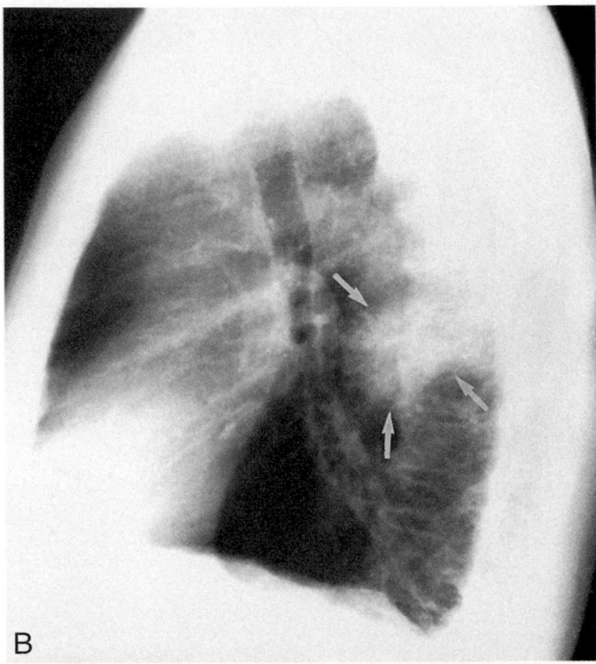

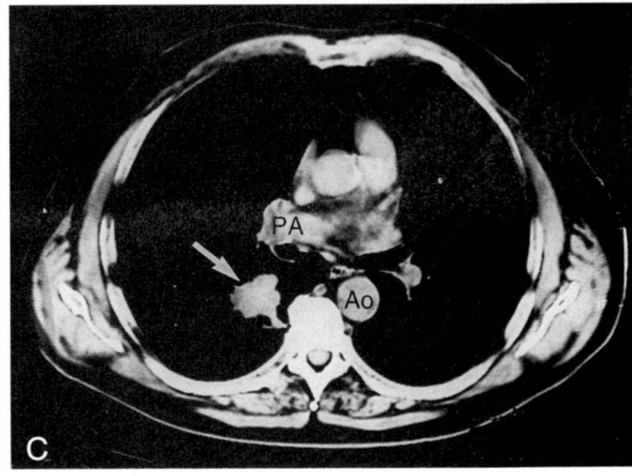

FIGURE 3-60 ■ Lung cancer. An ill-defined mass is noted on the posteroanterior chest x-ray *(arrows) (A)*. Although this appears to be located near the right hilum, the lateral chest x-ray *(B)* clearly shows the mass to be posterior to the hilum. Its shaggy appearance is very suggestive of carcinoma. Further evaluation by computed tomography scan *(C)* clearly shows the mass in relation to the mediastinal structures, such as the pulmonary artery (PA) and aorta (Ao).

done with nuclear medicine whole-body PET scans, as described earlier.

Two classic, although uncommon, appearances of lung carcinoma are seen on the chest x-ray. The first of these is the "Golden S sign," from a hilar tumor that has caused peripheral atelectasis (most commonly of the right upper lobe). Normally, as the right upper lobe collapses, an upward bowing of the minor fissure appears from the hilum out to the lateral aspect of the chest. With the presence of the hilar mass, now inferior and lateral bowing are seen near the hilum, and this creates an "S" shape to the inferior margin of the collapsing right upper lobe (Fig. 3-61). The second classic appearance is that of the Pancoast tumor, an upper lobe carcinoma that has eroded into the pleura and adjacent structures, such as the ribs (Fig. 3-62).

Lung cancers commonly metastasize to the opposite lung, liver, bones, brain, and adrenal glands. The liver is the most common site, and the adrenal glands are involved in about 30% of patients. For this reason, any chest CT scan done for a suspected lung cancer should be extended far enough down to visualize these organs.

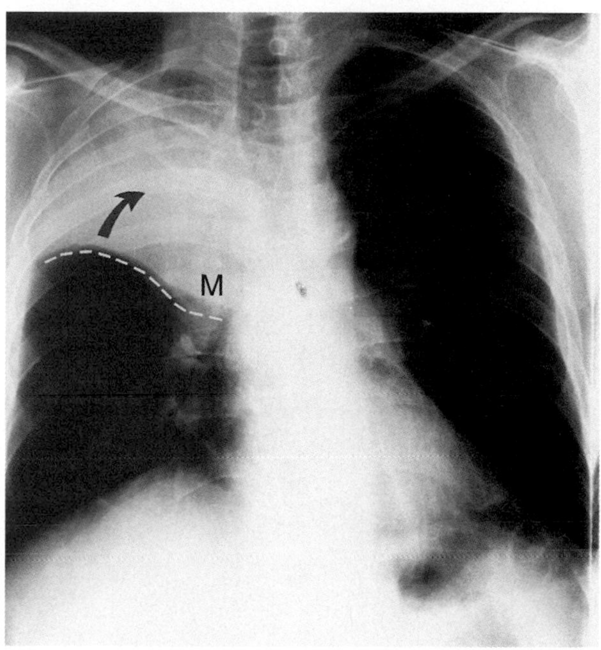

FIGURE 3-61 ■ **The "Golden S" sign of lung cancer.** Where a mass in the region of the hilum obstructs the upper lobe bronchus, the minor fissure collapses superiorly. With uncomplicated atelectasis, the minor fissure is simply bowed up, but with a mass near the hilum, the inferior margin of the upper lobe takes on an S shape as it goes around the mass.

When bony metastases are present, these are usually purely lytic or destructive. For peripheral lesions (that cannot be reached with a bronchoscope), a percutaneous biopsy can be performed with a thin needle guided by either fluoroscopy or a CT scan. The most common complication of this procedure is a pneumothorax (about 25% of cases); about 5% to 10% of patients will need a chest tube to correct this. Immunocompromised AIDS patients often have a higher incidence of Kaposi's sarcoma. This usually appears as indistinct focal pulmonary focal infiltrates rather than as well-defined discrete masses (see Fig. 3-47C).

Hilar Enlargement

Hilar enlargement may be seen on a chest x-ray. The three major etiologies are enlarged pulmonary arteries, lymphadenopathy, and a lung neoplasm. If the cause is unknown or a possibility of effective therapy exists, a contrasted chest CT scan is indicated for further evaluation.

Lymphomas, and particularly Hodgkin's disease, are most commonly visualized on the chest x-ray either as a large anterior mediastinal mass or as hilar adenopathy. If the lymphomatous mass is large and is up against the aorta, the mass can easily be mistaken for an aortic aneurysm. Hilar adenopathy is often difficult to distinguish from enlarged central pulmonary arteries. Extensive adenopathy can be recognized by multiple lumps or bumps rather than by the single one you might expect from a prominent main pulmonary artery. Adenopathy also may fill in the normal concavity between the left main pulmonary artery and the aortic arch. If any question remains, a CT scan can easily sort out the differences (Fig. 3-63). Lymphoma and Hodgkin's disease can cause pulmonary infiltrates or nodules, although this is a relatively uncommon presentation. Most lymphomas can be staged by using [^{18}F]FDG-PET scans.

Metastatic Disease

The pulmonary parenchyma is a very common site for metastatic deposits because the lungs act as a filter for large particles or cells. Most metastatic disease has two predominant patterns in the lung. One is the relatively familiar nodular lesion. Lesions are typically referred to as hematogenous metastases. Metastatic lesions in the pulmonary parenchyma vary from very small nodules to extremely large (cannonball) masses. The pulmonary metastases of thyroid cancer typically create a snowstorm of very small nodular lesions. Other tumors, such as colon and renal cell carcinomas, typically produce metastatic lesions that range from approximately 1 cm to several centimeters in diameter. When extremely large multiple masses (about the size of a tennis ball) are present, metastases from a sarcoma should be suspected. CT scans will show many more metastases than are suspected from the chest x-ray (Fig. 3-64).

A second variety of metastases is seen in which streaky or linear infiltrates appear throughout the lungs. This is referred to as lymphangitic spread of tumor. It is not really lymphangitic spread, but another appearance of

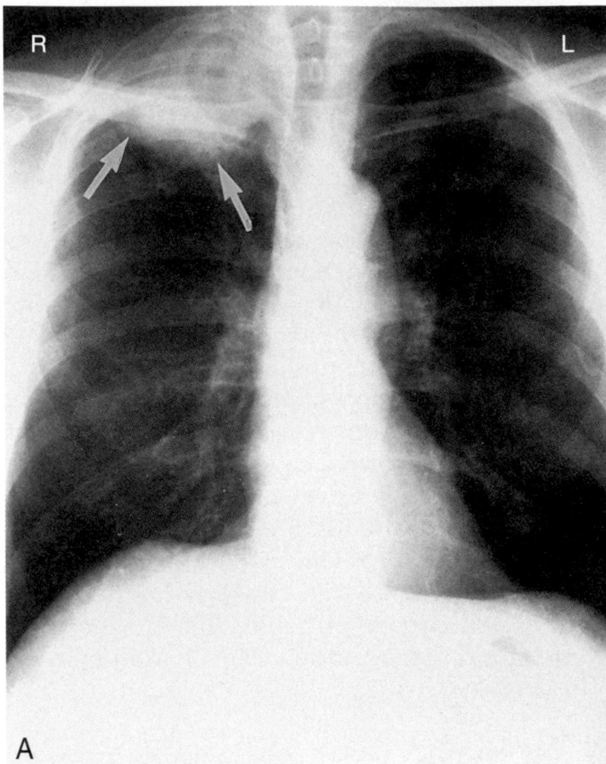

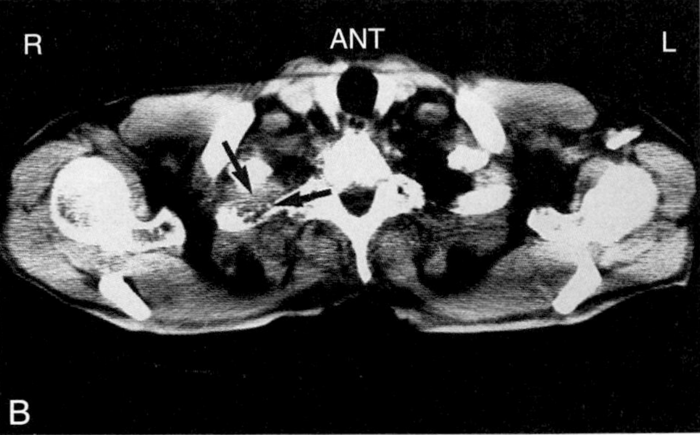

FIGURE 3-62 ■ Pancoast tumor. In this patient with shoulder pain, an ill-defined mass *(white arrows)* is seen in the right lung apex *(A)*. On a transverse computed tomography scan of the upper thorax *(B)*, permeative destruction of a right posterior rib by the tumor is identified *(black arrows)*.

hematogenously spread disease. This particular "lymphangitic" pattern occurs quite commonly with stomach cancer (Fig. 3-65). Breast cancer can produce either the rounded hematogenous metastases or the "lymphangitic" pattern. Of course, remember that, if you are looking for metastatic disease, you should carefully examine the mediastinum and hilar regions for evidence of lymphadenopathy, and you should examine the bony structures for evidence of lytic lesions (holes) as well as for sclerotic lesions (areas of ill-defined dense bone).

Clinicians commonly ask how often to get a periodic chest x-ray on a patient with a known cancer to exclude pulmonary metastases. It is rarely efficacious to order films monthly, and most oncologists will order chest x-rays only on a 6-month or annual basis and only if the results may affect therapy.

Hypertension

Most hypertension is idiopathic in origin. A small percentage is due to renal artery stenosis. Chest x-rays are not indicated on hypertensive patients because the yield of positive findings is very low. Chest pain in a hypertensive patient should suggest either a thoracic aneurysm or coronary artery disease. These conditions, in addition to an investigation of hypertension caused by renal artery stenosis, are discussed in Chapter 5.

Chest Pain and Dyspnea

Both chest pain and dyspnea can be due to a wide variety of causes including traumatic, infectious, neoplastic, and circulatory. A chest x-ray is almost always indicated if the patient has an

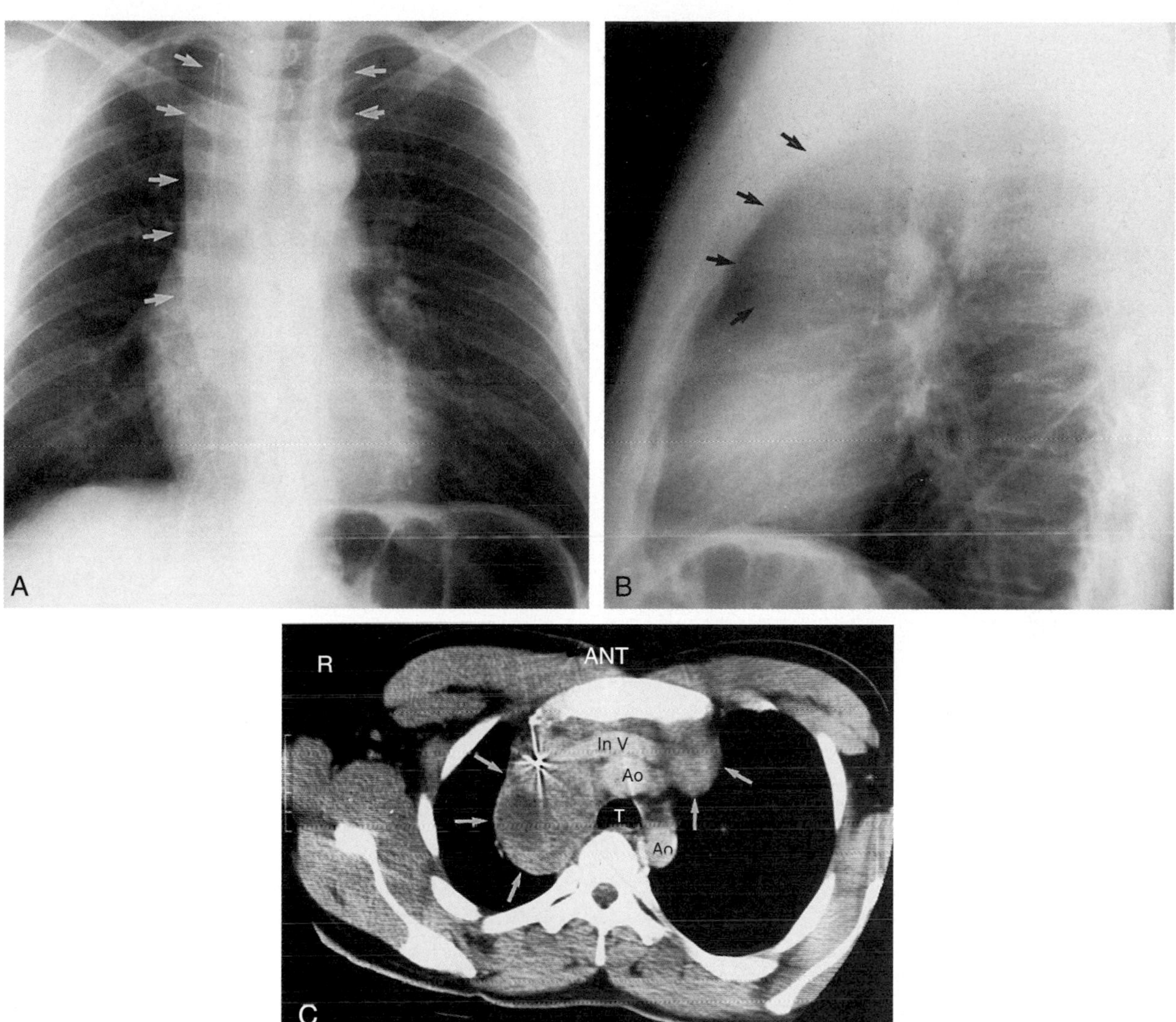

FIGURE 3-63 ■ Hodgkin's disease. In this 20-year-old man with low-grade fevers, a posteroanterior chest x-ray *(A)* shows marked widening of the middle and superior mediastinum *(arrows)*. On the lateral chest x-ray *(B)*, filling in of the retrosternal space by an ill-defined anterior mediastinal mass is seen *(arrows)*. The transverse contrast-enhanced computed tomography scan *(C)* through the upper portion of the chest shows the innominate vein (In V), ascending and descending aorta (Ao), and trachea (T). They are all enveloped by a mass of nodes *(arrows)*.

abnormal physical examination; has been traumatized; or has a fever, weight loss, or a cardiac condition. In a patient older than 40 years, a chest x-ray is usually done even if the physical examination is normal. For patients younger than 40 years who have a normal physical examination, no consensus exists about whether a chest x-ray is indicated. Issues related to cardiac conditions and angina are discussed in Chapter 5.

Congestive Heart Failure (CHF) and Pulmonary Edema

In the upright position, substantially more blood flows to the lung bases than to the apices. When you look at an upright chest x-ray, assess this normal difference in the pulmonary vascularity. The vessels should be distinct from the peripheral one third of the lung back centrally to the

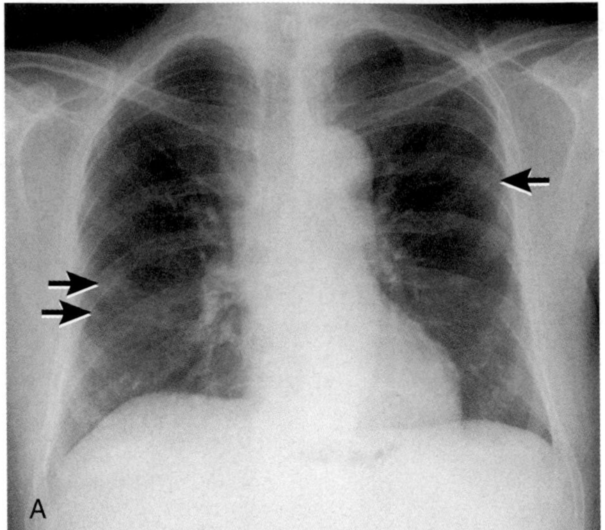

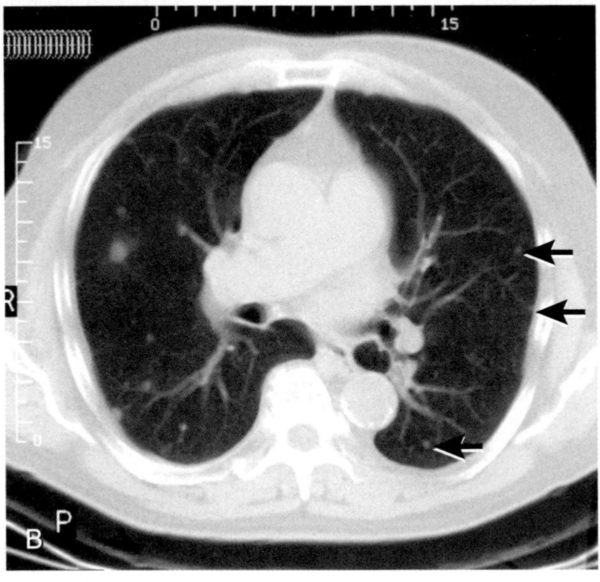

FIGURE 3-64 ■ Hematogenous metastases from renal cell carcinoma. The chest x-ray *(A)* shows a few nodules, but the computed tomography scan *(B)* shows many more metastases than are suspected (some are labeled with *arrows)*.

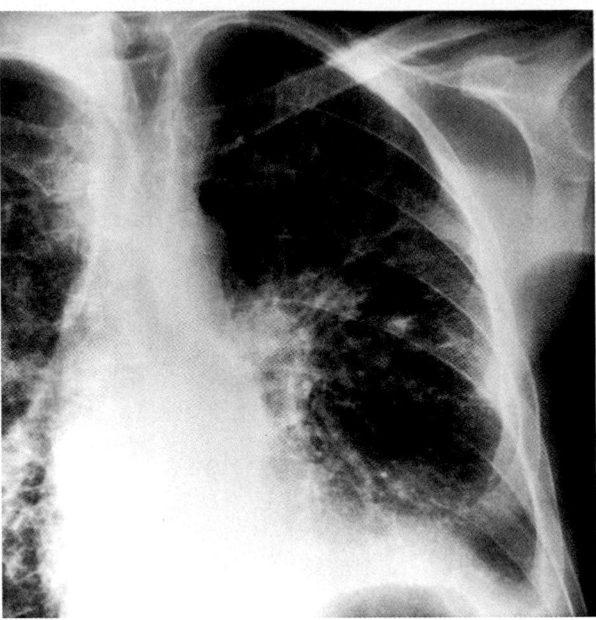

FIGURE 3-65 ■ Lymphangitic metastases. The streaky appearance in the lung parenchyma is due to metastatic disease, in this case, stomach carcinoma. The term *lymphangitic* is really a misnomer, because these actually do represent hematogenous metastases in the pulmonary interstitium.

hila, and they should be much more apparent in the lower lung zones than in the upper lung zones.

With CHF, a spectrum and a progression of findings are normally identified on an upright chest x-ray. In the early stages, minimal cardiomegaly and redistribution of the pulmonary vascularity may be seen, with almost equal flow to upper and lower lung zones (with mean capillary wedge pressures of 15 to 25 mm Hg). At this time, the diameter of upper lobe vessels will be equal to or greater than that of lower lobe vessels at the same distance from the hilum. Another way to tell is by the presence in the first intercostal space of pulmonary vessels that are greater than 3 mm in diameter. Remember that you cannot use these signs on a supine chest x-ray, because the pulmonary blood flow will change in a normal person as a result of gravity.

As CHF increases, fluid may be seen in the interlobular septa at the lateral basal aspects of the lung (25 to 30 mm Hg). These are referred to as Kerley B lines. They are always located just inside the ribs and are horizontal in orientation (Fig. 3-66). Remember, these cannot be blood vessels, because you should not normally see lung markings in the peripheral one fourth of the lungs.

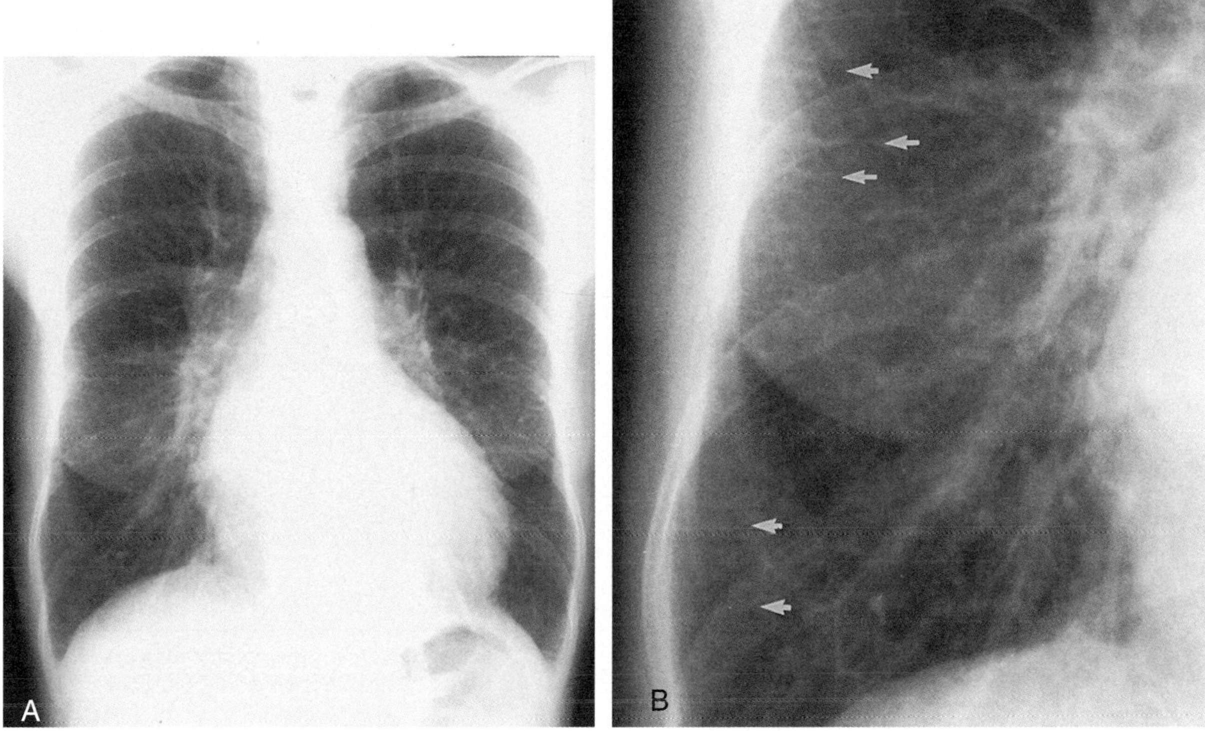

FIGURE 3-66 ■ Early findings of congestive heart failure. The major signs on upright posteroanterior chest x-ray *(A)* are cardiomegaly and redistribution of the pulmonary vascularity. Normally the vessels to the lower lobes are more prominent than those in the upper lobes; however, here they appear at least equally prominent. On a close-up view *(B)*, small horizontal lines can be seen at the very periphery of the lung *(arrows)*. These are known as Kerley B lines and represent fluid in the interlobular septa.

As CHF becomes more pronounced, vessels near the hila become indistinct because of fluid accumulating in the interstitium. Symmetrical and bilateral hilar indistinctness should immediately raise the possibility of CHF (Fig. 3-67*A*). Pleural effusions may be present, as evidenced by blunting of the lateral or posterior costophrenic angles. With pronounced CHF, fluid accumulates in the alveolar spaces, and frank pulmonary edema becomes apparent (Fig. 3-67*B*). This is seen as bilateral, predominantly basilar and perihilar alveolar infiltrates (>30 mm Hg). A note of caution is inserted here, because the changes of minimal cardiomegaly and the equalization of the pulmonary vasculature are essentially normal findings on a supine AP chest x-ray. Do not be fooled into making the diagnosis of minimal CHF on a supine chest x-ray.

Some common variations of CHF may be seen. In patients who have been lying down, on either their right or left side, relatively more accumulation of pulmonary edema occurs on the dependent side, because the fluid pressure is greater (Fig. 3-68). Patients who are in renal failure often look as though they are in CHF, particularly with a perihilar indistinctness and a sort of butterfly or bat-wing infiltrate centered about the hila. Typically, this is seen before dialysis, and after dialysis, the infiltrate resolves almost immediately (Fig. 3-69). Remember that pulmonary edema may occur from noncardiogenic causes. In the absence of cardiomegaly, consider drug overdose, head injury (with central nervous system depression), and acute inhalations of noxious agents as possible etiologies.

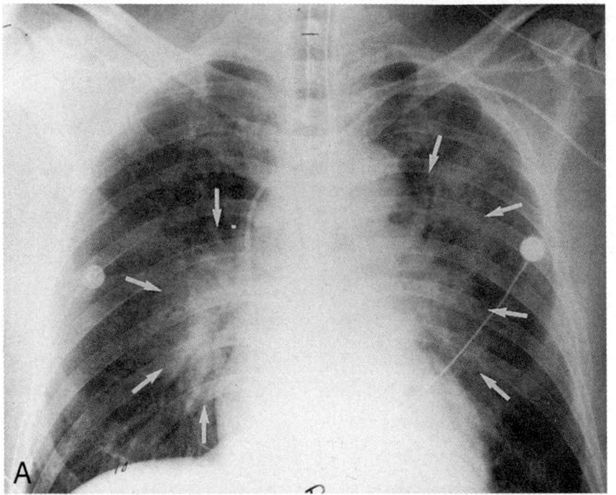

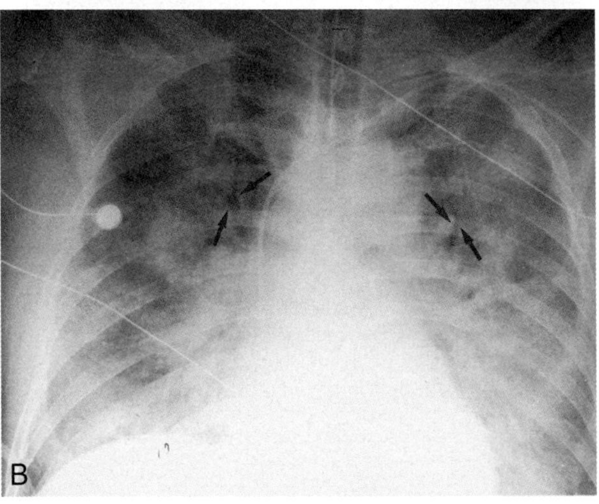

FIGURE 3-67 ■ Pulmonary edema. Pulmonary edema, or fluid overload, can be manifested by indistinctness of the pulmonary vessels as they radiate from the hilum *(A)*. This is sometimes termed a "bat wing" infiltrate. As pulmonary edema worsens *(B)*, fluid fills the alveoli, and "air bronchograms" *(arrows)* become apparent.

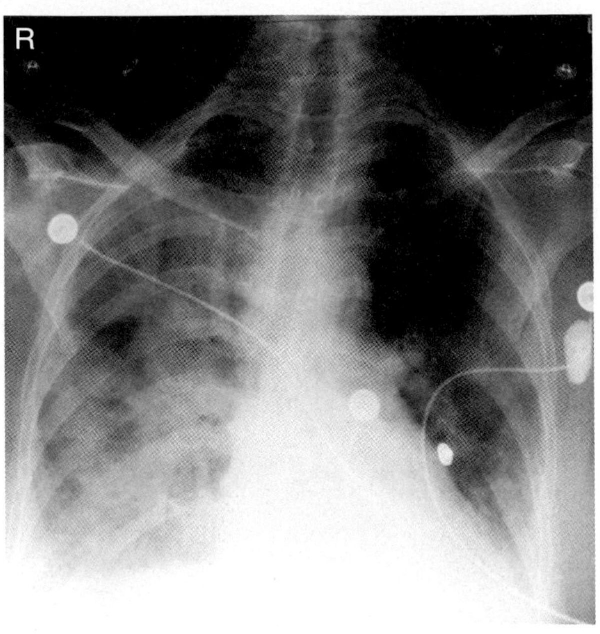

FIGURE 3-68 ■ Dependent pulmonary edema. In debilitated patients who are lying on one side, the increased hydrostatic pressure in the lung that is lower can produce pulmonary edema only in that one lung. In this intensive care unit patient, a right-sided alveolar infiltrate is due to dependent pulmonary edema.

PLEURAL PATHOLOGY

Pneumothorax

Pneumothorax refers to air in the pleural space. This is most often caused by trauma (such as a stabbing or motor vehicle accident). It also commonly results from attempted introduction of subclavian venous catheters or after liver biopsy (the pleural space extends down quite far between the liver and the lateral and posterior abdominal wall). A pneumothorax may occur spontaneously (as a result of bleb rupture) or even as a result of some unusual tumors, such as histiocytosis X or metastatic osteogenic sarcoma.

Because the pleural space is continuous around each lung, if the patient is in an upright or semi-upright position, air in the pleural space will typically go toward the apex. Thus, the first place to look for a pneumothorax is in the right and left upper hemithorax (Fig. 3-70). The most common appearance is an area adjacent to the ribs where no lung vascularity is seen and where a very thin white line represents the visceral pleura that has been separated from the parietal pleura by air. Look very carefully for this line, because it is often difficult to distinguish from the bony cortex of nearby ribs. If the pneumothorax is small and the pleural line is behind the rib, it can be almost impossible to see. In such circumstances, it may be useful to obtain an expiration chest x-ray in addition

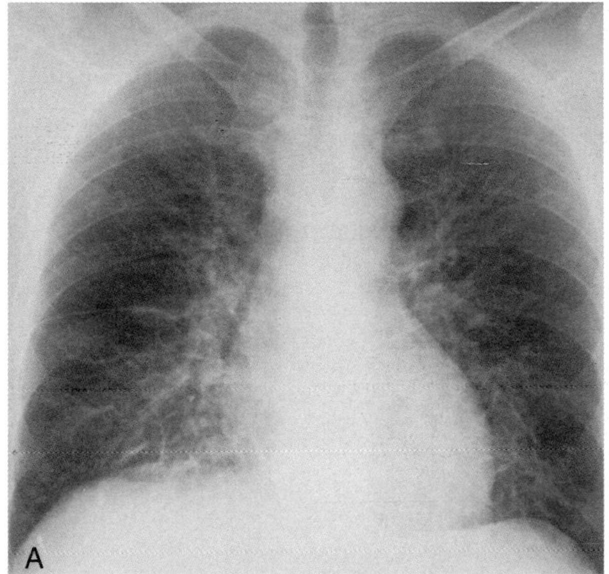

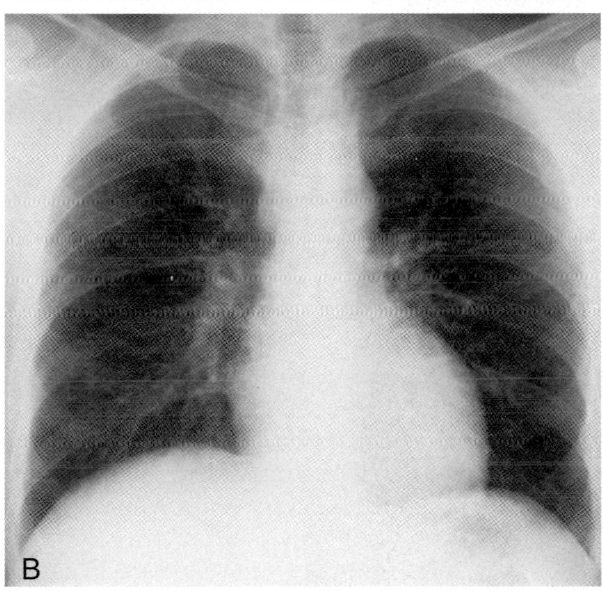

FIGURE 3-69 ■ Fluid overload in renal failure. A posteroanterior chest x-ray immediately before dialysis shows what appear to be many indistinct pulmonary vessels about the hila. Many of these are not vessels but interstitial fluid. Another chest x-ray obtained 1 hour after dialysis *(B)* shows that all these abnormalities have resolved.

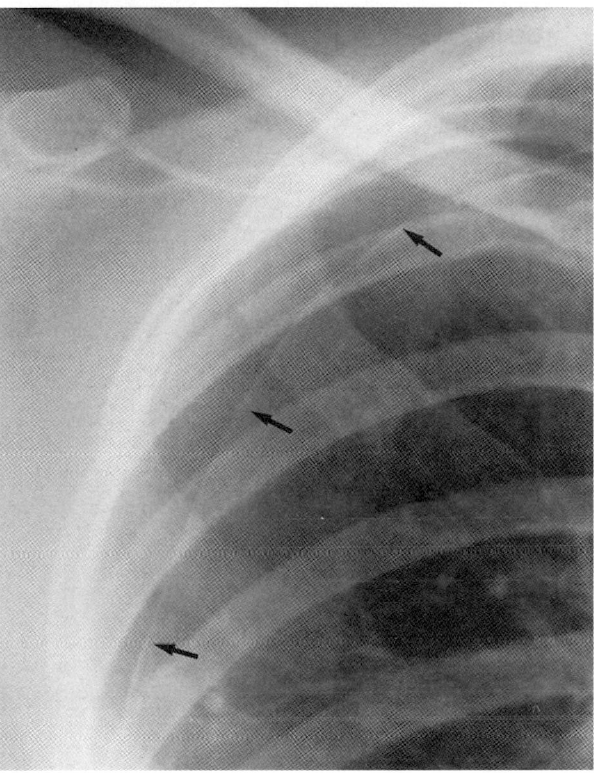

FIGURE 3-70 ■ Apical pneumothorax. A thin line caused by the visceral pleura is seen separated from the lateral chest wall *(arrows)*. Notice that no pulmonary vessels are seen beyond this line and that the line is curved. Notice also that the pleural line is white and that it is almost equally dark on the side of the pneumothorax and the side of the lung.

to the usual inspiration chest x-ray. On an expiration view, the lung becomes somewhat denser and smaller as expiration occurs. The amount of air in the pleural space will not change in size or density, and thus the pneumothorax will appear relatively larger during expiration (Fig. 3-71).

How much the lung collapses with a pneumothorax is a function of how much air can get into the pleural space. In patients who have adhesive pleural changes between the visceral and parietal pleura as a result of previous inflammatory disease or scarring, complete collapse of the lung is not possible, even if a large amount of air is available. The same is true of patients who have diffuse lung disease, because their relatively stiff lungs will not allow complete collapse.

Total lung collapse can occur in patients with normal lungs and without adhesions in the pleural space. This may or may not be

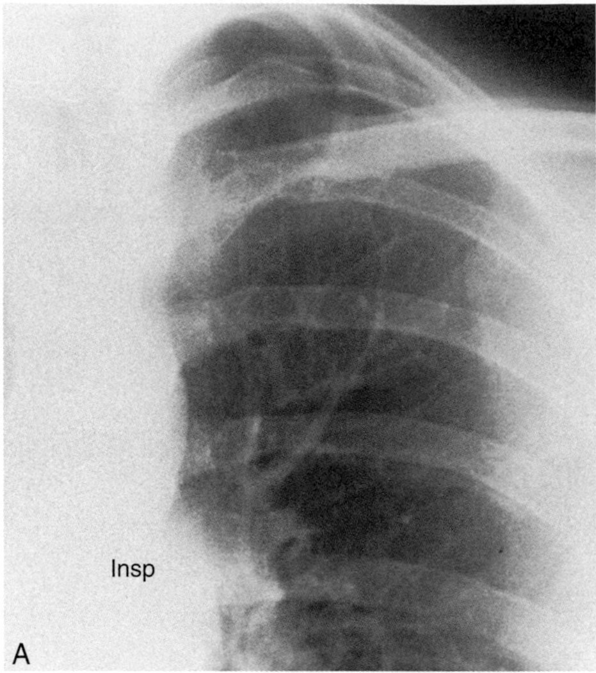

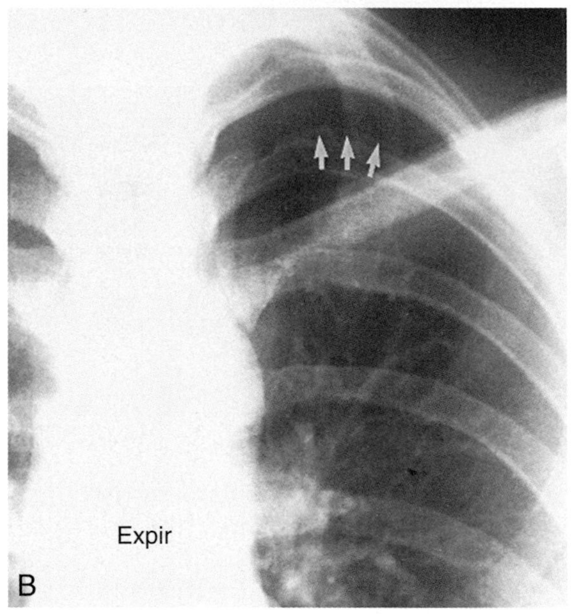

FIGURE 3-71 ■ Accentuation of the pneumothorax. In this young male patient with chest pain, on a typical inspiration chest x-ray *(A)*, no pneumothorax is identified. With expiration *(B)*, the lung becomes smaller, but the pneumothorax stays the same size; thus relatively it appears bigger and can sometimes be easier to see.

accompanied by mediastinal shift. If mediastinal shift occurs or if there is depression of the hemidiaphragm with displacement of the heart and trachea away from the side with the pneumothorax, your patient has a potentially lethal condition known as a *tension pneumothorax* (Fig. 3-72).

Occasionally a pneumothorax occurs when pleural fluid is present. This gives a rather characteristic, straight horizontal line as a result of the air/fluid level in the pleural space. This is termed a *hydropneumothorax*. Whenever you see a very straight horizontal line that extends to the chest wall, you should think of a hydropneumothorax (Fig. 3-73). Occasionally you will see an air/fluid level within a lung as a result of an abscess, but this almost always is surrounded by a thick wall and should be easy to distinguish from a hydropneumothorax.

Quite commonly, a skin fold may cause an artifact that looks very much like a pneumothorax. This artifact is caused by the patient's skin being folded over and pressed against the x-ray detector. The artifact is seen most often in patients who are either supine or semierect. It usually appears as an almost vertical line along the outer third of the upper lung zones. You must be able to recognize this artifact; otherwise, you will put a chest tube in a patient who does not need one. Three ways to recognize this artifact include the following.

1. A skin-fold line often extends above the lung apex into the supraclavicular soft tissues.
2. An increasing density or whiteness may become apparent as you look from the hilum toward the periphery of the lung, just before you reach the line that you think may be a pneumothorax. If there is increasing density (whiteness) as you proceed laterally, followed by sudden decrease in density, this probably represents a skin fold (Fig. 3-74). In the case of a small pneumothorax, both the lung and the pneumothorax are quite dark, and they are separated by a thin white line, which is the visceral pleura.
3. A skin-fold line often is relatively straight, whereas a pleural line follows the curve of the inner aspect of the chest wall.

Because air tends to go to the highest position that it can find in the pleural space, it can be difficult to appreciate a small or even a moderate-sized pneumothorax on a frontal chest x-ray of a

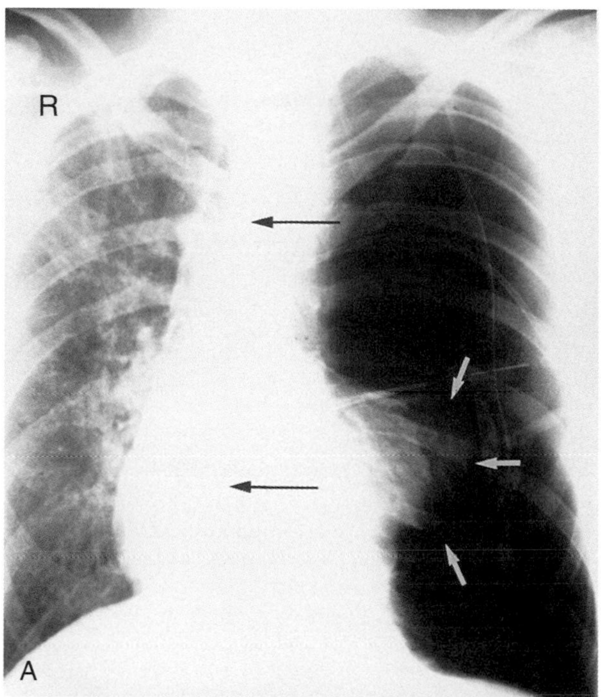

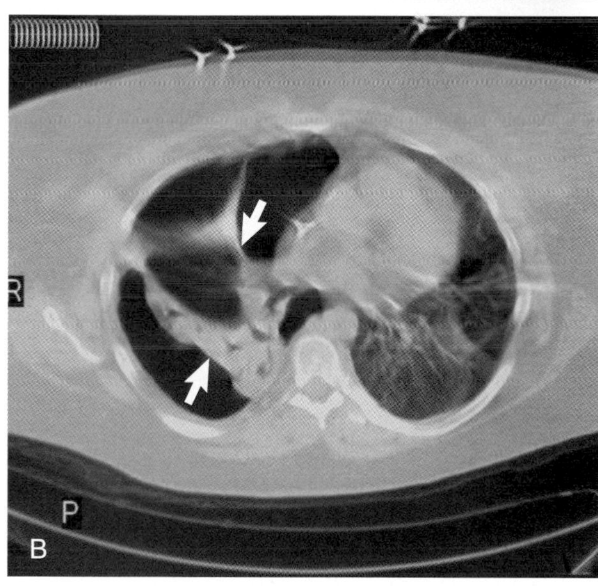

FIGURE 3-72 ■ **Tension pneumothorax.** On a posteroanterior chest x-ray *(A)*, the left hemithorax is very dark or lucent because the left lung has collapsed completely *(white arrows)*. The tension pneumothorax can be identified because the mediastinal contents, including the heart, are shifted toward the right, and the left hemidiaphragm is flattened and depressed. A computed tomography scan done on a different patient with a tension pneumothorax *(B)* shows a completely collapsed right lung *(arrows)* and shift of the mediastinal contents to the left.

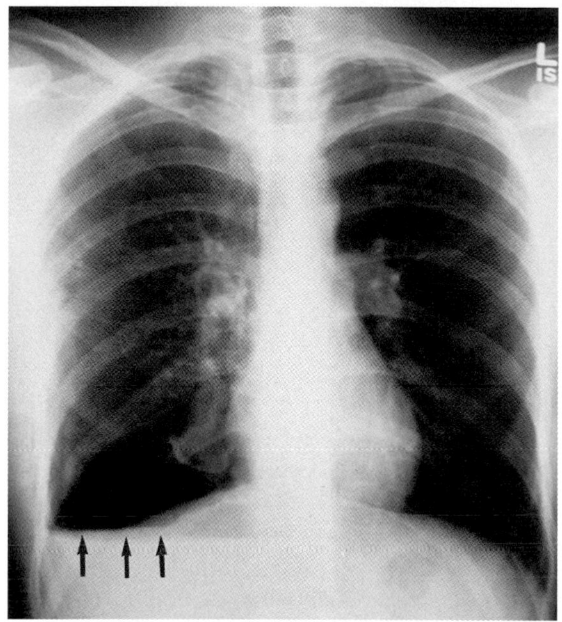

FIGURE 3-73 ■ **Hydropneumothorax.** When fluid and air are present in the pleural space on an upright chest x-ray, a perfectly straight horizontal line will extend all the way from the spine to the edge of the pleural cavity. In this patient, a loculated right basilar hydropneumothorax is present. The air/fluid interface is easily seen *(arrows)*. If this were a lung abscess, the air/fluid level would be very unlikely to extend all the way from the medial to the lateral aspect of the hemithorax.

supine patient. With a supine AP chest projection, the x-ray beam is vertical, and the pneumothorax is layered horizontally along the anterior portion of the chest and probably at least 500 cc of air must be in the pleural space. In supine infants and neonates, an anterior pneumothorax is common. Often the only way to see this pneumothorax is to obtain a supine lateral film and look for lucency (or a dark area) in the retrosternal region. As mentioned earlier, in severely traumatized patients, it is quite common to find, on a CT scan, a small anterior pneumothorax that was unappreciated on the chest x-ray (Fig. 3-75).

On the supine AP chest x-ray of an adult, one of the most reliable signs of a pneumothorax is what is known as the *deep sulcus sign*. Normally, the lateral costophrenic angles are quite sharp or acute. The pleural space, however, goes much farther down along the edge of the lateral aspect of the liver and spleen than most people think. If

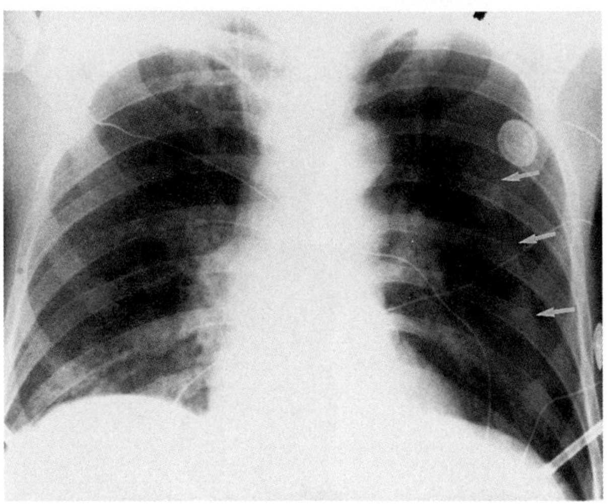

FIGURE 3-74 ■ Skin fold simulating a pneumothorax. A near-vertical line is seen projecting over the left hemithorax *(arrows)*. This is a fold of skin caused by the patient pressing up against the film detector or cassette. A skin fold can be recognized if it extends outside the normal lung area, by seeing pulmonary vessels beyond this line, or, as in this case, by noting that the lung is increasing in density or getting whiter from the hilum out to this line, and then becoming darker. A pneumothorax will be seen as a white line that is dark on both sides.

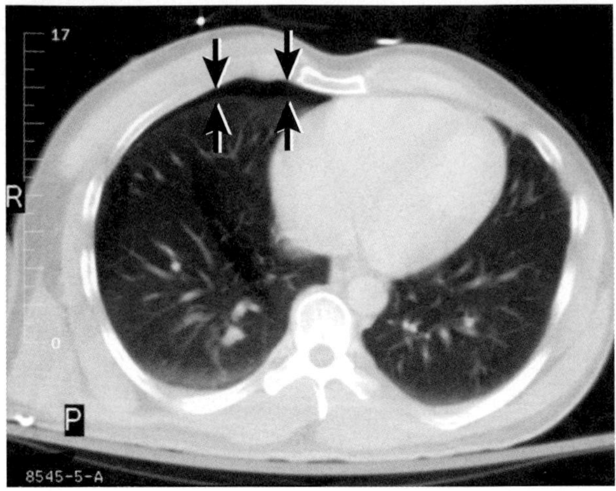

FIGURE 3-75 ■ Small anterior pneumothorax. A chest x-ray on this traumatized patient was thought to be normal, but a subsequent computed tomography scan of the chest revealed a small right anterior pneumothorax *(arrows)*, seen as a small dark crescentic band.

air is in the pleural space, it can easily track down, making the costophrenic angle or sulcus much deeper and the angle much more acute than is normally seen. Thus. be very careful to look for an extremely sharp or deep costophrenic angle or a costophrenic angle that becomes progressively deeper and sharper on sequential supine chest x-rays. If you see this, a pneumothorax is probably present (Fig. 3-76). Have the patient sit upright, and take another chest x-ray; you will often see an apical pneumothorax, because the air typically will move from the sulcus up to the apex.

Most of the findings that we have discussed describe the situation in which the air in the pleural space can move freely. In patients who have had prior inflammatory processes and adhesions in the pleural space, the air may not be able to move freely, and a loculated pneumothorax may be found. These can be difficult to appreciate, but if you see a dark area of lucency either around the edge of the lung or along the cardiac border, consider the possibility of a loculated pneumothorax (Fig. 3-76*B*).

A number of issues arise with regard to appropriate clinical management of a pneumothorax. Often clinicians want to know how big the pneumothorax is. A few radiologists will give the volume in terms of percentage, although this is very inaccurate. I refer to them as small, medium, large, and tension pneumothoraces. Experiments have been done on cadavers indicating that, on an upright film, if 50 cc of air has been placed in the pleural space, the apex of the lung will have dropped approximately to the level between the second and third posterior ribs. One centimeter of space lateral to the lung constitutes about a 10% pneumothorax. One inch of space between the lateral chest wall and the lung margin is about a 30% pneumothorax.

After a chest tube has been placed, note not only the size of residual pneumothorax and the position of the tip but also the side port of the chest tube, if it has one. This is seen as a discontinuity of the opaque line in the catheter; it should project inside the chest cavity and not be out in the soft tissues (see Fig. 3-27*B*). When a chest tube is properly placed, connected to a vacuum, and unobstructed, if there is persistence of the pneumothorax, consider the possibility of a bronchopleural fistula. This usually is a result of

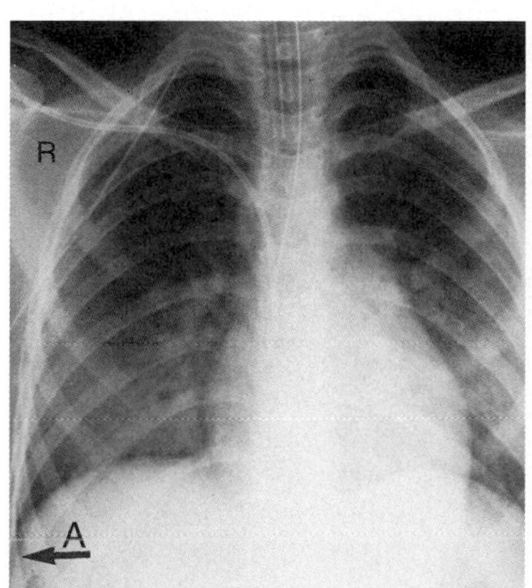

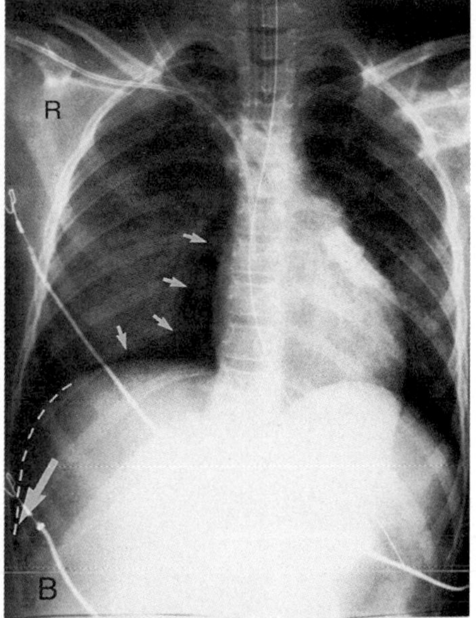

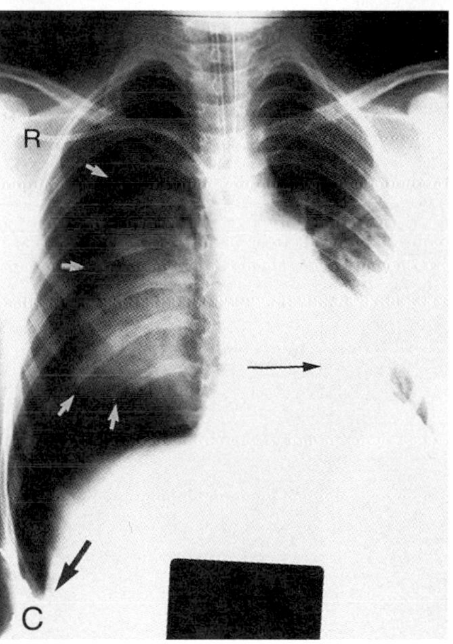

FIGURE 3-76 ■ Deep sulcus sign of pneumothorax. On a posteroanterior chest x-ray *(A)*, the costophrenic angle is normally acute *(arrow)*. In a supine patient, a pneumothorax will often be anterior, medial, and basilar. On a subsequent supine film *(B)*, the dark area along the right cardiac border and lung base appeared larger *(small arrows)*, and the costophrenic angle much deeper and more acute than normal *(large arrow)*. These findings were not recognized, and, as a result, a tension pneumothorax developed in the same patient *(C)* with an extremely deep costophrenic angle *(large black arrow)*, an almost completely collapsed right lung *(small white arrows)*, and shift of the mediastinum to the left.

blunt trauma with a tear in the region of a major bronchus. Other possibilities are a loculated pneumothorax or an anterior pneumothorax (with a posteriorly placed chest tube and the patient supine).

After a lung has been fully re-expanded and the chest tube remains in place, some slight compressive atelectasis is found in the lung that abuts the chest tube. As a result, for a day or so after the chest tube is withdrawn, you can see a linear track where the chest tube had been. This is normal, and it will resolve spontaneously in a day or so.

Pneumomediastinum

Air within the mediastinum often (although not always) is associated with a pneumothorax. With a pneumomediastinum, air collections that are typically vertical are found within the upper portion of the mediastinum and lower neck.

On the lateral view, you can sometimes see air in front of or behind the trachea (Fig. 3-77). A pneumomediastinum can be the result of a tracheobronchial tear. This entity carries up to a 50% mortality rate if not treated. You should suspect pneumomediastinum in a post-traumatic patient who has an abnormal air collection in the chest that does not resolve with placement of a chest tube.

It is sometimes difficult to distinguish between a pneumomediastinum and a pneumopericardium. Pneumopericardium in an adult is very rare, typically resulting from a stab wound. You should remember that the pericardium envelops the heart and reaches only as high as the level of the hila. It does not extend around the hila or over the ascending aorta. Thus in a pneumopericardium, air should be confined to the margins of the major chambers of the heart and not higher (see discussion in Chapter 5 and Fig. 5-4).

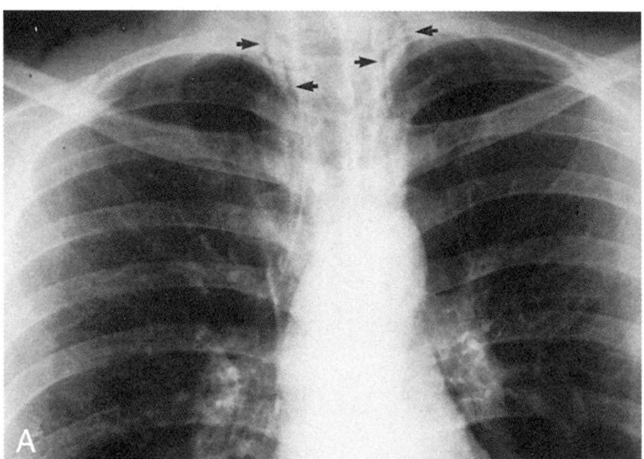

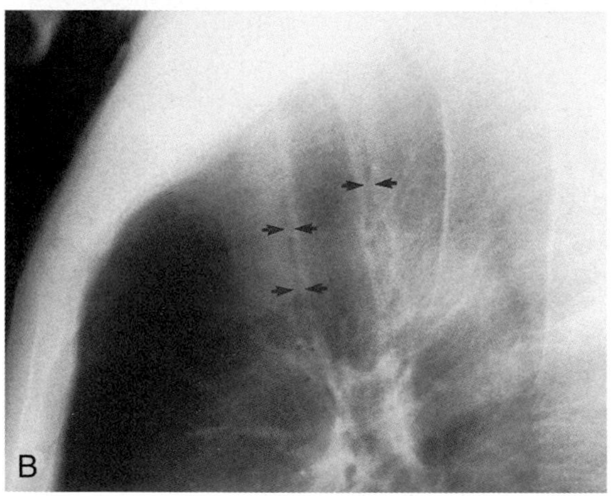

FIGURE 3-77 ■ **Pneumomediastinum.** Vertical dark (lucent) lines representing air within the mediastinum are usually seen at or above the level of the aortic arch. On the posteroanterior view *(A)*, these can be seen extending up into the lower cervical soft tissues *(arrows)*. On the lateral view *(B)*, dark linear air collections can be seen in front of and behind the trachea.

Subcutaneous Emphysema

Air in the soft tissues of the chest wall is often caused by blunt trauma, with a pneumothorax and some broken ribs, or by penetration, as with a stab wound or placement of a chest tube. Air in the soft tissues is seen as dark linear or ovoid areas. Subcutaneous emphysema can extend into the supraclavicular and lower cervical regions. When this happens, however, make very sure that you are seeing subcutaneous emphysema and not a pneumomediastinum that has extended up into the lower cervical area. When subcutaneous emphysema is extensive, it can dissect into the pectoral muscles, producing a bizarre fan-shaped appearance of the air as it outlines the muscle fibers (Fig. 3-78).

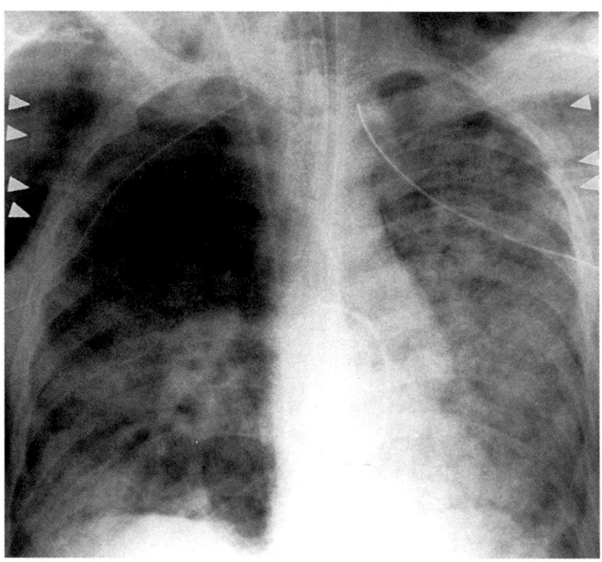

FIGURE 3-78 ■ **Subcutaneous emphysema.** Air is seen along the lateral soft tissues of the chest outside the rib cage dissecting into the pectoral muscles, creating fan-shaped dark lines over the upper chest *(arrowheads)*.

Pleural Effusions

The appearance of pleural effusions or other fluid collections depends on their size and location. Pleural effusions usually are at least 100 cc if they are seen on a routine upright chest x-ray. The most typical location of an effusion is in the dependent portions of the pleural space; therefore they are seen best on upright chest x-rays. Blunting of the lateral costophrenic angles will be identified on the anterior or posterior chest x-ray, and blunting of the posterior costophrenic angle will be seen on the lateral view. Somewhat larger effusions may extend into the inferior aspect of the major fissure (Fig. 3-79), and very large effusions displace and compress lung tissue.

The appearances of larger effusions vary according to the position of the patient when the x-ray was obtained. On the upright chest x-ray, increasing basilar density (whiteness) and loss of the normal lung/hemidiaphragm interface is noted (Fig. 3-80*A*). It can be difficult to figure out whether you are looking at a large or moderate-sized basilar pleural effusion or a basilar alveolar infiltrate. If the patient was supine when the x-ray was obtained, the effusion typically will be layered horizontally in the posterior pleural space. Because the x-ray beam is vertical for a supine chest x-ray, all you may see is a relatively increased density or whiteness of the affected hemithorax as compared with the normal side (Fig. 3-80*B*). In cases of doubt or to determine whether a pleural fluid collection is freely moving, you can obtain a decubitus chest x-ray. If you suspect that an effusion is present on the right, order a right lateral decubitus view, that is, with the right side down when the x-ray is taken (Fig. 3-80*C*). Pleural effusions are easy to see on chest CT scans and often have some associated air-space disease or atelectasis not easily appreciated on chest x-rays (Fig. 3-81).

Pleural effusions have two other appearances sufficiently common that you should be aware of them. The first is a subpulmonic pleural effusion. In my experience, this is more common on the right side. The tip-off to its existence is when it appears that the hemidiaphragm on the right is slightly higher than normal, with the highest portion of the dome more lateral than usual. The highest portion of the dome of the right hemidiaphragm is normally in the midclavicular line or slightly medial to this. If the

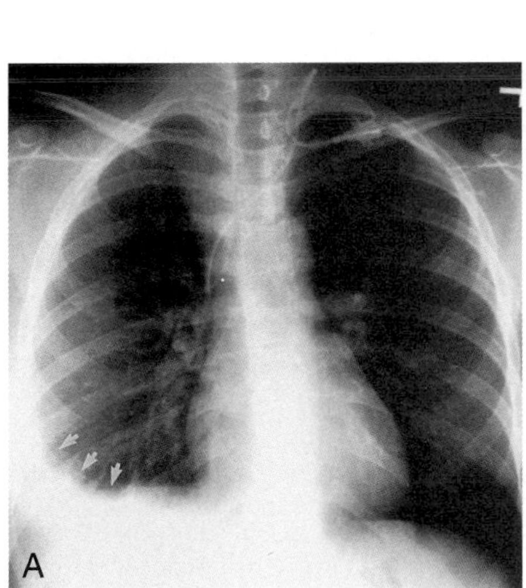

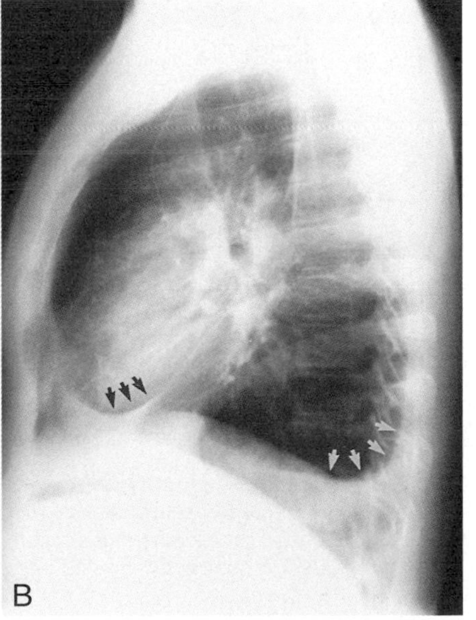

FIGURE 3-79 ■ Moderate-sized pleural effusion. On this upright posteroanterior chest x-ray *(A)*, blunting of the right costophrenic angle is due to pleural fluid. On the lateral view *(B)*, fluid can be seen tracking up into the major fissure *(black arrows)*, and blunting of the right posterior costophrenic angle is seen *(white arrows)*.

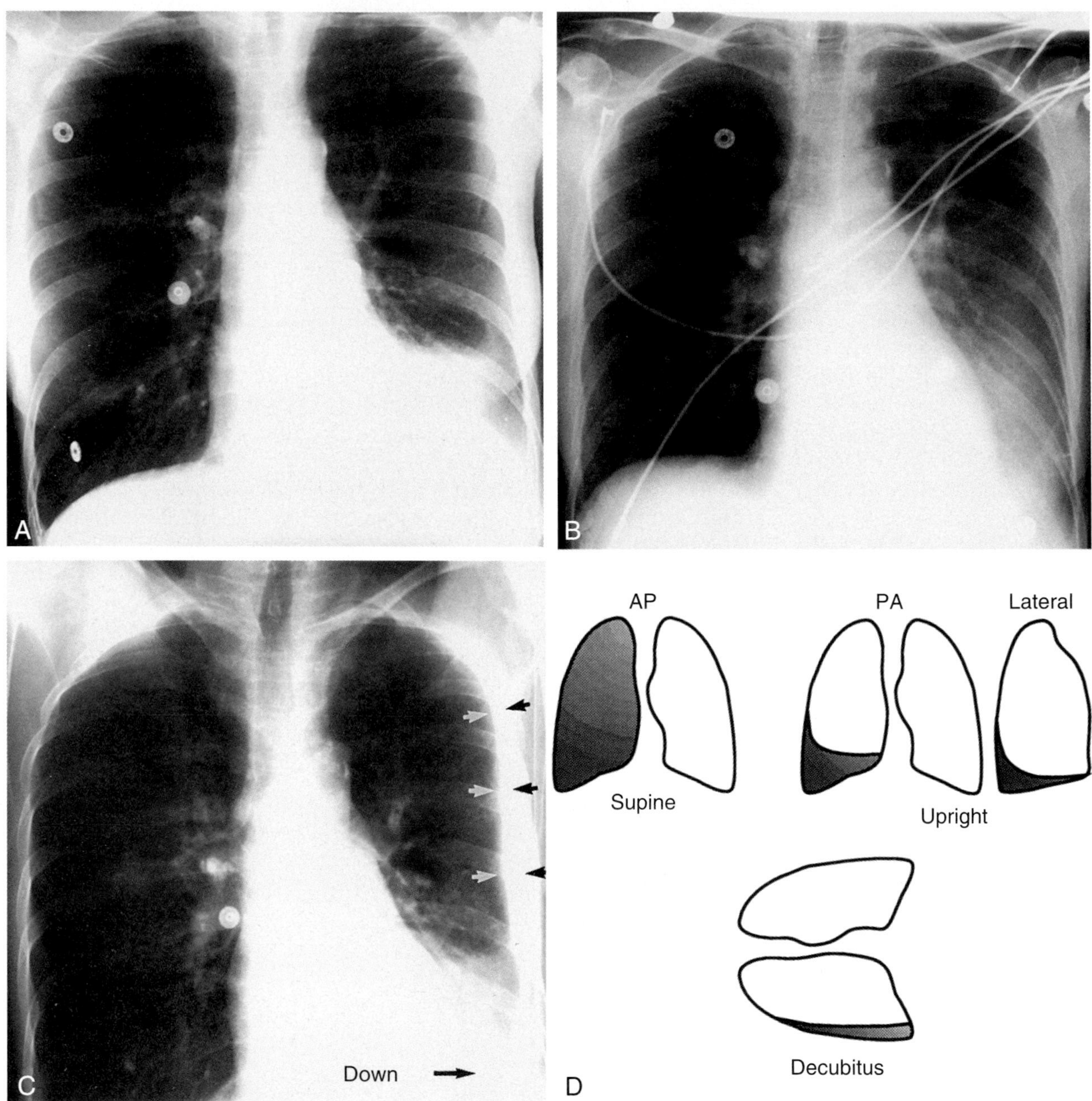

FIGURE 3-80 ■ The appearance of pleural effusions depending on patient position. On an upright posteroanterior chest x-ray *(A)*, a large left pleural effusion obscures the left hemidiaphragm, the left costophrenic angle, and the left cardiac border. On a supine anteroposterior view *(B)*, the fluid runs posteriorly, causing a diffuse opacity over the lower two thirds of the left lung; the left hemidiaphragm remains obscured. This can easily mimic left lower lobe infiltrate or left lower lobe atelectasis. With a left lateral decubitus view *(C)*, the left side of the patient is dependent, and the pleural effusion can be seen to be freely moving and layering *(arrows)* along the lateral chest wall. These findings are shown diagrammatically as well for a right pleural effusion *(D)*.

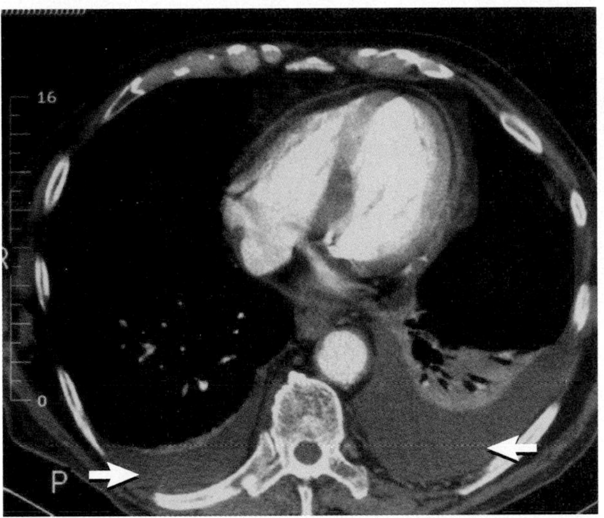

FIGURE 3-81 ■ Pleural effusions on computed tomography scan. The scan shows bilateral fluid collections posteriorly on both right and left sides *(arrows)*. The fact that the fluid is lower attenuation (darker) than the soft tissues and the pleura is not thickened implies that these are effusions rather than an empyema. Note that some adjacent lung density is seen from atelectasis. This is common secondary finding when moderate or large effusions are present.

highest portion is lateral, suspect a subpulmonic effusion (Fig. 3-82).

A loculated pleural effusion located within a fissure may be mistaken for an intrapulmonary lesion (a pseudotumor). On careful examination, loculated effusions in a fissure are typically lenticular or oval (not round) and are located in the expected position of the major or minor fissure (Fig. 3-83).

Chest x-rays cannot be used to differentiate between a transudate and an exudate. The cause of an effusion, however, can sometimes be inferred. Massive effusions are usually malignant in origin. Pancreatitis is associated with left-sided effusions, whereas cirrhosis is associated with right-sided effusions. Most cardiogenic effusions are bilateral and are associated with cardiomegaly and other signs of CHF. About 40% of pneumonias are associated with a small effusion. When a moderate or large pleural fluid collection occurs with a pneumonia, an empyema or malignancy should be suspected.

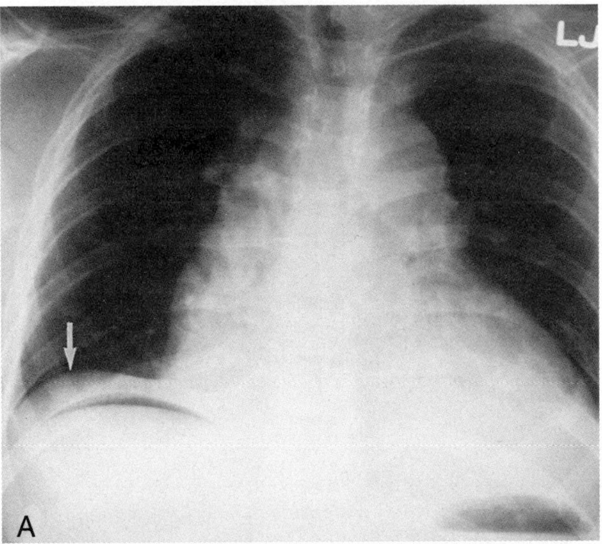

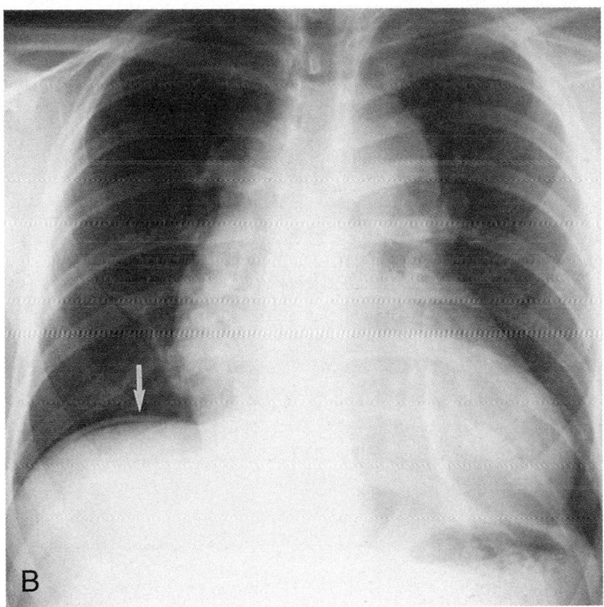

FIGURE 3-82 ■ Subpulmonic effusion. The only finding of a subpulmonic effusion on an upright chest film may be that what looks like the superior aspect of the right hemidiaphragm is quite lateral *(A)*. The actual hemidiaphragm can be seen here because this patient has a pneumoperitoneum, or free air, underneath the hemidiaphragm. The normal thickness of the hemidiaphragm and its position can be seen in a patient with a pneumoperitoneum without a subpulmonic effusion *(B)*.

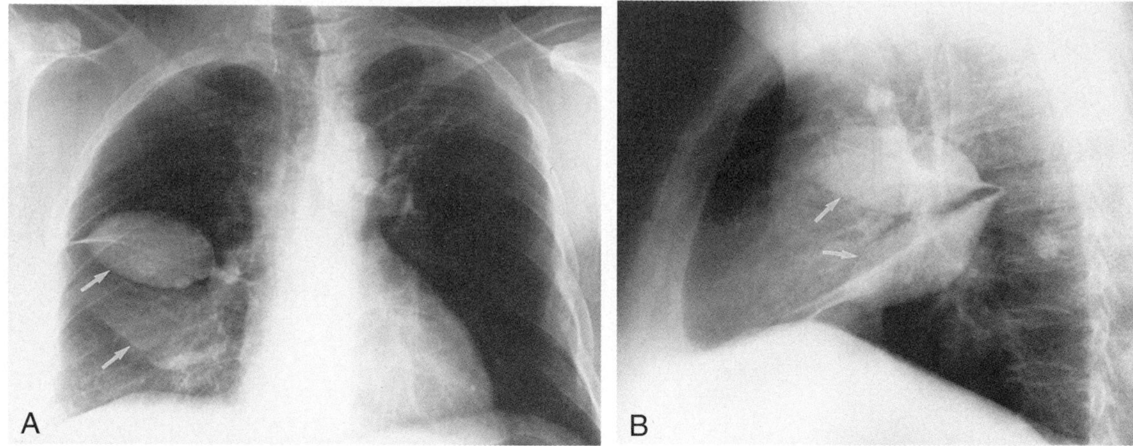

FIGURE 3-83 ■ **Loculated pleural effusions.** Occasionally, pleural effusions *(arrows)* may become loculated in the fissures. These can be seen on the posteroanterior view *(A)* as well as on the lateral chest x-ray *(B)*. These are lenticular, with a long axis oriented along either the major or the minor fissure.

Empyemas. An empyema is pus within the pleural space. It is the result of a postinfectious process 60% of the time, being postsurgical (20%) or post-traumatic (20%) the rest of the time. On a chest x-ray, an empyema may look very much like a pleural effusion or pleural thickening, but it does not move freely and will not layer on a decubitus chest x-ray. The process is often elliptical, with the long axis along the lateral chest wall, and the lung is compressed or displaced. Empyemas often are loculated and have septa. A CT scan is the easiest way to visualize empyemas and locate them for potential drainage (Fig. 3-84). Occasionally an empyema may contain gas or air. The gas is most commonly the result of a bronchopleural fistula and is much less frequently due to gas-forming bacteria or a prior thoracentesis. On a contrasted CT scan, an empyema also can be recognized by thickened or enhancing pleura.

Pleural Calcification and Pleural Masses. Most pleural calcifications are the result of an old calcified empyema or asbestosis. Calcification

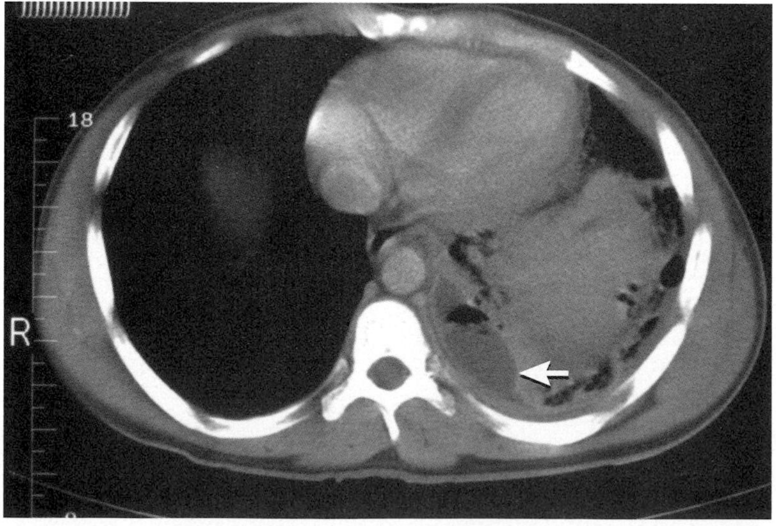

FIGURE 3-84 ■ **Empyema.** A computed tomography scan shows a posterior left pleural fluid collection *(arrow)* containing air *(dark)* and surrounded by thickened pleura. The thickened pleura appears to be split by the lenticular fluid collection.

from an empyema is almost always unilateral and can be quite dense, whereas after asbestos exposure, calcification is often bilateral and not quite so dense (Fig. 3-85). Asbestosis also can produce an interstitial or reticulonodular pulmonary parenchymal pattern and occasionally a "shaggy-looking" heart. Mesotheliomas occur after asbestos exposure, and a focal pleural mass or thickening should raise your suspicion of this tumor. You should remember, however, that the most common tumor after asbestos exposure is a lung cancer and not a mesothelioma.

MEDIASTINAL LESIONS

Masses

A large number of diseases initially occur in the mediastinum and are seen on the anterior chest x-ray as a widening or bulge in the central soft tissues of the chest. The differential diagnosis will change depending on the location of the lesion in the mediastinum. You must determine whether the problem is in the anterior, middle, or posterior mediastinum. The "silhouette sign" can be helpful in determining the site of a pathologic process. This was described earlier in this chapter.

Probably the next and simplest way to localize the lesion is to look at the lateral chest x-ray. Several classification schemes exist of the portions of the mediastinum and its contents. I use anterior, middle, and posterior, but some authors include a superior portion. If filling-in of the space behind the top of the sternum and the ascending aorta is seen, you are most likely dealing with an anterior mediastinal lesion. Basically four types of lesions tend to occur in the anterior mediastinum: substernal thyroid gland, thymic lesions, germ cell tumors (much more common in male patients) (Fig. 3-86), and lymphoma. Occasionally retrosternal and internal mammary lymph nodes can become enlarged from metastases of breast cancer or from leukemia. Students can remember most of the anterior mediastinal lesions by using the four Ts. This stands for *t*hymoma (Fig. 3-87), *t*hyroid lesions, *t*eratoma (Fig. 3-88), and *T*-cell lymphomas. A benign normal variant is the pericardial fat pad (Fig. 3-89). This almost always is found at the right cardiophrenic angle.

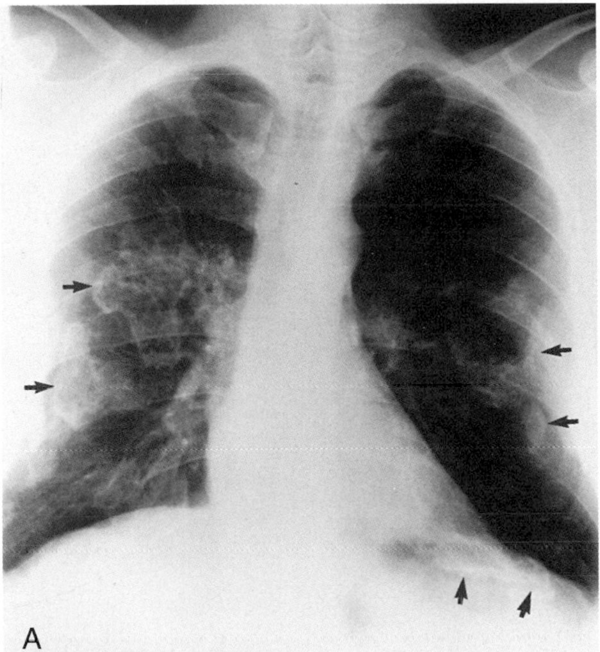

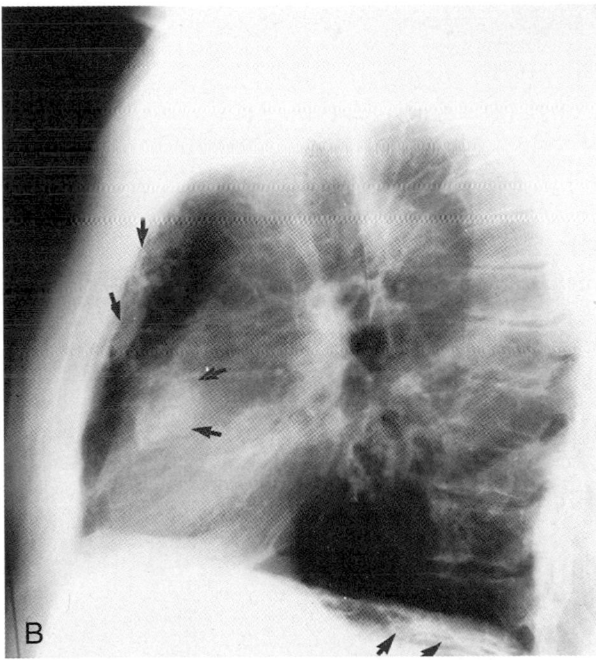

FIGURE 3-85 ■ **Asbestosis.** Both the posteroanterior chest x-ray *(A)* and the lateral view *(B)* show areas of plaquelike calcification along the pleura and the hemidiaphragms *(arrows)*. Pleural lesions often appear to project within the lung parenchyma.

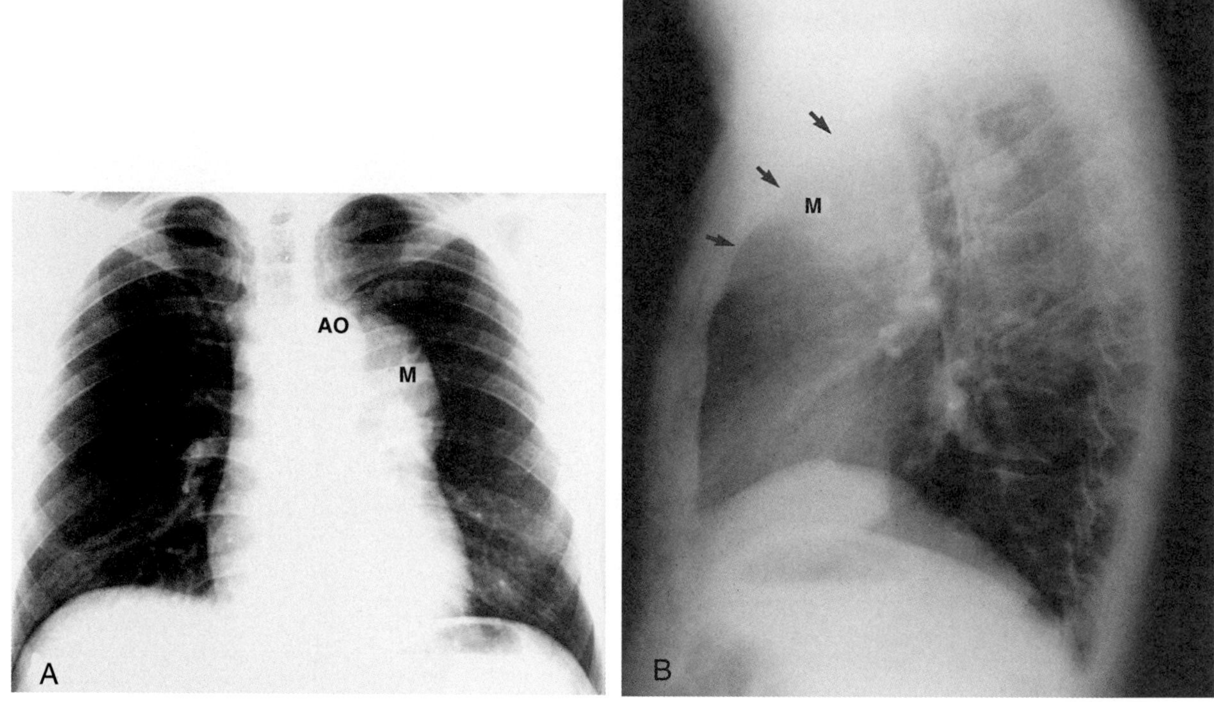

FIGURE 3-86 ■ Seminoma. On the posteroanterior chest x-ray *(A)* of a 25-year-old patient with testicular enlargement, a mass can be clearly seen (M). Note the outline of the aortic arch (AO), indicating that this mass must be either in front of or behind the aortic arch, but not next to it. A lateral view *(B)* shows an anterior mediastinal mass, in this case, metastatic seminoma.

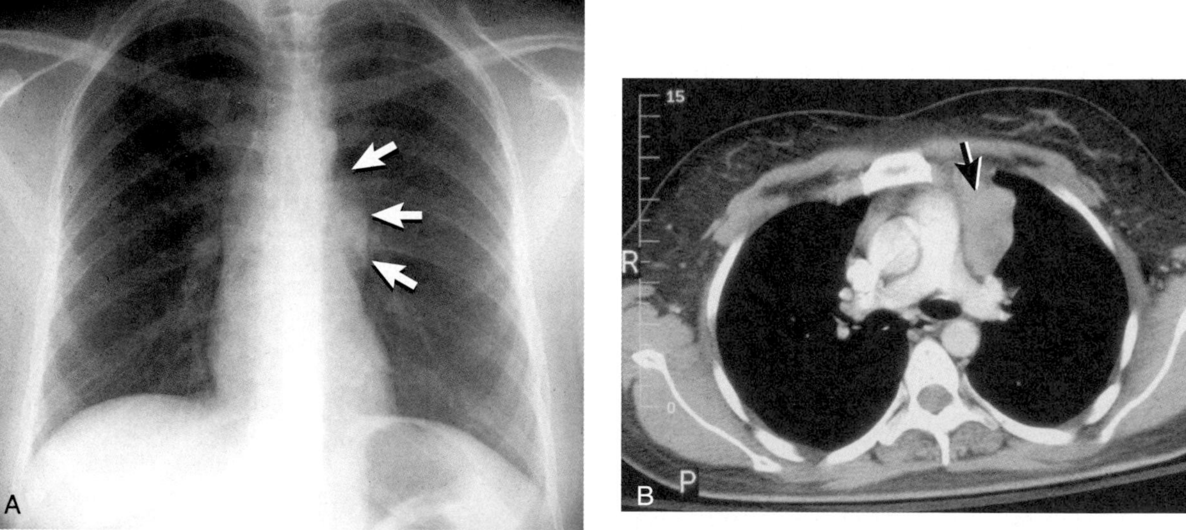

FIGURE 3-87 ■ Thymoma. A chest x-ray *(A)* reveals an unusual contour over the left hilum *(arrows)*. That the hilum is not obscured (no silhouette sign) indicates that the mass must either be in front of or behind the hilum. A computed tomography scan *(B)* reveals a soft tissue mass *(arrow)* just to the left of the aorta. This is the most common location of a thymoma.

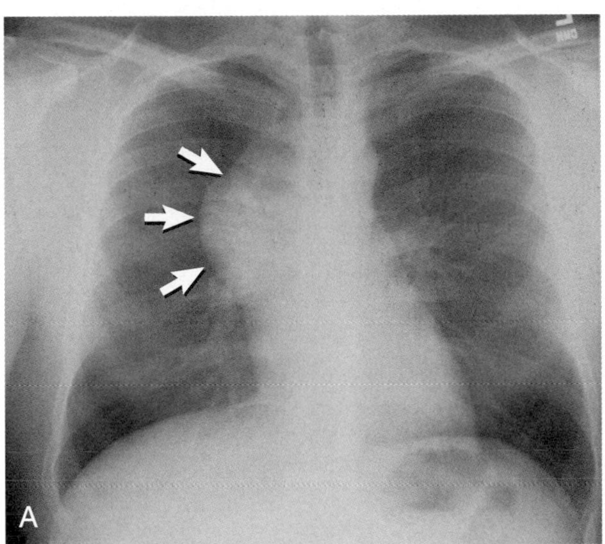

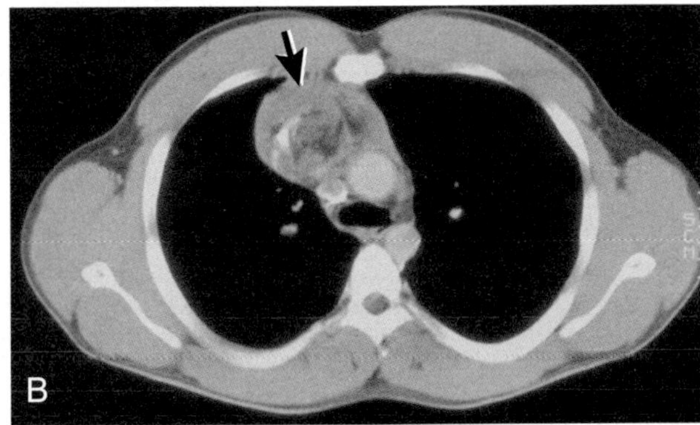

FIGURE 3-88 ■ Mediastinal teratoma. A chest x-ray (A) shows a large upper right mediastinal mass *(arrows)*, but no specific internal structure is apparent. A computed tomography scan *(B)* reveals that the mass contains multiple types of tissue elements including fat *(dark)*, soft tissue *(gray)*, and calcium *(white)*. This is essentially diagnostic of a teratoma.

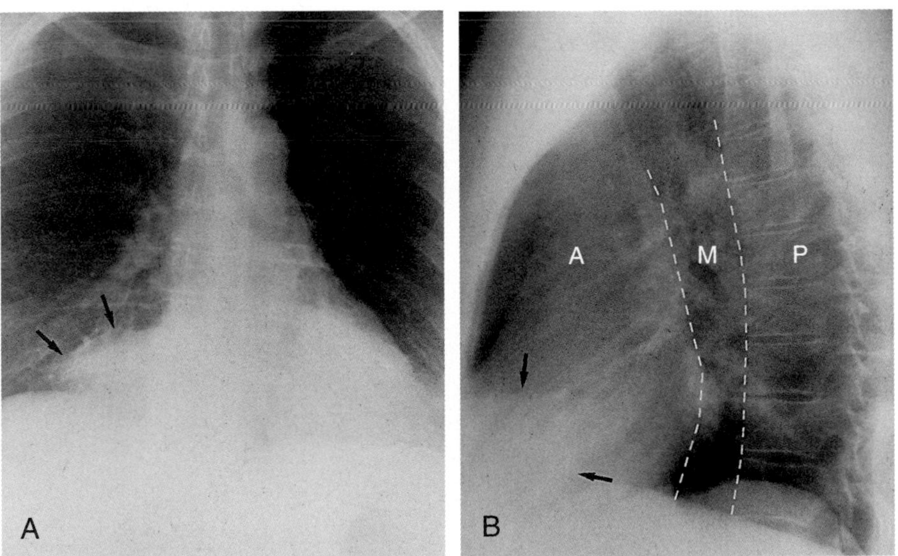

FIGURE 3-89 ■ Pericardial fat pad. *A,* A soft tissue mass *(arrows)* is seen in the right cardiophrenic angle on the frontal chest x-ray. *B,* It also is seen in the anterior mediastinum on the lateral view. On this view, the anterior (A), middle (M), and posterior (P) portions of the mediastinum have been identified.

Lesions in the middle mediastinum include thoracic aortic aneurysms, hematomas, neoplasms, adenopathy (Fig. 3-90), esophageal lesions, diaphragmatic hernias (hiatal or Morgagni type), and duplication cysts. Morgagni hernias tend to be on the right side. Any middle mediastinal lesion associated with the aorta should be considered an aneurysm until proven otherwise.

Posterior mediastinal lesions are seen on the lateral view projecting over the spine and are also paraspinous on the frontal chest x-ray. Most (90%) posterior mediastinal lesions are neurogenic. They may represent neuroblastomas in young children, but in adults are more likely to be neurofibromas, schwannomas, or ganglioneuromas. Other posterior mediastinal lesions include hernias (hiatal or Bochdalek type), neoplasms, hematomas, or extramedullary hematopoiesis. Bochdalek hernias are most often on the left side.

DIAPHRAGM

Diaphragmatic Rupture

Rupture of the diaphragm may occur after blunt trauma. The diaphragm most frequently is ruptured on the left side, perhaps because the liver may dissipate some of the force of an abdominal blow, lessening the likelihood of rupture of the right hemidiaphragm. The most common appearance is loops of bowel protruding into the lower chest cavity without the normal dome-shaped structure of the hemidiaphragm (Fig. 3-91). The manifestations of a ruptured diaphragm can be delayed, and sometimes the bowel herniates through the diaphragm only 1 or 2 weeks after the initial accident. The patient may remain asymptomatic for months or years.

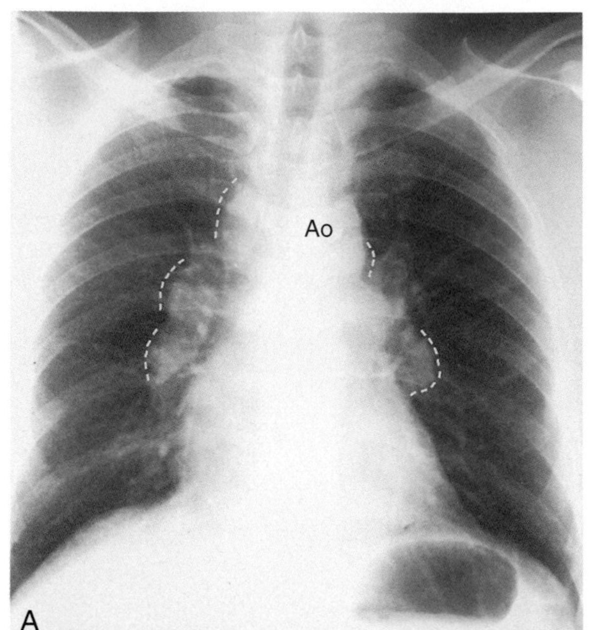

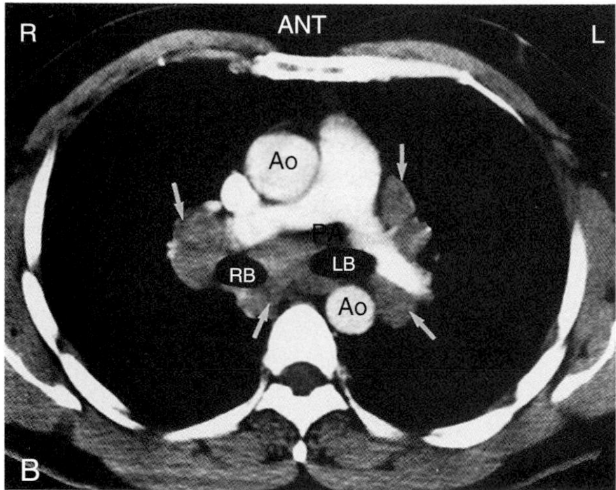

FIGURE 3-90 ■ Sarcoid. Marked lymphadenopathy *(dotted lines)* is seen in the region of both hila in the right paratracheal region *(A)*. The transverse contrast-enhanced computed tomography scan of the upper chest *(B)* clearly shows the ascending and descending aorta (Ao) as well as the pulmonary artery (PA) and superior vena cava. The right and left main-stem bronchus area also is seen. *Arrows,* the extensive lymphadenopathy. (See also Fig. 3-55 for the alveolar form of sarcoid.)

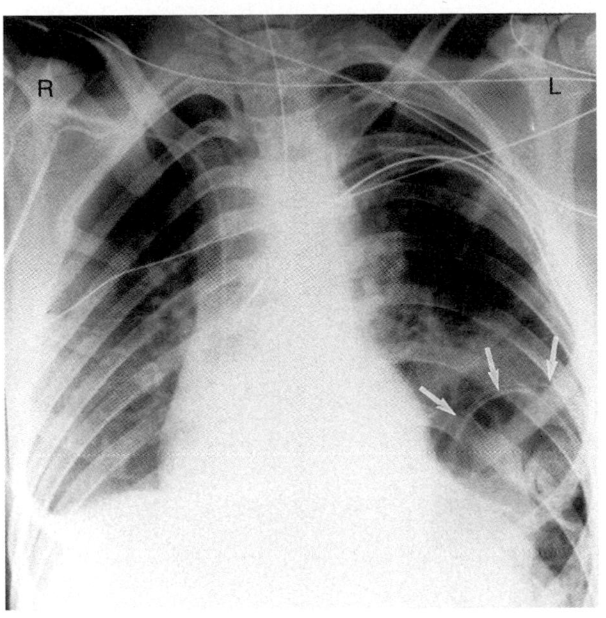

FIGURE 3-91 ■ Diaphragmatic rupture. Six days after an auto accident, bowel loops can be seen in the left lower chest (arrows). Diaphragmatic rupture is more common on the left than on the right.

Suggested Textbooks on the Topic

Fraser RS, Muller C, Pare J, Pare PD: Fraser and Pare's Diagnosis of Diseases of the Chest, 3rd ed. Philadelphia, WB Saunders, 1999.

Muller NL, Fraser RS, Coleman N, Pare PD: Radiologic Diagnosis of Diseases of the Chest, 1st ed. Philadelphia, WB Saunders, 2001.

Naidich DP, Webb R, Muller NL, Zerhouni EA, McGunness G, Webb WR, Krinsky GA, Siegelman SS: Computed Tomography and Magnetic Resonance Imaging of the Thorax, 3rd ed. Philadelphia, Lippincott Williams & Wilkins, 1999.

Reed JC: Chest Radiology: Plain Film Pattern and Differential Diagnosis, 5th ed. Philadelphia, WB Saunders, 2003.

Webb WR, Muller NL, Naidich DP: High Resolution CT of the Lung. Philadelphia, Lippincott Williams & Wilkins, 2000.

4 Breast

IMAGING METHODS

Breast imaging generally refers to mammography. Mammography is complementary to physical examination, and each can detect a significant number of tumors not found by the other. The primary purpose of mammography is to detect small breast cancers and, by so doing, to improve survival. In young women, the breast is extremely dense. The density of the normal parenchymal tissue is the same as the density of a carcinoma. In young women, not only is the incidence of breast cancer low, but it is also very difficult to tell whether a cancer is present amid the normal dense tissue. As women age, fatty infiltration of the breast and atrophy of the parenchyma occur. Because the fat is lucent (dark) on a mammogram and a cancer is dense (white), tumors are more easily visualized as a woman ages. The density of the breast is partly due to hormonal stimulation. In older women receiving estrogen replacement therapy, the density of the breast tissue increases, making tumors more difficult to see (Fig. 4-1).

Mammograms are usually obtained in what are referred to as the craniocaudal (top to bottom) and axillary oblique views. The latter, a somewhat tilted lateral view, allows better visualization of the tail of the breast tissue as it extends out toward the axilla than is possible on a straight lateral view. On the craniocaudal view, it is often not easy to tell which is the medial and which is the lateral aspect. By convention, the identifying markers or technologist's initials are placed along the lateral edge of the breast.

Ultrasound examination is often used as an adjunct to mammography to determine whether a lesion is cystic. Ultrasound can be a useful adjunctive method but should not be relied on as a screening method for breast cancer. Computed tomography (CT) scanning is not indicated for examination of the breast, and the role of magnetic resonance imaging (MRI) and nuclear medicine for evaluation of a suspicious mass or screening for breast cancer remains in the realm of research.

INTERPRETATION

Great variation is often found between women in the appearance of the breast tissue. Fortunately, most women have very symmetrical tissue when one breast is compared with the other. Any asymmetries in density should be examined carefully, because they may represent a cancer (Fig. 4-2). In addition to asymmetrical masses, another sign of breast cancer is very tiny grouped calcifications. Often called microcalcifications, these are usually very fine (approximately ≤1 mm) and sandlike and can sometimes be seen to have a branching structure. Most women, as they age, have benign calcifications within the breast. These are usually rounded calcifications greater than 2 mm in diameter (Fig. 4-3). In women over the age of 60, serpiginous calcifications can normally be seen within blood vessel walls. Associated indirect signs of malignancy also may be present. These include focal skin thickening or dimpling due to an

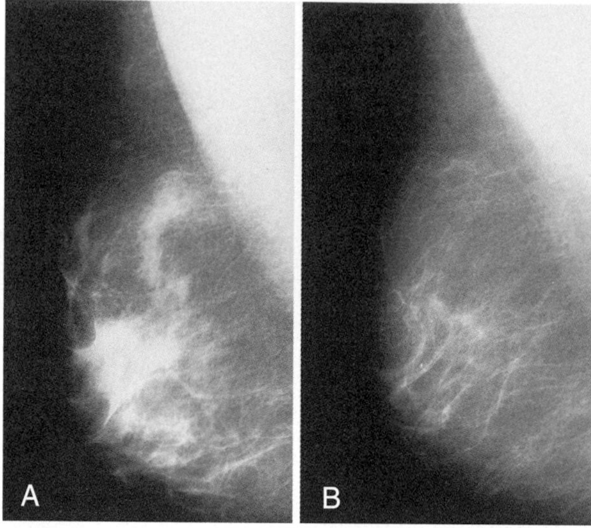

FIGURE 4-1 ■ Normal mammogram and the process of aging. On the axillary oblique view of the right breast *(A),* the normal breast parenchyma is seen as ill-defined white densities located predominantly behind the nipple. In young women, the breast tissue can be extremely dense with only a small amount of interspersed fat, making tumors hard to see. Another mammogram *(B)* on the same patient several years later shows fatty replacement of most of the breast tissue. The breast tissue can become dense again if the woman is given estrogen therapy.

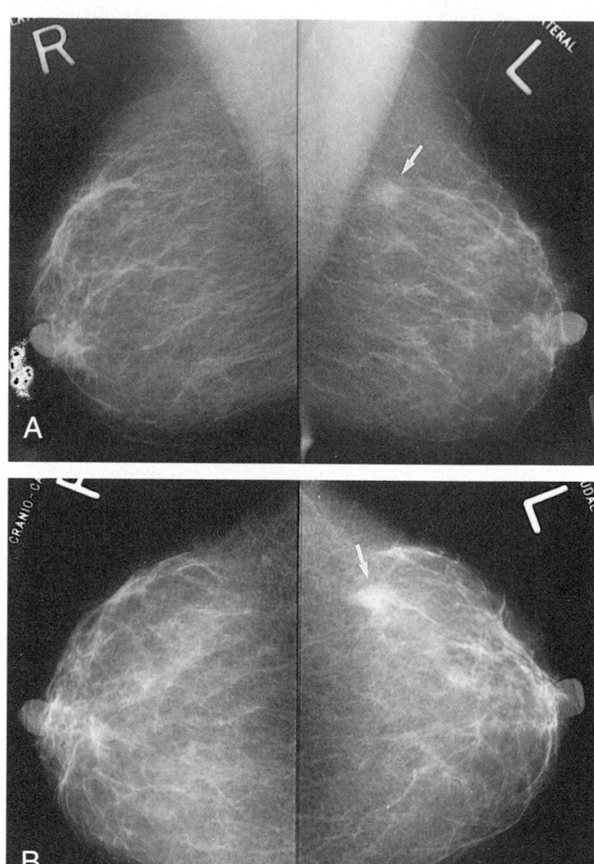

FIGURE 4-2 ■ Breast cancer. Axillary oblique views *(A)* and craniocaudal views *(B)* of the right and left breast show an asymmetrical density *(arrows)* in the upper outer aspect of the left breast. Any asymmetrical density should raise suspicion of a neoplasm.

underlying tumor, unilateral nipple retraction, and vascular asymmetry (increased vascularity due to the tumor).

Once a suspicious lesion is identified on both craniocaudal and axillary oblique views, further investigation usually ensues, in the form of a magnified mammogram, an ultrasound examination (Fig. 4-4), or a biopsy. If a lesion is solid, asymmetrical, or stellate, or if grouped microcalcifications are seen, an intensive search should be undertaken for prior mammograms that can be used for comparison. The reason for this is that a surgical biopsy will necessarily result in scar tissue, and scar tissue often leaves an asymmetrical radial density that can look like a neoplasm; hence you should obtain biopsies only when necessary. If the solid lesion is new or if old films are not available and the lesion is thought to be suspicious, a biopsy is recommended. If the lesion is palpable, the surgeon may simply proceed with a biopsy.

If the suspicious lesion is not palpable, a procedure called stereotactic needle biopsy, or needle localization, can be performed by the radiologist. In the stereotactic procedure, the patient is placed face down on a table with the breast suspended, and images are taken with coordinates. These coordinates are entered into a computer, and a core-biopsy gun is fired, taking a sample of the lesion for pathologic analysis.

The needle localization procedure is done for nonpalpable lesions immediately before surgery for excision or lumpectomy. The breast is compressed with a holder that has coordinates on the sides, and a mammogram is taken. A thin

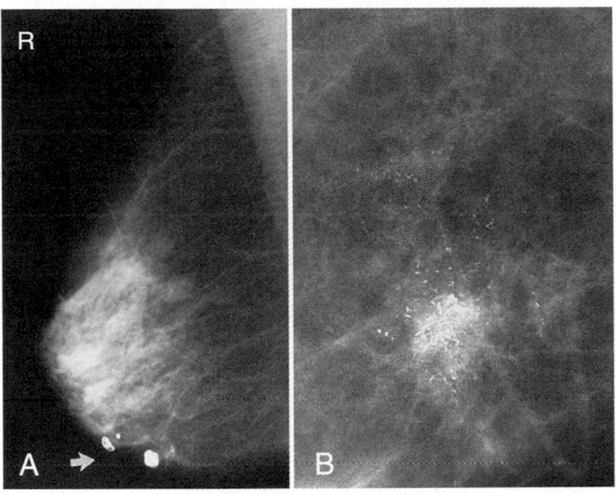

FIGURE 4-3 ■ **Breast calcifications.** A lateral view of the right breast *(A)* shows several well-defined rounded or lobular calcifications. These are almost always benign. Malignant calcifications *(B)* tend to be very small, sandlike, and clustered as seen in this very enlarged view from a mammogram in a different patient with breast cancer.

needle can then be inserted at the coordinates of interest until it is shown that the end of the needle is either at or slightly past the lesion. At this point, a small amount of blue dye is injected, and a thin, hooked wire is passed through the needle. As the wire exits the point of the needle, it opens and becomes fixed in the tissue. The needle is withdrawn, leaving the wire in place. The surgeon then removes the tissue near the end of the hooked wire (Fig. 4-5). The biopsy specimen is x-rayed to make sure that the lesion of interest has been removed.

The lymph node drainage of a breast cancer can be very variable. As a result, before surgery for a known breast cancer, many surgeons will want the patient to have a nuclear medicine procedure to localize the sentinel node. A small amount of radioactive substance is injected near the lesion site, and then the radioactivity migrates to the nearest draining lymph node. This node can be marked or localized at surgery, and in theory, it is the node that is most likely to contain metastases.

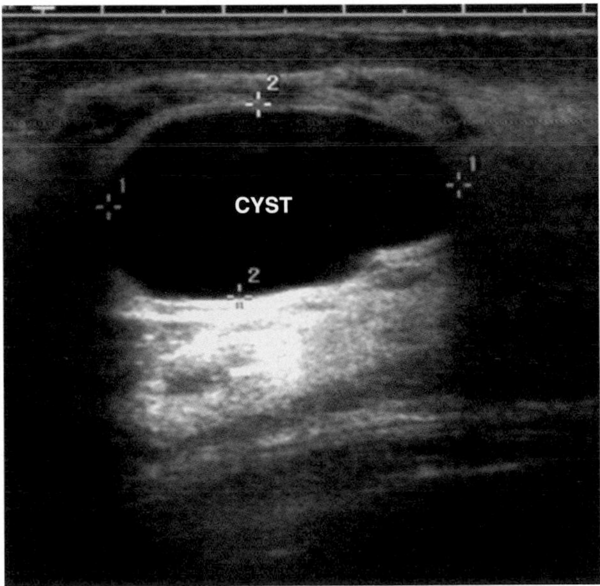

FIGURE 4-4 ■ **Breast cyst.** An ultrasound examination of a young woman with a palpable lesion shows an echo-free simple cyst.

SCREENING

Much discussion over the last decade has concerned the indications for screening mammography. Concerns about overutilization revolve about financial issues as well as the potential of radiation-induced breast carcinoma several decades later. Current guidelines are shown in Table 4-1.

The radiation cancer studies (such as those done for follow-up of atomic bomb survivors at Hiroshima and Nagasaki) show that the risk of breast cancer after radiation exposure is greatest when exposure occurs at a young age. Little, if any, risk ensues from mammograms performed after age 50. Present guidelines vary as to whether to perform a mammogram every 1–2 years or only a baseline study in women aged 40 to 50. Always remember that screening mammography is not a substitute for monthly breast examination by the woman herself.

Mammograms can be used in the evaluation of a breast prosthesis. Normally the prosthesis can be seen as an oval area of increased density in the central portion of the breast. Complications that arise include calcification, which can occur around the prosthesis, and this is sometimes visualized on chest x-rays (Fig. 4-6). Leakage of a prosthesis can be identified if the

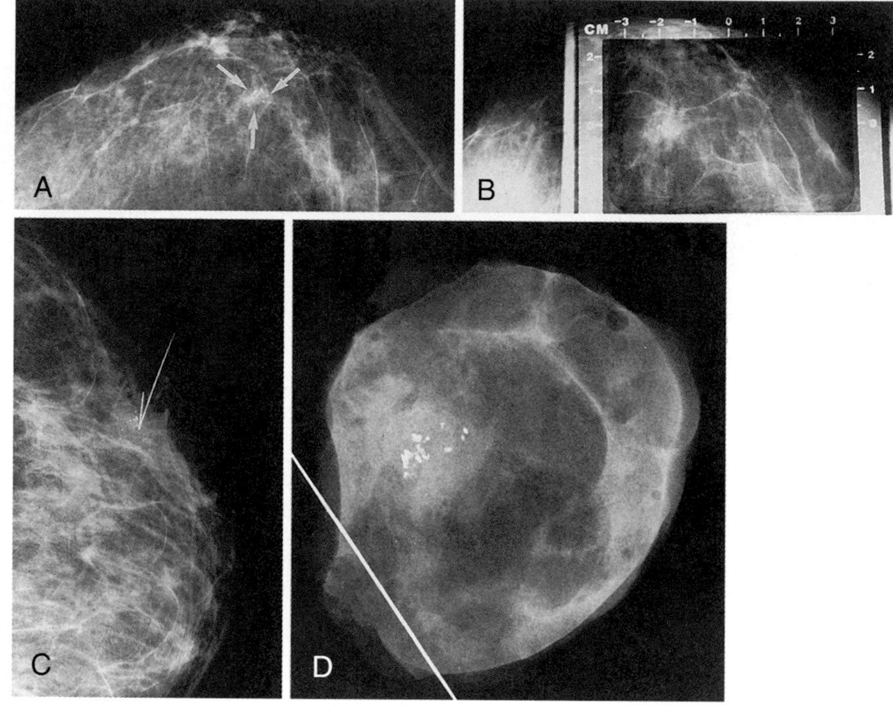

FIGURE 4-5 ■ Localization and biopsy of a breast cancer. A group of suspicious calcifications *(arrows)* is seen on a craniocaudal view of the left breast *(A)*. Needle localization is first performed by repeating the mammogram in the same projection but with an overlying grid that has coordinates *(B)*. A needle is then inserted straight down at the appropriate coordinates. A lateral view of the breast is obtained, and when it is clear that the tip of the needle is in the right location, a hooked wire is inserted through the needle, and the needle is withdrawn *(C)*. The patient is then taken to the operating room, and the specimen of concern at the end of the wire is removed. A magnified specimen x-ray is then obtained *(D)* to ensure that the suspicious calcifications have been removed.

TABLE 4-1 ■ **Breast Cancer Screening Guidelines for Various Organizations as of July 2003**

For Women Age 20–39

American Cancer Society

Monthly breast self-exam (BSE), clinical breast exam (CBE) every 3 yr. Women at higher risk should consult with their physician about beginning mammography before age 40

National Cancer Institute

No recommendation. Women at higher risk* should consult with their physician about beginning mammography before age 40.

For Women Age 40–49

American Cancer Society

Monthly BSE, begin annual mammography and CBE at age 40. Women at higher risk should consult with their physician to determine their mammography schedule in their 40s

National Cancer Institute

Mammography every 1–2 yr for women at average risk for breast cancer. Women at higher risk should consult with their physician to determine their mammography schedule in their 40s. CBE every 1–2 yr

For Women Age 50 or Order

American Cancer Society

Annual mammography and CBE, monthly BSE

National Cancer Institute

Mammography every 1–2 yr

*High risk includes those who have had breast cancer, have close relatives with breast cancer, have lumpy or dense breasts, or have first pregnancy after age 30.

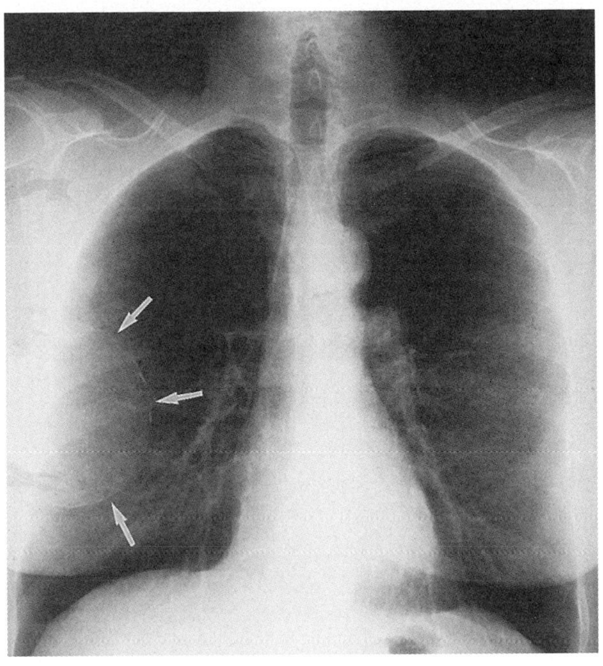

FIGURE 4-6 ■ Calcification around the breast prosthesis. On the chest x-ray, a rim of calcification *(arrows)* can occasionally be seen around a breast prosthesis.

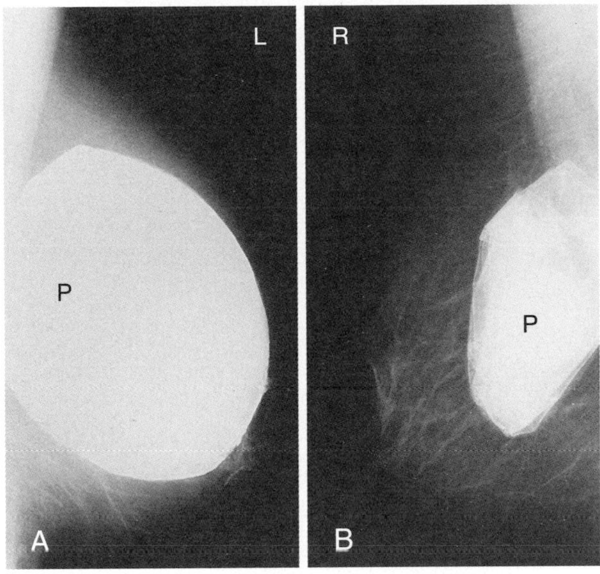

FIGURE 4-7 ■ Normal and ruptured breast prosthesis. A normal prosthesis is seen in the left breast. The right breast prosthesis is collapsed as a result of rupture. Actual extravasation of either saline or silicone is usually not visible on a mammogram.

leakage has been enough to cause deflation of the prosthesis (Fig. 4-7). Leaking silicone or saline cannot be visualized directly on a mammogram. Screening mammography for occult breast carcinomas can be quite difficult in patients with prostheses, because the prosthesis can obscure a small cancer.

Ultrasound examination of the breast should not be considered to be a primary screening tool, because it cannot differentiate carcinomas from fibroadenomas or other benign solid lesions. It is useful only to differentiate a solid lesion from a cyst.

Suggested Textbook on the Topic

Kopans D: Breast Imaging, 2nd ed. Philadelphia, Lippincott Williams & Wilkins, 1997.

5 Cardiovascular System

NORMAL ANATOMY AND IMAGING TECHNIQUES

The normal anatomy and configuration of the heart on a chest x-ray and on computed tomography (CT) scanning were discussed in Chapter 3. Imaging of the heart also can be done by using magnetic resonance imaging (MRI). This modality gives quite good visualization of the cardiac anatomy. The lungs are not well seen on these scans because respiratory motion causes image degradation. The anatomy of the heart at several different levels on an MRI scan is shown in Figure 5-1. Both MR and nuclear medicine images can be gated to the cardiac cycle, allowing images to be produced in systole and diastole as well as in the phases in between (Fig. 5-2). Transthoracic ultrasound (echocardiography) also can be used to image through those portions of the heart that are in contact with the chest wall. This method is generally considered the practice of cardiologists and is discussed here only when it is the appropriate test to order.

Imaging of the peripheral vascular system has changed dramatically over the last decade. Historically, good spatial resolution was achieved only with invasive techniques that used direct arterial access and injection of contrast material through a catheter. With the advent of faster CT and MRI scanners, both venous and arterial anatomy can be visualized adequately for most diagnostic purposes. Even though CT and MRI scans are typically displayed as "slice anatomy," the vascular image data are often manipulated to display rotating three-dimensional images of the vascular anatomy. Invasive procedures are normally reserved for therapeutic intervention (such as balloon dilatation of a stenosis or stent placement). Appropriate imaging indications for cardiovascular problems are shown in Table 5-1.

EVALUATION OF THE CARDIAC SILHOUETTE

Generalized Cardiomegaly

Examination of the shape of the heart on a chest x-ray can sometimes provide clues to the type of cardiac disease present. If the heart appears large in most dimensions, it is often difficult to tell whether multichamber enlargement, a myocardiopathy, or a pericardial effusion is present. If acute (within several days), marked enlargement of the cardiac silhouette is seen, the most likely diagnosis is a pericardial effusion. Under these circumstances, the heart has a very pendulous appearance and is much wider at the base. This is often referred to as a "water bag" appearance (Fig. 5-3). Pericardial effusions must be greater than 250 ml to be detectable radiographically. Effusions are sometimes visible on CT scans of the chest, but if you suspect a pericardial effusion, the imaging procedure of choice is echocardiography. After penetrating trauma or surgery, air may be seen within the pericardium (Fig. 5-4).

Constrictive pericarditis is most commonly due to tuberculosis and viral and pyogenic infections. It also may occur with radiation therapy. Ninety percent of patients with constrictive

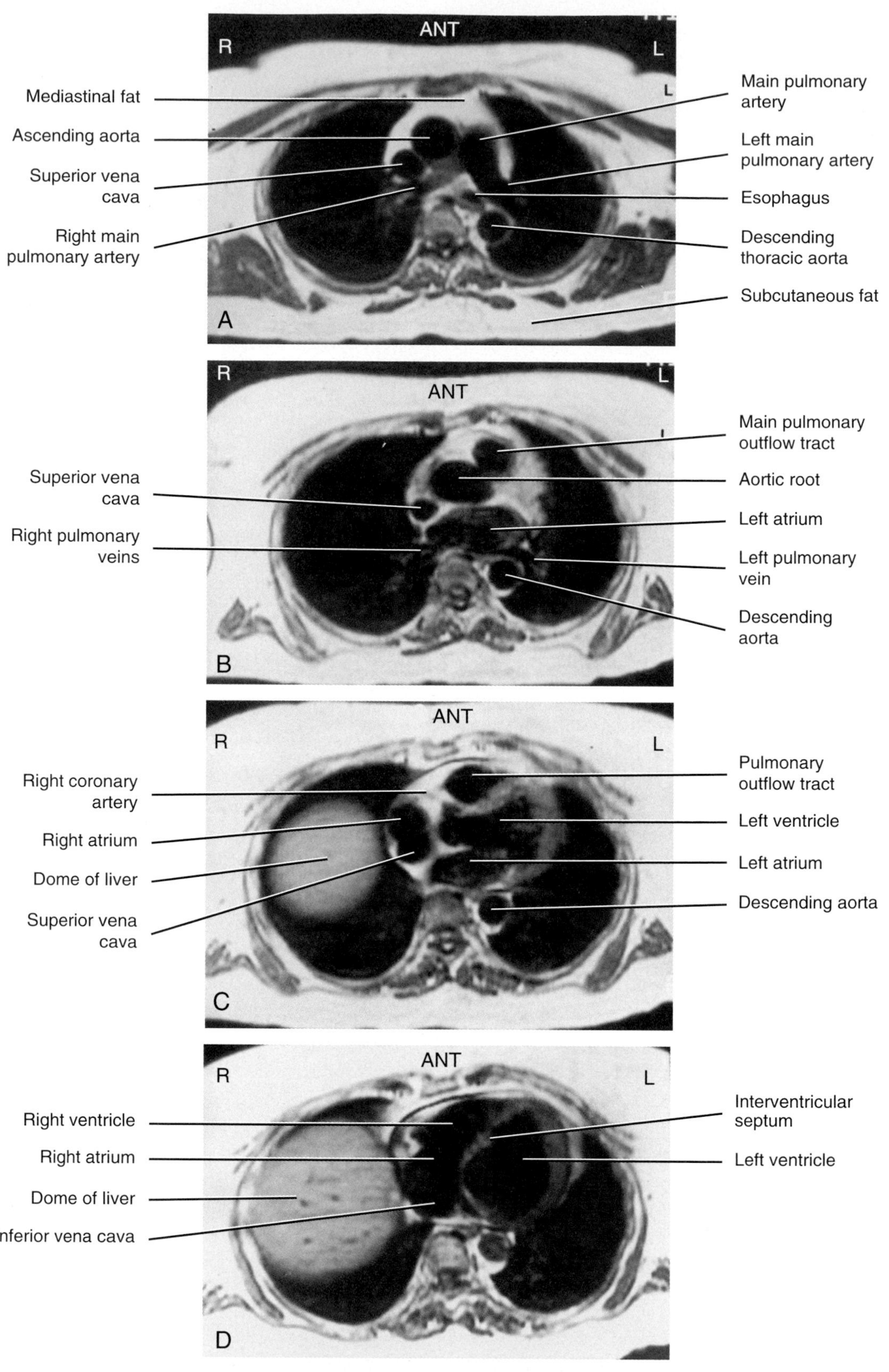

FIGURE 5-1 ■ Transverse (axial) T1-weighted magnetic resonance images *A* to *D* of the thorax in the transverse plane showing normal vascular anatomy.

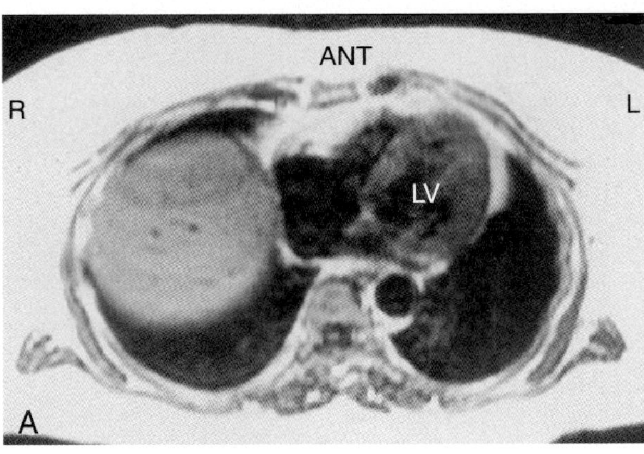

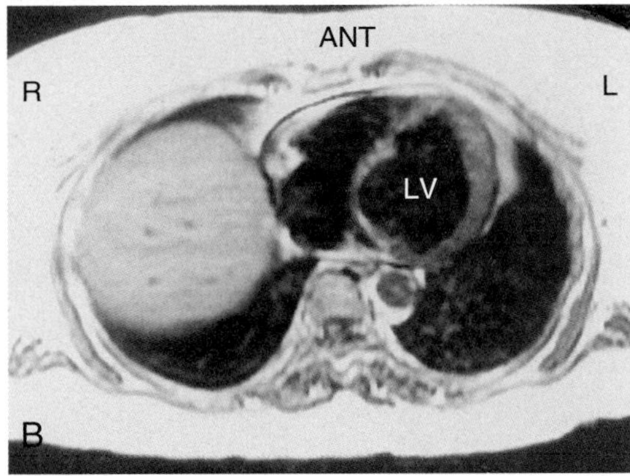

FIGURE 5-2 ■ Magnetic resonance (MR) images of the heart in systole and diastole. Transverse images obtained at the level of the right and left ventricle (LV) show the left ventricle in systole *(A)* and in diastole *(B)*.

TABLE 5–1 ■ **Appropriate Imaging and Other Studies for Cardiovascular Problems**

Clinical Problem	Imaging Study
Most cardiac problems	Initial posteroanterior and lateral chest radiography
Congestive heart failure (new or worse)	Chest radiography and ejection fraction; wall motion evaluation by nuclear medicine or echocardiography
Congestive heart failure (chronic)	Chest radiography
Hypertension (suspected essential)	No imaging indicated
Hypertension (suspected renal artery stenosis)	Nuclear medicine captopril renogram or magnetic resonance angiogram
Left ventricular ejection fraction	Gated nuclear medicine blood pool study or echocardiography
Chest pain or shortness of breath (suspected pulmonary embolism)	Chest radiography and nuclear medicine ventilation/perfusion scan
Shortness of breath (suspected cardiac origin)	Chest radiography and echocardiography or nuclear medicine myocardial perfusion study
Acute chest pain (suspected myocardial infarction [6 hours])	Electrocardiography, chest radiography, and coronary angiography
Chronic chest pain (suspected cardiac origin)	Electrocardiography, chest radiography, nuclear medicine myocardial perfusion or coronary angiogram
Coronary ischemia	Electrocardiography; if negative then stress electrocardiogram, nuclear medicine, myocardial perfusion study, or stress echocardiogram; if positive, then coronary angiogram
Congenital heart disease	Chest radiography, echocardiography, or cardiac catheterization
Endocarditis	Echocardiography
Valvular disease	Echocardiography
Pericardial effusion	Echocardiography
Constrictive pericarditis	Echocardiography, if equivocal then computed tomography
Aortic trauma	Angiography or computed tomography with contrast
Thoracic aortic dissection	Computed tomography with contrast or transesophageal ultrasonography
Abdominal aortic aneurysm	Computed tomography with contrast if symptomatic; ultrasonography for screening or follow-up
Deep venous thrombosis	Duplex ultrasonography
Carotid bruit	Duplex ultrasonography; if high-grade stenosis, then contrast angiography
Claudication	Doppler ultrasonography of lower extremity

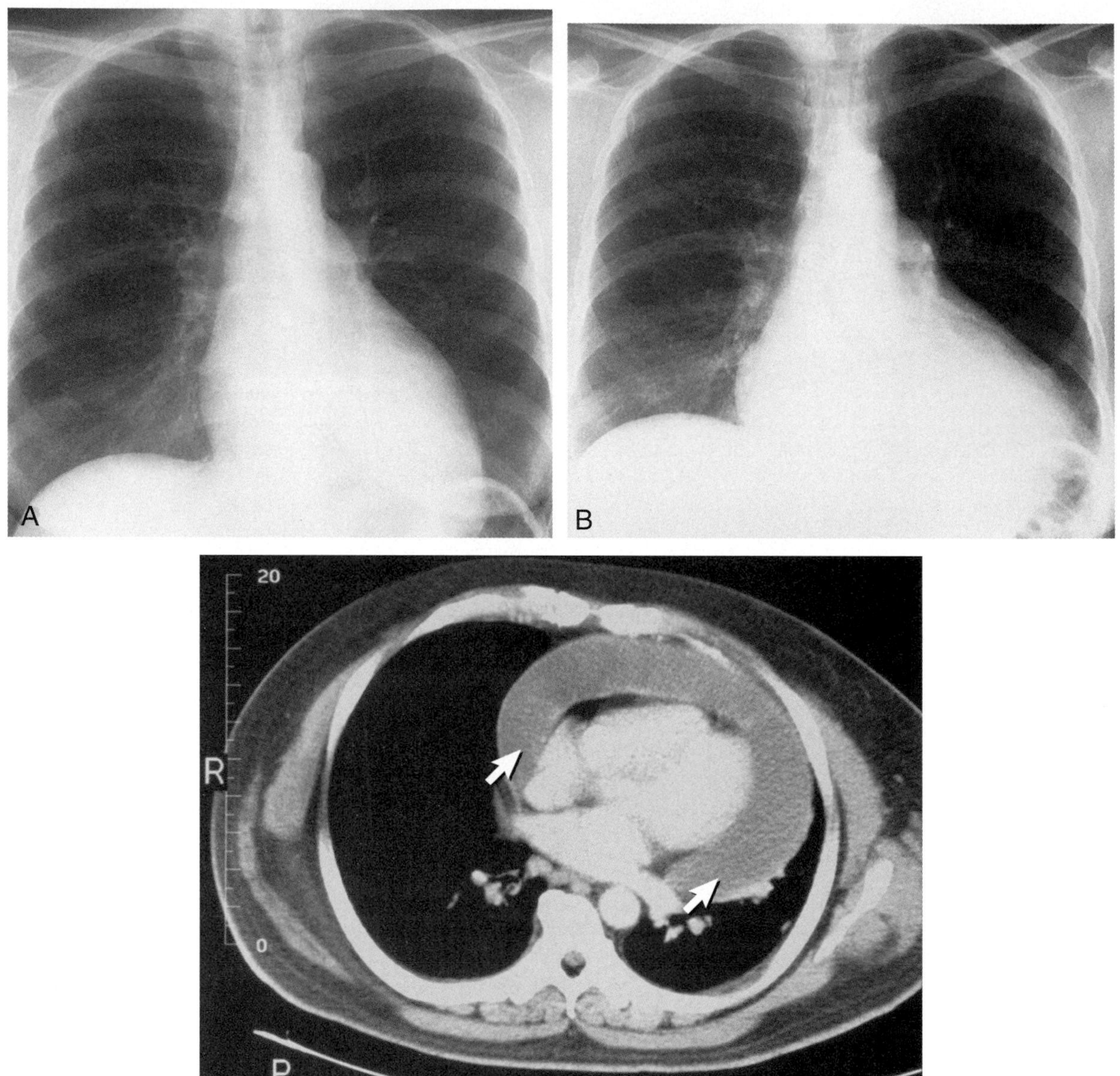

FIGURE 5-3 ■ Pericardial effusion. In a patient with a viral syndrome, a posteroanterior chest x-ray *(A)* shows mild cardiomegaly with prominence of the left cardiac border. One week later *(B)*, a marked and sudden increase in the transverse diameter of the heart due to a pericardial effusion is apparent. A definitive diagnosis is best made by using cardiac ultrasound. Pericardial effusions also can be seen on computed tomography (CT) scans *(C)* as a fluid density surrounding the heart.

pericarditis will have pericardial calcification (which may be visible only on CT), and 60% will have a pleural effusion. Of those patients with pericardial calcification, 50% also will have constrictive pericarditis.

Cardiomegaly can be due to valvular disease, cardiomyopathy, congenital heart disease, pericardial effusion, and mass lesions. Cardiomyopathies and pericardial effusions both generally lead to symmetrical enlargement, whereas valvular disease and congenital heart disease often have specific chamber enlargement. The dilated cardiomyopathies are caused by ineffective contraction during systole and most commonly result from infections and metabolic disorders. They also may be caused by collagen vascular disease and

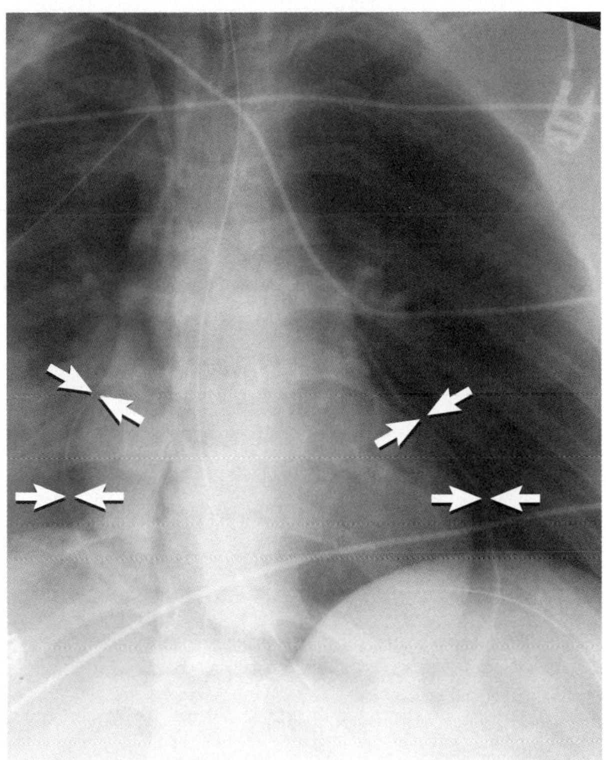

FIGURE 5-4 ■ Pneumopercardium. On this chest x-ray, the pericardium *(arrows)* is outlined by air between the pericardium and heart and air in the lungs. Note that the pericardium does not extend above the level of the pulmonary arteries. This helps distinguish pneumopericardium from pneumomediastinum.

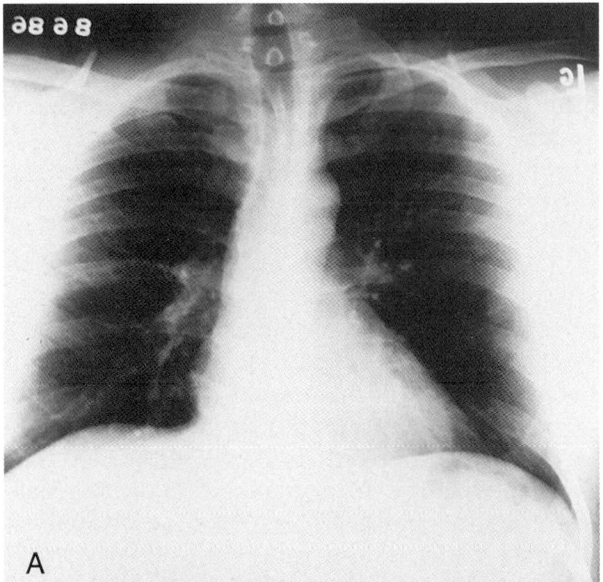

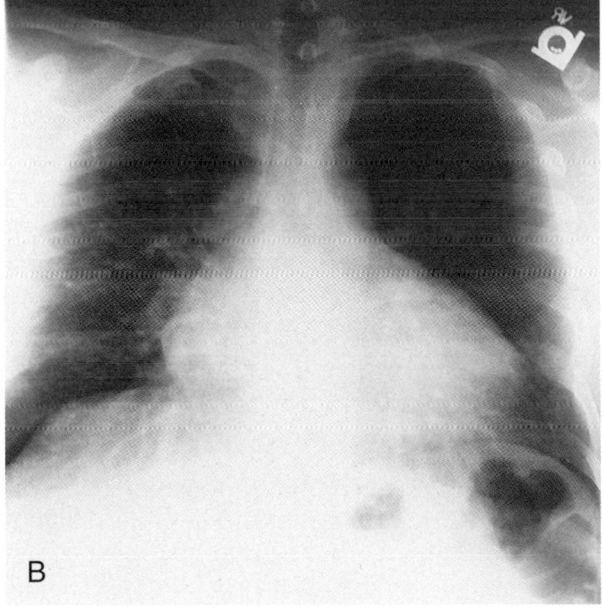

FIGURE 5-5 ■ Cardiomyopathy. In this case, cardiomyopathy is due to cancer chemotherapy with doxorubicin. An initial chest x-ray *(A)* demonstrates a normal-sized heart. After several therapeutic courses of doxorubicin *(B)*, marked enlargement in the cardiac silhouette is due to multichamber dilatation.

toxic agents such as alcohol and chemotherapeutic drugs. An example of the latter is doxorubicin, one of the most widely used chemotherapeutic agents (Fig. 5-5).

Use of the cardiothoracic ratio to assess heart size and the effect of cardiac failure on the appearance of the pulmonary vessels and lungs was discussed in Chapter 3. The width of the heart should not exceed half the width of the chest at its widest point. This measurement is reliable only on an upright posteroanterior (PA) chest film; on an anteroposterior (AP) chest x-ray, the heart will often exceed this measurement owing to magnification. On a supine film, even more magnification and high position of the hemidiaphragms occur. This high position will push the heart upward and outward, making it appear wide. A note of caution should be inserted here about patients who have chronic obstructive pulmonary disease (COPD). The shape of the heart is determined by external forces and by internal factors. One factor relates to the level of the hemidiaphragms. The measurement of cardiothoracic ratio assumes that the hemidiaphragms are in normal position. With COPD, the hemidiaphragms are driven inferiorly (often to the level of the posterior twelfth rib). The heart then sags and elongates. This can make an enlarged heart appear normal in size, especially considering the cardiothoracic ratio. It follows, then, that if the heart appears too wide in a patient who has COPD, it is really very large.

Because assessment of cardiac function by chest x-ray is rather poor, quantitative evaluations of cardiac ejection fraction are usually made by nuclear medicine gated blood pool (MUGA) or gated single-photon emission CT (SPECT) studies or by echocardiography. In the nuclear medicine MUGA procedure, red cells are labeled with radioactive material, and images of the heart are obtained in a gated fashion. Computer analysis enables construction of a time/activity curve showing the amount of activity in the left or right ventricle in both diastole and systole, allowing calculation of an ejection fraction. The normal left ventricular ejection fraction (LVEF) is between 55% and 75%. In older persons, the lower limit of LVEF is probably about 50%. With both the nuclear medicine gated SPECT study (Fig. 5-6) and echocardiography, visualization of the myocardium occurs. The ventricular cavity is then measured at various portions of the cardiac cycle, and the ejection fraction is calculated. All of these studies also can detect regional wall-motion abnormalities.

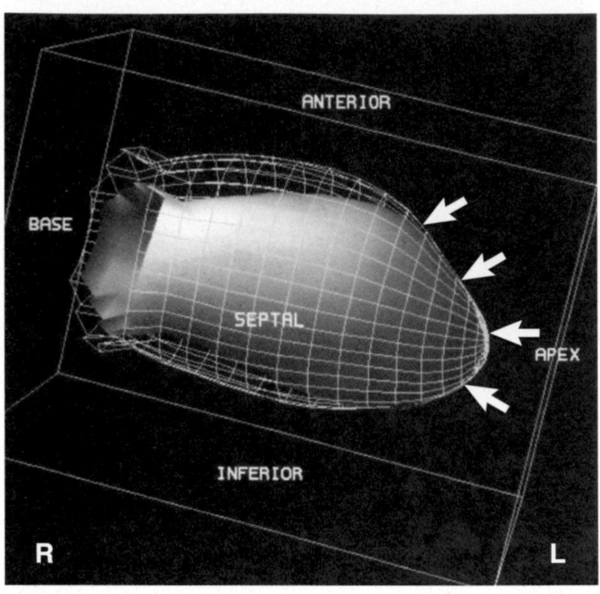

FIGURE 5-6 ■ Measurement of cardiac ejection fraction and regional wall motion. A nuclear medicine technique in which myocardium is visualized allows the computer to construct a view of the heart and, by inference, the cavity of the left ventricle. When the data are acquired in conjunction with an electrocardiogram, an image can be derived that shows the outline of the ventricular cavity at diastole *(the mesh outline)* and at systole *(the gray center)*. In this patient, poor wall motion of the distal anterior wall and apex is seen *(arrows)*.

Left Atrial Enlargement

Isolated left atrial enlargement occurs most commonly in mitral stenosis. The earliest sign is displacement of the esophagus posteriorly (Fig. 5-7*A*). Enlargement of the left atrial appendage on the PA view is the next sign to appear (Fig. 5-7*B*). As the left atrium enlarges further, the esophagus becomes more posteriorly displaced; splaying or widening of the inferior carinal angle is seen; and the enlarged left atrium can be seen on the PA x-ray as a double density behind the heart and below the carina (Fig. 5-7*C*). The normal inferior carinal angle should not exceed 75 degrees.

Rheumatic heart disease most often affects the mitral valve and to a lesser extent the aortic valve. The classic appearance of a mitral heart on a PA chest x-ray is easily recognized by four bumps along the left cardiac border. This also is sometimes called the "ski mogul" heart. Going from superior to inferior, the bumps represent the aortic arch, pulmonary artery, left atrium, and left ventricle (Fig. 5-7*B*). Left atrial enlargement also is seen with congenital cardiac lesions that have intracardiac shunts, as well as in patients who have left ventricular failure.

As rheumatic heart disease progresses, mitral stenosis and mitral insufficiency develop. The heart becomes very large because of dilatation and hypertrophy of the left ventricle. In the combined form of mitral disease, the left atrium becomes even larger than is seen in mitral stenosis alone. Typical findings are a straightening of the left cardiac border due to left atrial enlargement; left ventricular enlargement as evidenced by leftward and downward displacement of the cardiac apex; and, if left ventricular dilatation becomes massive, rightward displacement of the

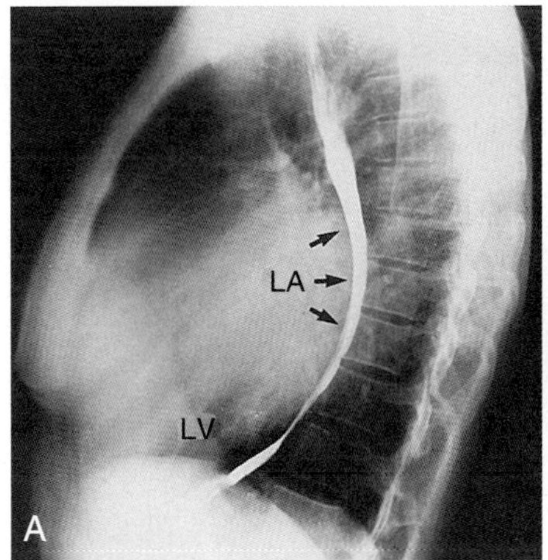

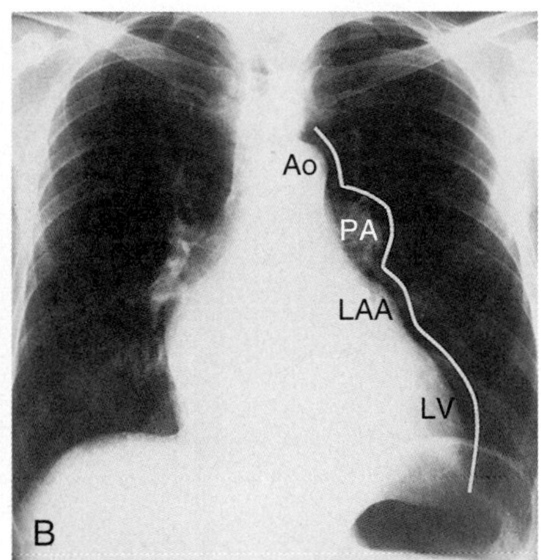

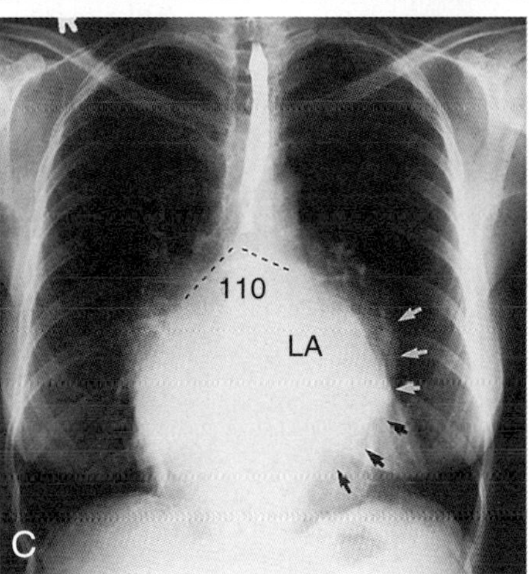

FIGURE 5-7 ■ Mitral stenosis. One of the earliest signs of mitral stenosis is left atrial (LA) enlargement, which can be seen on the lateral view of the chest *(A)*. The left atrium can be seen displacing the barium-filled esophagus posteriorly. A somewhat later finding on a posteroanterior chest x-ray *(B)* is the four-bump or "ski mogul" heart. The four bumps are created by the aorta (Ao), pulmonary artery (PA), left atrial appendage (LAA), and left ventricle (LV). The left atrial appendage normally does not bulge out. Very late findings of left atrial enlargement on the posteroanterior chest x-ray *(C)* are a double density behind the heart *(arrows)* and splaying of the subcarinal angle, which normally does not measure more than 75 degrees.

right ventricle. On the lateral view, in addition to the obvious left atrial enlargement, the posterior displacement of the heart continues down inferiorly, indicating left ventricular enlargement as well. In severe mitral disease, the mitral valve and the aortic and tricuspid valves are affected. In general, the manifestations of the more proximal valve lesion are the most prominent. With mitral and tricuspid disease, enlargement of the left atrium and left ventricle and also of the right atrium and right ventricle occurs.

Many radiologists say that you cannot differentiate right atrial from right ventricular enlargement on a chest x-ray, and this is probably true. Fortunately, in most adults, when one of the right chambers is enlarged, so is the other. On the frontal chest x-ray, right atrial enlargement is suggested by an increased convexity of the right heart border. Isolated right ventricular enlargement is very difficult to appreciate, because it overlaps the right atrium and left ventricle on the frontal view. On the lateral view, both right ventricular and right atrial enlargement will cause a filling in of the anterior clear space behind the sternum (Fig. 5-8). Normally on the lateral view, the anterior portion of the heart fills in only approximately one third or less of the anterior clear space, unless enlargement of the right atrium or right ventricle is found.

Prosthetic tricuspid and mitral valves are often used in treatment of rheumatic heart disease. You should be able to recognize these valves by their size, location, and orientation (Fig. 5-9). The valve with the largest area is the tricuspid valve; the mitral valve is intermediate sized, and the smallest is the aortic valve. You

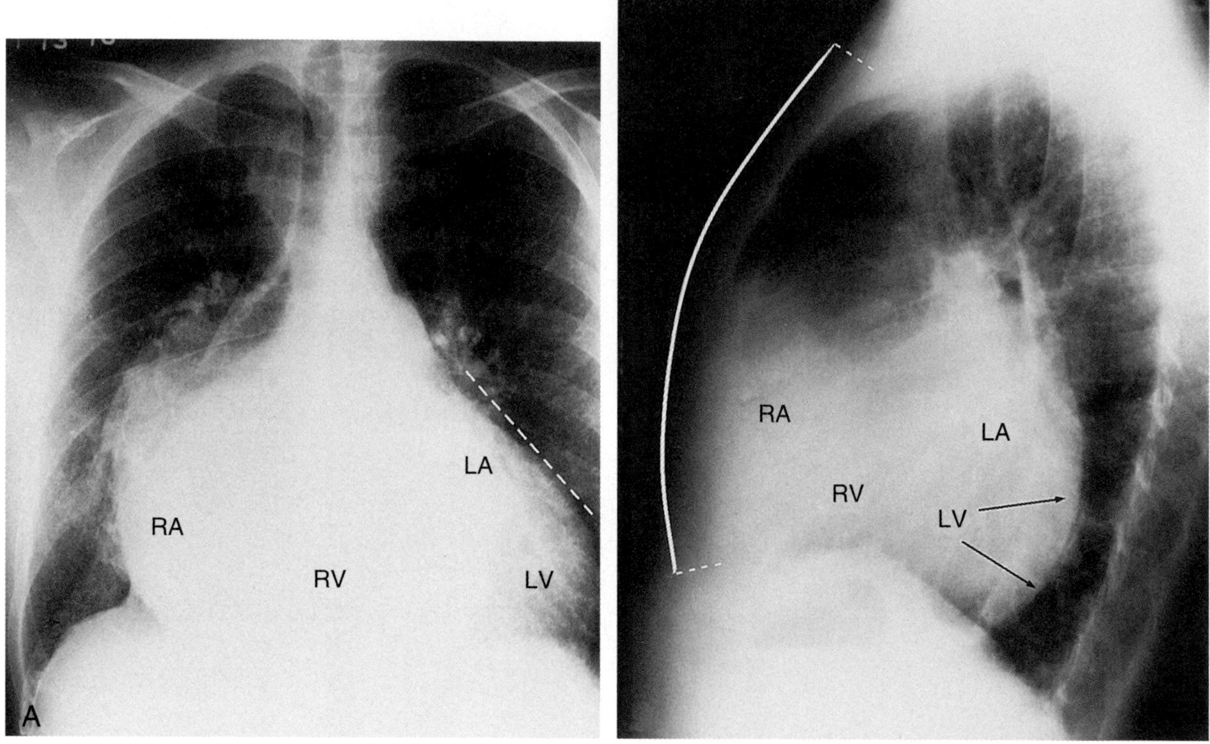

FIGURE 5-8 ■ Mitral and tricuspid insufficiency. As a late finding in rheumatic heart disease, mitral and sometimes tricuspid insufficiency develops. On the posteroanterior chest x-ray *(A),* there is marked enlargement of not only the left atrium (LA) but also the left ventricle (LV; seen as straightening of the left cardiac border) as well as right-sided enlargement, particularly of the right atrium (RA; seen by marked prominence of the right cardiac border). On the lateral view of the chest *(B),* the left ventricle can be seen overlapping the spine, and the right atrium and right ventricle (RV) have filled in the retrosternal space to more than the usual lower one third.

also should be able to recognize prosthetic mitral and tricuspid valves. As expected, the mitral valve is located posteriorly and to the left in the heart, and the tricuspid valve is anterior and toward the right side.

Left Ventricular Enlargement

On a frontal chest x-ray, left ventricular enlargement, as already mentioned, produces a round left cardiac border as well as downward displacement of the apex. On the lateral view, the posterior aspect of the heart, where it intersects the hemidiaphragm, is usually posteriorly displaced behind the inferior vena cava. The Hoffman-Rigler sign also can be used. To use this, find the intersection of the inferior vena cava with the hemidiaphragm on the lateral film, and then measure 2 cm up and 2 cm back. If the heart projects posteriorly, left ventricular enlargement probably is present. A note of caution should be inserted here because an enlarged right heart can sometimes push the left ventricle back. To exclude this, look at the space behind the sternum: only the lower one third should be filled by soft tissue.

Left ventricular dilatation can be due to a number of causes, including coronary artery disease, aortic stenosis, and aortic regurgitation. You should take care to consider the possibility of a left ventricular aneurysm before you suggest left ventricular enlargement and quit. Ventricular aneurysms most commonly occur near the apex and anteriorly and have a high rate of mortality. Left ventricular hypertrophy is difficult to detect radiographically. It may be

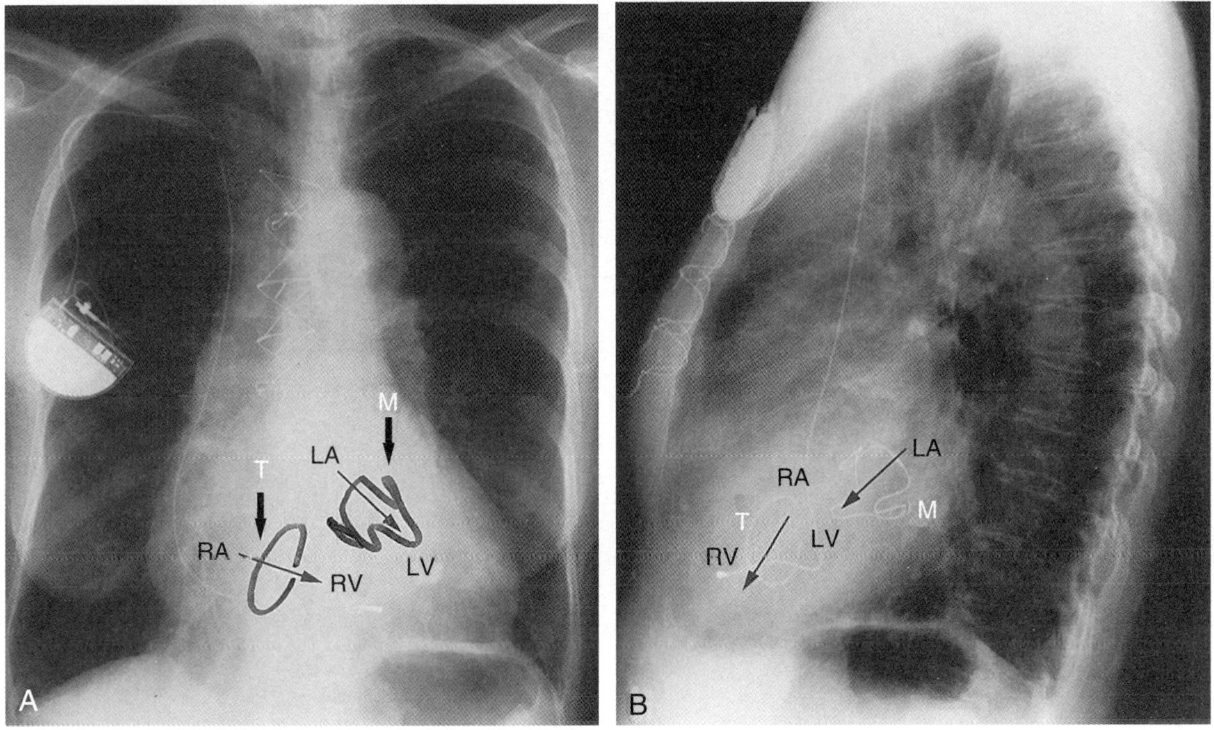

FIGURE 5-9 ■ Prosthetic mitral and tricuspid valves. Both the mitral (M) and the tricuspid (T) valves were difficult to appreciate on the posteroanterior view of the chest *(A)* and were, therefore, drawn in. They are easily seen on the lateral view *(B)* in the expected regions between the left atrium (LA) and left ventricle (LV) and the right atrium (RA) and right ventricle (RV). Also note that a cardiac pacer comes down the superior vena cava through the right atrium and into the right ventricle. These two valves are normally relatively large because of relatively low pressure gradients across these valves.

present in patients who have a normal cardiac configuration on chest x-ray. If this is suspected, a cardiac echo (ultrasound) is the test of choice.

Aortic Stenosis and Insufficiency

Aortic stenosis is most commonly valvular, although in a smaller number of patients, it may be either subvalvular or supravalvular. Valvular stenosis can be due to rheumatic heart disease, a bicuspid (rather than tricuspid) aortic valve, or degenerative changes (usually in patients older than 70 years). It may be difficult to detect this condition from findings on a plain film of the chest, and sometimes the only finding is a calcified aortic valve. Initially, with aortic stenosis, left ventricular hypertrophy is noted. The heart will be normal in size and may show slight rounding of the cardiac apex. When left ventricular dilatation occurs, the left cardiac border elongates, and the apex of the heart moves downward toward the left hemidiaphragm. The aortic knob will be normal in size, although the ascending aortic arch is enlarged, causing a convexity of the right upper cardiac margin. The enlargement of the ascending aorta is due to poststenotic dilatation.

With aortic insufficiency, the left ventricle becomes much larger, and on a PA chest x-ray, the apex of the heart may project below the most superior portion of the left hemidiaphragm. The ascending aorta still shows some enlargement (Fig. 5-10). Prosthetic aortic valves are relatively easy to recognize by their relatively small size and the fact that they are located at the root of the ascending aorta (Fig. 5-11).

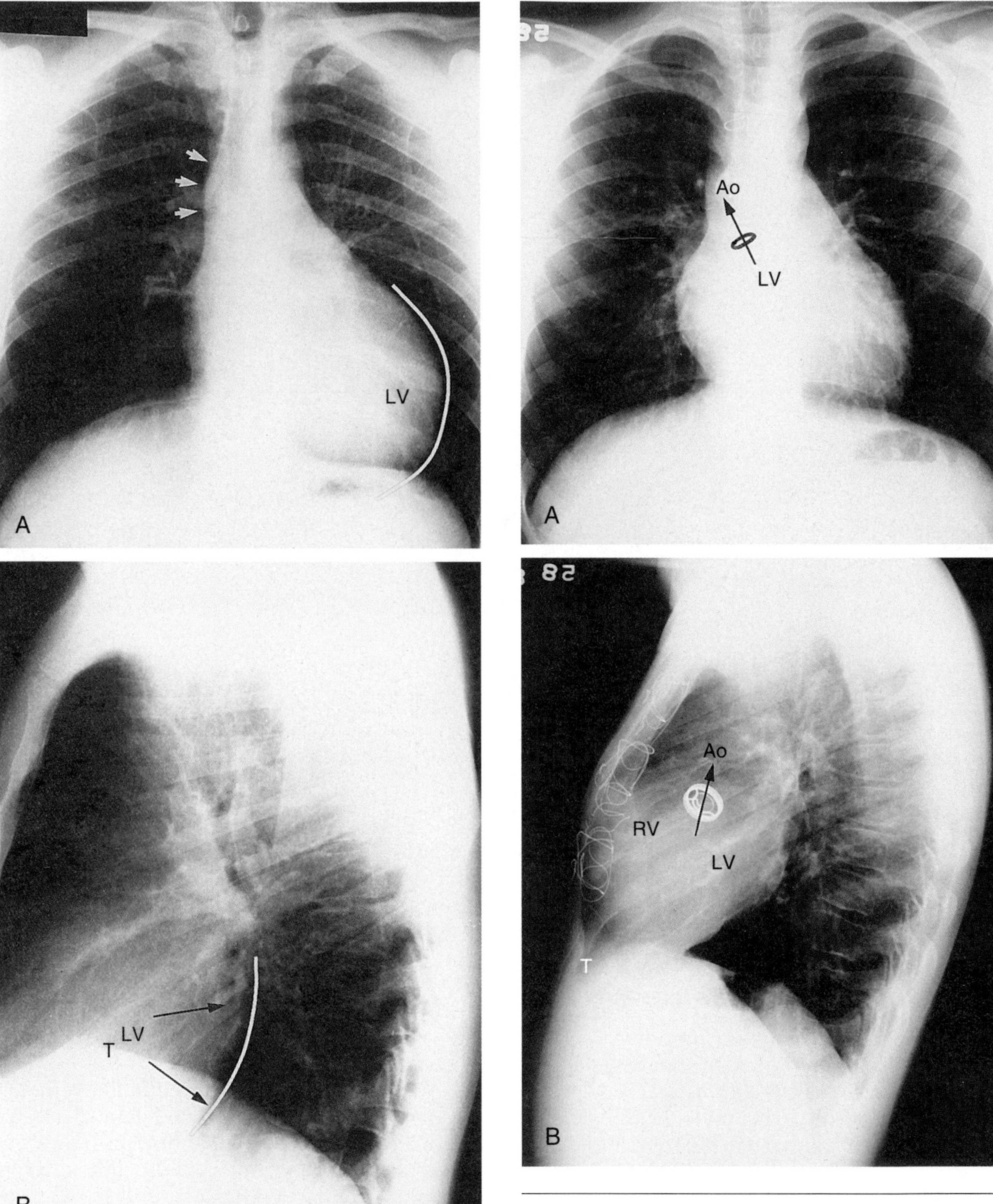

FIGURE 5-10 ■ **Aortic insufficiency.** A very prominent left ventricle (LV) is seen both on the posteroanterior view *(A)* and the lateral view *(B)*. In addition, a convexity appears in the region of the ascending aorta *(arrows)* because of poststenotic dilatation.

FIGURE 5-11 ■ **Prosthetic aortic valve.** The prosthetic valve was not easily visible on the posteroanterior view *(A)* and was, therefore, drawn in. On the lateral view *(B)*, the valve is easily seen in the expected region between the left ventricle (LV) and the ascending aorta (Ao). Also note its relatively small size. The *arrows* indicate the direction of blood flow.

Pulmonary Artery Enlargement

Enlargement of the pulmonary artery is fairly easy to recognize on the PA chest x-ray by a bulging along the left cardiac border just below the aortic arch (Fig. 5-12). Pulmonary artery enlargement can be due to a number of causes, but probably the three most common are pulmonic stenosis (with poststenotic dilatation), pulmonary artery hypertension, and abnormalities in which increased flow through the pulmonary artery occurs, such as a patent ductus arteriosus or an atrial septal defect (ASD).

If enlargement of both the left and the right main pulmonary arteries is present, consider the diagnosis of pulmonary arterial hypertension. In this entity, in addition to the very large central pulmonary arteries, rapid "pruning" of the vessels occurs as they proceed peripherally in the lung. Even though the central vessels are very large, it is unusual to be able to see vessels at the very edge of the lung. Pulmonary hypertension may be due to a number of causes, including atrial septal defect (ASD) and ventricular septal defect (VSD), patent ductus arteriosus, arteriovenous shunt, left ventricular failure, mitral valve disease, pulmonary emboli, parenchymal lung disease, COPD, and other less common entities.

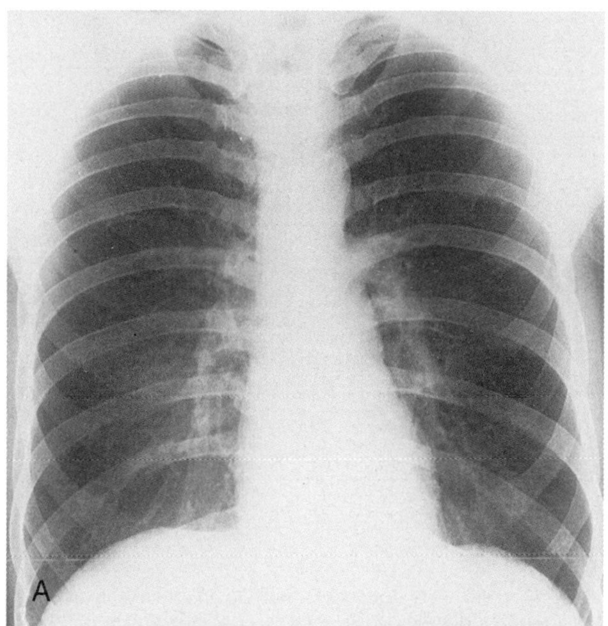

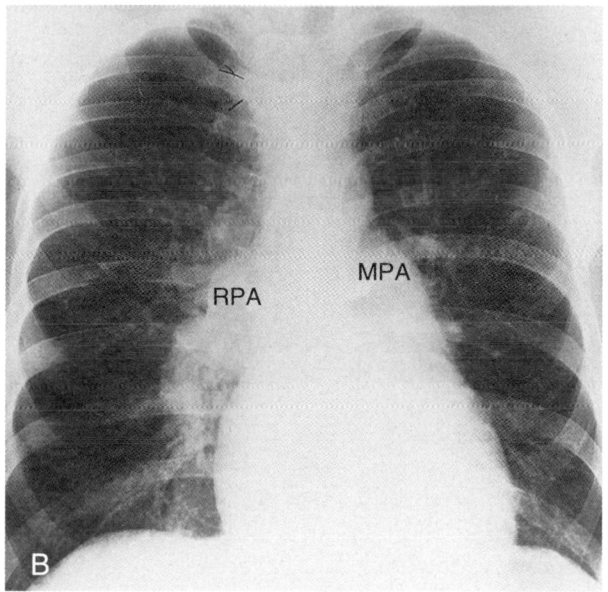

FIGURE 5-12 ■ Progressive pulmonary arterial hypertension. This patient initially was seen with a relatively normal chest x-ray *(A)*. However, several years later *(B)*, increasing heart size as well as marked dilatation of the main pulmonary artery (MPA) and right pulmonary artery (RPA) is noted. Rapid tapering of the arteries as they proceed peripherally is suggestive of pulmonary hypertension and is sometimes referred to as "pruning."

CONGENITAL CARDIAC DISEASE

Rather than including every entity, I present a few examples here to give you an approach to interpretation. Several very important factors to assess in the evaluation of congenital cardiac disease include the age of the individual; the clinical findings, such as murmurs; whether the patient is cyanotic or acyanotic; specific chamber enlargement; and pulmonary vascularity (increased, decreased, or normal).

Probably the easiest place to begin is in the determination of whether or not the individual is cyanotic. A cyanotic infant who has normal or decreased pulmonary vascularity and a normal heart size probably has a tetralogy of Fallot. Tetralogy of Fallot includes pulmonic stenosis, VSD, an overriding aorta, and right

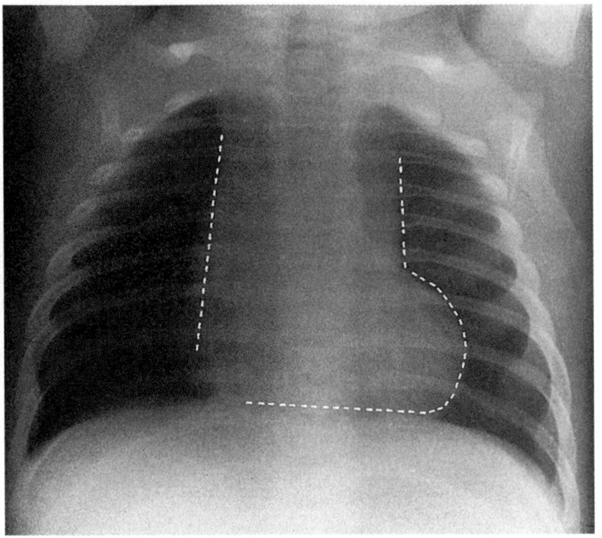

FIGURE 5-13 ■ **Tetralogy of Fallot.** On an anteroposterior view of the chest, the heart is shaped like a boot seen from the side. This is due to the uplifted apex of the heart. Also note that a concavity appears on the left cardiac border and decreased pulmonary vascularity.

ventricular hypertrophy. On the x-ray, usually decreased pulmonary vascularity and a boot-shaped heart with an uplifted apex and a concavity along the left cardiac border is seen (Fig. 5-13). If cardiomegaly with the right atrium enlarged is noted, the differential diagnosis includes Ebstein's malformation, tricuspid atresia, and pulmonic atresia. In Ebstein's anomaly, a giant right atrium appears, with a shoulder along the right side of the heart and a very small pulmonary artery. In this entity, downward displacement of the tricuspid valve occurs, with the right ventricle being partially atrialized (Fig. 5-14).

Cyanotic heart disease with increased pulmonary vascularity includes transposition of the great vessels (which is most common), truncus arteriosus, total anomalous pulmonary venous return (TAPVR), tricuspid atresia, and a single ventricle. Radiographic features of transposition of the great vessels include a heart that is said to have an "egg-on-side" shape and a narrow superior mediastinum secondary to a hypoplastic thymus (Fig. 5-15).

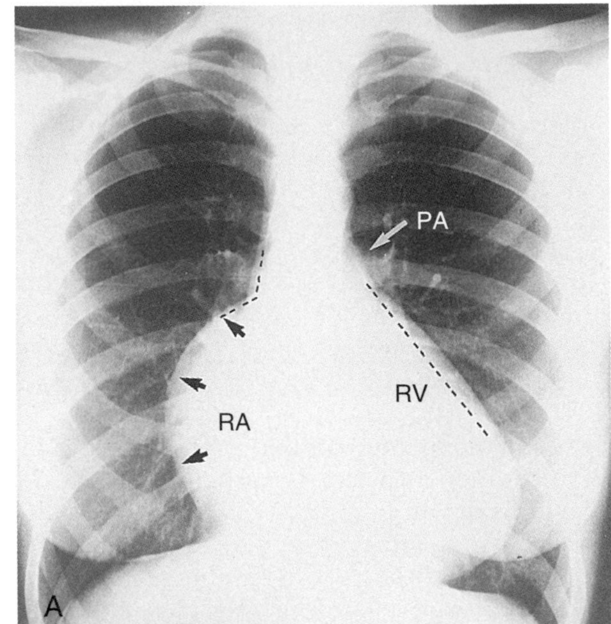

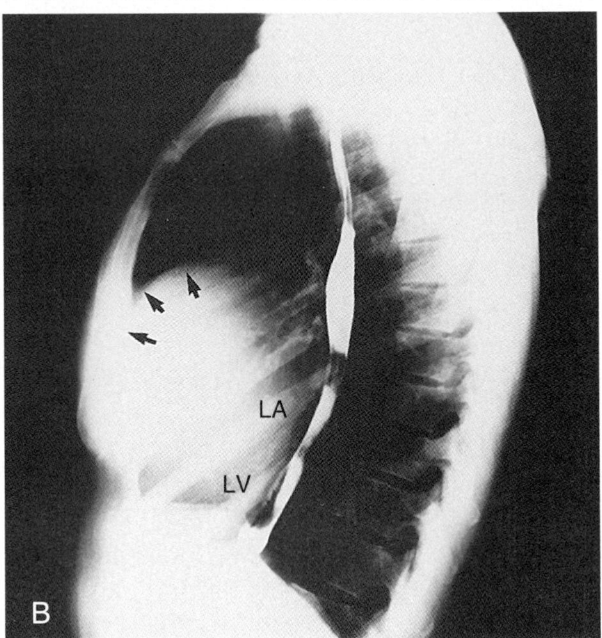

FIGURE 5-14 ■ **Ebstein's anomaly.** On the posteroanterior view of the heart *(A),* a giant right atrium (RA) causes a shoulder along the right cardiac silhouette. A giant right ventricular (RV) outflow tract causes the left cardiac border to be straight, and the pulmonary artery (PA) is very small. On the lateral view *(B),* the left atrium (LA) and left ventricle (LV) are essentially normal, but the right atrium and right ventricle are filling in the retrosternal space *(arrows).*

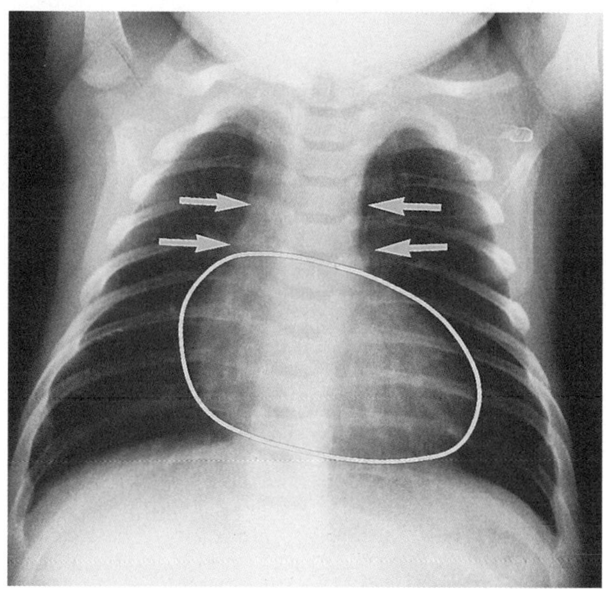

FIGURE 5-15 ■ Transposition of the great vessels. With this entity, the heart is classically described as looking like an "egg lying on its side." A very narrow vascular pedicle or upper mediastinum *(arrows)* is seen, and pulmonary vascularity is usually increased.

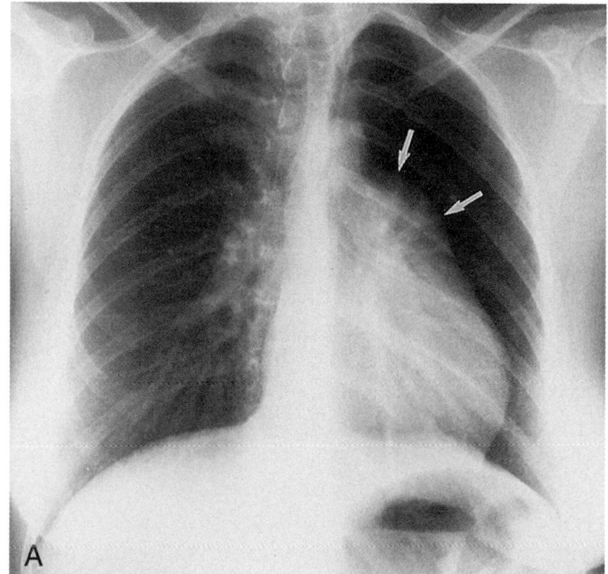

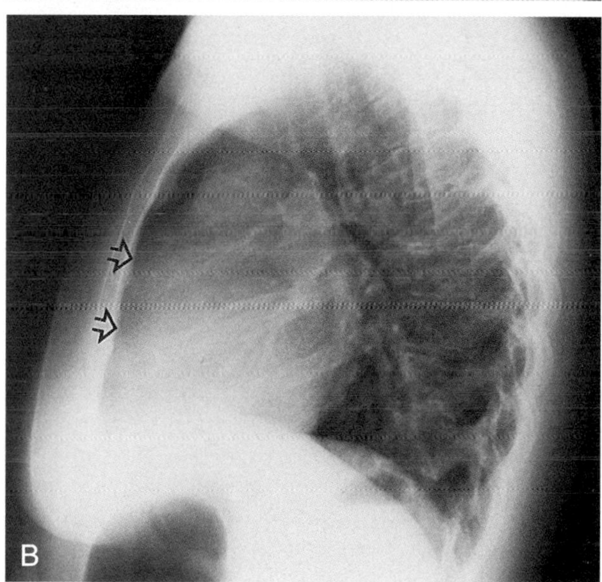

FIGURE 5-16 ■ Atrial septal defect. Extra blood flow from the left side of the heart back to the right side increases the size of the main pulmonary artery (seen best on the posteroanterior chest x-ray) *(A)*. An increase in the size of the right ventricle is noted (seen best on the lateral view [*B*] as soft tissue filling in the lower and middle retrosternal space).

Acyanotic congenital heart disease similarly should initially be evaluated by determination of pulmonary vascularity. In those with normal vascularity, aortic stenosis, pulmonic stenosis, coarctation, and interruption of the aortic arch should be considered. Acyanotic heart disease with increased pulmonary vascularity should next be investigated by looking for left atrial enlargement. This is not present in ASD, and an endocardial cushion defect may be considered.

An ASD is the most common congenital cardiac anomaly in adults and rarely is symptomatic in infancy or childhood. The common radiologic findings in an ASD, in addition to enlargement of the pulmonary artery, are an increase in the size of the right atrium and right ventricle. This is often best seen as filling in of the retrosternal clear space on the lateral view (Fig. 5-16). The imaging modality of choice, if an ASD is suspected, is echocardiography.

If acyanotic heart disease with increased pulmonary vascularity and left atrial enlargement is found, next look at the aorta. If the aorta is enlarged, a patent ductus arteriosus should be suspected, because excess blood flow through the aortic arch is shunted to the pulmonary arteries. If the aorta is not enlarged, consider a VSD.

PULMONARY EMBOLISM

Pulmonary embolism (PE) is a potentially fatal entity. Typical symptoms include dyspnea (80%), tachypnea (>16 respirations per minute, 80%) pleuritic chest pain (70%), rales (60%), fever (45%), tachycardia (40%), and hemoptysis (20%). Patients who initially have no dyspnea, pleuritic chest pain, or tachypnea are unlikely to have a PE. A low-grade fever may occur with PE, but a high-grade fever and leukocytosis suggest a pneumonia. About 35% of patients with PE will also have clinically evident phlebitis. The converse is more important, however; that is, about two thirds of patients with PE will not show evidence of phlebitis.

The chest x-ray findings in a patient with PEs are relatively nonspecific, and the major reason for ordering a chest x-ray is to exclude other causes of the patient's symptoms. Occasionally a small pleural effusion, atelectasis, or an elevated hemidiaphragm may be present. If infarction of a portion of the lung is a result of the embolism, a wedge-shaped infiltrate may be noted (Fig. 5-17).

After a chest x-ray, the next study to be performed is a nuclear medicine ventilation/perfusion (V/Q) lung scan or a contrasted CT scan. In the nuclear medicine study, ventilation is assessed by having the patient inhale and then exhale a radioactive gas or an aerosol containing radioactive particles (Fig. 5-18*A*). Perfusion is assessed by intravenously injecting a number of biodegradable radioactive particles that are unable to pass through the pulmonary capillary bed. These are trapped in the capillary bed, and because they give off radiation, images of the lungs can be obtained in various projections (Fig. 5-18*B*). The V/Q lung scans are then compared. You are looking for a defect on the perfusion scan that is not seen on the ventilation scan (a mismatch). The reason is that a PE generally does not interfere much with ventilation. Abnormalities such as tumors and bullae would cause both a ventilation abnormality and a perfusion abnormality (a matched defect).

If a number of segmental defects are seen on the perfusion scan and are not identified on the ventilation scan, the images will be interpreted as high probability for PE. Under these circumstances, it is more than 80% likely that the patient has PE. Rarely is there any need to perform pulmonary angiography on a patient with a high-probability scan, unless a significant contraindication to anticoagulation exists.

A correlation can be made between the likelihood of PE based on the size of an infiltrate seen

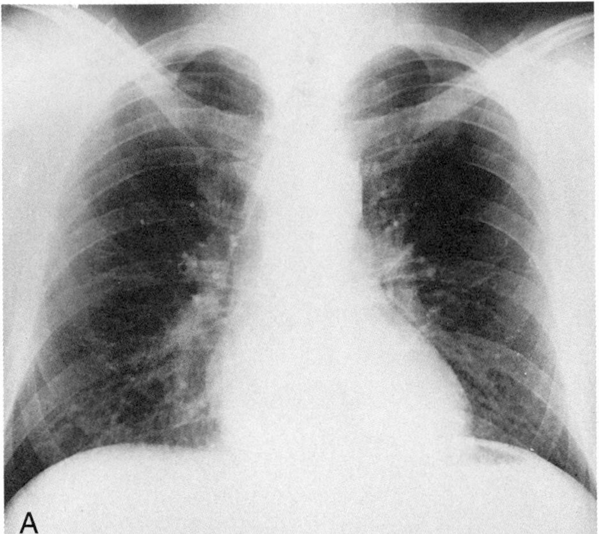

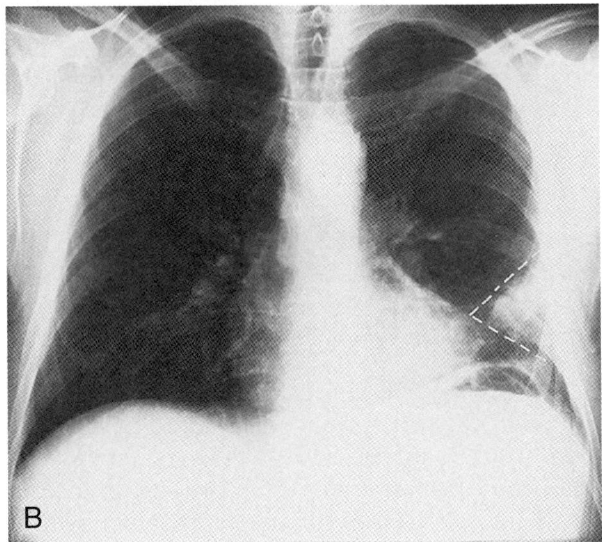

FIGURE 5-17 ■ Pulmonary embolism and infarction. Immediately after an acute episode of shortness of breath due to a pulmonary embolism, the posteroanterior chest x-ray is essentially normal *(A)*. If the pulmonary embolism actually leads to infarction, a peripheral wedge-shaped infiltrate develops *(B)*.

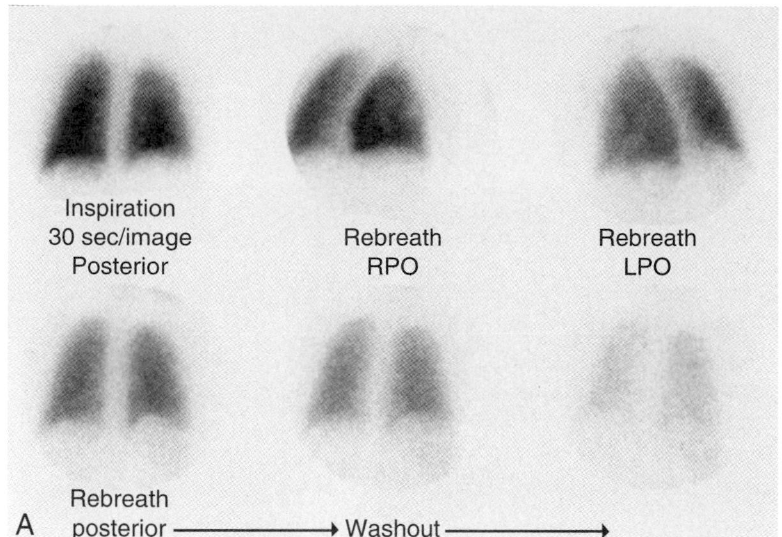

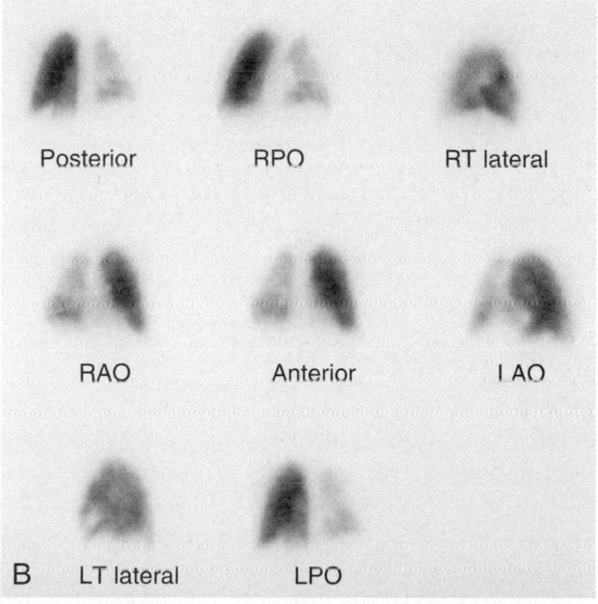

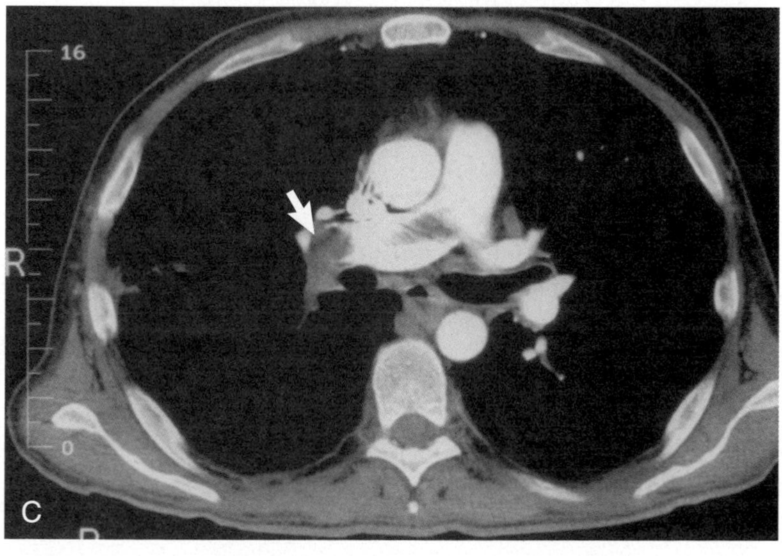

FIGURE 5-18 ■ Large central pulmonary embolism. A nuclear medicine ventilation scan *(A)*, done with a short-lived radioactive gas, shows normal ventilation of both lungs. This was followed with a nuclear medicine perfusion scan *(B)* that shows decreased perfusion of the right lung compared with the left. A contrast-enhanced computed tomography (CT) scan of the chest *(C)* shows the pulmonary artery with a large clot *(arrow)* obstructing the right main pulmonary artery. RPO, right posterior oblique; LPO, left PO.

on the chest x-ray and the size of a defect seen on a nuclear medicine lung-perfusion study. An embolus typically has a larger area of nonperfusion than the size of the resultant infiltrate. If an infiltrate is seen on the chest x-ray, it represents infarcted lung. With a pneumonia, usually a large area of infiltrate is noted on the chest x-ray, but on the perfusion lung scan, the area of decreased perfusion is relatively smaller. If the perfusion defect and the infiltrate are almost the same size, the probability of PE is intermediate.

The advent of fast spiral and multidetector CT scanners has allowed evaluation of PEs. Scanning is done with a bolus of intravenous contrast. The images must be correctly timed to have contrast in the pulmonary arteries at the time of imaging. Hard-copy images are somewhat difficult to interpret, and usually the radiologist will view the images on a workstation to allow rapid paging back and forth. Large emboli are easily seen (Fig. 5-18*C*), but small peripheral emboli are significantly more difficult to diagnose.

If nuclear medicine scans or CT scans are equivocal and if a patient has positive tests for deep venous thrombosis, and clinical suspicion is high, the individual usually is treated. If tests for deep venous thrombosis are negative, yet clinical suspicion remains high, then pulmonary angiography is sometimes performed (Fig 5-19). Some clinicians believe that in a patient with severe COPD, a ventilation scan should not be performed. Their reasoning is that the V/Q scan will most likely be interpreted as intermediate.

Septic PEs are common in drug addicts. They are usually seen as ill-defined pulmonary nodules, but they can cavitate (Fig. 5-20). Differentiation from metastatic disease is made mostly on the basis of patient history, and, in the case of septic emboli, positive blood cultures and presence of fever.

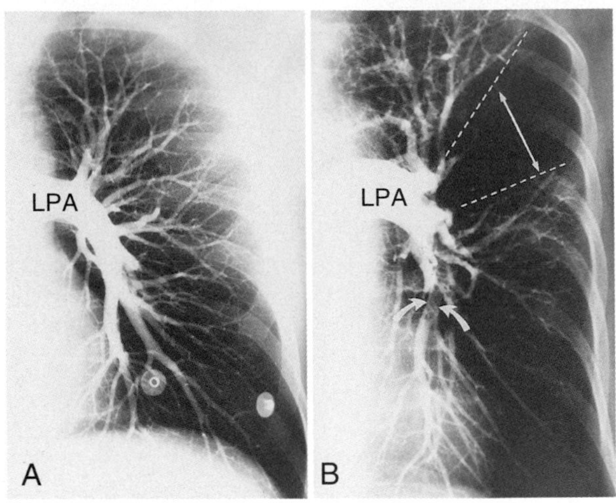

FIGURE 5-19 ■ Pulmonary emboli. The gold standard for evaluation of pulmonary emboli is pulmonary angiography. In this, contrast is injected directly into the left main pulmonary artery (LPA). A normal angiogram *(A)* shows the typical branching structures of the pulmonary artery. The pulmonary arteriogram in a patient with pulmonary emboli *(B)* shows a large area of nonperfusion. This is suggestive of, but not specific for, pulmonary emboli. Much more specific is the filling defect seen within the lumen of the left lower lobe pulmonary artery *(curved arrows)*.

ISCHEMIC CARDIAC DISEASE

Congestive Failure

The pulmonary imaging findings of congestive heart failure (CHF) are discussed in Chapter 3. The diagnosis of CHF is made on the basis of the patient's medical history and physical examination; a chest x-ray is confirmatory. Accurate measurements of left ventricular ejection fraction and regional wall motion are made using previously discussed nuclear medicine techniques or echocardiography. If exercise treadmill, nuclear medicine, or echocardiography results are positive or if the LVEF is less than 35%, a coronary angiogram may be indicated.

Coronary Artery Disease and Angina

Coronary artery disease can be asymptomatic, associated with stable or unstable angina, or evident as the result of a myocardial ischemic event. Angina is considered stable if it occurs with a predictable level of exertion and has not changed pattern for more than 60 days. It usually lasts 0.5 to 10 minutes and quickly subsides with rest or nitroglycerin. Unstable angina is pain at rest or with minimal exertion, typically lasting 20 to 30 minutes or increasing in fre-

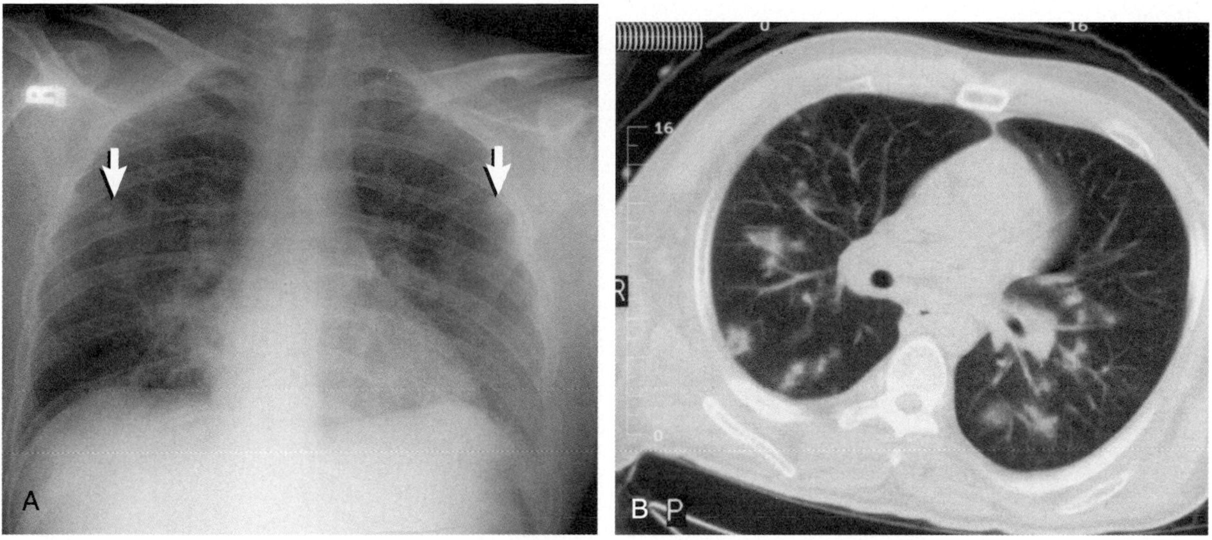

FIGURE 5-20 ■ Septic emboli. In this patient, who is a drug abuser with a fever, the initial chest x-ray *(A)* shows ill-defined patchy infiltrates *(arrows)*. A computed tomography scan *(B)* of the same patient shows these to be predominantly peripheral.

quency, duration, or severity. It is caused by insufficient oxygenation of the myocardium. Laboratory abnormalities [e.g., elevated creatine kinase, myocardial bound (CK-MB) levels] of a myocardial infarction (MI) are not present.

Most patients with coronary artery disease have relatively normal chest x-rays. As coronary artery disease progresses, however, cardiac decompensation may occur, with enlargement of the cardiac silhouette and signs within the pulmonary parenchyma of congestive failure. Although it is quite rare, occasionally calcifications in the coronary arteries can be seen on a plain film (Fig. 5-21). Coronary artery calcification is associated with intimal atheroma. Although calcification is a reliable marker for atherosclerosis, it does not indicate a significant coronary artery stenosis. Calcification is seen best on CT scans and is not seen on a chest x-ray unless it is very extensive. With conventional CT, about 90% of patients who have coronary artery calcification have some stenosis, although not necessarily of significant size (>50% reduction in diameter).

Evaluation of coronary artery disease usually involves a determination of whether the patient simply has angina, a significant stenosis and ischemia, or a myocardial infarction (MI). The normal initial workup includes tests of cardiac enzymes and an electrocardiogram (ECG). A stress ECG also frequently is performed. Indications for an initial noninvasive cardiac stress test are shown in Table 5-2. The least invasive imaging methods for evaluation of coronary artery disease are echocardiography and nuclear medicine myocardial perfusion studies. Echocardiography is based on stressing the patient and then looking for a regional wall-motion abnormality, caused either by induced ischemia or by a previous infarction. Although this method is used in many institutions, it is very operator dependent, and therefore nuclear medicine studies are commonly performed.

A nuclear medicine study can use a number of radioactive myocardial perfusion agents (such as thallium and sestamibi) to image the musculature of the left ventricle. Images are typically obtained in "slice" or tomographic cuts. With computer analysis, these images may be displayed in the short axis, that is, looking down the barrel of the left ventricle; in the horizontal long axis, essentially slicing the left ventricle horizontally lengthwise; or in the vertical long axis (e.g., slicing the left ventricle from top to bottom in the long axis). Patients are typically imaged with and without the heart having been stressed either by exercise or by chemical agents. If a defect is seen

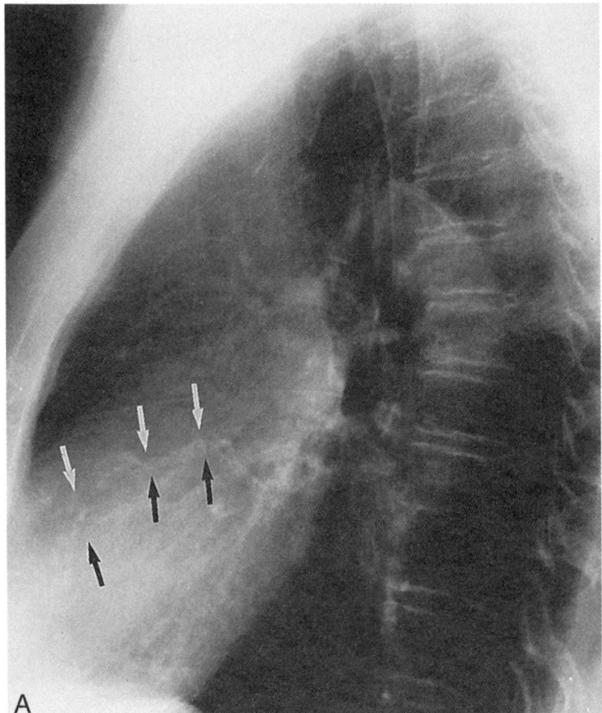

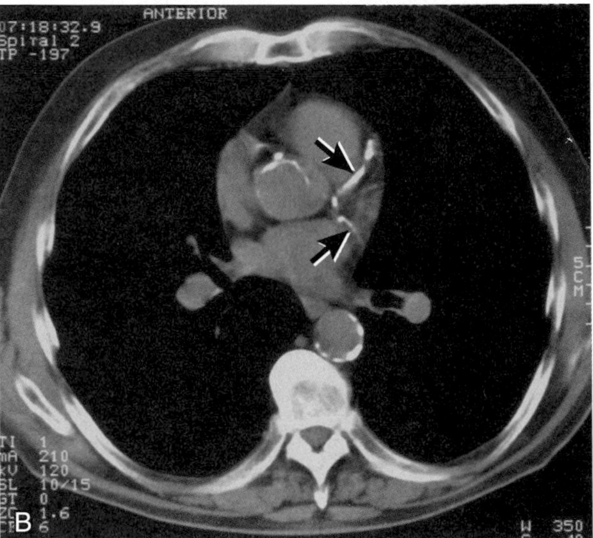

FIGURE 5-21 ■ Coronary artery calcification. On this lateral view of the chest *(A)*, calcification of the coronary arteries can be easily seen *(arrows)*. Computed tomography (CT) scanning *(B)* is much more sensitive for detection of calcification in the coronary arteries *(arrows)*. Unfortunately, calcification is not well related to the presence of a significant stenosis. In this CT, calcification also is seen in the ascending and descending thoracic aorta.

on both exercise and rest images, a high probability of MI exists; if a defect is seen only on stress images, this implies ischemia (Fig. 5-22).

Coronary artery stenosis occurs most commonly in the left anterior descending artery, next most commonly in the right coronary artery, and least commonly in the left circumflex artery. The degree of stenosis is directly related to the amount of blood-flow reduction. A decrease of less than 50% in the diameter of a vessel or less than 75% in the cross-sectional area is not considered significant. A greater than 75% decrease in the diameter of a vessel is equivalent to a greater than 95% decrease in cross-sectional area, and this is regarded as a severe stenosis. As a rule of thumb, a decrease of 50% or more in diameter of a vessel is equivalent to a 75% or greater decrease in cross-sectional area and flow, and this level or more is regarded as significant.

TABLE 5–2 ■ **Indications for an Initial Noninvasive Cardiac Stress Test**[*†]

Patients with a known history of coronary artery disease
A male older than 60 yr or a female older than 70 yr with definite angina
Patients experiencing hemodynamic changes or electrocardiographic changes during an episode of pain
Patients who describe a change in angina pattern
Patients with an electrocardiogram that reveals ST-segment elevation or depression of ≥1 mm
Patients with an electrocardiogram that reveals marked symmetric T-wave inversion in multiple precordial leads

*In patients with chest pain in whom a myocardial infarction has been excluded.
†Exercise stress test, pharmacologic stress test, nuclear medicine myocardial stress test, or echocardiographic stress test.

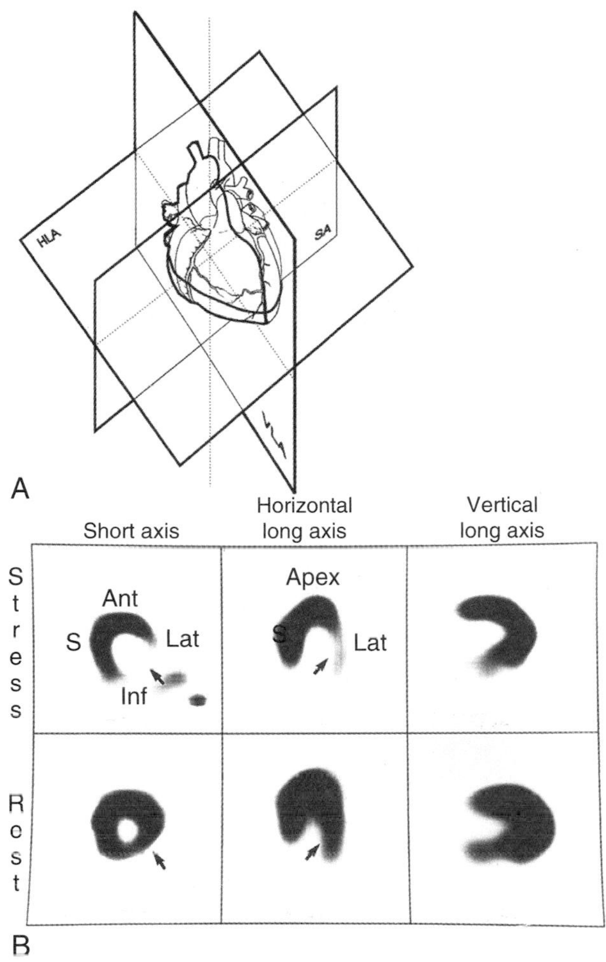

FIGURE 5-22 ■ Assessment of myocardial perfusion. A number of nuclear medicine agents can label the myocardium. With computer techniques, images of the left ventricular wall can be obtained in the short axis, horizontal long axis, and vertical long axis *(A)*. By imaging during stress and rest, it is possible to tell whether an area of reversibility (ischemia) exists, or whether a fixed defect (scar or infarction) is present. In this case *(B)*, the *arrows* show that the defect during stress reverses or "fills in" during the rest images, indicating ischemia of the inferolateral wall of the left ventricle.

Visualization of the individual coronary arteries is best done with coronary angiography. Because this is an invasive, expensive procedure and the radiation dose is high, it is not used as a screening test. It often is done only after positive results of nuclear medicine study or echocardiogram are found. Obviously, it also must be done if bypass surgery is contemplated. Coronary angiograms are performed and interpreted by cardiologists. Cardiologists can now use coronary angiography to place a catheter either to dilate a particular area of coronary stenosis (angioplasty) or to infuse a clot-lysing agent in an area of recent occlusion. After dilatation, a wire mesh stent can be placed in the coronary artery to retard and, hopefully, to prevent restenosis. These can sometimes be seen on chest x-rays (Fig. 5-23).

Computed Tomography (CT) Coronary Artery Screening and Calcium Scoring

In the last several years, evaluation of older patients for the amount of calcium in the coronary arteries has become popular. This rather quick examination is done with either a multidetector spiral CT (see Fig. 5-21*B*) or an electron-beam CT scanner. No intravenous contrast is used. The CT scan is used to detect, count, and measure calcifications in the coronary arteries. Calcification indicates atherosclerosis and may

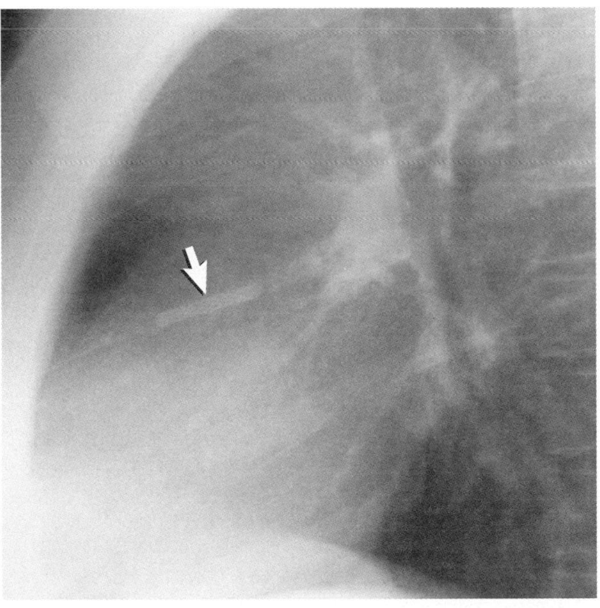

FIGURE 5-23 ■ Coronary artery stent. After balloon dilatation of a coronary artery, a tubular wire mesh stent *(arrow)* can be seen on the lateral chest x-ray. The stent was placed to retard reocclusion.

be one of the first signs of coronary artery disease. The presence of calcification alone does not indicate significant coronary artery disease. For example, detectable calcification is found in 30% to 40% of persons in their 40s and in 70% to 80% of persons in their 60s. In general, a multidetector CT calcium score of 0 to 10 indicates very low risk; 11 to 100, moderate risk; 101 to 400, moderately high risk; and more than 400, high risk. The calcium score for an individual is measured against age and gender norms. Usually only those at 75% or greater on age- and sex-specific calcium score go on for additional workup. Remember that a patient can have significant coronary artery disease without calcifications. As many as 50% of persons with an MI (often due to a "soft" plaque) will not have significant calcification.

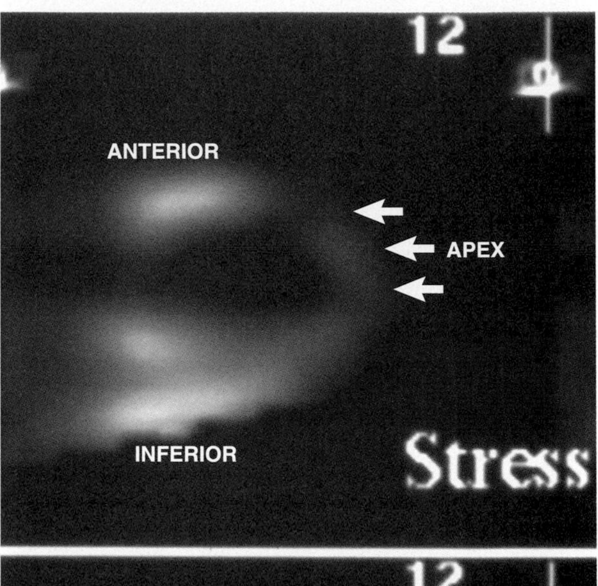

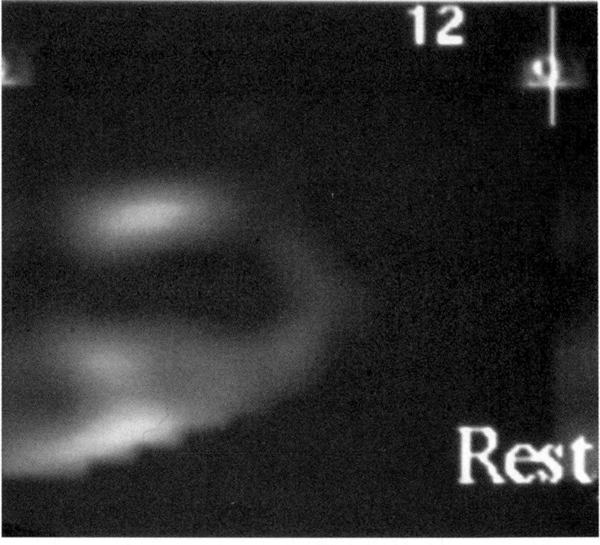

FIGURE 5-24 ■ **Myocardial infarction.** Here the left ventricle is viewed from the side. Clearly, less perfusion exists in the distal anterior wall and apex *(arrows)*. This did not change at rest, indicating a permanent lack of perfusion (infarct). This is the same patient shown in Figure 5-6, who had abnormal wall motion in the same area.

Myocardial Infarction

An acute MI is usually diagnosed by history, ECG changes, and laboratory abnormalities (elevated CK-MB levels). If the patient is within 6 hours of the onset of chest pain, a coronary angiogram is indicated in a facility where balloon angioplasty, stent placement, or thrombolytic therapy is performed. Coronary angiography also is indicated if cardiogenic shock, papillary muscle rupture, LVEF less than 35%, or an ischemic VSD is present, or if the patient has an arrhythmia and is a cardiac arrest survivor. If the patient is initially seen later than 6 hours with evidence of an MI, initial evaluation is done either by a rest or stress ECG, nuclear medicine myocardial perfusion scan (Fig. 5-24), or echocardiogram.

AORTA

Anatomy and Imaging Techniques

A number of anomalies of the aortic arch are found, the most common of which is a right-sided aortic arch (Fig. 5-25). There are several different types. Some have the arch on the right, with simple mirror-image branching of the innominate, common carotid, and right subclavian arteries. This type also descends along the right side of the spine and can be associated with tetralogy of Fallot or truncus arteriosus. Right aortic arches are associated with congenital heart disease in 5% of cases. Other variants of right-sided aortic arch include anomalous origins of the pulmonary artery off the ascending or descending aorta; however, these are impossible to differentiate on plain chest x-ray.

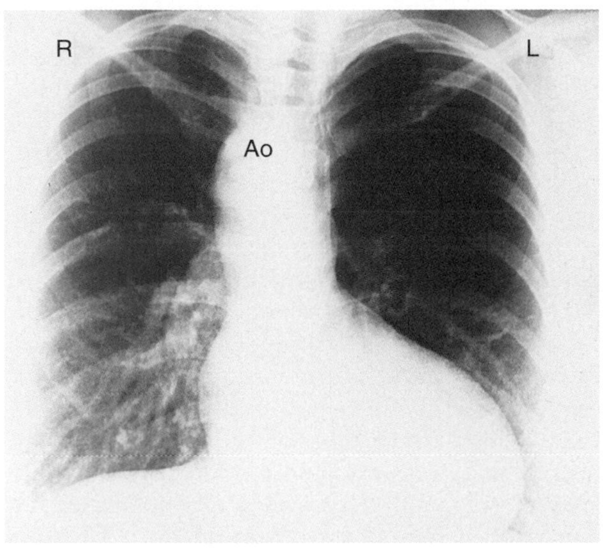

FIGURE 5-25 ■ Right-sided aortic arch. Although the heart is in its normal left-sided configuration, the ascending, transverse, and descending thoracic aorta (Ao) are on the right side.

Calcification of the aortic arch is very common in persons older than 60 years. It is fairly unusual between the ages of 40 and 50 years, and calcification suggests a higher than average incidence of atherosclerotic disease. Calcification can be seen in the aortic arch and also often in the great vessels (Fig. 5-26).

Injection of contrast directly into the aorta (contrast angiography) yields the most definitive evaluation of normal and anomalous anatomy (Fig. 5-27). The left anterior oblique view is the most useful, because this lays out the anatomy better without much overlap of the great vessels or of the ascending and descending aorta. Imaging also can be done with CT or MR scanning.

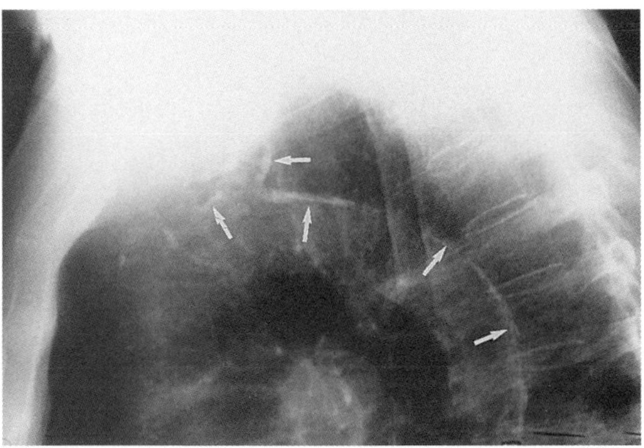

FIGURE 5-26 ■ Calcification of the aortic arch and great vessels. The lateral view of the upper chest clearly shows areas of increased density in the walls of the aortic arch *(white arrows)* and in the great vessels.

Coarctation of the Aorta

Coarctation is a congenital narrowing of the proximal descending thoracic aorta, which usually occurs in the vicinity of the ductus arteriosus. Symptoms are rarely, if ever, present during childhood. The diagnosis is usually arrived at by

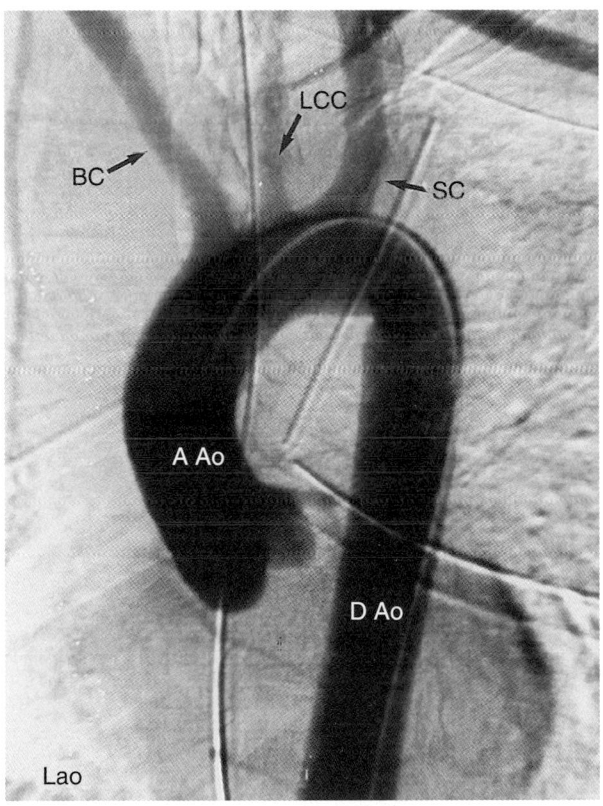

FIGURE 5-27 ■ Normal thoracic aortogram. This angiogram was done with a catheter in the aortic arch and contrast injection. Digital subtraction computer techniques were used to eliminate the bony structures. The ascending (A Ao) and descending thoracic aorta (D Ao) as well as the brachiocephalic (BC), left common carotid (LCC), and left subclavian arteries (SC) are clearly shown. The projection used here is a left anterior oblique because the great vessels do not project over each other in this view.

accident during a physical examination by noting diminished or absent femoral pulses or by finding that the patient has hypertension of the upper extremities.

On the chest x-ray, the heart may be normal or may have slight left ventricular enlargement with prominence of the ascending aorta. Occasionally the actual site of the coarctation can be visualized as narrowing in the proximal portion of the descending aorta. In addition, often prominence along the left paratracheal region is seen in continuity with the outline of the aortic knob, caused by dilatation of the left subclavian artery. A rather characteristic finding is notching of the inferior aspect of the ribs due to erosion by tortuous and dilated intercostal arteries (Fig. 5-28). The actual site of stenosis is best visualized by either CT or MR angiography (Fig. 5-29).

Aortic Tears

Traumatic disruption of the aorta usually occurs as a result of an automobile accident, with the driver's chest striking the steering wheel. Rupture of the aorta causes 15% to 40% of the fatalities in motor vehicle accidents. Rapid deceleration can cause the aorta to tear, usually in the proximal portion of the descending aorta at the level of the attachment of the ligamentum arteriosum. Ninety-five percent occur at this level, and approximately 5% occur at the level of the aortic root. Signs of a tear on a frontal chest x-ray include a mediastinal width of more than 8 to 10 cm at or above the level of the aortic arch, apical pleural density (capping) due to blood above the apical portion of the lung, and deviation of the trachea or nasogastric tube to the right. Usually poor definition of the aortic arch and opacification of the aortopulmonary window also are seen (Fig. 5-30). Tears should be suspected if a mediastinal hematoma is found on a CT scan done on a traumatized patient (Fig. 5-31).

Thoracic Aortic Aneurysms

Aneurysms may be the result of atherosclerosis; inflammatory, mechanical, traumatic, or congenital causes; fibromuscular dysplasia; and cystic medial necrosis. An aneurysm of the

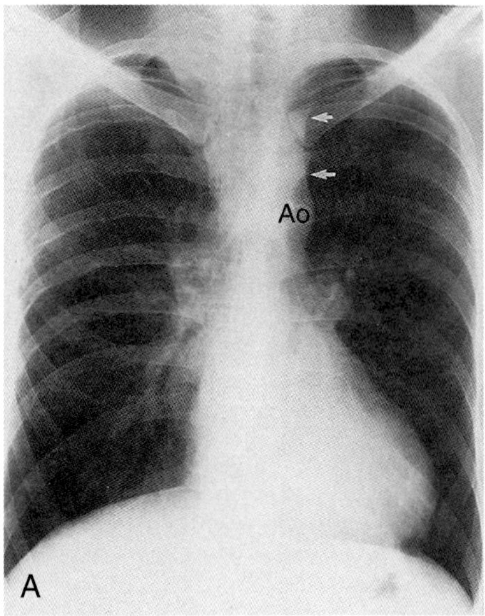

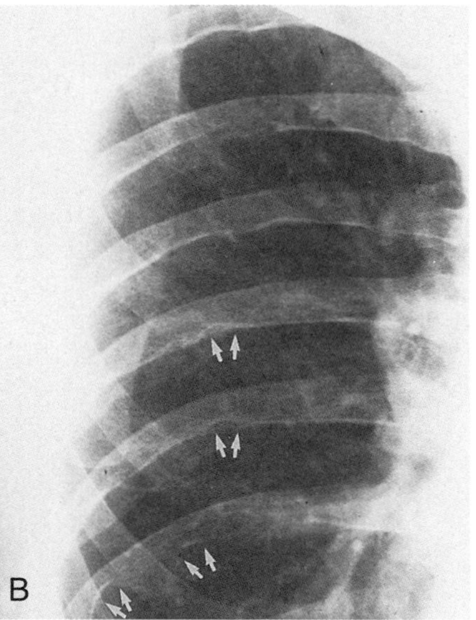

FIGURE 5-28 ■ **Coarctation of the aorta.** A chest x-ray was obtained in this patient, who had very high blood pressure in both upper extremities *(A)*. It demonstrates prominence of the left cardiac border (due to left ventricular hypertrophy). A dilated left subclavian artery *(arrows)* is due to increased flow, because blood has difficulty getting down the descending aorta (Ao). A close-up view *(B)* of the chest shows notching along the inferior aspects of the ribs *(arrows)* due to dilated intercostal arteries.

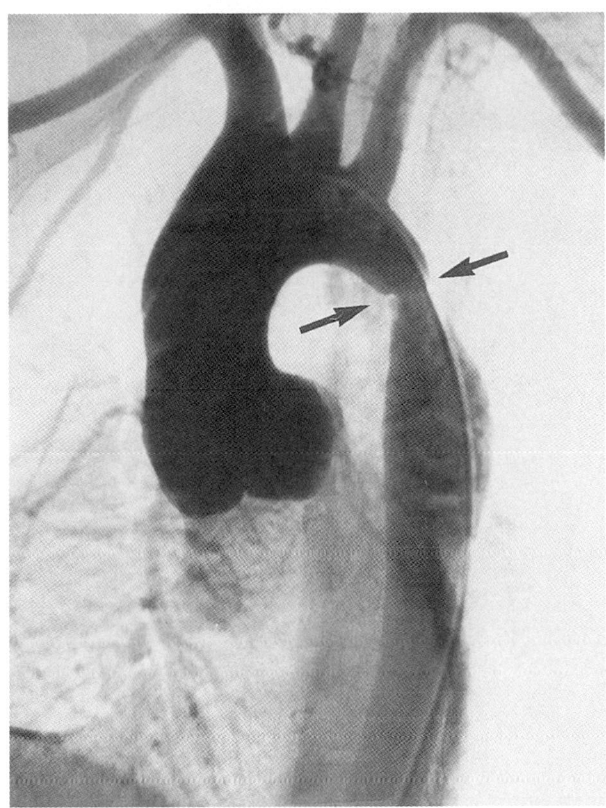

FIGURE 5-29 ■ Coarctation of the aorta. A digital subtraction contrast aortogram clearly shows the area of coarctation, or narrowing, distal to the left subclavian artery.

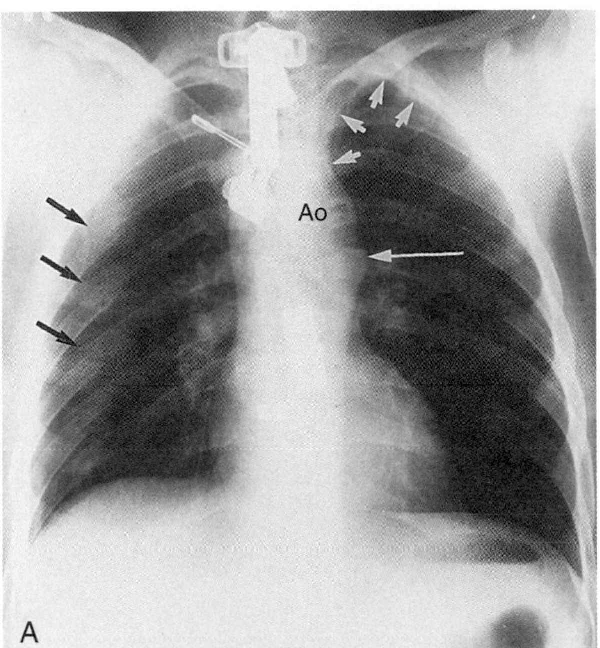

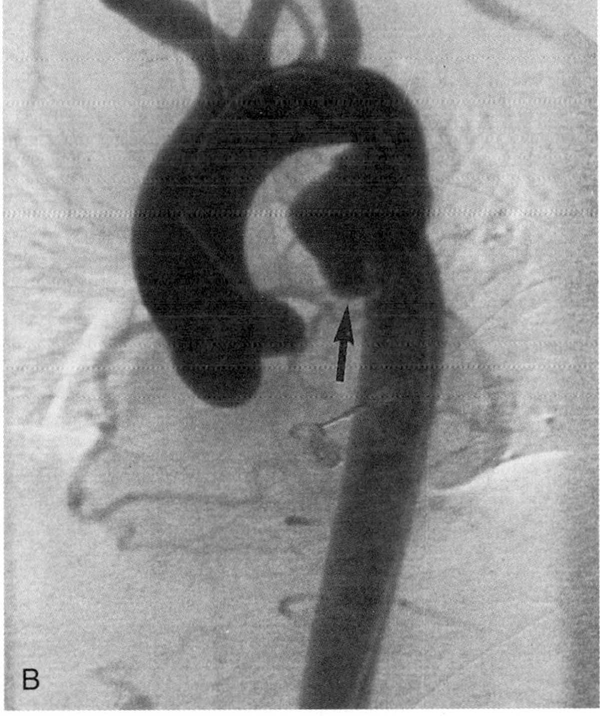

FIGURE 5-30 ■ Aortic tear. A chest x-ray *(A)* obtained in an individual who was in a motor vehicle accident shows multiple rib fractures *(black arrows)*, filling in of the normal concavity of the anteroposterior window *(long white arrow)*, and fluid over the apex of the left lung. These latter two findings are suggestive of mediastinal hemorrhage. A digital subtraction contrast aortogram *(B)* shows a bulge of contrast *(arrow)* due to a tear in a very typical location.

ascending aorta historically was most likely due to syphilis. This is very rare now, and Marfan's syndrome is a more likely cause.

With aneurysms of either the thoracic or the abdominal aorta, surgery or endograft placement is often performed, because a marked increase in risk of aortic rupture is found. Aneurysms may be discovered incidentally, or the patient may present with pain, rupture, or thromboembolic complications. Aneurysms of the thoracic aorta are fairly easy to identify on chest x-rays as widening of the ascending aorta or aortic arch (Fig. 5-32). Sudden onset of chest pain in a patient with an aneurysm should suggest rupture or ongoing dissection.

Detailed evaluation of an aneurysm can be easily performed by using CT scanning with a bolus of intravenous contrast. This will allow the lumen to be visualized as well as clot along the

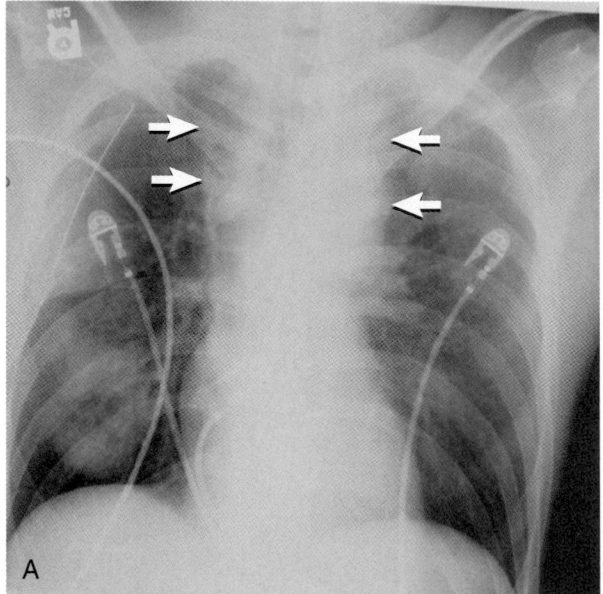

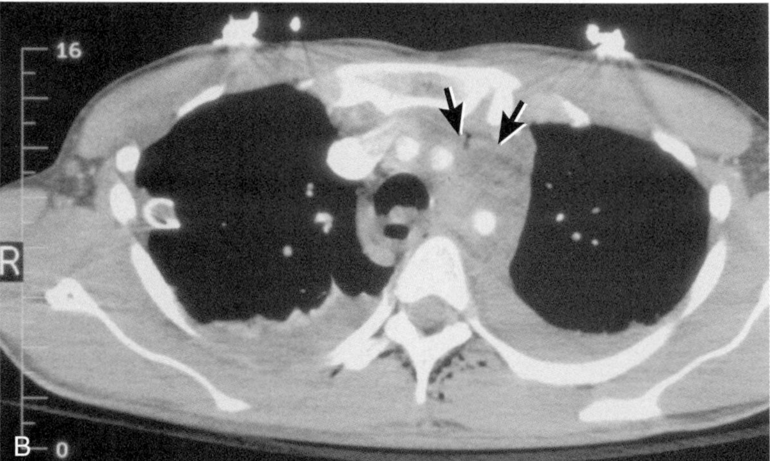

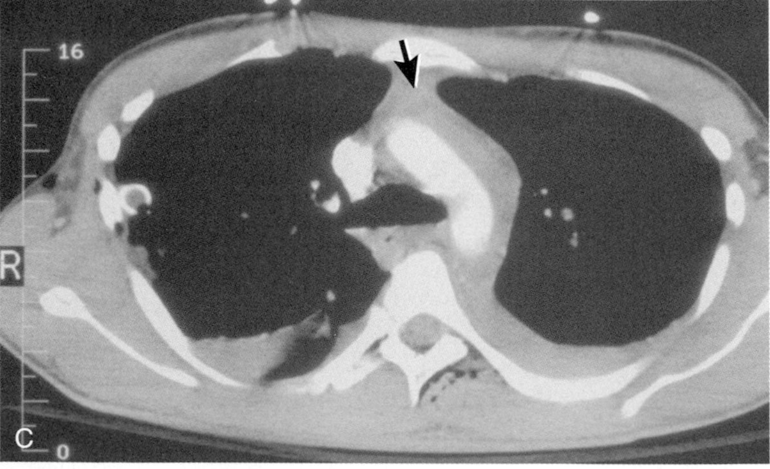

FIGURE 5-31 ■ Mediastinal hematoma. The chest x-ray *(A)* in a traumatized patient shows a widened upper mediastinum. A contrast-enhanced computed tomography (CT) scan at the level of the thoracic inlet *(B)* and at the level of the aortic arch *(C)* shows gray soft tissue density surrounding the vessels, indicating hemorrhage *(arrows)* and vascular damage.

inner wall of the aneurysm. In many patients, portions of the clot come loose and lead to distal thromboembolic events (Fig. 5-32*C*). An arteriogram is not the best initial method for evaluation of aneurysms, because usually all that is visualized is the patent lumen and not the outer wall or the thickness of intraluminal clot. In addition, a catheter in the aorta raises the possibility of knocking loose portions of clot. MRI can be used, but imaging times are longer than those of CT scanning. Further, if the patient is unstable, it is difficult to manage life support because of the high magnetic field strength and the inability to bring ferromagnetic materials into the room.

Aortic Dissection

Aortic dissection is the result of an intimal tear causing separation of the layers of the wall of the aorta. It is more common in men than in women and usually occurs between the ages of 45 and 70 years. The incidence is higher in patients with Marfan's syndrome, coarctation of the

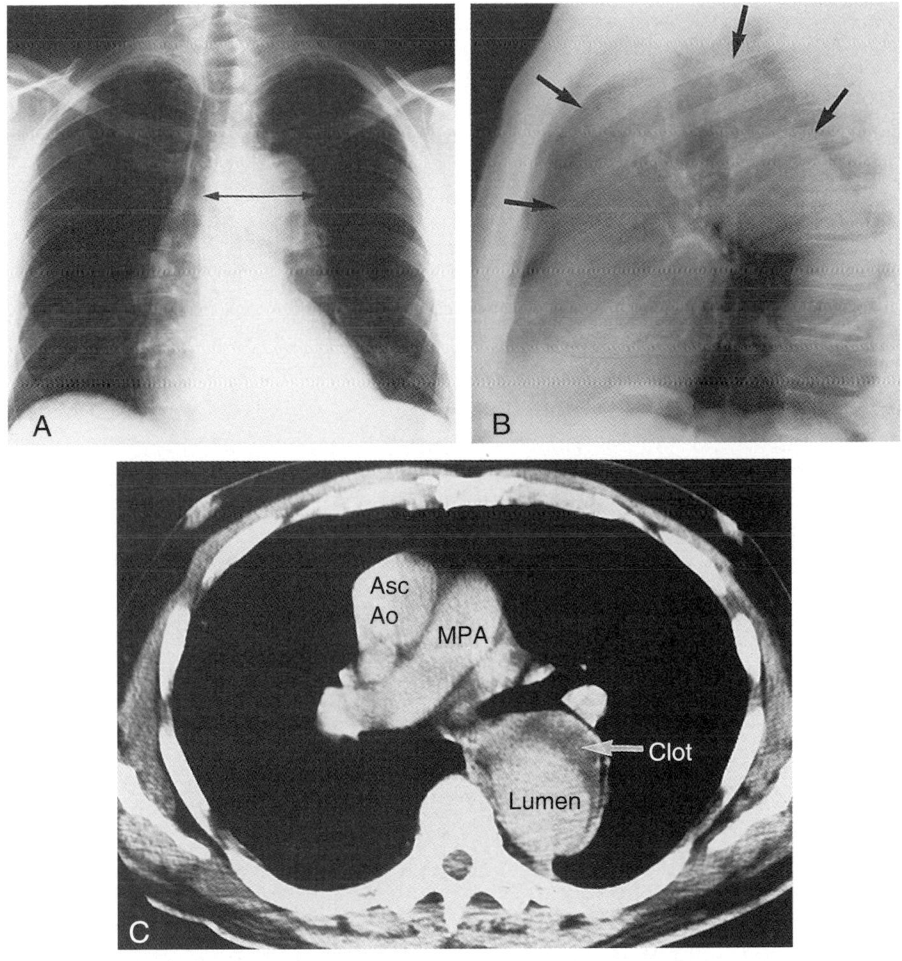

FIGURE 5-32 ■ Aortic aneurysm. A posteroanterior chest x-ray *(A)* demonstrates a markedly widened aortic arch *(double-ended arrow)*. The lateral view *(B)* also shows marked dilatation of the entire aortic arch *(arrows)*. A contrast-enhanced transverse computed tomography (CT) scan *(C)* shows the ascending aorta (Asc Ao), the main pulmonary artery (MPA), and marked dilatation of the proximal portion of the descending thoracic aorta. The contrast-enhanced lumen is seen, as well as mural clot.

aorta, and bicuspid aortic valve disease. Aortic dissection also commonly occurs in patients with aortic atherosclerosis, particularly those who are hypertensive. Dissection carries a very high mortality if undiagnosed and untreated. Dissection of the thoracic aorta proximal to the left subclavian artery is a surgical emergency, whereas dissections of the descending thoracic aorta are usually managed by medical treatment of the patient's hypertension.

The dissection can allow blood to flow between the layers of the aortic wall, causing a false lumen. Sometimes this false lumen will reenter the true lumen farther down the aorta. Generally, aortic dissection begins either in the ascending aorta or in the descending aorta just distal to the left subclavian in the upper back and chest. About one third of patients will have extremity pain, and another one third will have a central nervous system (CNS) abnormality if the dissection involves the ascending aorta and great vessels.

Aortic dissection should be suspected on a chest x-ray if a double contour of the aortic arch is seen, if progressive serial enlargement is noted, or if displacement of intimal calcification more than 6 mm from the outer aortic margin is found. This last sign must be interpreted with caution, because a minor degree of rotation of the chest may cause anterior arch calcification to project eccentrically over the posterior arch. On chest x-ray, most patients with a dissection will have a dilated aorta with a widened mediastinum and cardiomegaly.

Enlargement of the aortic arch on a single film is not specific for a dissection, inasmuch as the aortic arch can frequently be enlarged in patients with hypertension or atherosclerosis. Lack of enlargement of the aortic arch should not be taken as evidence that a dissection is not present, because the arch is of normal size in 25% of dissection cases (Fig. 5-33).

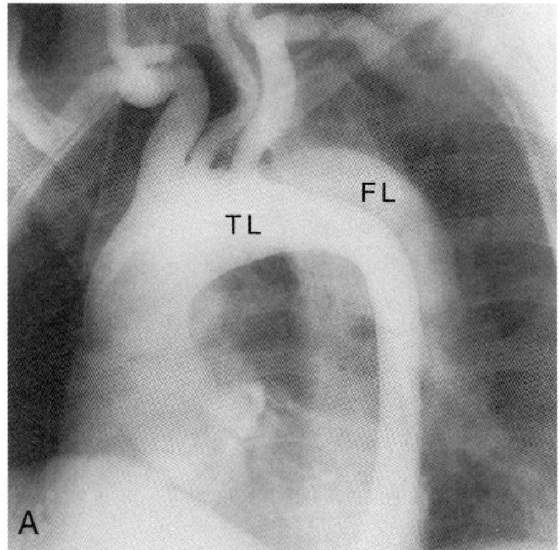

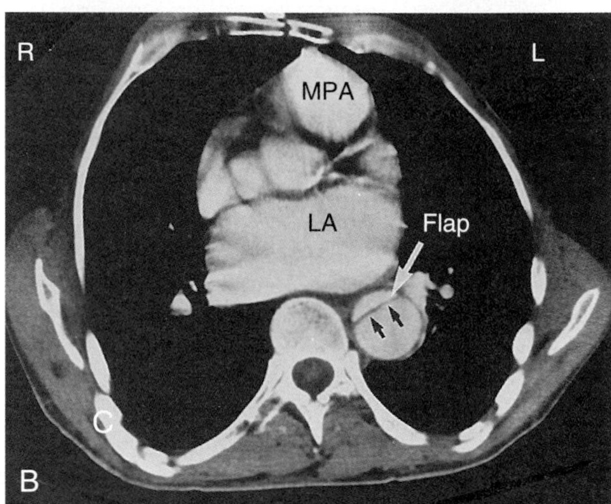

FIGURE 5-33 ■ **Aortic dissection.** A standard contrast aortogram in the left anterior oblique projection *(A)* shows contrast in the true lumen (TL) as well as the great vessels. Contrast also is seen in the false lumen (FL), which is a channel within the wall of the aorta. A contrast-enhanced transverse computed tomography (CT) scan *(B)* easily shows the intimal flap between the true lumen and the false lumen. MPA, main pulmonary artery; LA, left atrium.

The diagnosis of dissection can be made with a contrasted CT or an MRI study. CT scanning is somewhat quicker, and it is easier to manage a patient who may suddenly decompensate. Demonstration of an intimal flap on CT is conclusive evidence of a dissection. An intimal flap and the false lumen can be seen in 70% of patients. Transesophageal ultrasound can be used to evaluate dissections or aneurysms of the descending thoracic aorta, because the esophagus is in such close proximity. Generally, however, surgeons want a more complete evaluation, such as that provided by CT, before they will operate on a patient.

PERIPHERAL VESSELS

Head and Neck

A carotid bruit may be identified as part of a stroke or transient ischemic attack workup or as an incidental result of a physical examination done for other reasons. Carotid bruits are not sufficiently predictive of high-grade symptomatic carotid stenosis to identify those that are amenable to surgery. As a result, both asymptomatic and symptomatic patients with a bruit should be evaluated with duplex ultrasonography to determine the degree and extent of stenosis. Interpretation is based on the image of the vessel walls and the flow across the area in question. Patients with a high-grade (>60% to 80%) stenosis may benefit from carotid endarterectomy. The role of surgery in low-grade stenoses or in asymptomatic patients remains debatable. Surgery is considered in those patients with recurring transient ischemic attacks while receiving medical therapy and in those with severe carotid ulceration. Carotid ultrasound also is indicated in patients with other vascular disease and before carotid surgery or aortic aneurysm repair. It also is widely done in patients with other peripheral vascular disease, for example, in those with foot pain at rest, nonhealing foot ulcers, gangrenous changes of the feet, or a resting ankle-brachial index of 0.5 or less.

Evaluation of vessels of the head and neck classically was done by using contrast angiography. This involves percutaneous access to the femoral artery and placement of the catheter up the aorta with selective catheterization of the individual great vessels, including the carotid and vertebral arteries. The typical contrast angiogram shows exquisite detail of the vessels of the neck, face, and brain, and can easily demonstrate areas of stenosis or aneurysm (Fig. 5-34).

All contrast angiography of the vessels of the head and neck carries a small risk of stroke, due to injection of air bubbles, or of vascular spasm or clotting, due to the catheter. Recently,

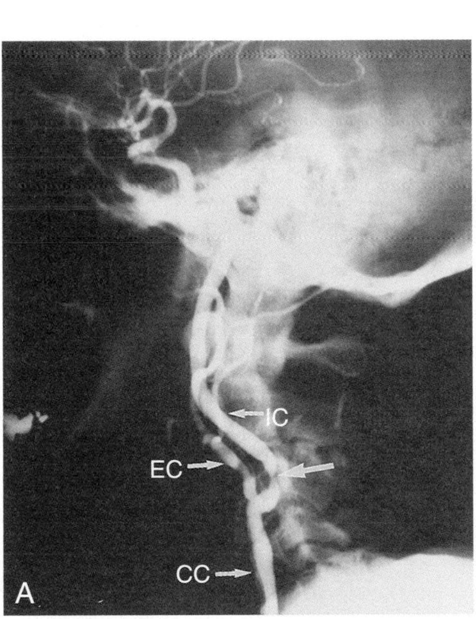

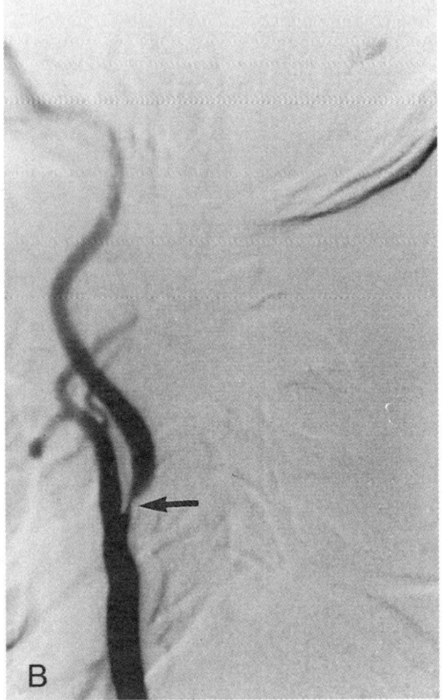

FIGURE 5-34 ■ Carotid artery stenosis. A lateral projection *(A)* from a standard contrast arteriogram shows the common carotid (CC), the external carotid (EC), and the internal carotid (IC) arteries. An area of stenosis can be identified at the base of the internal carotid artery *(large arrow)*. A digital subtraction angiogram *(B)* makes areas of stenosis much easier to see, because the bones have been subtracted off the image.

advances in CT and MRI scanning have allowed MR and CT angiography to be performed as noninvasive procedures.

Abdominal Aorta and Iliac Vessels

In patients with extensive atherosclerosis, striking calcification of the abdominal aorta and iliac arteries may occur (Fig. 5-35*A*). Remember that atherosclerosis is a common cause of aneurysm formation, and you should therefore be assessing the diameter of the vessels. Because on the AP view of the abdomen the aorta overlies the spine, it can be difficult to assess calcification in the aortic wall. The lateral view of the abdomen or of the lumbar spine often gives a better appreciation of the calcified abdominal aorta (Fig. 5-35*B*). The abdominal aorta should not exceed 2.5 cm in diameter; as with the thoracic aorta, once the diameter exceeds 5 cm, an increased likelihood of rupture exists. The diameter of the aorta should be measured from the anterior wall back to the vertebral bodies and not just to the posterior calcified wall. Sometimes the calcification in an abdominal aneurysm can be somewhat subtle and, on the AP view, may be seen as curvilinear streaks along the lateral aspects of the vertebral bodies (Fig. 5-36).

A very easy noninvasive examination of the abdominal aorta can be done using abdominal ultrasound. Not only the aorta but also other vessels can be visualized, such as superior mesenteric artery and vein (Fig. 5-37). Abdominal ultrasound is the imaging test of choice if follow up is needed on a patient who has a dilated aorta that has not yet reached 5 cm in diameter. In a symptomatic patient whose condition raises fear of clot within the aorta, dissection, or rupture, a

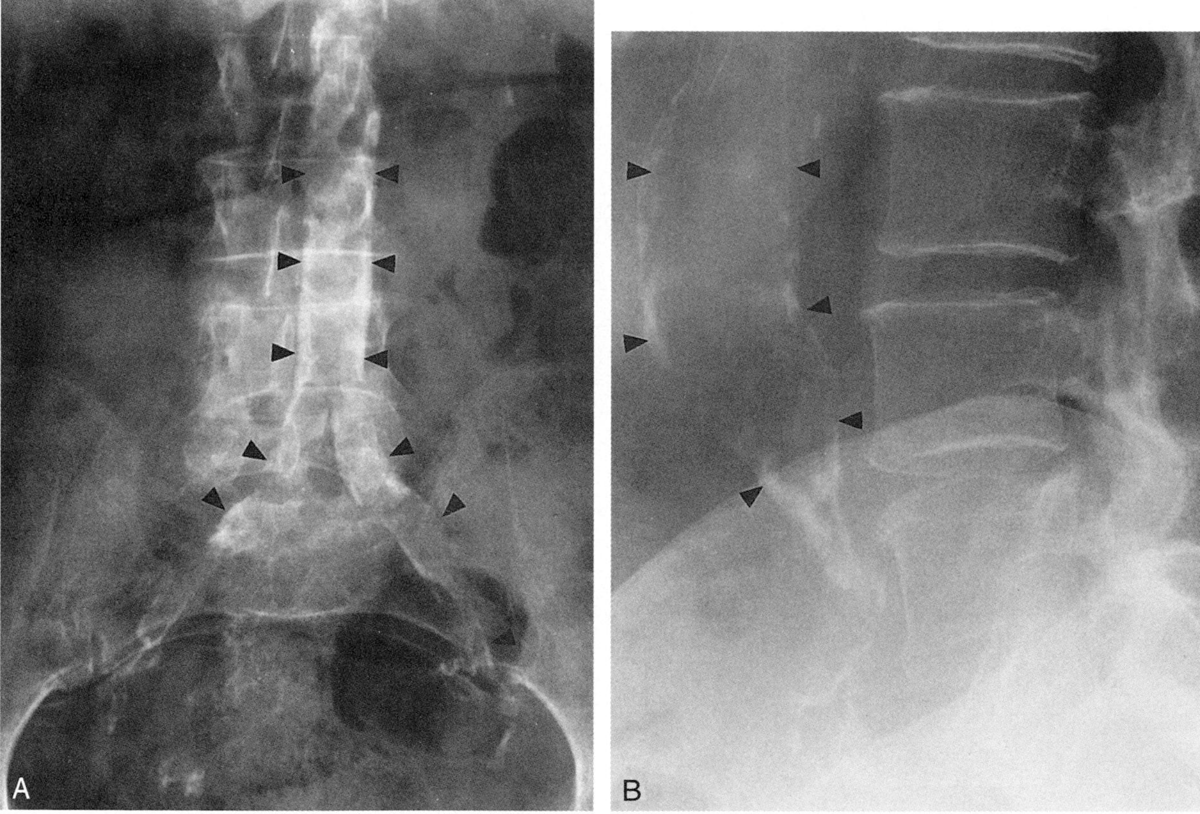

FIGURE 5-35 ■ Calcification of the abdominal aorta. A plain x-ray of the abdomen *(A)* shows extensive calcification of the abdominal aorta and iliac vessels. Calcification of the abdominal aorta is usually much easier to see on the lateral view *(B)*. If the distance from the anterior calcified wall back to a vertebral body exceeds 5 cm, an abdominal aortic aneurysm is present.

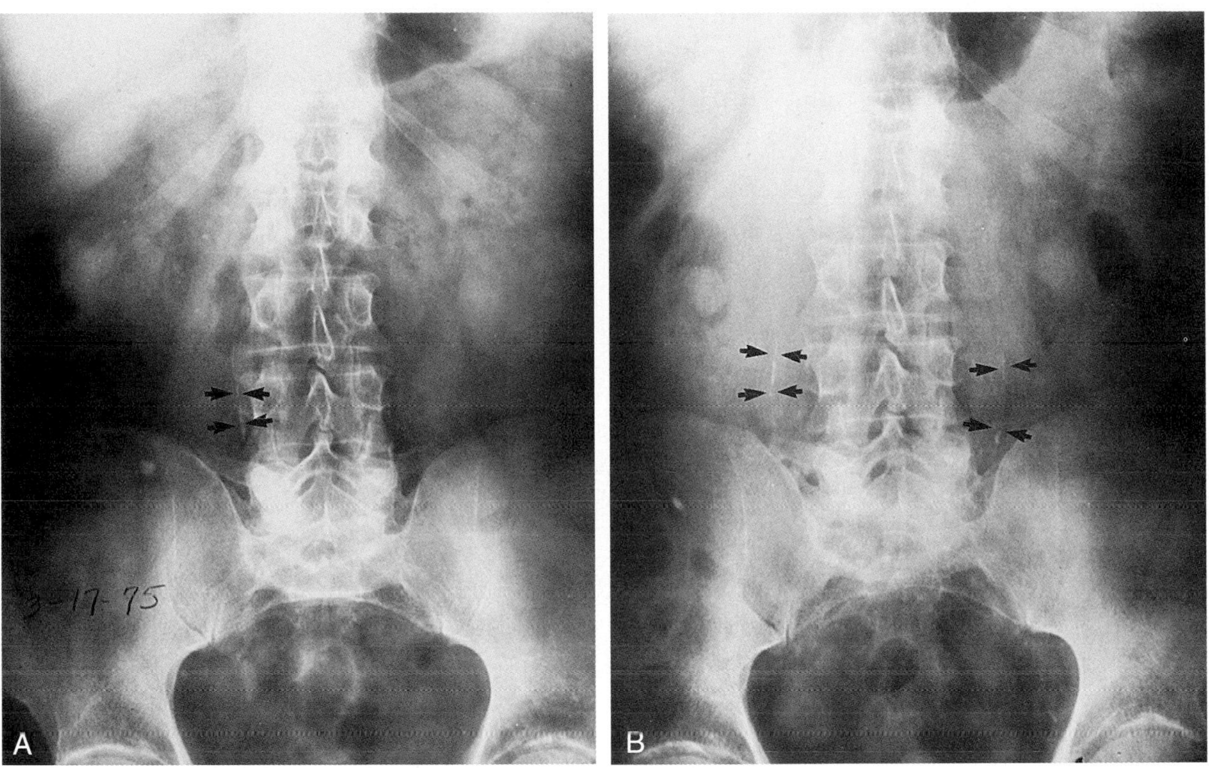

FIGURE 5-36 ■ Progressive development of an abdominal aortic aneurysm. A plain x-ray of the abdomen of a patient done in 1975 *(A)* showed a small area of linear calcification overlying the right side of L5 *(arrows)*. This represents calcification within the wall of the aorta. A repeated x-ray 10 years later *(B)* showed bilateral linear areas of calcification *(arrows)*. The distance between these two linear calcifications represents the width of the aneurysm.

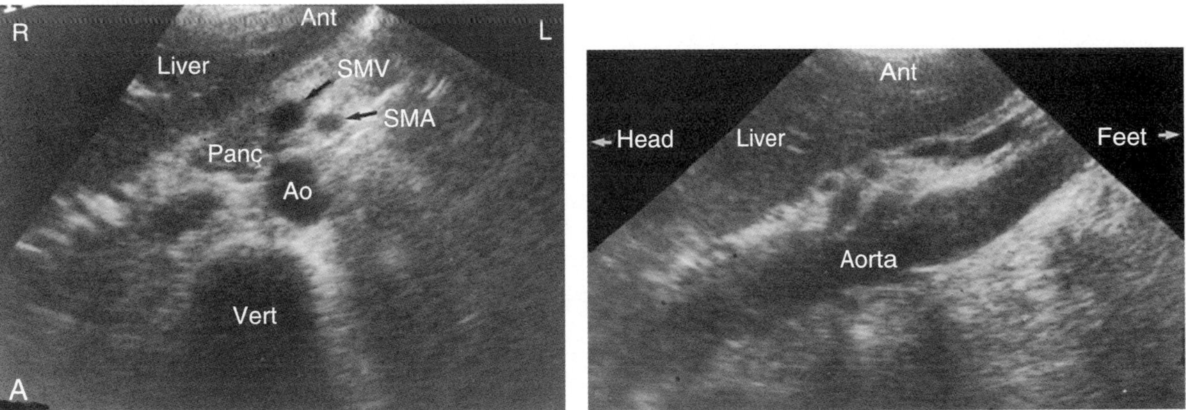

FIGURE 5-37 ■ Ultrasound demonstration of normal vascular anatomy in the upper abdomen. A transverse sonogram *(A)* shows structures such as the liver and pancreas (Panc) and vertebral body (Vert), but also the superior mesenteric artery (SMA), vein (SMV), and abdominal aorta (Ao). A longitudinal view just to the left of midline *(B)* shows the liver and abdominal aorta as well as the origin of the celiac axis and superior mesenteric artery.

CT scan with an intravenous bolus of contrast material is the test of choice (Fig. 5-38). Some physicians recommend that abdominal ultrasound be used as a screening procedure for abdominal aortic aneurysm in nonsmoking men older than 65 years, in male smokers older than 50 years, and in all persons older than 50 years who had a parent with abdominal aneurysm. Recent treatment of abdominal and iliac aneurysms involves the use of large endoluminal endografts. These are typically placed via catheter access in the femoral artery (Fig. 5-39). Follow-up of these endografts to exclude progression of the aneurysm, leakage, or occlusion is usually done with CT (Fig. 5-40).

Historically, evaluation of abdominal and pelvic vessels other than the aorta was best done by contrast angiography. Not only can the major vessels, such as hepatic artery and renal arteries, be identified, but also all their branches can be seen in great detail. Even small lumbar arteries can be visualized (Fig. 5-41). Atherosclerotic changes and areas of stenosis also are easily identified. After identification of areas of stenosis, it is possible to insert a catheter that has a balloon on the end and to dilate the areas of stenosis. This is called percutaneous transluminal angioplasty. The success rate actually depends on the vessel, and the success of angioplasty is greatest in the larger

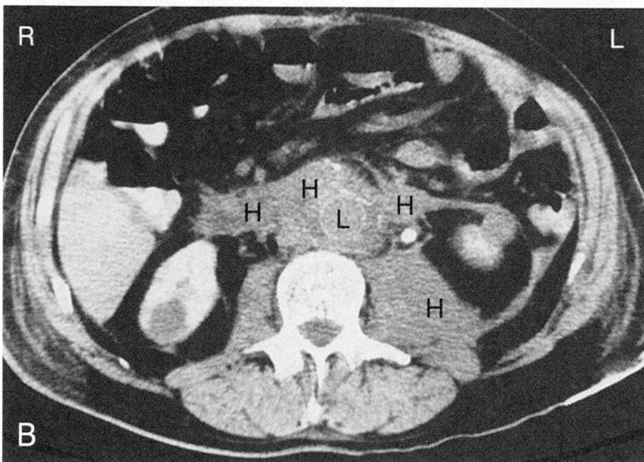

FIGURE 5-38 ■ Abdominal aortic aneurysm and rupture. A transverse contrast-enhanced computed tomography (CT) scan *(A)* of the lower portion of the abdomen shows the aorta with a calcified rim and the lumen (L) filled with contrast and mural clot (C). In a different patient who had abdominal pain, a non-contrasted CT scan *(B)* shows the true lumen of the aorta (L), which is visible because of the calcified aortic wall. What looks like soft tissue surrounding the aorta and extending into the left psoas region is hemorrhage (H) due to a leak.

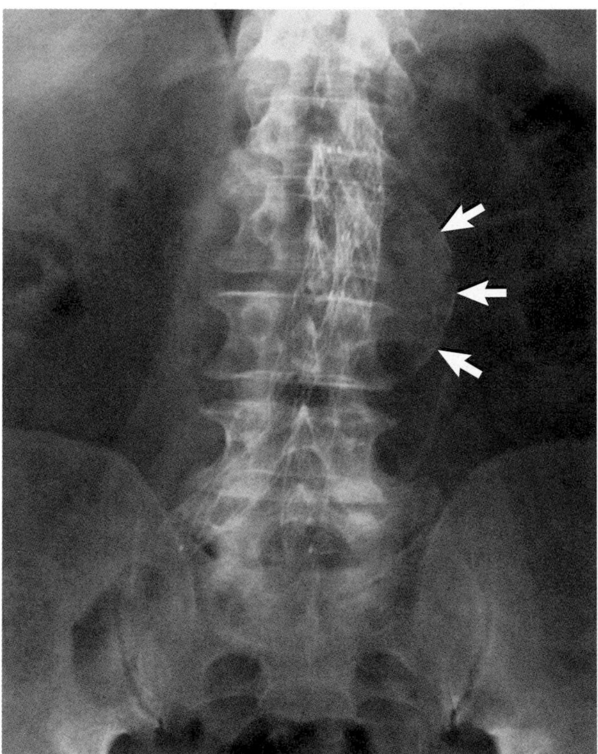

FIGURE 5-39 ■ Aortic aneurysm endograft repair. Here wire mesh stents with a lining have been inserted into the abdominal aorta and proximal iliac arteries. They can be seen projecting over the lumbar spine and sacrum. These endografts are inserted though the femoral arteries, and an open surgical procedure is not required. The calcified rim of the aneurysm is visible on the left *(arrows)*.

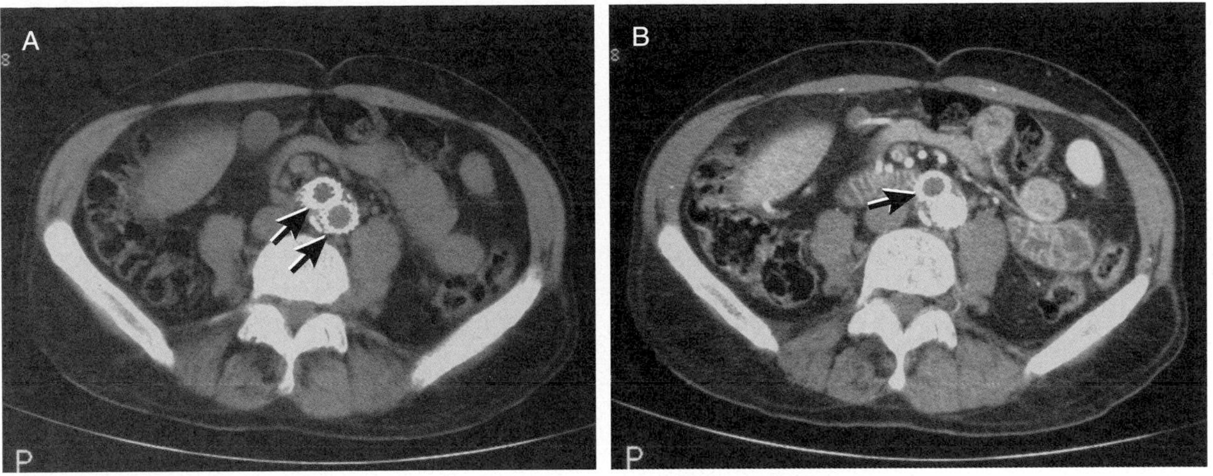

FIGURE 5-40 ■ **Occluded endograft repair.** Evaluation and follow-up of aortic and iliac stents is done with computed tomography (CT) scanning. In the noncontrasted CT scan *(A),* the wire mesh stents in the iliac vessels can be seen. On the contrast-enhanced CT scan *(B),* only one of the limbs of the repair is patent, and the other *(arrow)* is occluded and does not fill with contrast.

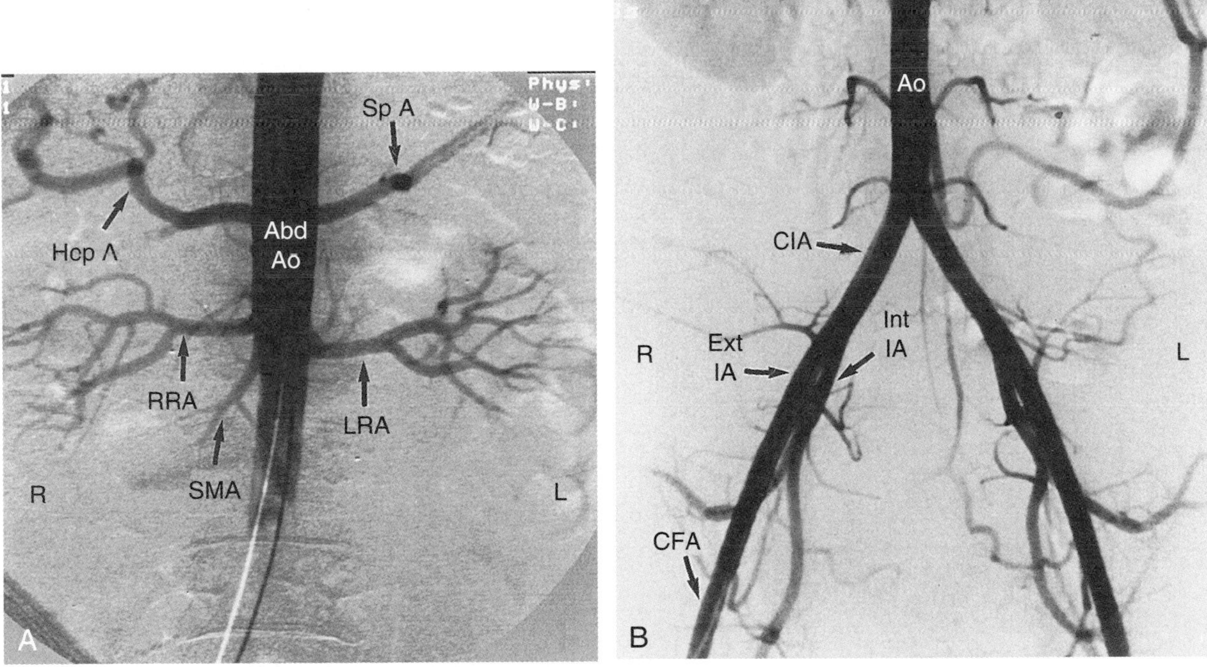

FIGURE 5-41 ■ **Normal vascular anatomy of the abdomen and pelvis.** A digital subtraction angiogram in an anteroposterior projection of the upper abdomen *(A)* shows the abdominal aorta (Abd Ao), the hepatic (Hep A) and splenic arteries (SpA), the right (RRA) and left renal arteries (LRA), and the superior mesenteric artery (SMA). A subsequent image over the lower abdomen and pelvis *(B)* taken a few seconds later shows the distal abdominal aorta with small lumbar branches, the common iliac artery, the internal and external iliac arteries, and the common femoral artery.

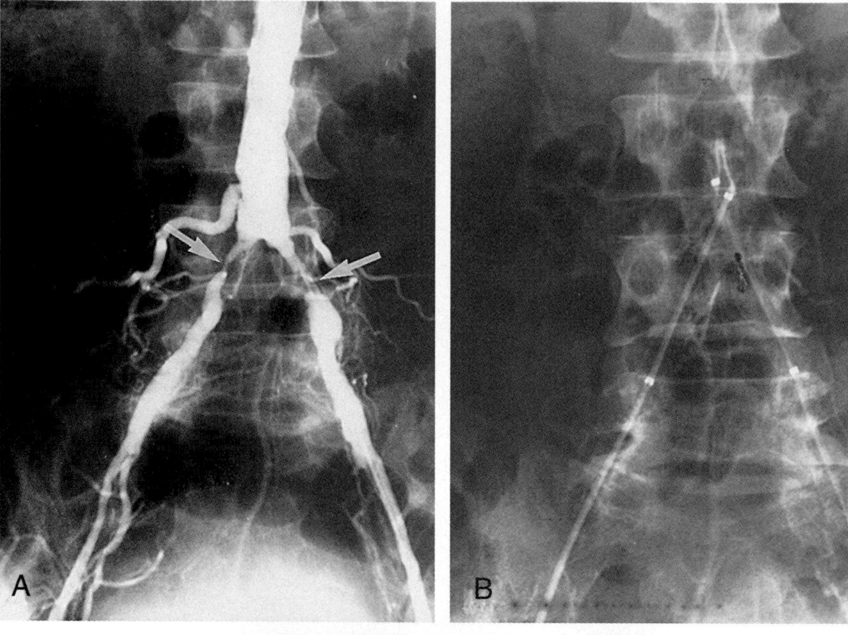

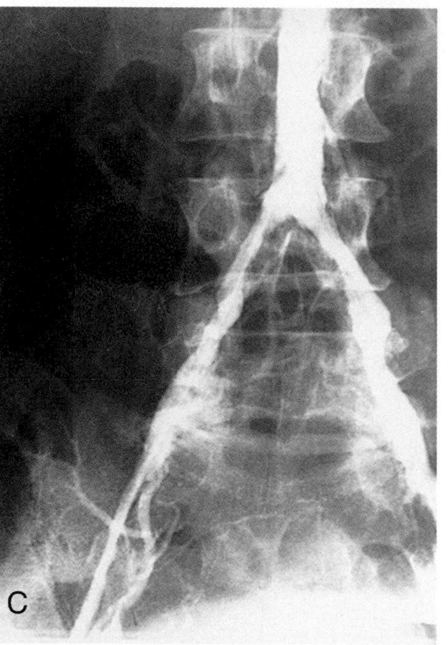

FIGURE 5-42 ■ Bilateral iliac artery stenosis and angioplasty. A standard contrast angiogram *(A)* shows two areas of very high grade stenosis in both common iliac arteries *(arrows)*. A catheter was placed across each area of stenosis. These catheters have balloons that can be inflated along the length of the catheter between the two metallic markers *(B)*. After balloon dilatation *(C)*, there has been some, although not complete, relief of the stenoses.

vessels, such as the iliac arteries (Fig. 5-42). Five-year patency rates are usually quoted as 70% to 90%. Often it also is possible to insert a metallic stent, an expandable wire mesh tube that is placed inside the vessel to keep it from restenosing.

Another relatively new procedure is the creation of an intrahepatic portal shunt. This method is used on patients with end-stage cirrhosis and portal hypertension who are not candidates for surgery. The approach involves puncturing the right jugular vein and passing a catheter down the superior vena cava into the inferior vena cava and then into the hepatic vein. A needle is pushed through the liver into the portal system; the needle tract is dilated with a balloon; and a stent is placed in the dilated tract. This is called a transjugular intrahepatic portal shunt (TIPS) procedure.

Renal Artery Stenosis and Hypertension

Only 1% to 2% of hypertension is due to renal artery stenosis. The clinical features that help distinguish this from other forms of hypertension are occurrence at an unusual age (younger than 30 and older than 50 years) or poor response to medical therapy. Physical examination may reveal a bruit in the flank or upper abdomen. Laboratory evaluation may rarely yield evidence of hyperaldosteronism, including hypokalemia and metabolic acidosis. An appropriate initial imaging test is a nuclear medicine captopril renogram. The captopril causes the affected kidney to have poor function temporarily. If this occurs, the study is repeated without captopril, and, if this is normal (because the kidney compensates for the renal artery stenosis), an angiogram and possible angioplasty are indicated. Another choice is to perform an MR angiogram (Fig. 5-43) or a CT angiogram.

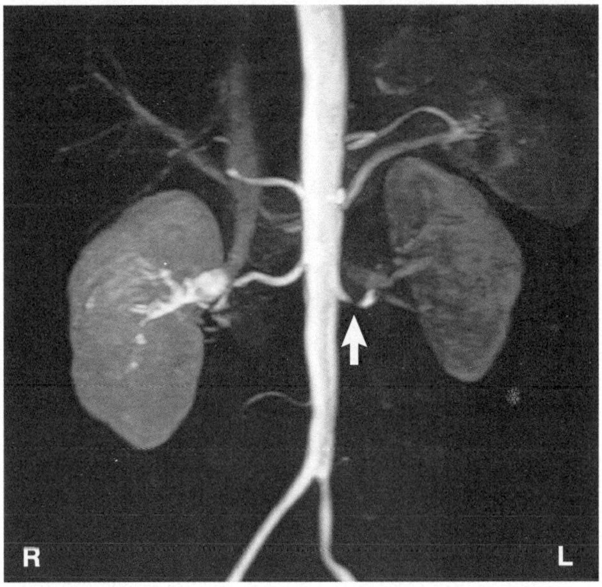

FIGURE 5-43 ■ **Renal artery stenosis.** In this case, a young woman had a blood pressure of 220/140 mm Hg and was referred for a magnetic resonance angiogram (MRA). The MRA showed an area of stenosis *(arrow)* of the left renal artery as well as a slightly smaller and poorly perfused left kidney. After balloon dilatation angioplasty, her pressure returned to normal almost immediately.

Deep Venous Thrombosis

Evaluation of the veins of the lower extremities is particularly important, because this is a very common site for development of thrombi that can lead to potentially fatal pulmonary emboli. Deep venous thrombosis fails to produce clinical signs in half the patients who have it. Thrombosis in calf veins is usually insignificant; however, in the femoral veins and pelvic veins, thrombi are significant. Risk factors include prolonged bed rest, immobilization of an extremity, pregnancy, oral contraceptives, malignancy, and postoperative and traumatic circumstances.

The historical approach for imaging veins was contrast venography. With this approach, contrast material is injected into the veins on the dorsum of the foot, and the contrast is visualized as it proceeds up the veins of the leg and into the pelvis. Contrast venography allows visualization of the deep venous system but not of the superficial venous system. Clots can be seen as intraluminal defects with contrast material surrounding them. Total obstruction with visualization of collateral veins also can be seen with thrombosis. One of the problems with contrast venography is that it involves the use of iodinated and intravenously administered contrast material. Sometimes venous access is difficult in patients who have a grossly swollen leg. It is possible that the contrast itself may cause some inflammation of the vein and may carry a low but real complication rate of thrombophlebitis. As a result, the use of contrast venography has markedly declined.

The initial imaging test of choice for a patient with suspected deep venous thrombosis is ultrasonography. Ultrasound examination has a sensitivity and specificity of approximately 95%. The femoral artery and vein can both easily be visualized by using ultrasound. With pressure, the femoral vein will normally be compressed. If a clot exists within the vein, echoes will be seen

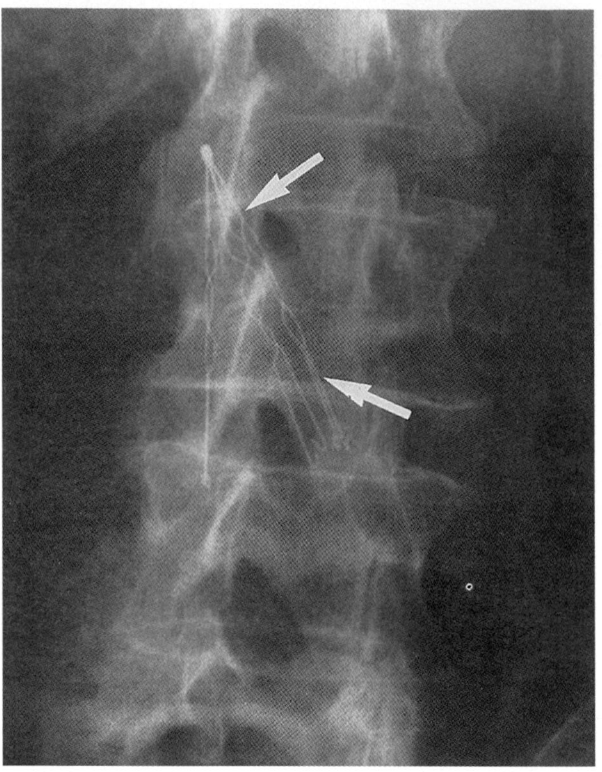

FIGURE 5-44 ■ Inferior vena caval filter. An expandable wire mesh basket *(arrows)* has been placed in the inferior vena cava. This can be done by pushing the device out of a catheter and allowing it to expand in place. This will keep the large clots from traveling from the lower extremities and pelvis up the inferior vena cava and into the lung.

within the lumen, and no compression will be identified. Color Doppler ultrasound can be used to classify flow in the vein into no flow or partial flow.

Recurrent deep venous thrombosis or deep venous thrombosis that is not successfully treated with heparin can result in multiple episodes of PEs. Because of the life-threatening nature of this problem, methods have been developed to keep the thrombi from migrating into the lung. Probably the most frequently used method is placement of a filter in the inferior vena cava. Access is gained through the femoral vein, and contrast is injected to make sure that no clot is in the iliac vein or inferior vena cava itself. After this, a catheter is advanced to the level just below the renal veins, and an expandable wire net or basket is pushed out the end of the catheter. The most commonly used device now is a Greenfield filter, and if it is present, it is easily seen on an AP x-ray of the abdomen projecting over the right side of the upper lumbar vertebra (Fig. 5-44).

Workup of Claudication

Claudication is most commonly caused by chronic arterial ischemia from atherosclerosis. The atherosclerosis can involve any site from the aortoiliac region distally. The simplest method to document lower extremity arterial occlusive disease is with ultrasonography. This is most commonly done in a vascular laboratory, and Doppler ultrasonography is used to measure the ankle-brachial index. A normal ankle-brachial index is 1.0 or greater. Before any type of surgical intervention, an arteriogram that includes visualization of the aortoiliac, femoral, popliteal, and tibial arteries is required. Few imaging tests are useful in evaluating extremity pain caused by venous or small vessel insufficiency, or for neurologic or muscular pain.

Suggested Textbooks on the Topic

Higgins CB, de Roos A: Cardiovascular MRI and MRA. Philadelphia, Lippincott Williams & Wilkins, 2002.

Manning WJ, Pennell DJ: Cardiovascular Magnetic Resonance. Philadelphia, WB Saunders, 2002.

Remy-Jardin M, Remy J, Mayo JR, Muller NL: CT Angiography of the Chest. Philadelphia, Lippincott Williams & Wilkins, 2001.

6 Gastrointestinal System

INTRODUCTION

Imaging Techniques and Anatomy

The most common imaging study of the abdomen is referred to as a KUB, or plain image of the abdomen. The term *KUB* is historical nonsense. It stands for *k*idneys, *u*reter, and *b*ladder, none of which is usually seen on a regular x-ray of the abdomen; nevertheless, the term remains widely used. A KUB is usually done with the patient supine (Fig. 6-1). When examining this image, you should look at the bony structures, the lung bases, and then at the soft tissue and gas patterns (Table 6-1). The soft tissue–pattern analysis should include evaluation of the lateral psoas margins. Whether you see them bilaterally, only faintly, or throughout their length depends on the shape of the psoas and the amount of retroperitoneal fat in that individual. It is all right if you do not see the psoas margin on either side. If you see the psoas margin on one side but not on the other, this is most commonly due to normal anatomic variation. In about 25% of cases, however, pathology will be found on the side of the obscured psoas margin.

Even though it is difficult to see, you should look for the outlines of the kidneys. Again, if you cannot see the outlines, you should not be terribly concerned, because they are often obscured by overlying bowel gas and fecal material. The liver is seen as a homogeneous soft tissue density in the right upper quadrant. The spleen can sometimes be seen as a smaller homogeneous density in the left upper quadrant. Although you will be able to appreciate massive enlargement of either one of these organs, minimal to moderate enlargement is very difficult to ascertain, and you should think twice before you suggest it. Clinical palpation and percussion are at least as accurate as x-rays in this situation.

Evaluation of the gas pattern also is important (Table 6-2). Because people routinely swallow air and drink lots of carbonated beverages, the stomach almost always has some gas within it. When a person is lying on his or her back, the air will go to the most anterior portion of the stomach, which is the body and antrum. This is seen as a curvilinear air collection, just along the left side of the upper lumbar spine (Fig. 6-2). If the person has swallowed a lot of air, you may see gas bubbles within the entire gastrointestinal (GI) tract extending from the stomach to the rectum. The origin of almost all these bubbles is swallowed air and not gas produced by intestinal bacteria. You should be able to identify the air patterns in the stomach, small bowel, colon, sigmoid, and rectum. Gas in the small bowel usually can be identified, because small bowel mucosa has very fine lines that cross all the way across the lumen. Most small bowel gas is located in the left midabdomen and the lower central abdomen. The colon often can be traced from the cecum in the right lower quadrant to both the hepatic and the splenic flexures and down to the sigmoid. The cecum and the colon often have a bubbly appearance representing a mixture of gas and fecal material. Colonic air often has a somewhat cloverleaf-shaped appearance caused by the haustra of the colon. Normal small bowel diameter should not exceed 3 cm,

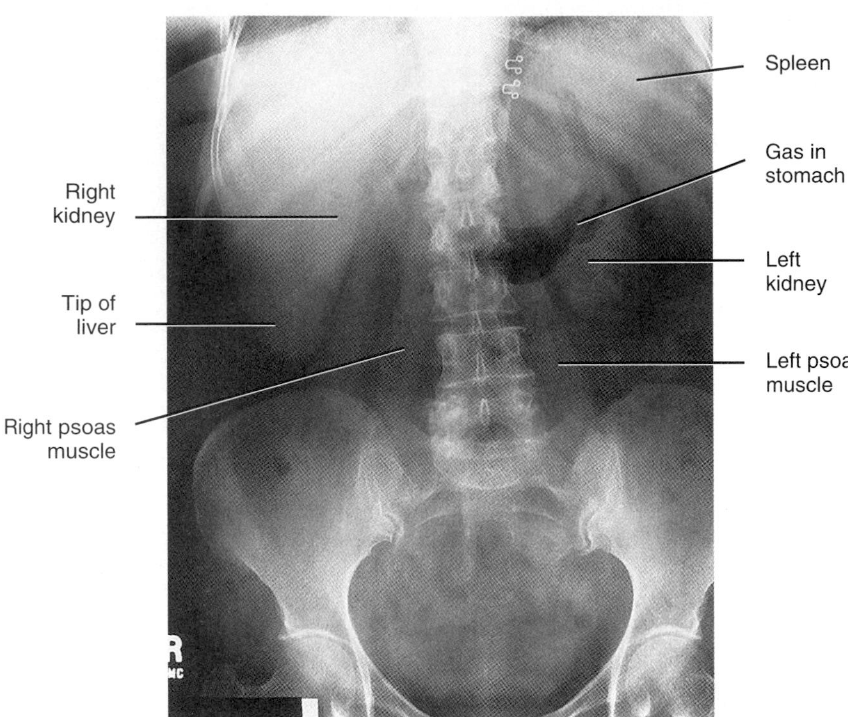

FIGURE 6-1 ■ Normal anatomy seen on a supine x-ray (KUB) of the abdomen.

and the colon should not exceed 6 cm. The cecum can normally be somewhat larger than the rest of the colon and may be up to 8 cm in diameter.

In addition to a supine abdominal image, a "three-way" view of the abdomen is often obtained. The additional two views are an upright posteroanterior (PA) chest x-ray and a view of the abdomen taken with the patient standing upright. The PA view of the chest is taken to look for chest pathology that may be mimicking or causing abdominal symptoms as well as to look for free air underneath the hemidiaphragms. The reason for the standing view of the abdomen is to look at the air/fluid levels within the bowel to differentiate between an obstruction and ileus.

TABLE 6–1 ■ **Items to Look for on a Plain Abdominal Image (KUB)**

Gas Patterns
Stomach, small bowel, and rectosigmoid
Abnormal or ectopic collections
Organ Shapes and Sizes
Liver
Spleen
Kidneys
Soft tissue pelvic masses
Calcification
Asymmetric psoas margins
Skeleton
Basilar lung abnormalities

KUB, kidneys, ureter, bladder.

TABLE 6–2 ■ **Evaluation of Gas Patterns on a Plain Image of the Abdomen**

Collections Normally Present
Look for dilatation of structure and assessment of wall or mucosal thickness in stomach, small bowel, colon, and rectosigmoid
Collections Not Normally Present
Free air under the diaphragm (upright film)
Free air on supine films (double bowel wall sign)
Right upper quadrant: Portal vein (peripheral in liver), biliary system (central in liver)
Small bubbles in an abscess
Emphysematous cholecystitis, pyelonephritis, or cystitis

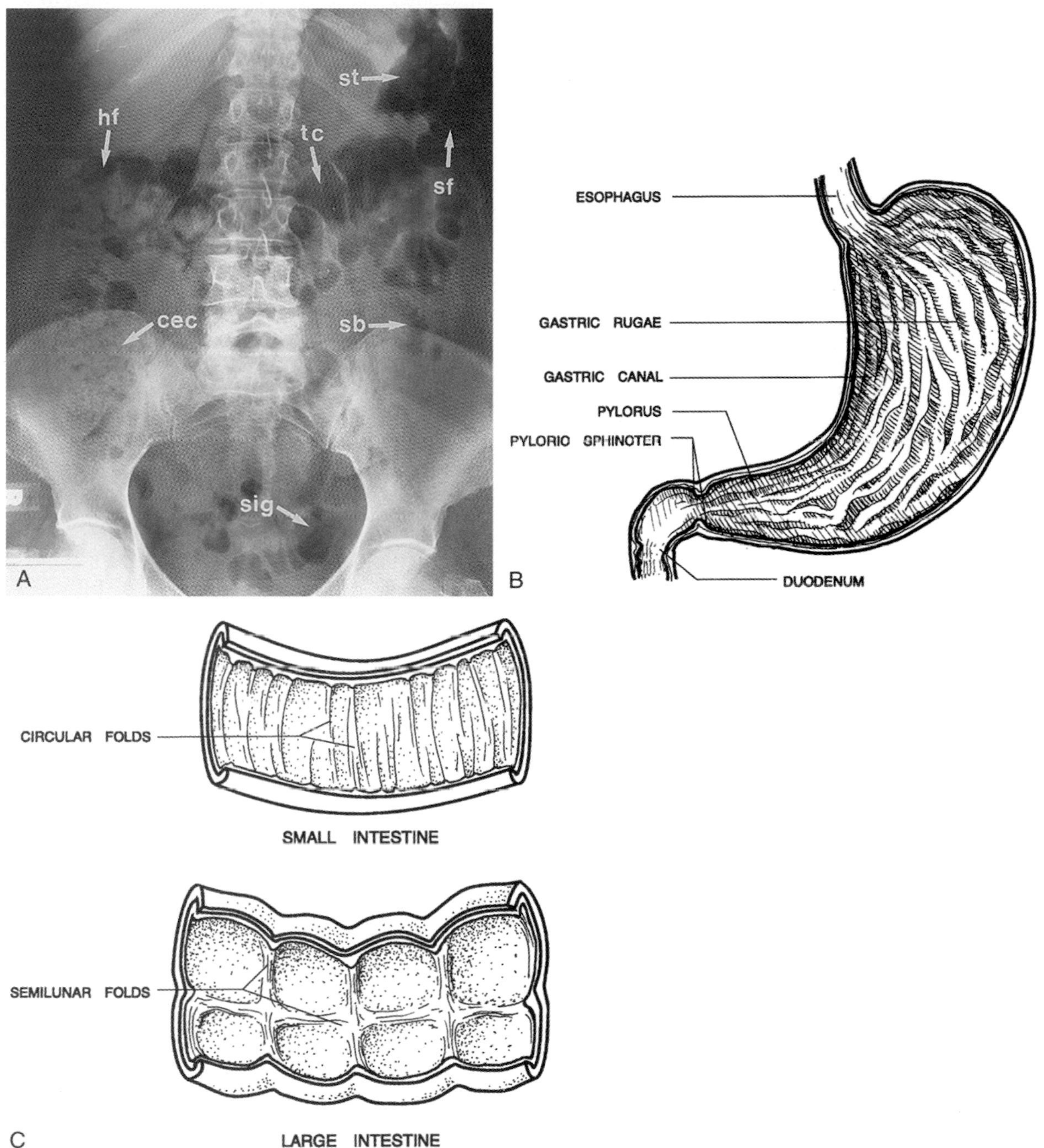

FIGURE 6-2 ■ Normal bowel gas pattern. Gas is normally swallowed and can be seen in the stomach (st). Small amounts of air normally can be seen in the small bowel (sb), and this is usually in the left midabdomen or central portion of the abdomen. In this patient, gas can be seen throughout the entire colon, including the cecum (cec). Where the air is mixed with feces, a mottled pattern appears. Cloverleaf-shaped collections of air are seen in the hepatic flexure (hf), transverse colon (tc), splenic flexure (sf), and sigmoid (sig).

A common variant is called *colonic interposition* (also called Chilaiditi syndrome). In this normal variant, the hepatic flexure of the colon can slip up between the superior aspect of the liver and the dome of the right hemidiaphragm (Fig. 6-3). This should not be mistaken for free air. When colonic interposition occurs, you can almost always see the haustral markings of the colon.

Computed tomography (CT) scanning is the most common procedure used to image nonintestinal abdominal pathology. The visualization of the solid organs, peritoneum, and retroperitoneum that is obtained with CT means that CT is being ordered as much as or more than abdominal plain films. CT anatomy is presented in Figure 6-4. With new scanners, the entire pelvis and abdomen can be imaged in a few minutes. The patients commonly prepare by drinking oral contrast for about 1 to 3 hours before the examination. This is important because it allows differentiation of bowel tissue from other soft tissues. If pelvic pathology is suspected, rectal contrast also should be given at the time of the examination. For most examinations, if renal function is normal, intravenous contrast also is given. This clearly outlines the vascular structures and provides excellent visualization of the kidneys, ureters, and bladder. Recently CT "virtual colonoscopy" was introduced. With this technique, a three-dimensional reconstruction of the abdomen is generated and the computer is used to create images that track the inside of the colon. The technique requires that the colon be well cleaned so that small bits of fecal material are not mistaken for polyps. True colonoscopy has the advantage that if a lesion is seen, a biopsy can be performed.

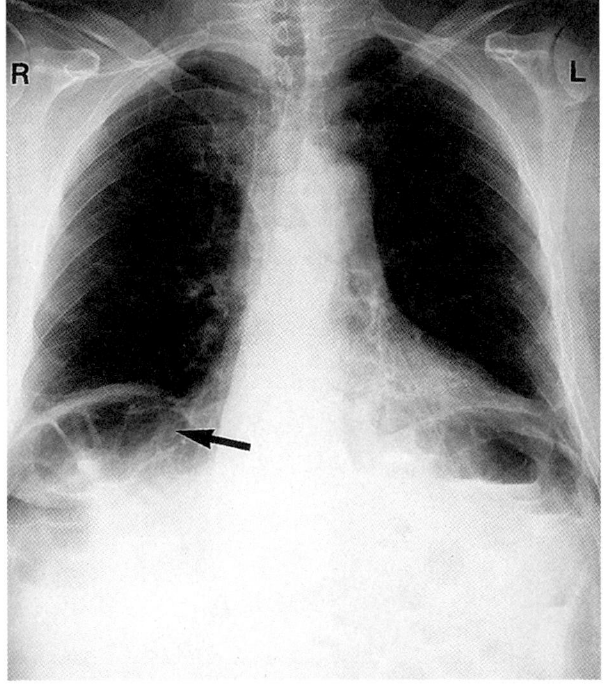

FIGURE 6-3 ■ **Colonic interposition.** This is a normal variant in which the hepatic flexure can be seen above the liver. This is seen as a gas collection under the right hemidiaphragm *(arrow)*, but it is clearly identified as colon, owing to the transverse haustral markings.

Ultrasound examination is used primarily to image the liver, kidneys, gallbladder, common bile duct, and, to a much lesser extent, the pancreas and appendix. Ultrasound is often limited by the inability of the sound to penetrate air and by large loops of bowel that may obscure underlying pathology. Ascites is easily detected and localized for paracentesis.

Nuclear medicine scans provide physiological information that is often not available using other imaging techniques. It is often used to quantitate gastroesophageal reflux and gastric emptying times, to diagnose acute cholecystitis and bile leaks, to determine the site of GI bleeding, and to stage tumors.

Pneumoperitoneum

It is easiest to identify small amounts of free air in the peritoneal cavity by doing an upright chest x-ray. In this manner, as little as 3 or 4 cc of air may be visualized (Fig. 6-5*A*). An upright abdominal film is usually not very useful to look for free air, because the domes of the diaphragms are often off the upper edge of the film. It is very difficult to appreciate even relatively large amounts of free air within the peritoneal cavity by looking at a supine (KUB) view of the abdomen. If a lot of free air is present, you may be able to see the bowel wall outlined by air (Fig. 6-5*B*). If the patient is too sick to stand, and you suspect a small

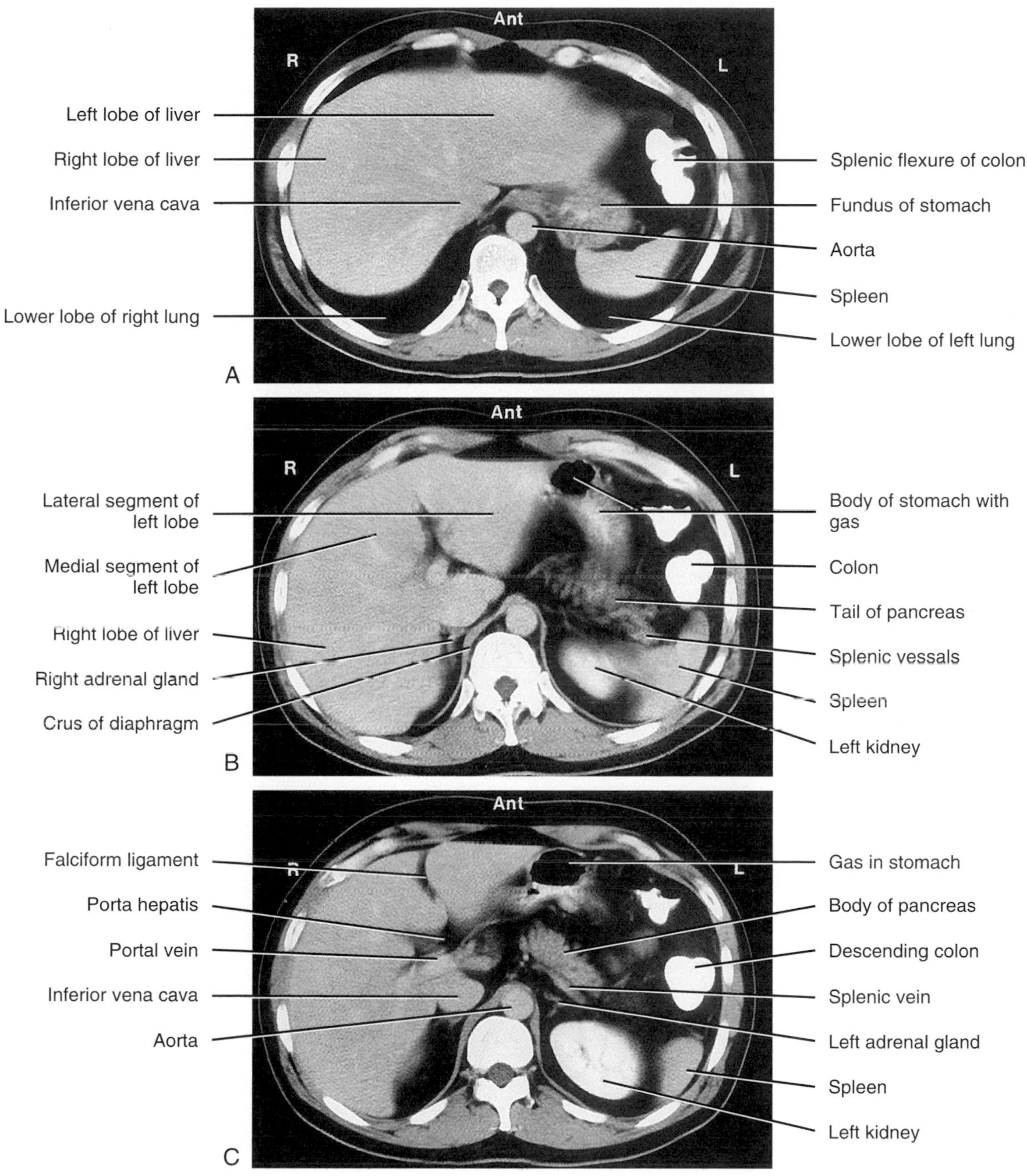

FIGURE 6-4 ■ Normal transverse computed tomography (CT) anatomy of the abdomen and pelvis. The patient has been given oral, rectal, and intravenous contrast media.

Continued

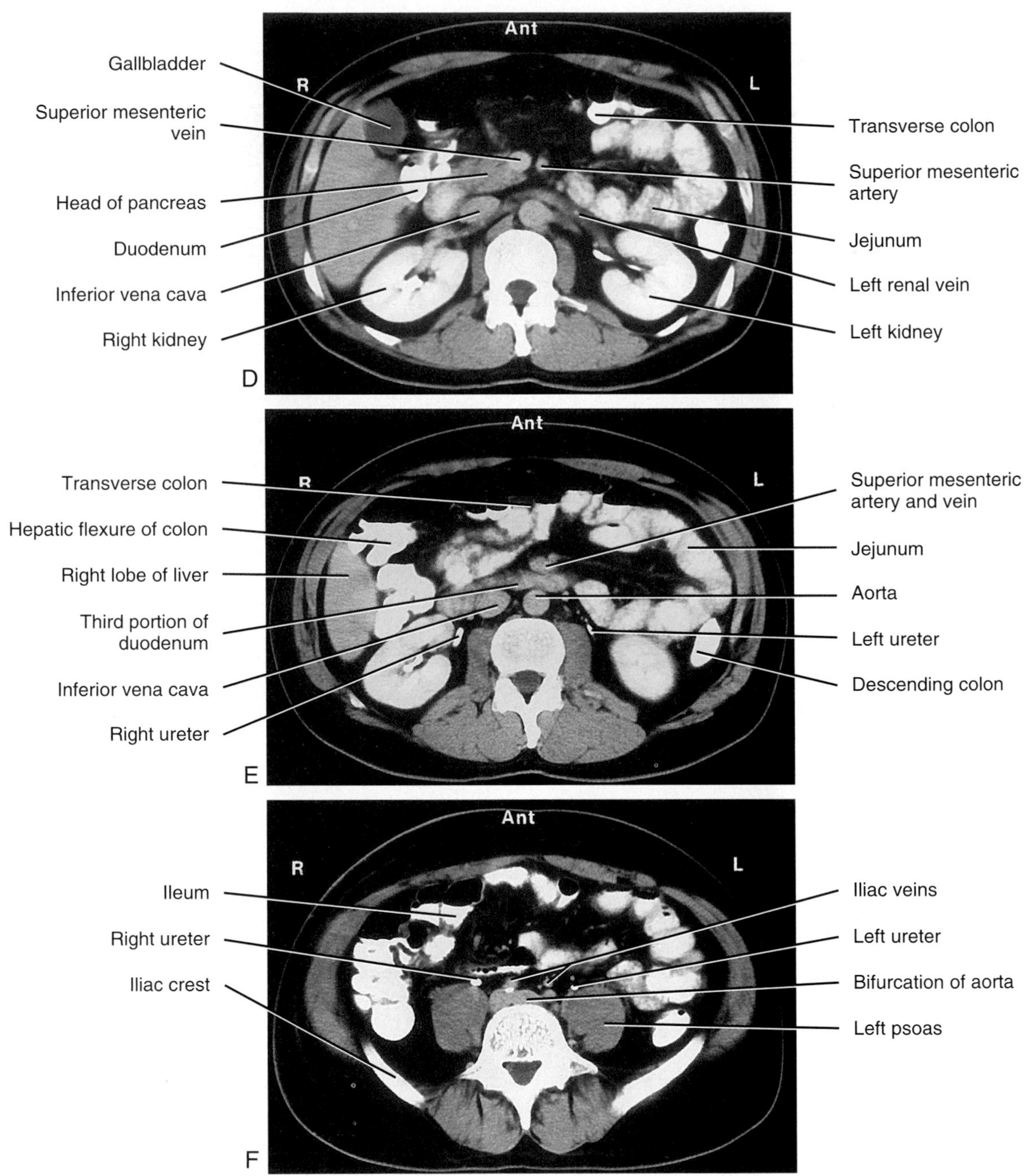

FIGURE 6-4 cont'd

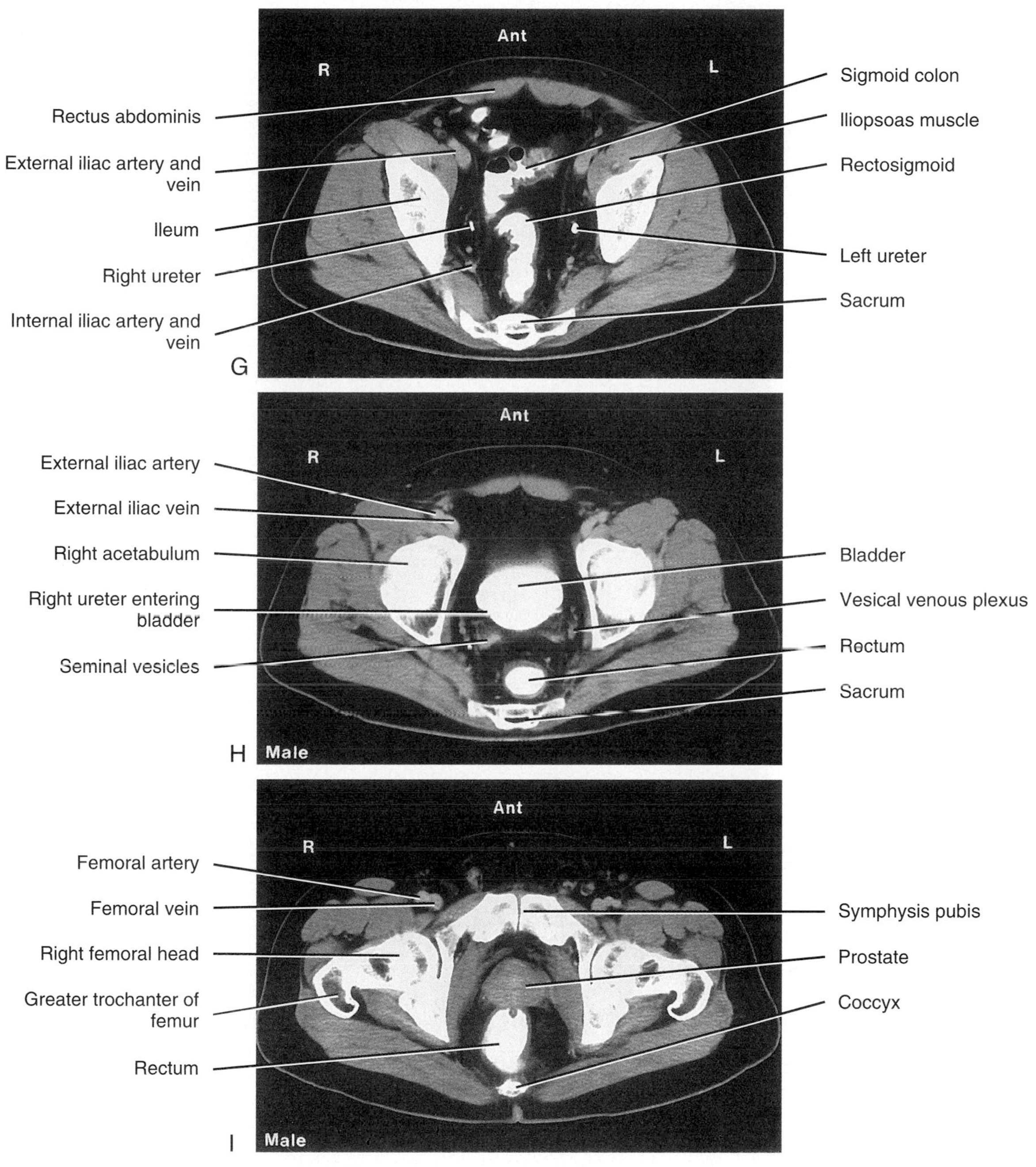

FIGURE 6-4 cont'd

Continued

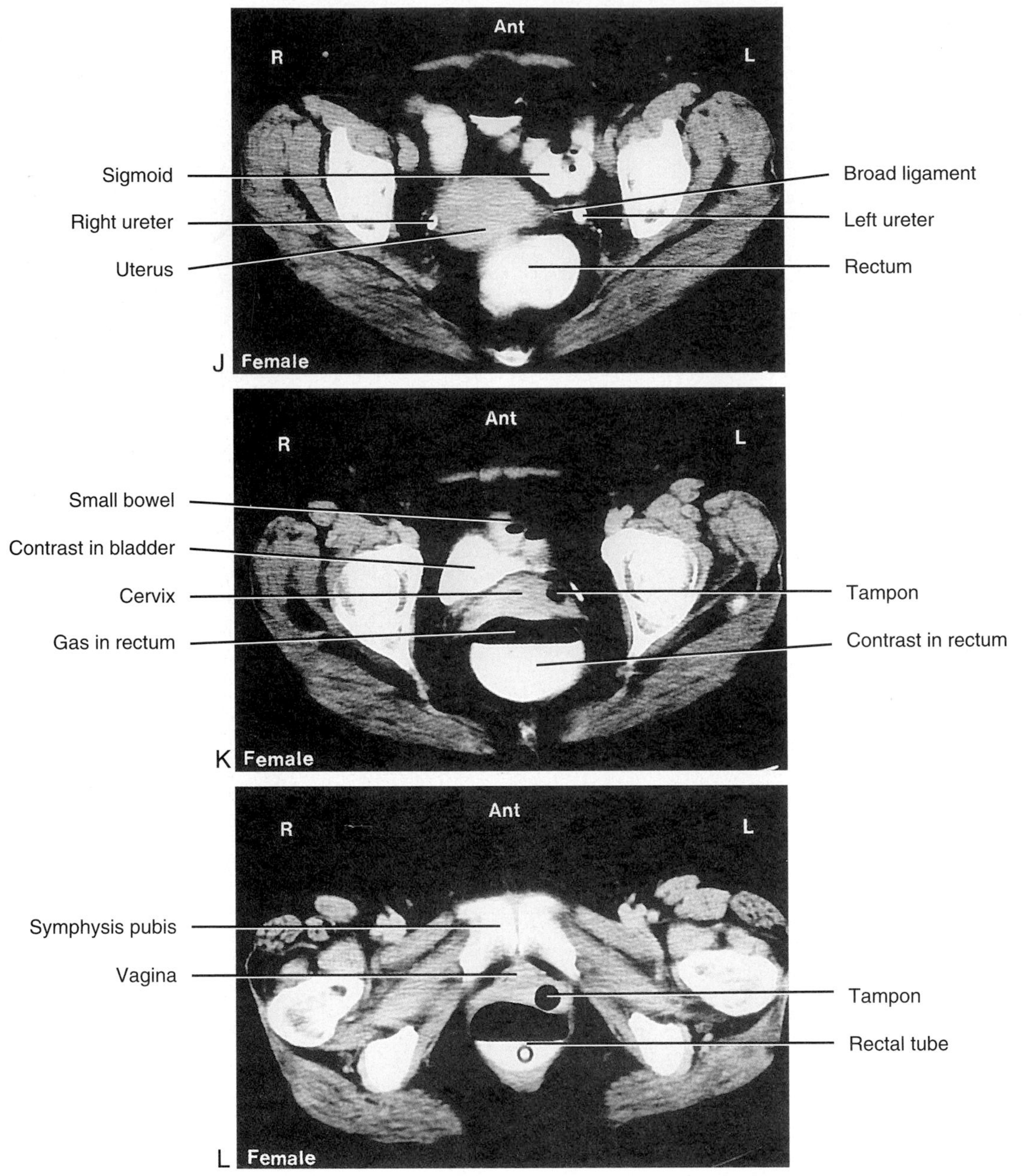

FIGURE 6-4 cont'd

pneumoperitoneum, order a left lateral decubitus view of the abdomen. In this manner, with the patient lying on the left side (for 10 to 15 minutes), small amounts of air can be seen tracking up over the lateral aspect of the right lobe of the liver.

Intraabdominal Abscesses and Fever of Unknown Origin

Air can be seen within some, but by no means all, abscesses. Although a very large abscess may be appreciated on a plain film, it is often difficult to tell whether you are looking at air in

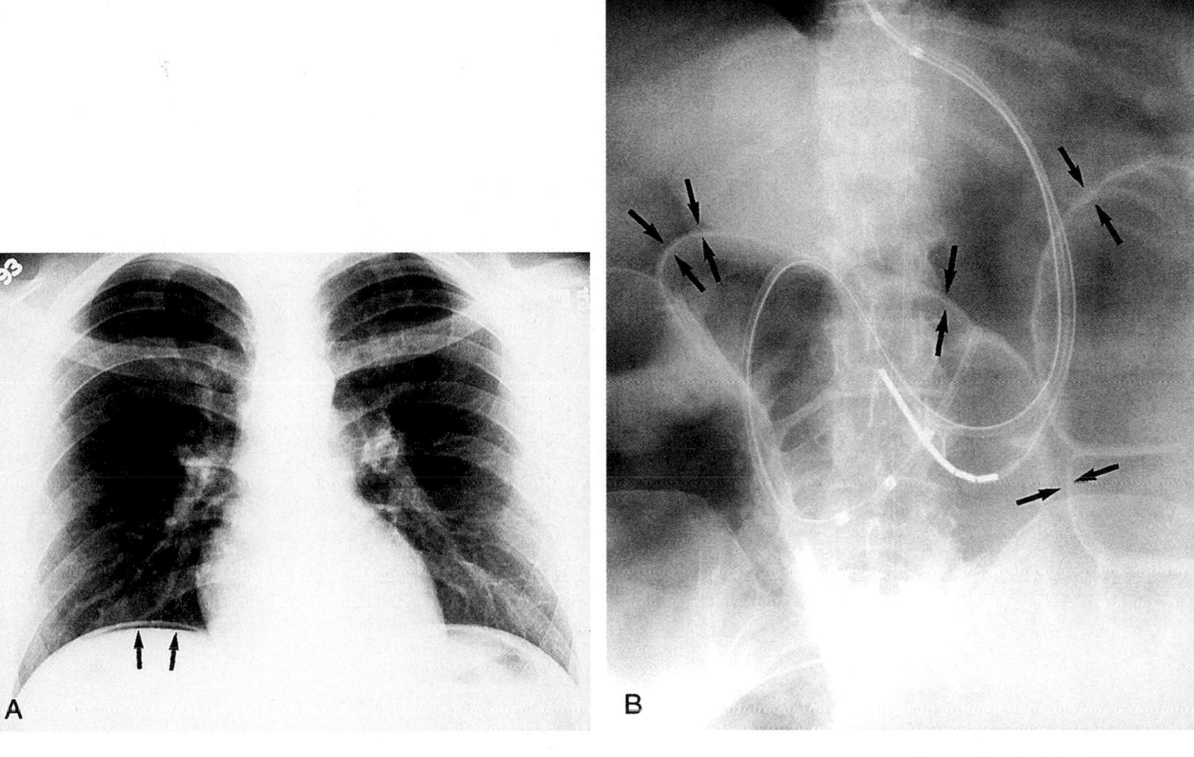

FIGURE 6-5 ■ Pneumoperitoneum. *A,* A few milliliters of free air can be identified *(arrows)* under the right hemidiaphragm on this upright posteroanterior (PA) chest x-ray. *B,* A supine abdominal film obtained on a different patient with massive pneumoperitoneum shows the bowel wall *(arrows)* outlined on both sides by air.

the bowel or in some other structure. For this reason, the imaging test of choice when an abdominal or pelvic abscess is suspected is a CT scan (Fig. 6-6). It is very important that under these circumstances, you order a CT scan with GI contrast so that the entire bowel can be filled with contrast. If this is not done, it may be difficult, even on a CT scan, to differentiate a collection of bowel that has air and fluid within it from an abscess.

The imaging workup of a patient with a fever of unknown origin usually begins with a chest x-ray. Most infectious processes of the chest are quite obvious. Once intrathoracic pathology has been excluded, the next place to look is the abdomen and pelvis. Assuming that the physical examination of the abdomen and pelvis is negative, a CT scan is usually ordered.

Feeding Tubes

As mentioned in Chapter 3, feeding tubes or nasogastric tubes are particularly recalcitrant medical devices. Not only can they inadvertently be passed into the trachea and major bronchus, but also they love to coil within the pharynx and stomach. On the plain film, a well-placed enteric (Dobbhoff) feeding tube can be seen coming down the esophagus, passing in an arc through the stomach toward the right of midline, and then progressing downward in a reverse arc through the duodenum, back to the left, across the vertebral column. It is best to have the tip of these feeding tubes near the junction of the duodenum and jejunum (ligament of Treitz) (Fig. 6-7). An unacceptable position of a feeding tube tip is in the esophagus or at the gastroesophageal

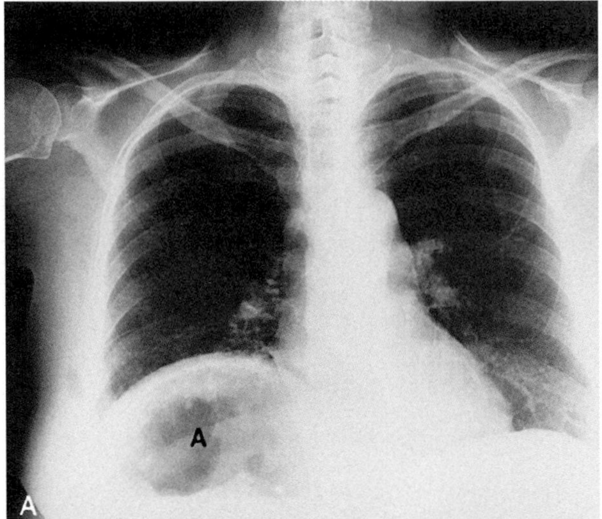

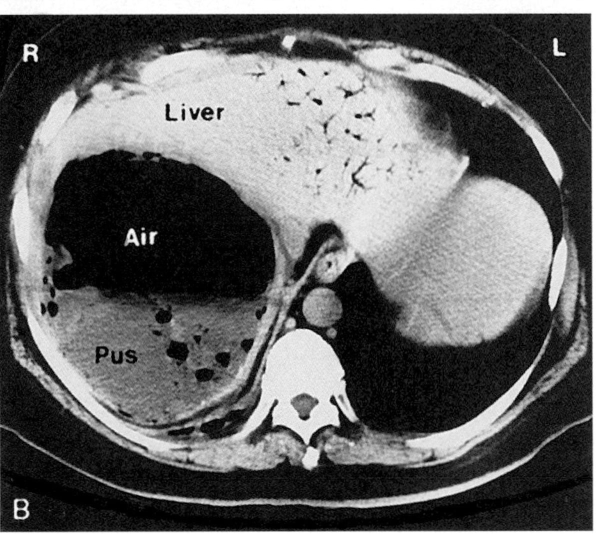

FIGURE 6-6 ■ Hepatic abscess. This drug abuser initially was seen with right upper quadrant pain and fever. On the upright chest film *(A)*, a collection of air is seen in the right upper quadrant. Notice the thick and irregular margin between the air and the hemidiaphragm, indicating that this is not free air. A transverse computed tomography (CT) scan *(B)* shows an air and pus collection due to a large abscess in the right lobe of the liver.

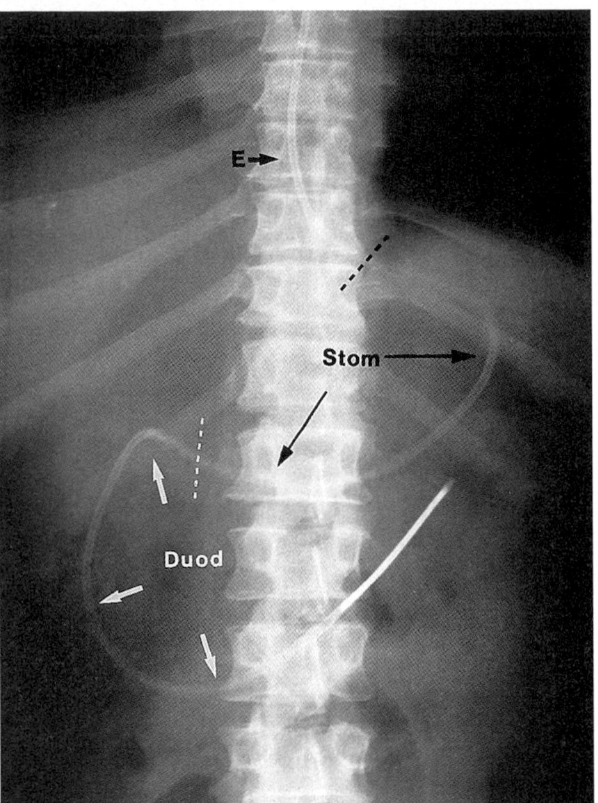

FIGURE 6-7 ■ Optimal positioning for an enteric feeding tube. On an anteroposterior (AP) film of the upper abdomen, the feeding tube should be seen extending down the esophagus (E) slightly to the left of midline, taking a gentle curve to the right through the stomach (Stom), and then reversing its curve through the duodenum (Duod) and going back to the left across the spine to the junction of the fourth portion of the duodenum and the jejunum (ligament of Treitz).

junction (Fig. 6-8). If you feed patients with a tube in these positions, esophageal reflux and the potential for aspiration can occur.

Abdominal Calcifications

Abdominal calcifications are quite common, and you should be familiar with them so that you know which are important and which to discount (Table 6-3). Fortunately, most of them have some characteristics that make this task relatively easy. Calcifications in the right upper quadrant are usually gallstones or kidney stones. If the calcifications are multiple, are very close together, and lie outside the normal expected area of the kidney, you can be reasonably assured that they are gallstones (Fig. 6-9). A single calcification in the right upper quadrant may be due either to a kidney stone or to a gallstone. A simple way to tell the difference is to take a right posterior oblique view. A gallstone will rotate anteriorly and will not move with the outline of the kidney. Another way to tell the differ-

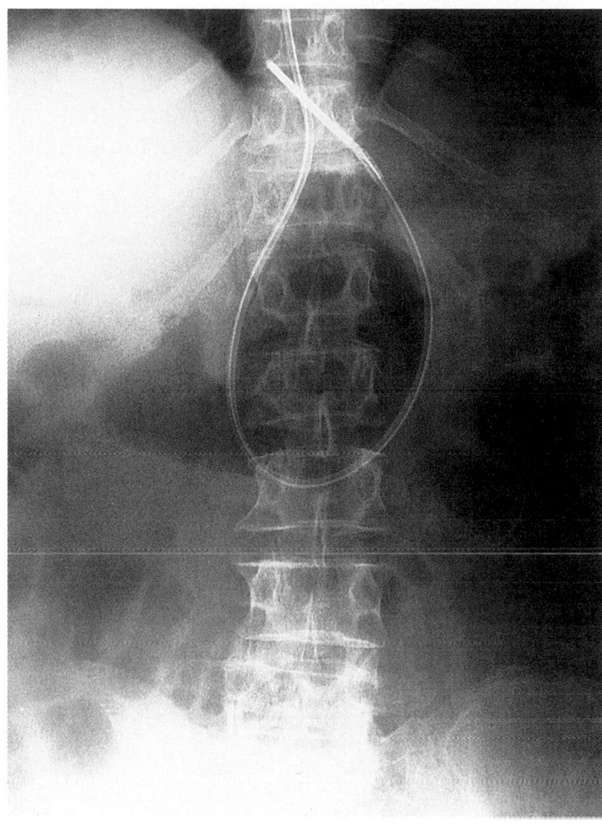

FIGURE 6-8 ■ Unacceptable position of feeding tube. In this case, the tip of the feeding tube is in the distal esophagus, with the remainder coiled within the body of the stomach. Feeding with the tube in this position is likely to cause aspiration.

TABLE 6–3 ■ **Differential Diagnosis of Abdominal Calcifications**

Right Upper Quadrant
- Gallstones
- Renal calculus, cyst, or tumor
- Adrenal calcification

Right Midabdomen or Right Lower Quadrant
- Ureteral calculi
- Mesenteric lymph node
- Appendicolith

Left Upper Quadrant
- Splenic artery
- Splenic cyst
- Splenic histoplasmosis (multiple and small)
- Renal calculus, cyst, or tumor
- Adrenal calcification
- Tail of pancreas

Central Abdomen
- Aorta or aortic aneurysm
- Pancreas (chronic pancreatitis)
- Calcified metastatic nodes

Pelvis
- Phleboliths (low in pelvis)
- Uterine fibroids (popcorn appearance)
- Dermoid
- Bladder stone
- Calcifications in buttocks from injections
- Prostatic (behind symphysis)
- Vas deferens (diabetic)
- Iliac or femoral vessels

ence is to order a right upper quadrant ultrasound study, on which gallstones are very easily identified (Fig. 6-10). In addition, if the patient has right upper quadrant pain or jaundice, the ultrasound image will allow you to assess whether the common bile duct is dilated and to look at the internal architecture of the liver and pancreas.

Left upper quadrant calcifications are essentially always related to the spleen. Multiple small punctate calcifications are the result of histoplasmosis (Fig. 6-11). Serpiginous or rounded calcifications in the left upper quadrant usually are related to splenic artery calcification or to a splenic artery aneurysm (Fig. 6-12).

With chronic pancreatitis, calcification of the pancreas often is found. This can be seen as spotted or mottled calcification, usually lying in a somewhat horizontal distribution over the vertebral bodies of L1 and L2 and extending to the left. Remember, however, that on a plain abdominal x-ray, most persons with chronic pancreatitis do not have visible calcifications. CT scanning can identify calcifications much more easily than can a standard x-ray (Fig. 6-13*A*), but you should rely on clinical and laboratory history, not on a CT scan (Fig. 6-13*B*), for the diagnosis of chronic pancreatitis.

Calcification of mesenteric lymph nodes can occur as a result of previous infections. These are usually seen as somewhat rounded or popcorn-shaped calcifications in the right midabdomen. A tip-off is the significant downward movement of these calcifications on the upright views, because the mesentery is very mobile (Fig. 6-14).

In a patient who has right lower quadrant pain, look very carefully in this area for calcifications. A stone within the appendix (appendicol-

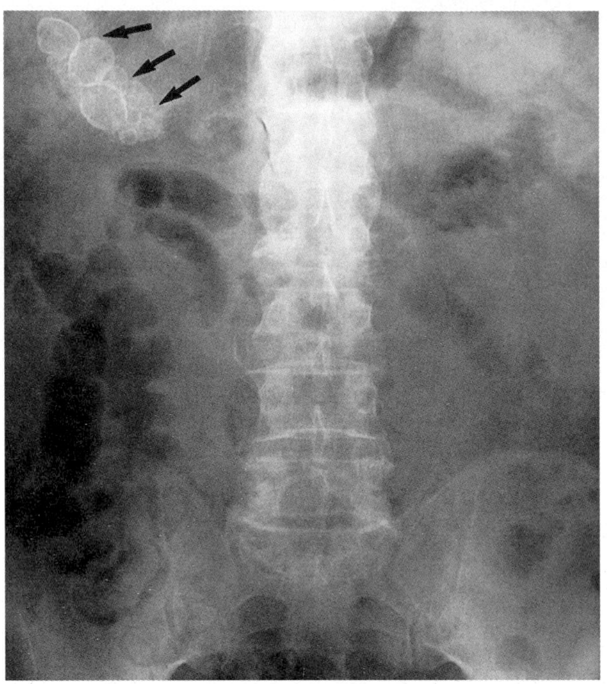

FIGURE 6-9 ■ Multiple gallstones. Any collection of grouped calcifications in the right upper quadrant *(arrows)* is most likely due to gallstones but does not indicate acute cholecystitis.

ith) often projects over the right side of the sacrum (Fig. 6-15) and can be difficult to see unless you look carefully. An appendicolith is present in approximately 10% of patients with appendicitis, and if you see an appendicolith, a very high probability of appendicitis exists. Other signs of appendicitis are a bubbly gas collection (appendiceal abscess) in the right lower quadrant or a focal ileus (dilatation) of the nearby small bowel caused by the inflammatory reaction.

In adults, it is very common to see rounded calcifications in the lower half of the pelvis. These almost always are 1 cm or less in diameter, and they are phleboliths (calcifications within pelvic venous structures). They are easy to identify because they often have a lucent or dark center (Fig. 6-16). They can occasionally be confused with stones in the distal ureter, and if a patient has symptoms of renal colic or obstruction, it is often necessary to perform a noncontrasted CT or intravenous pyelogram (IVP) to determine which of the calcifications in the lower pelvis may be a phlebolith or a calculus.

Uterine fibroids can often be calcified. This type of calcification is very similar to the popcorn type seen in the mesenteric lymph nodes. The difference is that fibroids are located in a suprapubic position and centrally in the pelvis. On occasion, these can be quite large and spectacular (Fig. 6-17).

Two special types of calcification can be seen in the male pelvis. The first, prostatic calcifications, are found immediately behind the symphysis pubis. They are quite common and are the result of benign inflammatory disease. They are not associated with prostate cancer (Fig. 6-18). The second, and more rare, type of calcification looks like a little set of antlers in the middle of the pelvis, projecting slightly above the symphysis pubis. This represents calcification of the vas deferens and almost always indicates that the patient has diabetes (Fig. 6-19).

Acute Abdominal Pain

Acute atraumatic abdominal pain requires urgent evaluation. Evaluation of the location, onset, progression, and character of abdominal pain is necessary to begin development of a reasonable differential diagnosis. A thorough medical history and physical examination are necessary because abdominal pain may be associated with GI, genitourinary, cardiovascular, or respiratory disorders. An electrocardiogram may be necessary to exclude myocardial causes. In addition to physical examination of the chest and abdomen, pelvic and rectal examinations also may yield useful information. Sudden onset of pain is often associated with bowel perforation, ruptured ectopic pregnancy, ovarian cyst, aneurysm, or ischemic bowel. Gradually increasing and localizing pain is more common in appendicitis, cholecystitis, and bowel obstruction.

After the patient has been assessed clinically, a reasonable approach to imaging can be formulated. In most cases of acute abdominal pain, the best initial imaging study is an upright posteranterior (PA) chest x-ray and a supine and upright view of the abdomen (the so-called "three-way abdomen"). CT scanning is used when abscess, aneurysm, or retroperitoneal pathology is sus-

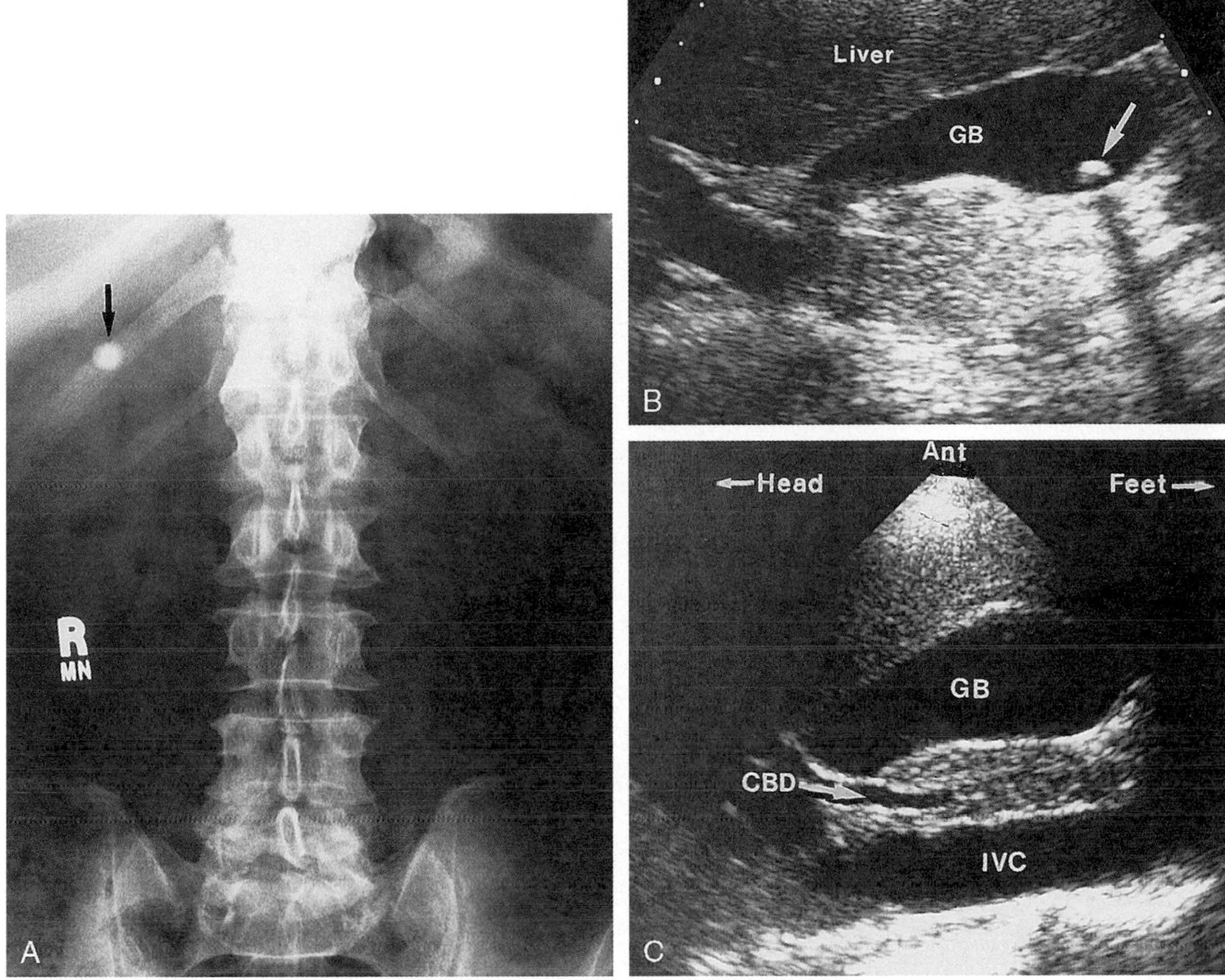

FIGURE 6-10 ■ Single gallstone. *A,* On the KUB (plain film of the abdomen), a single calcification is seen in the right upper quadrant. It is not possible to tell from this one picture whether this is a gallstone, kidney stone, or calcification in some other structure. *B,* A longitudinal ultrasound image in this patient clearly shows the liver, gallbladder, and an echogenic focus *(arrow)* within the gallbladder lumen, representing the single gallstone. Also note the dark shadow behind the gallstone. *C,* Another longitudinal ultrasound image slightly more medial also shows the inferior vena cava (IVC) and the common bile duct (CBD), which can be measured. Here it is of normal diameter.

pected. Ultrasound is the best initial examination if gallbladder, obstetric, or gynecologic etiologies are suspected.

Acute Gastroenteritis

A diagnosis of acute gastroenteritis is made on the basis of clinical history and the presence of diarrhea. The patients also may have vomiting, nausea, and abdominal pain. Dehydration is a common complication. The only procedure recommended is flexible sigmoidoscopy if blood is present in the stool.

Abdominal Masses

Abdominal masses can arise from any organ or structure in the peritoneal space, retroperitoneum, aorta, pelvis, or abdominal wall. As a general rule, most abdominal masses do not

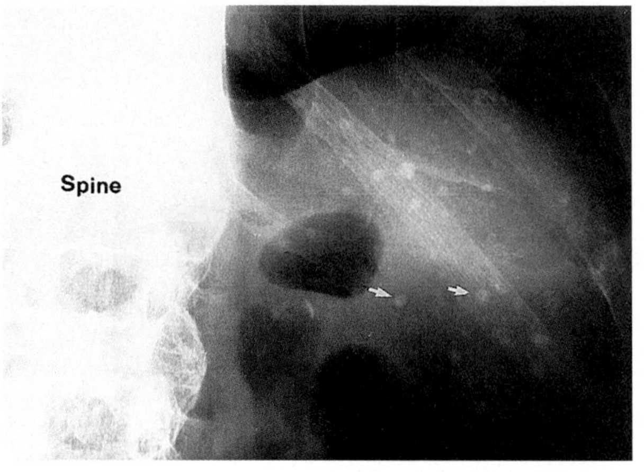

FIGURE 6-11 ■ Splenic histoplasmosis. Multiple small rounded calcifications in the left upper quadrant (some of which are shown with *small arrows*) are very specific, representing previous infection with histoplasmosis. These are of little, if any, clinical significance.

grow down into the pelvis, but pelvic masses (being largely confined) often grow up into the abdomen. The initial imaging study should be a three-way view of the abdomen to look for associated thoracic pathology (such as metastases or effusions) abnormal gas collections, displacement of the bowel, renal outlines, or associated calcification. Although ultrasound imaging can be used to characterize an abdominal mass, CT scanning of the abdomen and pelvis with intravenous and oral contrast is usually obtained.

ESOPHAGUS

Anatomy and Imaging Techniques

The appropriate initial imaging study for a number of suspected clinical problems is shown in Table 6-4. Imaging of the esophagus for many

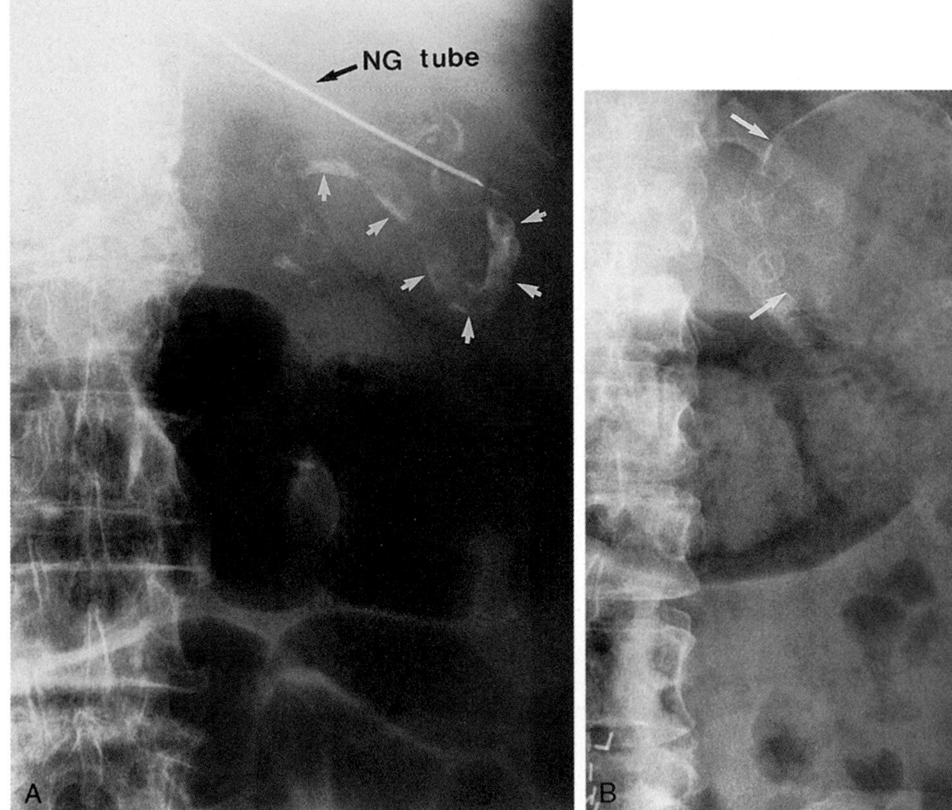

FIGURE 6-12 ■ Splenic vascular calcifications. Serpiginous calcifications in the left upper quadrant *(A)* are almost always due to splenic artery calcification. This finding is of no clinical significance. Occasionally, splenic artery aneurysms may cause a shell-like, rounded, left upper quadrant calcification *(B)*. NG, nasogastric tube.

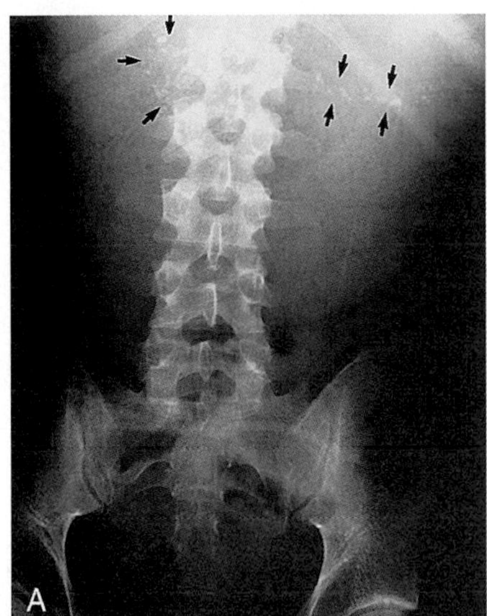

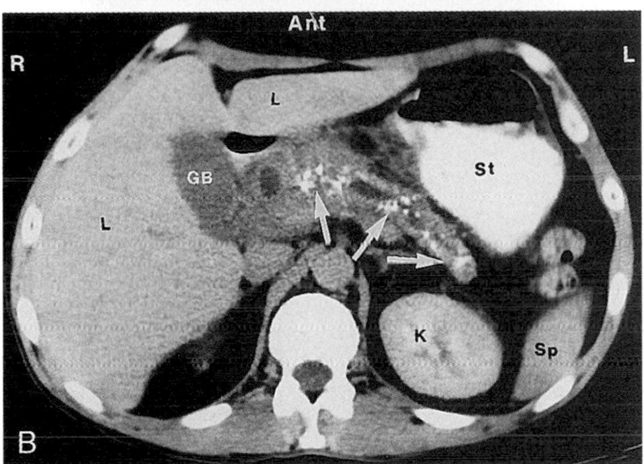

FIGURE 6-13 ■ Calcification in chronic pancreatitis. Rarely, on a plain film of the abdomen *(A)*, a horizontal band of calcifications can be seen extending across the upper midabdomen *(arrows)*. Calcification within the pancreas is much easier to see on a transverse computed tomography (CT) scan of the upper abdomen *(B)*. Calcification is seen as white speckled areas within the pancreas *(arrows)*. The darker areas within the pancreas represent dilated common and pancreatic ducts.

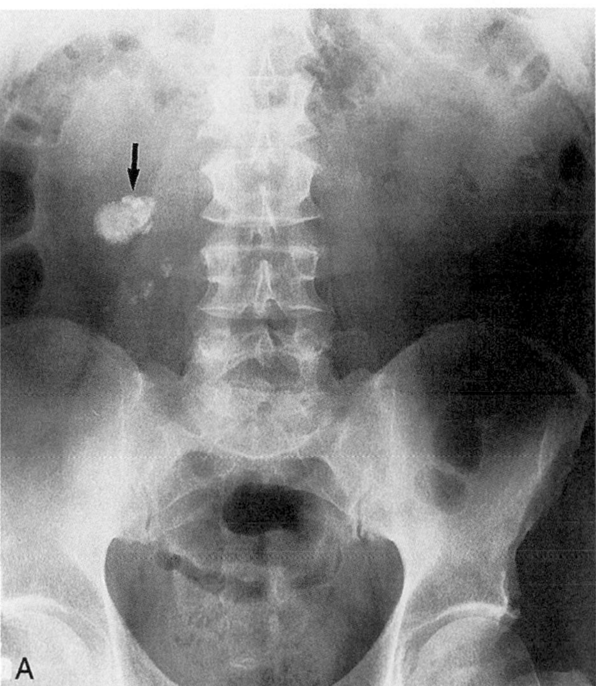

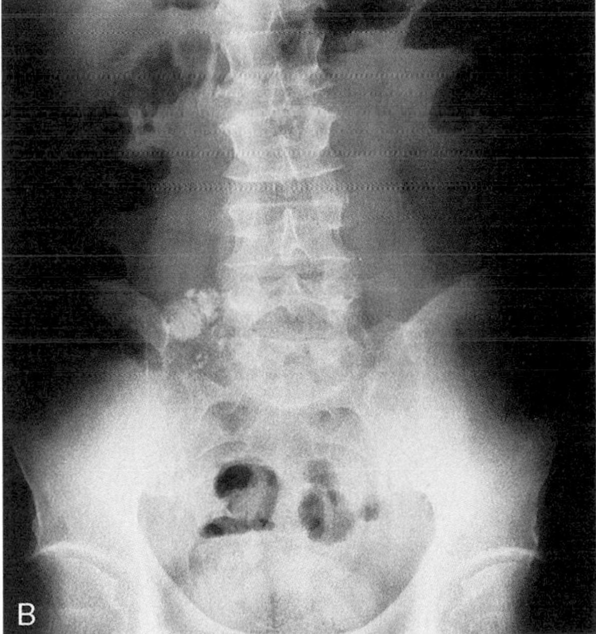

FIGURE 6-14 ■ Calcification in the mesenteric lymph nodes. This is a benign finding. The calcifications are typically located in the midabdomen to the right of midline, are somewhat popcorn shaped *(arrow)*, and are relatively easy to see on a supine KUB *(A)*. On an upright view of the abdomen *(B)*, these calcifications drop substantially, owing to the mobility of the mesentery.

problems is best done by direct visualization (endoscopy). Because this is a major procedure requiring sedation, many physicians begin by ordering an upper gastrointestinal (GI) examination or a contrast esophagogram. In addition to barium, other water-soluble contrast materials can be used. If a tear or perforation of the esophagus is suspected, it is best initially to use

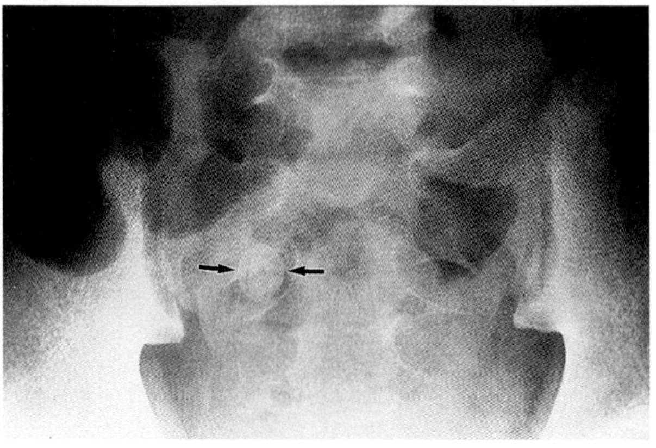

FIGURE 6-15 ■ Appendicolith. This calcification within the appendix can be seen almost anywhere in the right lower quadrant but is especially difficult to see when it overlies the sacrum *(arrows).* A right lower quadrant calcification in a patient with pain in this area should carry an extremely high clinical suspicion of acute appendicitis.

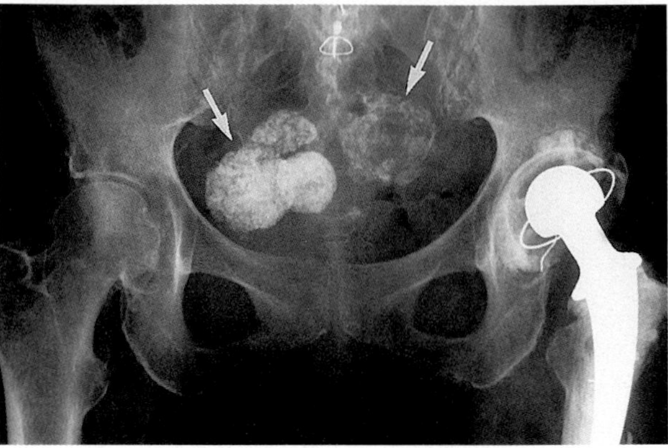

FIGURE 6-17 ■ Calcified fibroids. Central pelvic calcifications, which are somewhat amorphous, most commonly represent fibroids *(arrows).*

water-soluble contrast material rather than barium. If aspiration is suspected, barium is used, because water-soluble contrast can irritate the lung.

The normal esophagus has a rather smooth lining. Two indentations, due to impression by

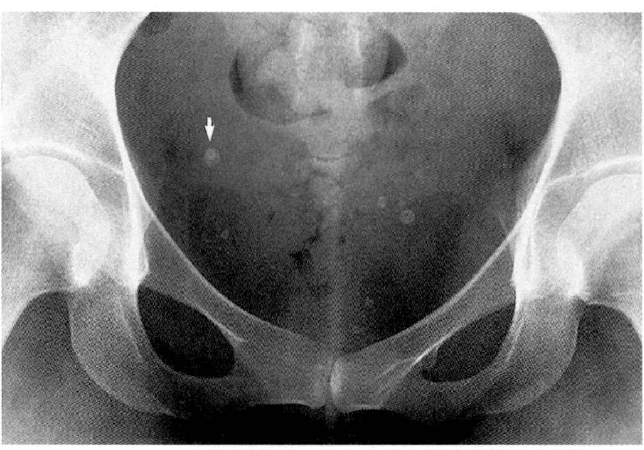

FIGURE 6-16 ■ Phleboliths. These rounded vascular calcifications within the pelvis *(arrow)* are very common and are of no clinical significance. They are usually round and less than 1 cm in diameter. They often have a lucent or dark center. They are typically seen in the lower half of the pelvic brim and can occasionally be difficult to differentiate from a ureteral calculus without an intravenous pyelogram.

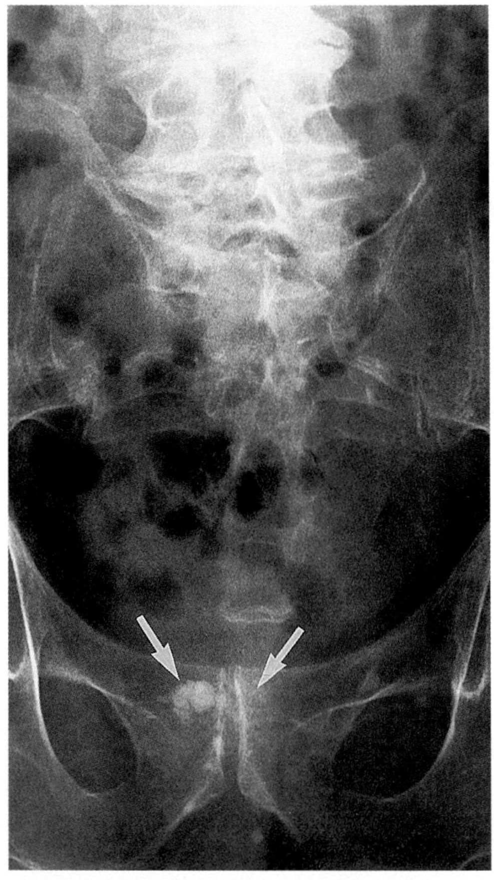

FIGURE 6-18 ■ Prostatic calcification. Calcification situated immediately behind the pubis *(arrows)* in a male patient usually represents the sequelae of previous prostatitis.

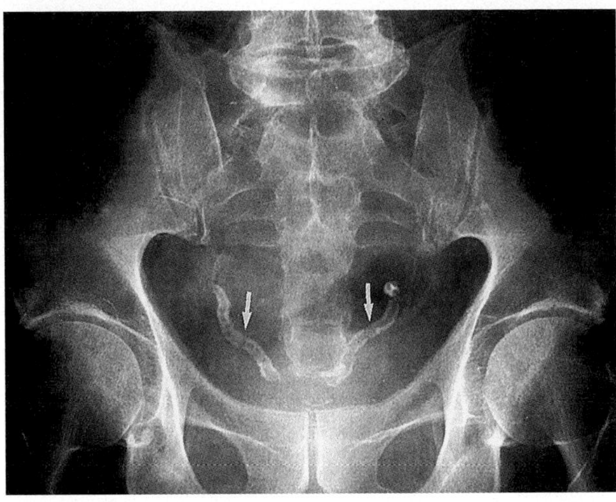

FIGURE 6-19 ■ Calcification of the vas deferens. These bilateral asymmetric calcifications occur in the lower to middle portion of the male pelvis. When they are seen, they almost always indicate that the patient has diabetes.

the aortic arch and the left main-stem bronchus, can be seen along the left side (Fig. 6-20). Normally a peristaltic wave, initiated by swallowing, propels food down the esophagus. You should not diagnose a stricture on the basis of one image alone, because you may be looking at a normal area of peristaltic contraction. Sometimes in the distal portion of the esophagus, a "Z" line can be seen going across the esophagus. This represents the junction between the mucosa of the esophagus and the stomach (Fig. 6-21).

Dysphagia and Odynophagia

Initially, it is important to differentiate dysphagia (difficulty swallowing or sticking of food) from odynophagia (pain with swallowing). The most common cause of dysphagia is hiatal hernia with gastroesophageal reflux disease (GERD). Patients with mild dysphagia do not need imaging or endoscopy, but they should have a trial of GERD medical therapy. Patients with severe symptoms should be investigated with endoscopy or barium swallow.

Of patients in the age range from 60 to 80 years, many have dysmotility and do not pass food properly. They generally have vague symptoms. A barium swallow is indicated to exclude other pathology. Patients who complain of food getting stuck often have a benign or malignant stricture. These usually require endoscopy with biopsy.

Difficulty swallowing also can be the result of central nervous system pathology. Pharyngeal paresis with ineffective constriction of muscles may be due to abnormalities involving cranial nerves IX and X, stroke, or degenerative changes. In these patients, failure to close the glottis often results in aspiration.

Odynophagia is usually due to an infection or a medication that produces esophagitis. In these patients, a barium swallow can visualize ulcerations or other characteristic mucosal patterns (such as herpes). Endoscopy also can be used, with the advantage of biopsy of visualized abnormalities.

Esophageal Diverticula

In the lower cervical region, sometimes a pharyngeal diverticulum (Zenker's diverticulum) projects posteriorly. Food can be caught in this, causing dysphagia (Fig. 6-22). In the middle of the esophagus (near the carina), a traction diverticulum may be caused by scarring from mediastinal granulomatous disease. Just above the stomach, a pulsion diverticulum can sometimes be found. The two latter types are rarely symptomatic.

Presbyesophagus

As a function of aging, tertiary deep contractions may develop within the esophagus. These are usually disordered and can interfere with the normal peristaltic process and swallowing. These tertiary contractions are easily visualized as multiple transverse or ringlike contractions of the esophagus (Fig. 6-23). No specific therapy is indicated for this condition, and it is very common in persons older than 60 years.

Hiatal Hernia and Gastroesophageal Reflux Disease

A large number of people suffer from "heartburn" or dysphagia as a result of reflux of gastric

TABLE 6–4 ■ **Initial Study to Order for Various Clinical Problems**

Suspected Clinical Problem	Imaging Study
Gastroesophageal reflux	
Mild or transient symptoms	Medical therapy
Severe or persistent symptoms	Endoscopy with biopsy
Esophageal obstruction	Barium swallow
Esophageal tear	Gastrografin swallow
Bowel perforation or free air	Upright chest and supine abdominal plain film; supine and left lateral decubitus, if patient is unable to stand
Hematemesis	Endoscopy (less preferred, contrast UGI series)
Gastric or duodenal ulcer	Test for *Helicobacter pylori;* if medical therapy fails, endoscopy or double contrast upper GI series
Trauma, blunt or penetrating	Supine/upright abdomen and CT
Abdominal aortic aneurysm	Supine and lateral abdomen, then ultrasound or contrasted CT
Pancreatic mass or inflammation	CT (intravenous and GI contrast)
Pancreatic pseudocyst follow-up	CT or ultrasound
Abscess	CT (intravenous and GI contrast)
Acute cholecystitis	Ultrasound or nuclear medicine hepatobiliary scan
Chronic cholelithiasis	Right upper quadrant ultrasound
Common duct obstruction	Right upper quadrant ultrasound
Jaundice	
Painful	Ultrasound and ERCP
Painless, suspect biliary obstruction	CT or ERCP
Painless, suspect liver	Ultrasound
Suspected bile leak	Nuclear medicine hepatobiliary study
Small bowel stricture or polyp	Enteroclysis with barium
Intestinal obstruction	Supine and upright film of abdomen as an initial study, followed by those listed below
Esophagus or stomach obstruction	UGI and small bowel series or endoscopy
Small bowel obstruction	CT
Distal small bowel or colon obstruction	Barium enema
Right upper quadrant pain (+ Murphy's sign, fever)	Nuclear medicine hepatobiliary scan or ultrasound
Right lower quadrant pain	Supine and upright film of abdomen; ultrasound, if female < 45 yr; CT, if suspect inflammatory process
Appendicitis	
Adults	CT
Children	Ultrasound
Abdominal abscess	Supine and upright plain film of abdomen, then CT with GI and intravenous contrast
Suspected pelvic abscess	CT or ultrasound
Ulcerative colitis	Colonoscopy (see text for screening); if incomplete or unavailable, barium enema
Ischemic colitis (without signs of peritonitis)	Plain radiograph, three-way view of abdomen, then colonoscopy or contrast enema (see text)
Suspected ureteral stone	Noncontrast CT or IVP
Pelvic pain (female)	Ultrasound
Bladder pathology	Cystoscopy; if not available, CT cystogram
Uterine or ovarian pathology	Ultrasound
Abdominal tumor	CT
Colon cancer	Colonoscopy (see text for screening); if incomplete or unavailable, barium enema
Abdominal trauma	CT
Acute diverticulitis	Plain film, CT
Rectal bleeding (obvious)	
Dark red	Esophagogastroduodenoscopy; if not available, UGI series
Bright red	Colonoscopy
Unknown source or colonoscopy nondiagnostic	Nuclear medicine bleeding study
Positive fecal occult blood test	
Older than 40 yr	Colonoscopy or barium enema
Younger than 40 yr with GI symptoms	*Helicobacter pylori* test, therapeutic trial; if fails, endoscopy or UGI series

CT, computed tomography; ERCP, endoscopic retrograde cholangiopancreatography; GI, gastrointestinal; IVP, intravenous pyelography; UGI, upper gastrointestinal.

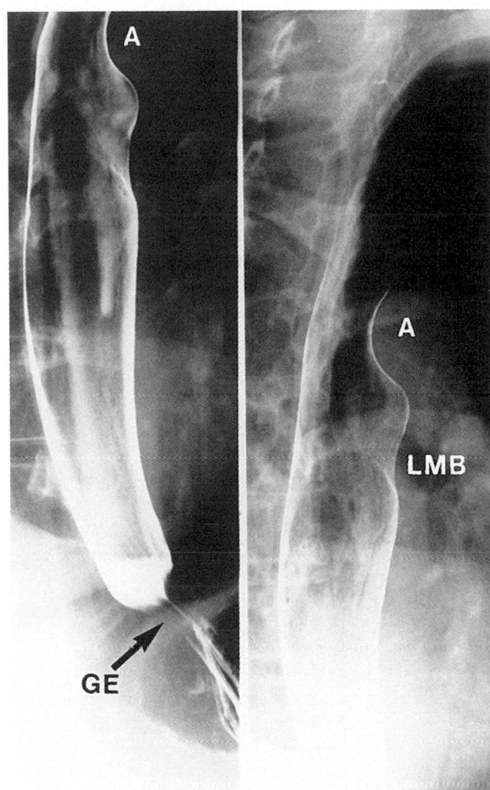

FIGURE 6-20 ■ Normal anatomy of the esophagus. The upper portion of the esophagus is seen on the image on the right and the lower half in the image on the left. An indentation along the left side of the esophagus occurs from the aorta (A) and another less significant one from the left main-stem bronchus (LMB). As the distal aspect of the esophagus goes through the diaphragm, the gastroesophageal junction (GE) also can be identified.

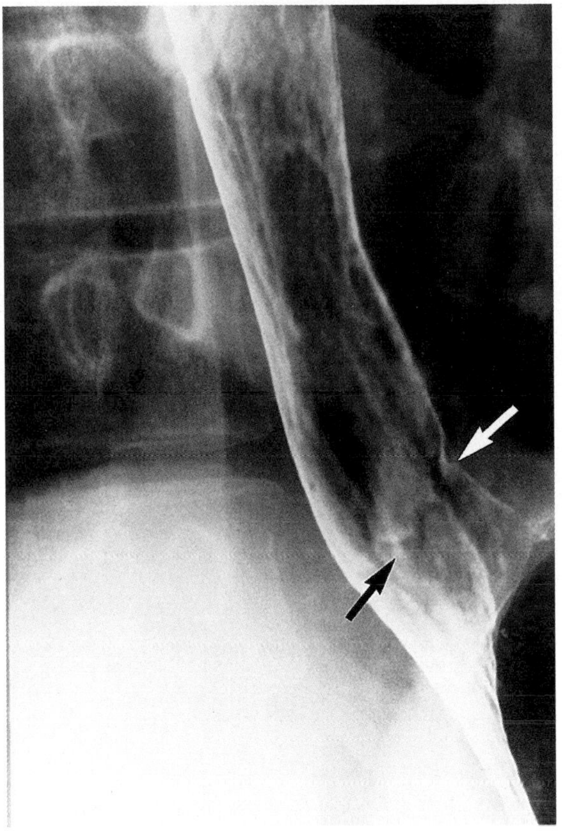

FIGURE 6-21 ■ Junction of the esophageal and gastric mucosa. In the distal esophagus, it is sometimes possible to see a dark horizontal zigzag line (between the two *arrows*). This is called the Z line and represents the normal junction between the two different types of mucosa.

contents into the esophagus. This may occur because of esophageal motility problems, incompetence of the lower esophageal sphincter, hiatal hernia, delayed gastric emptying, or increased intragastric or intra-abdominal pressure. In adults, the most common cause appears to be transient relaxation of the lower esophageal sphincter with reflux esophagitis.

With mild or transient symptoms, a trial of medical therapy is usually instituted without any imaging procedures being performed. If the symptoms are persistent or severe, endoscopy with biopsy is usually performed. In patients with swallowing difficulties, a barium swallow can demonstrate a mass or a stricture, which then requires endoscopic biopsy. A biopsy also is indicated in immunocompromised patients and those with known Barrett's esophagus. GERD can be documented by use of an intraesophageal pH probe or less sensitive imaging or nuclear medicine reflux studies.

The most common type of hiatal hernia is the sliding type, in which the gastroesophageal junction and a portion of the fundus of the stomach slide upward into the thorax. Small hiatal hernias can be identified by noting an indentation at the distal esophagus (Schatzki's ring), as well as longitudinal gastric mucosa folds distal to the ring (Fig. 6-24). Large hiatal hernias can be identified by seeing the fundus of the

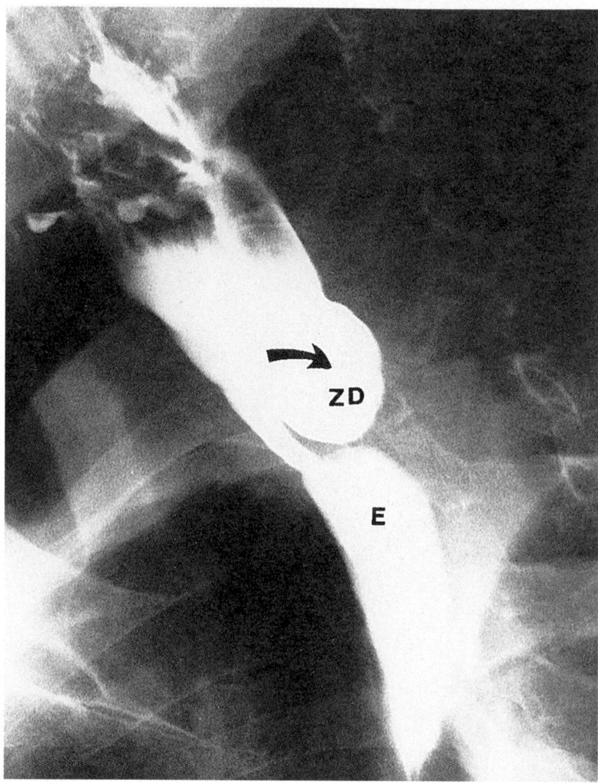

FIGURE 6-22 ■ **Zenker's diverticulum.** This is basically an outpouching of mucosa (ZD) in the pharynx. Food can be caught in this and cause symptoms. The esophagus (E) can be seen distally.

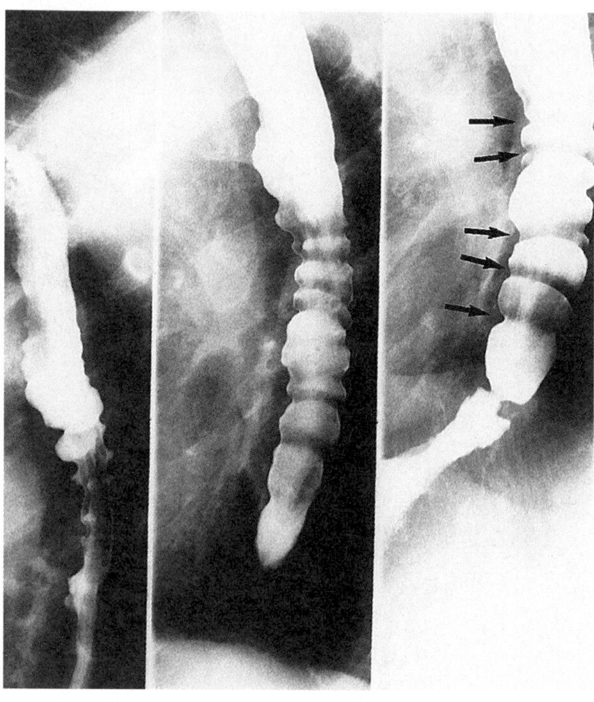

FIGURE 6-23 ■ **Presbyesophagus.** These tertiary or ringlike contractions are commonly seen in older persons, and they can disrupt the normal peristaltic motility of the esophagus.

stomach projecting up into the retrocardiac space (Fig. 6-25). Another type of hiatal hernia occurs more rarely. This is the paraesophageal type, in which the fundus of the stomach slips up past the gastroesophageal junction, which remains in the normal location. Large hiatal hernias can be seen on the chest x-ray, even without the use of barium. The typical finding is an air/fluid level or soft tissue mass located behind the heart but in front of the spine (Fig. 6-26).

Esophageal reflux can sometimes be seen on an upper GI examination, but if it is not seen, the patient may still be refluxing at other times and under other conditions. A more sensitive imaging method uses nuclear medicine. A small amount of radioactive material is mixed with orange juice, which the patient drinks. A computer region of interest is set up over the chest, abdominal compression is applied, and the patient is monitored for about 1 hour. If the study is positive, reflux occurs, but if it is negative, the same caveat applies. A more invasive but more accurate method used by gastroenterologists is to put a pH probe on the end of a tube and station this for some time above the gastroesophageal junction.

Foreign Bodies of the Esophagus

The foreign bodies lodged in the esophagus of children are most commonly coins. They often stick just above the level of the aortic arch (Fig. 6-27). A number of other foreign bodies lodge at the gastroesophageal junction (Fig. 6-28). In adults, the most common object is a piece of unchewed meat. Meat will not be visualized on a plain x-ray but can easily be seen during a contrast esophagogram.

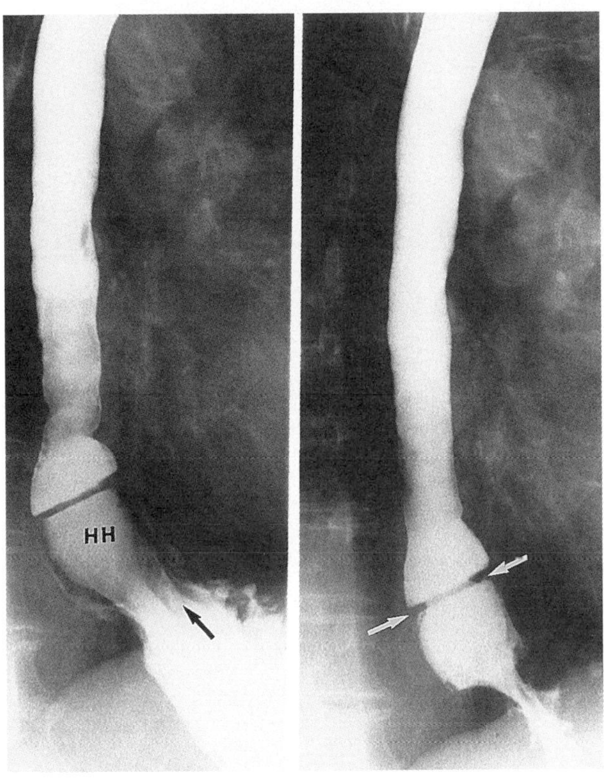

FIGURE 6-24 ■ Small sliding-type hiatal hernia. When a small portion of the fundus of the stomach slips up through the hemidiaphragm, a small hiatal hernia (HH) can be identified. The two keys to identification are (1) a very sharp ringlike construction (called Schatzki's ring, which is seen between the two *white arrows*); and (2) the normal longitudinal lines of gastric mucosa *(black arrow)*, which can be seen projecting up above the hemidiaphragm.

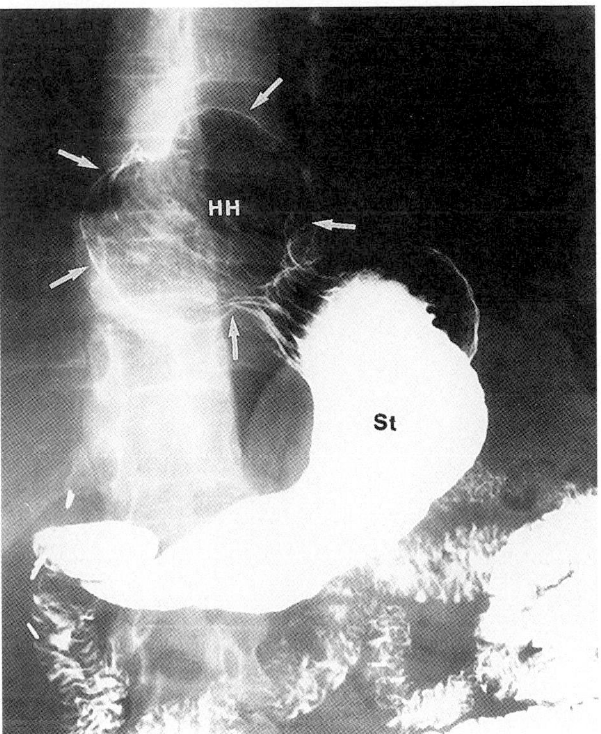

FIGURE 6-25 ■ Large sliding-type hiatal hernia (HH). A large portion of the fundus of the stomach (St) has slipped up through the hemidiaphragm into the retrocardiac region *(arrows)* and can easily be identified on an upper gastrointestinal examination.

Strictures and Dilatation

Strictures in the esophagus are a common cause of food lodging at a specific level. High esophageal strictures can occur as a result of scarring after suicide attempts in which the individual swallowed lye or corrosive alkaline material (Fig. 6-29). Middle and distal esophageal strictures may develop from scarring due to gastroesophageal reflux or may result from a tumor. Most benign strictures have a smooth appearance. The diameter of a stricture can be assessed during a barium swallow by giving the patient a radiopaque pill of known diameter. These pills will quickly dissolve (Fig. 6-30). Strictures due to carcinomas most commonly are irregular and have overhanging edges (Fig. 6-31). Biopsies are usually performed, even of benign-appearing strictures, to exclude malignancy.

Two entities can cause marked dilatation of the esophagus: achalasia and scleroderma. The esophagus may be so dilated that it can be visualized on chest x-ray as a tortuous structure in the post-tracheal and retrocardiac regions, and often a horizontal air/fluid level can be seen in the upper esophagus. Air/fluid levels within the esophagus are definitely abnormal.

In achalasia (Fig. 6-32), the gastroesophageal sphincter fails to relax. The esophagus becomes massively dilated and tapers distally to a beaklike shape. Usually no evidence of gastroesophageal reflux is found. A massively dilated esophagus that looks like achalasia can also be seen in Chagas' disease, which is caused

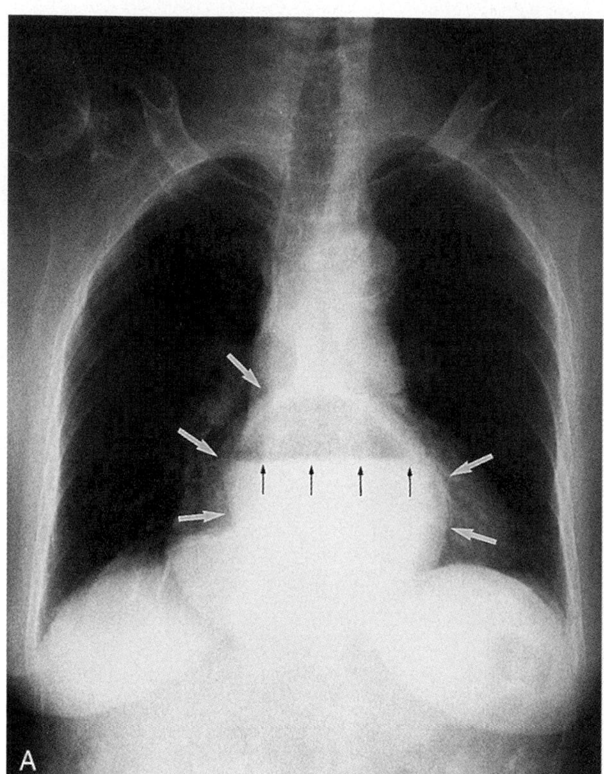

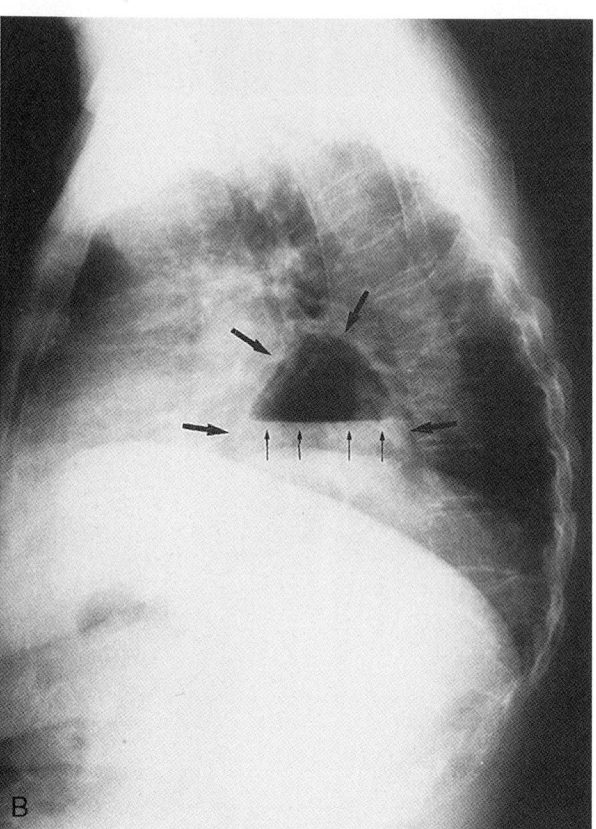

FIGURE 6-26 ■ **Large hiatal hernia.** Hiatal hernias can sometimes be seen on a plain chest x-ray. On an upright posteroanterior (PA) chest x-ray *(A)*, a mass with an air/fluid level within it can be seen behind the heart *(large arrows)*. This also can be easily seen on the lateral chest x-ray *(B)*.

by an infection with *Trypanosoma cruzi*. This parasite releases a neurotoxin that destroys ganglion cells in the myenteric plexus.

Scleroderma is a collagen vascular disease involving the smooth muscle. The esophagus is usually only mildly dilated and has no primary contractions. Gastroesophageal reflux can occur with this condition, causing stricture and ultimately proximal dilatation.

Esophagitis and Tears

Ulceration and irregularity of the esophageal mucosa can be the result of reflux esophagitis, and in these circumstances, the irregularities are very fine. In patients who are immunocompromised, *Candida albicans (Monilia)* infection of the esophagus may create a very coarse irregular pattern (Fig. 6-33).

Tears of the esophagus occur in Boerhaave's syndrome as well as in Mallory-Weiss syndrome. In Boerhaave's syndrome, spontaneous perforation of the esophagus occurs because of a sudden increase in intraluminal esophageal pressure, and, clinically, the patient has severe epigastric pain. Overall mortality in this syndrome is approximately 25%, but it approaches 100% if diagnosis is delayed 24 hours. Severe epigastric pain and dyspnea are common. An erect chest film is useful, because it may demonstrate a left pleural fluid collection, left pneumothorax, or mediastinal air.

A Mallory-Weiss tear is usually a longitudinal non-transmural tear in the lesser curvature

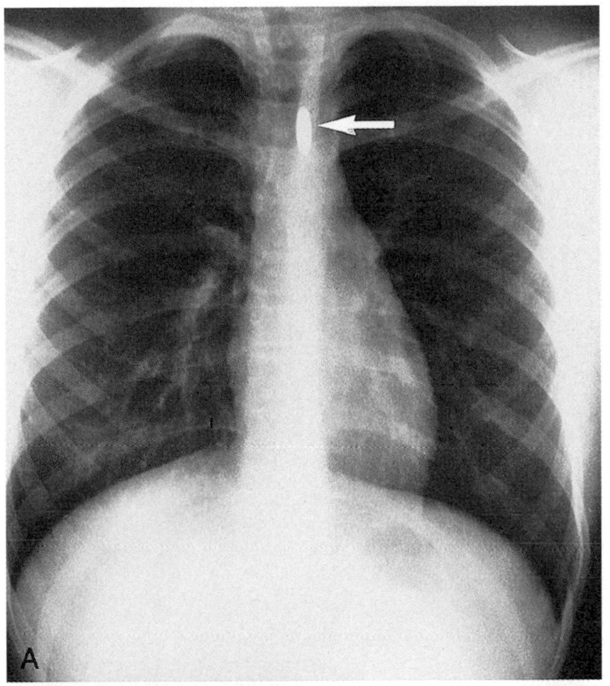

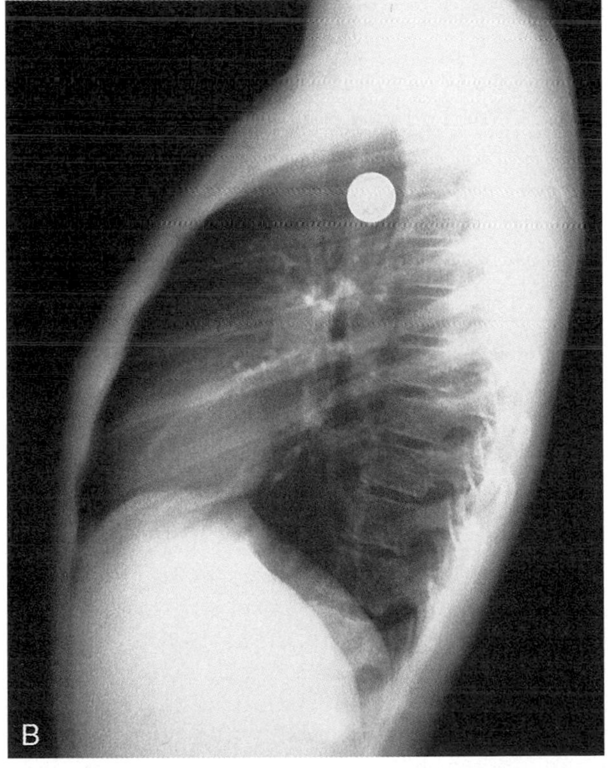

FIGURE 6-27 ■ Coin in the esophagus. The coin can easily be seen in both the posteroanterior (PA) chest x-ray *(A)* and the lateral view *(B)*. Objects often stick at this level because the esophagus is somewhat narrowed here by the impression of the aortic arch.

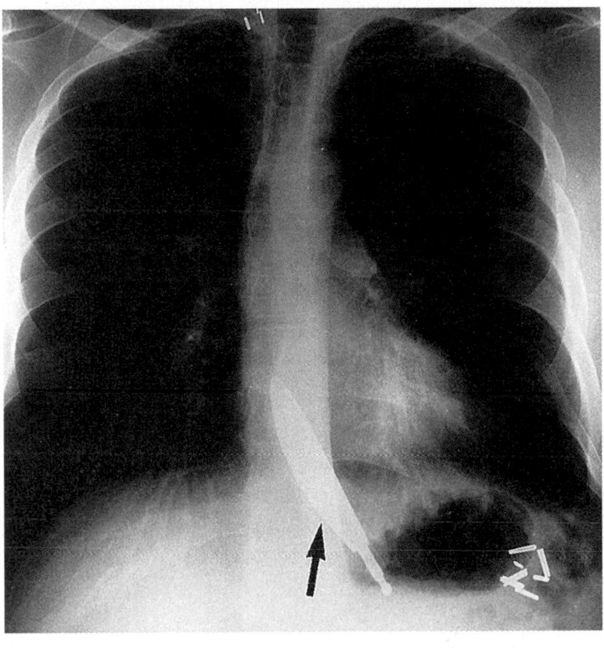

FIGURE 6-28 ■ Steak knife lodged at the esophagogastric junction. This mentally ill patient claimed to have swallowed his steak knife at dinnertime. The chest x-ray shows the metallic blade *(arrow)* at the gastroesophageal junction. The wooden handle of the knife, which is down in the stomach, is not seen because wood typically is not visible on a x-ray. Metallic surgical clips are seen to the left of the stomach gas bubble. These are from a previous surgery to remove other swallowed objects.

of the stomach, often extending across the gastroesophageal junction. These tears are produced by prolonged vomiting in alcoholics, are usually self-limited, and are not painful. There should be no evidence of a pneumomediastinum, although hematemesis is present.

Varices

Long, tortuous, longitudinal or vertical worm-like filling defects in the distal esophagus can be the result of varices. The large vascular channels in the esophageal wall are large enough to displace barium (Fig. 6-34*A*). The best way to appreciate varices is by endoscopy or CT scanning (Fig. 6-34*B* and *C*), because only when the varices are large and extensive can they be seen on a barium swallow.

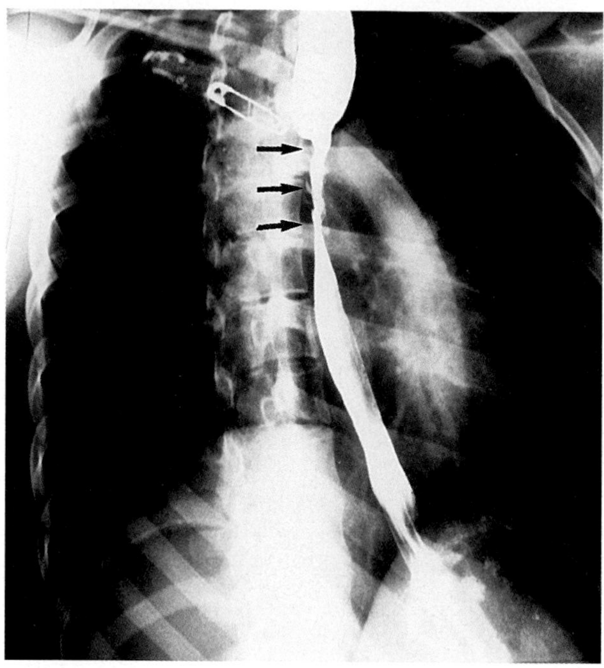

FIGURE 6-29 ■ Benign esophageal stricture. This upper esophageal stricture *(arrows)* was due to attempted suicide by lye ingestion. Notice that the stricture does not have any overhanging edges and is relatively smooth and tapered. Essentially all patients with esophageal strictures should have esophagoscopy and biopsy to rule out malignancy.

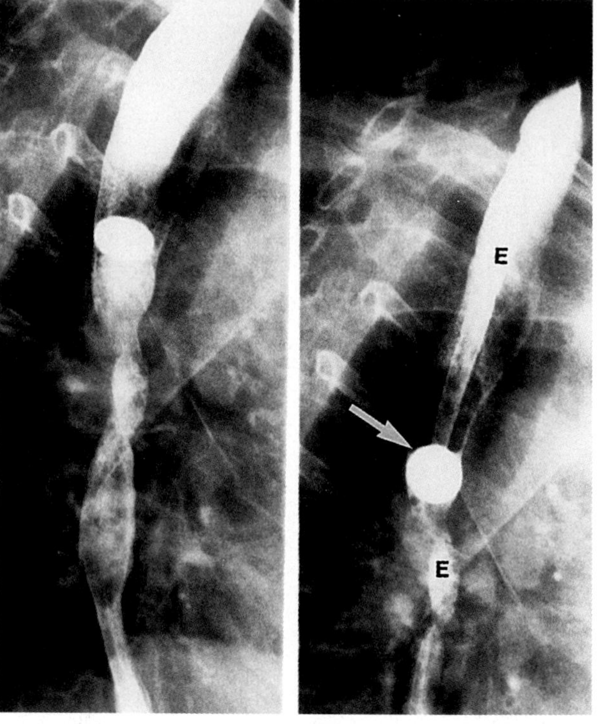

FIGURE 6-30 ■ Measurement of an esophageal stricture. During a barium swallow, a radiopaque pill of known diameter *(arrow)* can be given. This will lodge above a stricture, but it will quickly dissolve. Knowing the size of the pill allows measurement of a stricture.

Tumors

Malignant tumors of the esophagus are squamous cell carcinoma 95% of the time and adenocarcinoma about 5% of the time. Adenocarcinomas usually arise in the region of the gastroesophageal junction or have grown out of the stomach to involve the lower esophagus (see Fig. 6-31). Adenocarcinomas also occur somewhat higher in the esophagus in patients with chronic gastroesophageal reflux, in whom islands of columnar mucosa develop (Barrett's esophagus).

STOMACH AND DUODENUM

Anatomy and Imaging Techniques

Lesions of the stomach and duodenum are most appropriately visualized with an upper GI examination or endoscopy. If a perforated viscus is suspected, Gastrografin (meglumine diatrizoate) or another water-soluble material should be used as a contrast agent rather than barium. CT scanning is usually not an appropriate initial imaging modality for most stomach or intestinal pathology.

The appearance of the stomach on an upper GI study can be variable depending on whether the patient is prone or supine. With the patient supine, barium collects in the most dependent position, which is the fundus of the stomach, and the normal mucosal patterns of the body and antrum are easily visualized (Fig. 6-35). In the prone position, the body and antrum of the stomach are the most dependent, and barium will collect there. The duodenal bulb projects upward to the right and posteriorly relative to the gastric antrum. It is important to obtain images with the bulb distended. Radiologists

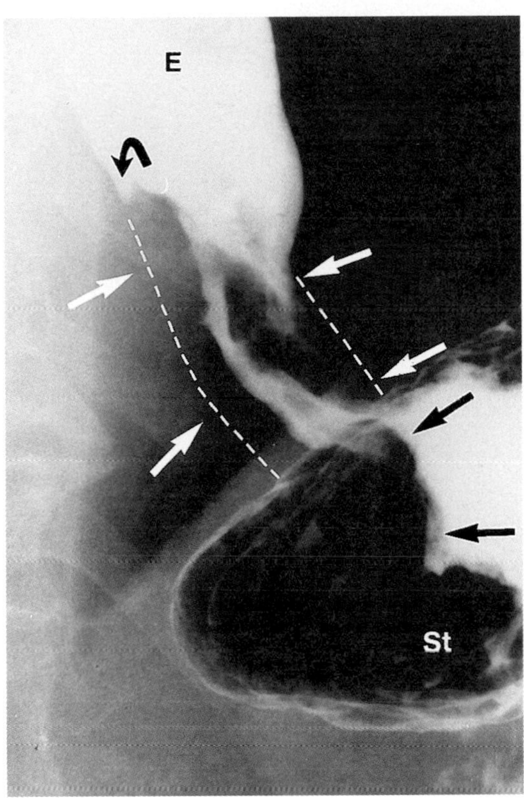

FIGURE 6-31 ■ **Esophageal carcinoma.** On this barium swallow, a spot image at the gastroesophageal junction clearly shows a dilated distal esophagus (E) as well as the fundus of the stomach (St). A thin, irregular column of barium is seen joining the two, and overhanging beaklike edges *(dark curved arrow)* suggest a malignancy. The normal contour of the esophagus is outlined, and the *dark straight arrows* indicate a mass protruding into the fundus of the stomach.

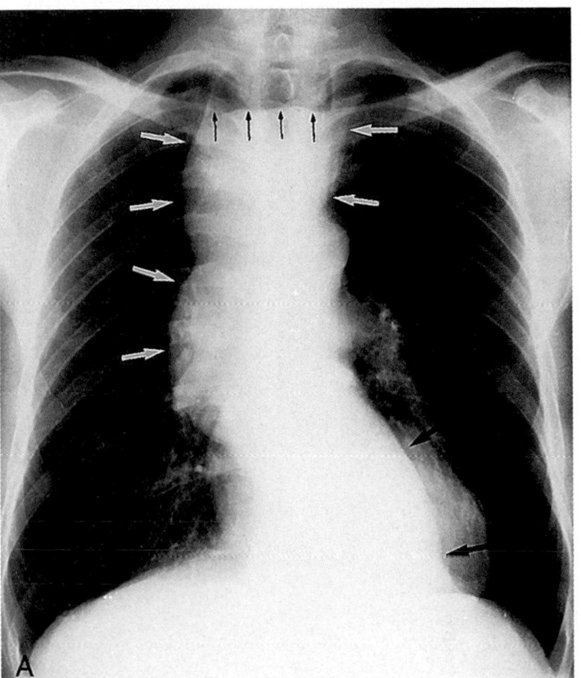

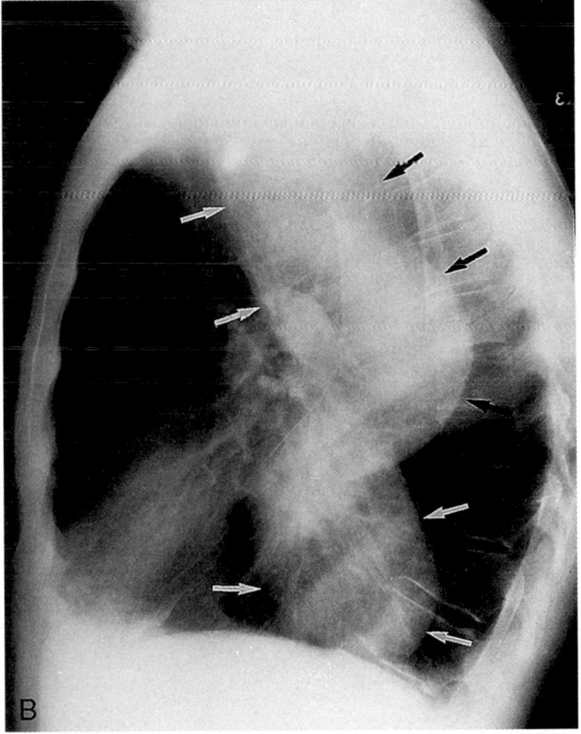

FIGURE 6-32 ■ **Achalasia.** On the frontal chest x-ray *(A)*, a tortuous structure is seen extending from the cervical region down into the retrocardiac region *(arrows)*. An air/fluid level also is seen near the top *(small arrows)*. This represents a massively dilated esophagus due to achalasia. The dilated esophagus also is seen on the lateral chest x-ray *(B)*, because it is dilated and filled with fluid.

will almost always take several pictures of the bulb in different stages of peristalsis (Fig. 6-36).

The duodenum has a C-loop configuration and extends to the ligament of Treitz near the body of the stomach. The jejunum is usually located in the left midabdomen, and the ileum, in the lower central and right abdomen. A normal variant is malrotation of the small bowel, with a number of variations. The stomach and duodenal bulb may be in a normal position, but the third and fourth portions of the duodenum may be on the right side of the spine rather than swinging across the spine and behind the stomach in the region of the ligament of Treitz (Fig. 6-37). Sometimes the duodenum is positioned normally,

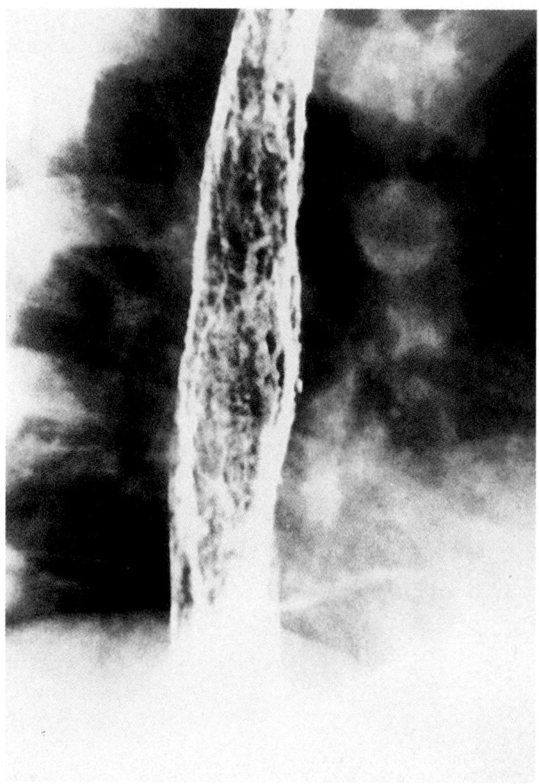

FIGURE 6-33 ■ **Candida esophagitis.** In this immunocompromised patient with acquired immunodeficiency syndrome (AIDS), the normal smooth esophageal mucosa has been replaced by a rough and irregular ulcerated mucosa extending the length of the esophagus. Very tiny ulcerations can be seen in tangent along the edge of the esophagus.

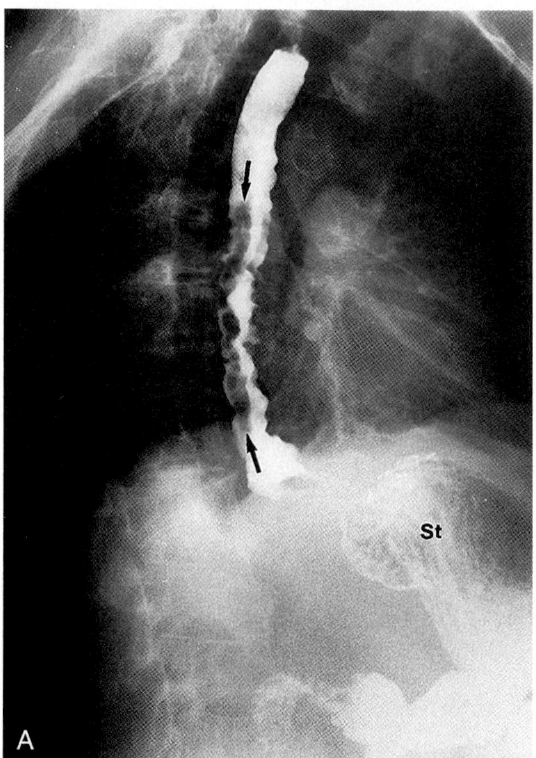

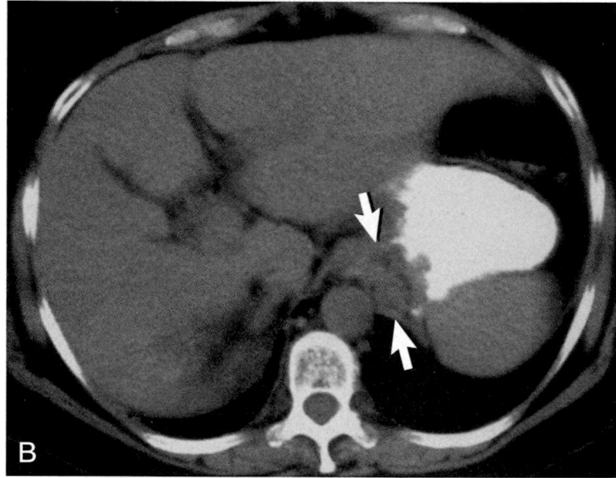

FIGURE 6-34 ■ **Esophageal varices.** In an oblique view from an upper gastrointestinal (GI) examination *(A)* performed on an alcoholic patient, a large, dark, wormlike filling density *(arrows)* is seen in the distal esophagus. It is caused by varices protruding into the lumen of the esophagus. The stomach (St) also is seen. Varices also can be seen on computed tomography (CT) scan. On a CT scan without intravenous contrast *(B),* they are seen as small rounded structures *(arrow),* and they may indent the fundus of the stomach.

Continued

but all of the small bowel is on the right side, and the cecum and colon are on the left side. Another much less common variant is situs inversus, in which the liver, stomach, and all abdominal organs are reversed between right and left, and the heart is on the right (Fig. 6-38).

Gastritis and Gastric Ulcer Disease

Helicobacter pylori is a bacterium responsible for about 80% of gastritis and gastric or duodenal ulcers. The presence of *H. pylori* is detected noninvasively with immunoglobulin G antibody serology or a urea breath test. Appropriate antibiotic therapy (such as bismuth, metronidazole, and tetracycline) usually cures 95% of

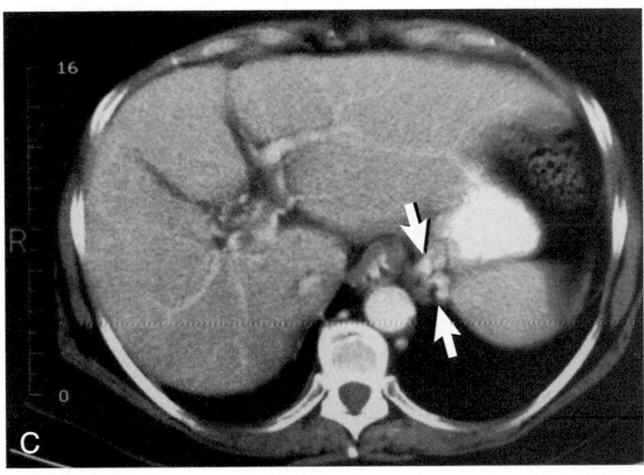

FIGURE 6-34 cont'd ■ When intravenous contrast is given *(C)*, they enhance and become whiter *(arrow)*.

patients. Symptomatic patients should also be treated and discouraged from using alcohol, aspirin, or nonsteroidal anti-inflammatory drugs, and asked to refrain from smoking. If symptoms persist or a fecal occult blood test (FOBT) is positive, an endoscopy or a barium upper GI series is indicated.

Large gastric folds may be the result of simple gastritis, although they also are seen with lymphoma, Ménétrier's disease (giant hypertrophic gastritis), and Zollinger-Ellison syndrome. Simple gastritis may be present without ulceration, and the only finding on an upper GI examination may be enlarged gastric folds (Fig. 6-39). Ulcers are unusual in Ménétrier's disease but are quite common in Zollinger-Ellison syndrome.

The detection rate of gastric ulcers with upper GI examination is only approximately 70%. The nondetectable ulcers are often too superficial or too small to be seen. Occasionally the ulcers are so large that the crater is overlooked. Ulcers identified on upper GI examination should be characterized as benign, indeterminate, or malignant. In general, benign ulcers decrease to half their original size with several weeks of therapy and should show almost complete healing within 6 weeks. Unless an ulcer has all benign features,

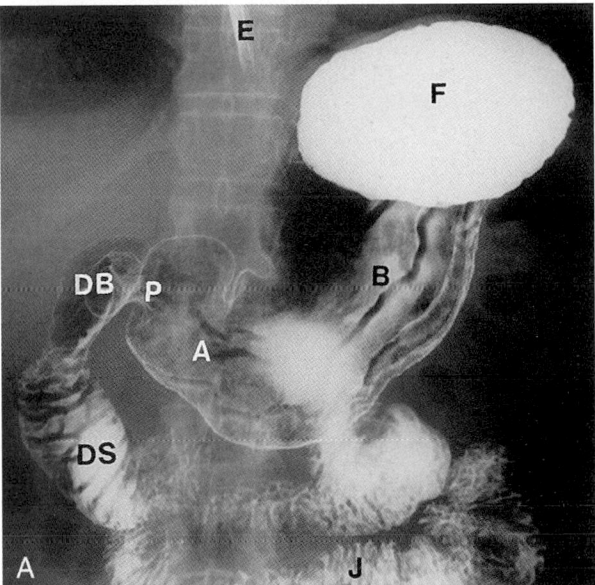

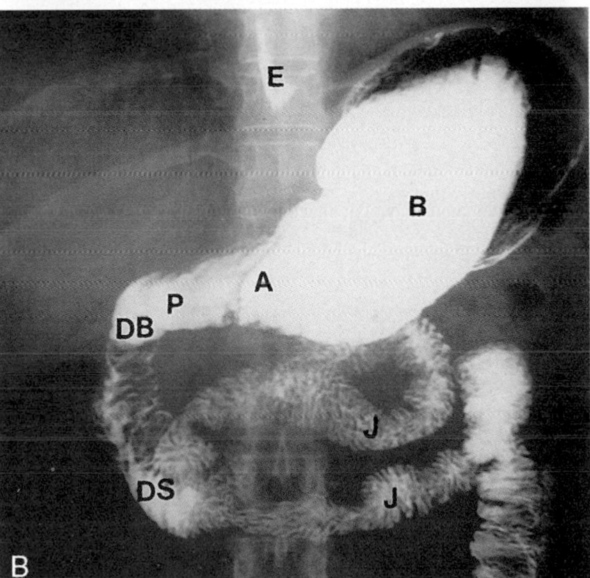

FIGURE 6-35 ■ **Normal upper gastrointestinal contrast examination.** On the supine view *(A)*, the barium layers in the most dependent portions. The esophagus (E), fundus (F), body (B), antrum (A), and pylorus (P) of the stomach are all easily identified. The normal longitudinal gastric mucosa also is seen. The duodenal bulb (DB), duodenal sweep (DS), and jejunum (J) also are identified with their predominantly transverse mucosal pattern. On a prone view *(B)*, the barium collects in the body and antrum of the stomach, because these are more dependent in that projection.

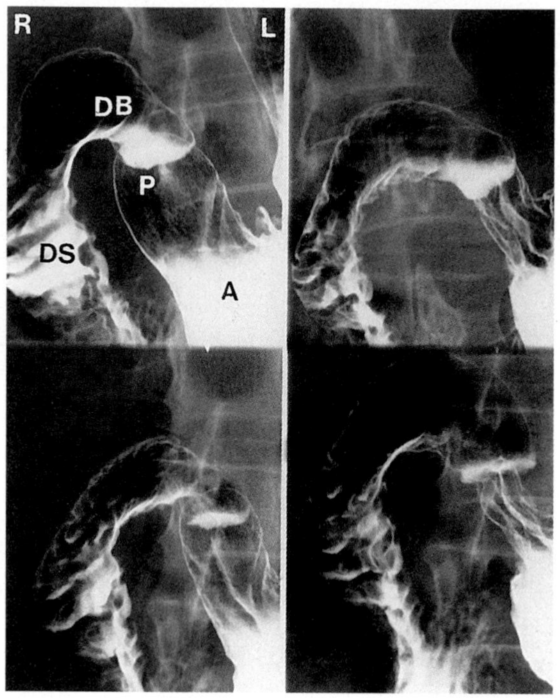

FIGURE 6-36 ■ Spot views of the duodenal bulb. Several views of the duodenal bulb are typically obtained, because it is undergoing active peristalsis during examination. Here, four similar spot views taken several seconds apart indicate the antrum (A), pylorus (P), duodenal bulb (DB), and duodenal sweep (DS).

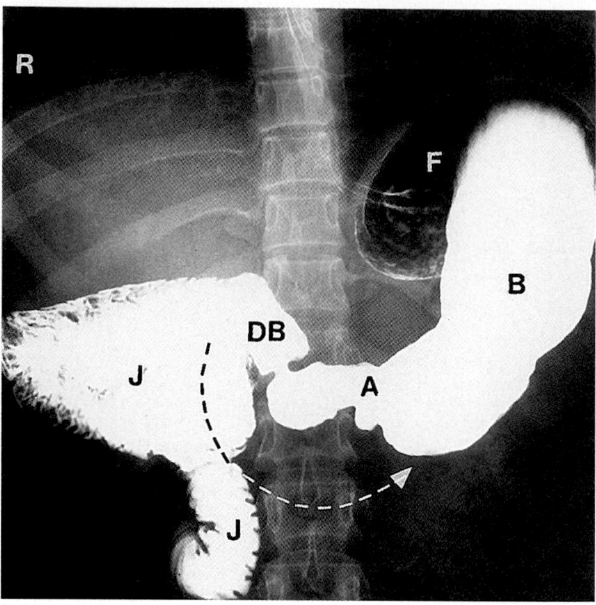

FIGURE 6-37 ■ Malrotation of the small bowel. On this barium contrast examination, the fundus (F), body (B), and antrum (A) of the stomach as well as the duodenal bulb (DB) are in normal position. However, the duodenal sweep and jejunum (J) should normally sweep across in the direction of the *dotted arrow* to the left behind the gastric antrum. In this case, because of a congenital malrotation, the jejunum is on the right side of the spine.

endoscopy with biopsy is usually recommended. There are four radiographic signs of a benign ulcer: (1) If the mucosal folds are thin and regular and extend up to the margin of the ulcer crater, the lesion is probably benign; (2) Benign ulcers typically extend beyond the projected margin of the stomach (Fig. 6-40*A*); (3) A 1- to 2-mm lucent line may be seen around the mouth of the ulcer on a tangential view of a benign ulcer; and (4) Normal peristalsis in the region and invagination of the wall opposite the ulcer are helpful signs to indicate benignity. Historically, a treatment for recurrent ulcer disease was a Billroth II operation. In this surgery, resection of the distal aspect of the stomach is performed, with an anastomosis made between the fundus of the stomach and the small bowel at the level of the ligament of Treitz. This leaves a blind-ending afferent loop composed of second, third, and fourth portions of the duodenum (Fig. 6-40*B*). Most benign ulcers now are treated with H_2-blocking agents.

Of all ulcers, 95% are benign, and 5% are malignant. Of the malignant ulcers, 90% are due to carcinoma and, to a lesser extent, to lymphoma and other rare malignancies or metastases. With a cancer, usually a thickened and markedly irregular wall is noted. Peristalsis is limited or decreased. The stomach may have decreased distensibility, and the mass or ulcer tends to lie within the projected outline of the stomach, rather than projecting beyond it (Fig. 6-41). If the tumor becomes large enough to involve most of the stomach, the stomach becomes rigid and nondistensible, and this is termed *linitis plastica* (leather bottle stomach) (Fig. 6-42).

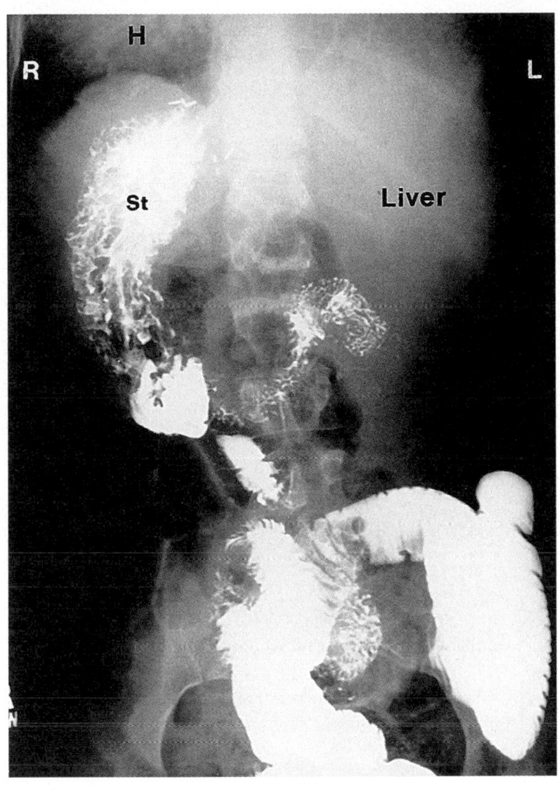

FIGURE 6-38 ■ **Situs inversus.** A complete situs is identified, with the heart (H) and stomach (St) on the right and the liver on the left.

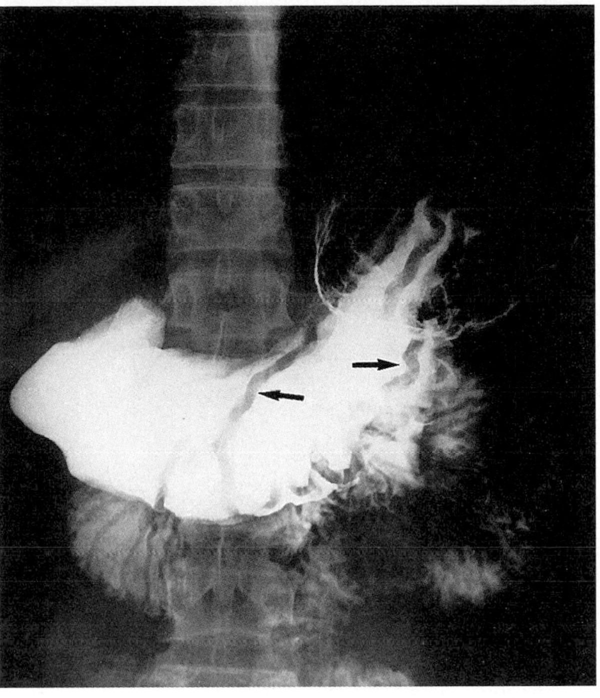

FIGURE 6-39 ■ **Gastritis.** In the body of the stomach, thickened mucosal folds *(arrows)*, the result of inflammation, can be seen.

Duodenal Ulcers

Ulcers that arise within the first portion of the duodenum are benign at least 90% of the time. These may have an infectious origin, and the spiral organism *H. pylori* has been implicated. Ulcers that occur distal to the duodenal bulb should be considered malignant until proved otherwise. Duodenal ulcers are 2 to 3 times more common than gastric ulcers. Their location is bulbar in 95% of cases and postbulbar in 5%. In the duodenal bulb, the anterior wall is the most common site of ulceration, and these anterior ulcers can lead to perforation, peritonitis, and pneumoperitoneum. Ulcers in the posterior wall of the duodenal bulb may penetrate into the pancreas. Duodenal ulcers can be difficult to appreciate if you have not seen many upper GI examinations. The key to identification is a duodenal defect that contains barium and remains essentially unchanged on the multiple spot films that are obtained. Generally, edema or thickening of the mucosal folds occurs in the proximal duodenum. Duodenal ulcers often heal with a scar that is accompanied by deformity and shrinking of the duodenal bulb. This is sometimes referred to as an "hourglass" or "cloverleaf" deformity (Fig. 6-43).

A duodenal diverticulum should not be confused with a duodenal ulcer. Duodenal diverticula are reasonably common and typically are seen as an outpouching of barium along the inner curvature of the duodenal sweep. The most common location is near the ampulla of Vater. No associated mucosal thickening or spasm is seen, and these diverticula are almost always are asymptomatic.

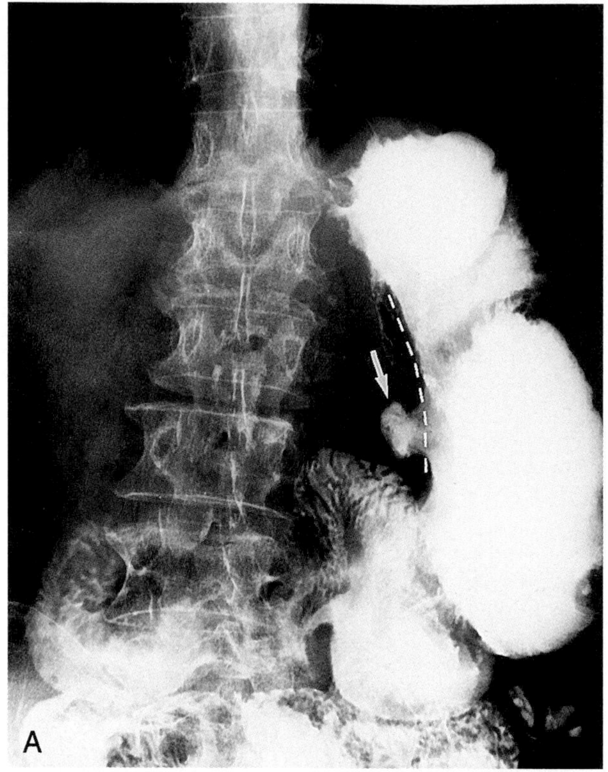

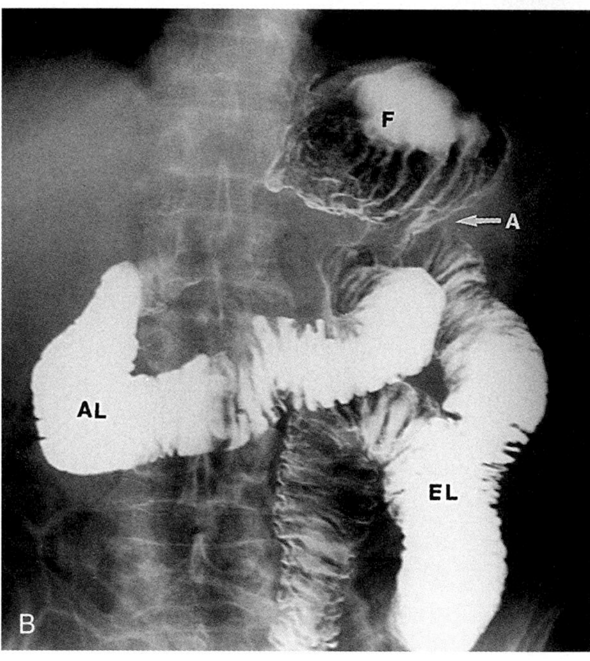

FIGURE 6-40 ■ Benign gastric ulcer. *A,* A large ulcer *(arrow)* is seen along the lesser curvature of the stomach. Notice that the ulcer projects out beyond the normal expected lesser curvature *(dotted line)*; this is one sign that the lesion is benign. *B,* A Billroth II operation was performed for recurrent ulcers and shows the residual fundus (F) of the stomach as well as the anastomosis (A) and the afferent (AL) and efferent (EL) loops of small bowel.

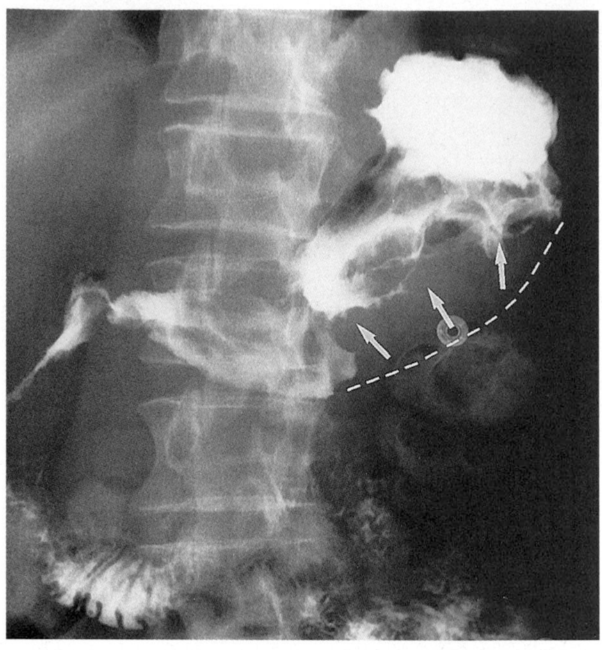

FIGURE 6-41 ■ Malignant gastric ulceration. A large series of ulcers is seen along the greater curvature of the stomach. Notice that, in addition, a mass projects into the lumen from the expected normal greater curvature *(dotted line)*. This is a sign of malignancy.

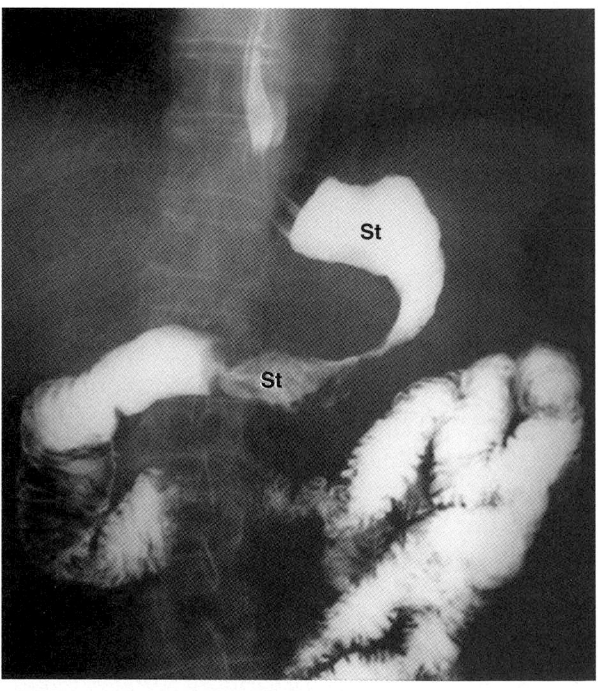

FIGURE 6-42 ■ Linitis plastica. On this upper gastrointestinal (GI) examination, the stomach (St) is small, deformed, and narrowed. It never changed appearance on later additional images. This so-called "leather bottle" stomach or linitis plastica is due to advanced infiltrative gastric cancer.

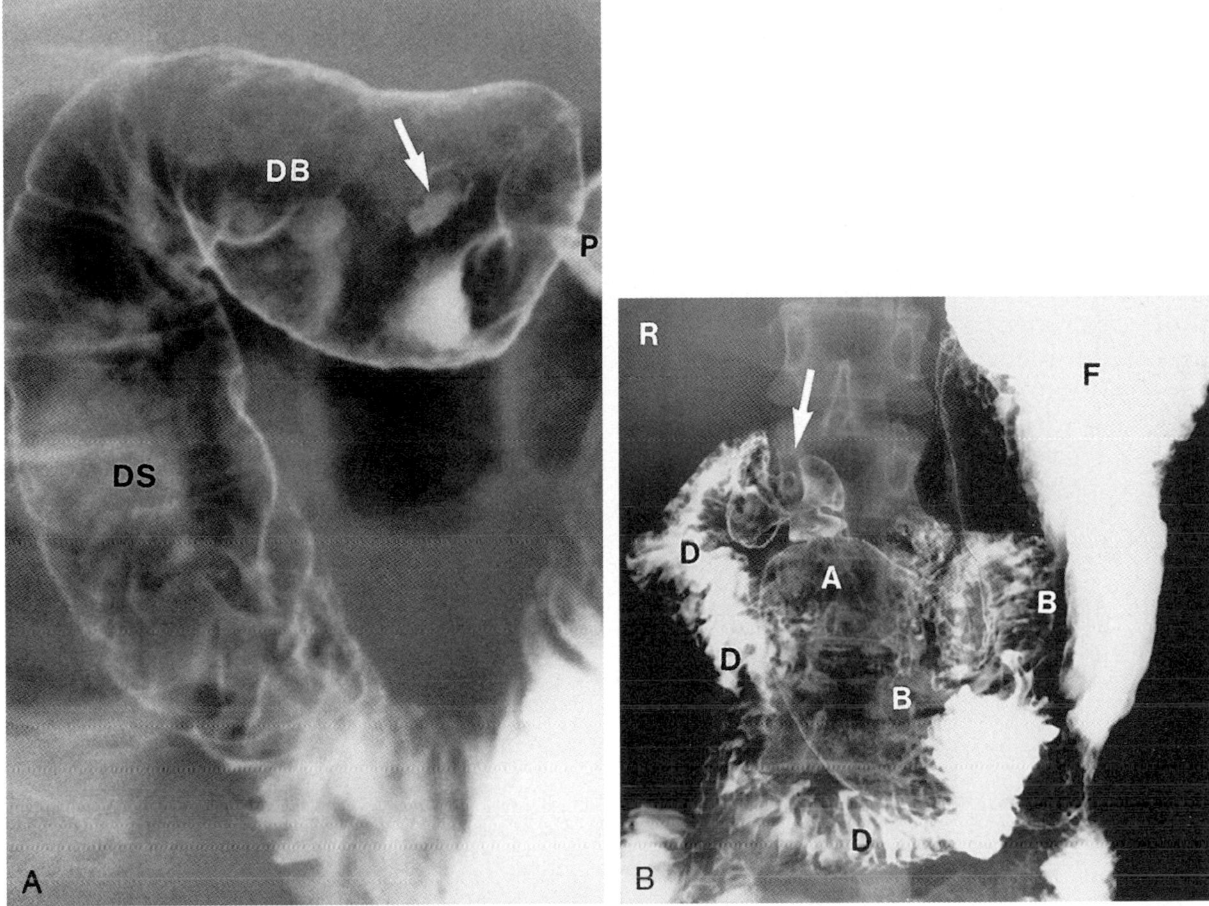

FIGURE 6-43 ■ Duodenal ulceration. A spot view from an upper gastrointestinal (GI) examination *(A)* shows the duodenum. An acute ulcer is seen as a persistent barium collection *(arrow)* just distal to the pylorus in the duodenal bulb (DB). This was seen on multiple views. A different patient with a healed ulcer and scarring had an upper GI examination *(B)*. The fundus (F), body (B), and antrum (A) of the stomach are normal, as is most of the duodenal sweep (DS). The duodenal bulb, however, has a cloverleaf deformity *(arrow)* due to scarring.

Gastric Emptying

Patients with abnormal gastric motility may have either accelerated emptying of gastric contents (dumping) or delayed gastric emptying. The latter is quite common in diabetics. Because barium is not physiologic, nuclear medicine studies that tag food or liquid with a small amount of radioactive material are used to quantitate gastric emptying. Computer regions of interest are drawn over the stomach, and the emptying rate is calculated. For solid foods, half the material should leave the stomach in less than 90 minutes.

Gastric Dilatation or Outlet Obstruction

Gastric distention can be due to a number of causes that can be divided into physiologic and metabolic or obstructive. An enlarged stomach may be seen on a plain abdominal x-ray in a patient with vomiting or loss of appetite. If causes of gastric dilatation and poor motility, such as diabetes, narcotic drugs, and others are not evident, obstructive causes such as neoplasms must be excluded. Either a barium upper GI series or endoscopy is indicated. If an abdominal mass other than the stomach can be palpated, a CT scan is indicated.

LIVER

Today the most common method of imaging the liver and spleen is with a CT scan. In many institutions, CT scans are done with and without the use of intravenous contrast. For most situations, however, a single CT scan with intravenous contrast is often adequate and less expensive. The liver or spleen also can be imaged by using ultrasound or nuclear medicine, but there is less anatomic resolution and less complete imaging of other nearby structures.

Cirrhosis and Alcoholic Liver Disease

Probably the most common imaging manifestation of alcoholic liver disease is fatty infiltration. On a noncontrasted CT scan, the liver and spleen should be of the same density. If the liver is darker than the spleen or muscle, you can suspect fatty infiltration. Often the fatty infiltration is focal and not uniform, especially because portal venous flow delivers more alcohol to the right lobe of the liver than to the left lobe (Fig. 6-44).

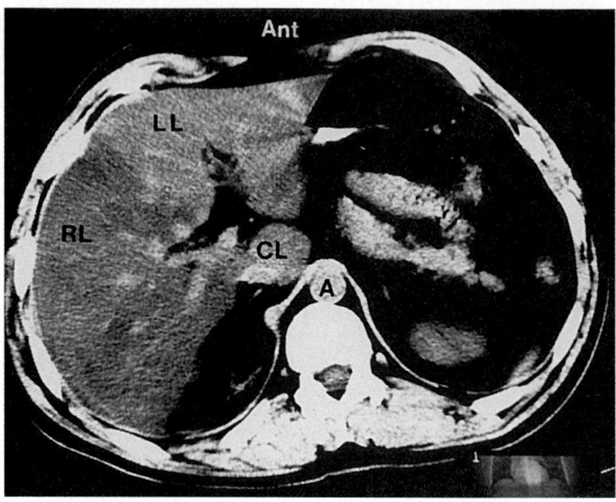

FIGURE 6-44 ■ Focal fatty infiltration of the liver. On this transverse computed tomography (CT) scan (done without intravenous contrast), the right lobe of the liver (RL) is darker than the left lobe (LL). This is due to fatty infiltration of the right lobe. Notice also that the sparing of the caudate lobe (CL). Normal vascular structures are seen in the right lobe, even without contrast enhancement, because they are surrounded by fat.

Obesity is the most common cause of a fatty liver. The low density in the area can usually be differentiated from low density due to malignancy or other abnormality, because fatty infiltration is usually geographic or has straight borders in its distribution. Lack of a mass effect also may be noted, with normal vessels and architecture being preserved in the areas of the fat. Finally, the periportal region or medial segment of the left lobe is often spared. Even without the use of intravenous contrast, the hepatic and portal veins in the area of fatty infiltration will appear prominent (whiter) because of the surrounding low density.

Ascites is another common manifestation of alcoholic liver disease. If ascites is massive, gas in the small bowel will be seen floating centrally or concentrated in the middle and anterior abdomen on a supine plain film of the abdomen. You also may see a generalized gray haziness overlying the whole abdomen (Fig. 6-45). Small amounts of ascites can easily be visualized on a CT scan along the edge of the liver and in the pericolic gutters. If your only interest is in determining whether the patient has ascites or in locating a suitable area to tap the ascites, ultrasound is a very efficient and much less expensive modality (Fig. 6-46).

Trauma

In penetrating abdominal injuries, the liver is the most commonly injured intra-abdominal organ, and it is the second most commonly injured organ in blunt abdominal trauma. Blunt abdominal trauma can cause hepatic lacerations, subcapsular hematomas, and intraparenchymal hemorrhage. Usually, in cases of blunt abdominal trauma, a CT scan is ordered to assess not only the liver but also the spleen, kidneys, and other organs. Hepatic laceration and hemorrhage usually manifest as an area of low density compared with the liver, although very acute hemorrhage can be denser (whiter) than the liver (Fig. 6-47). Hepatic lacerations are often treated conservatively if possible, because removal of a large portion of liver carries a high

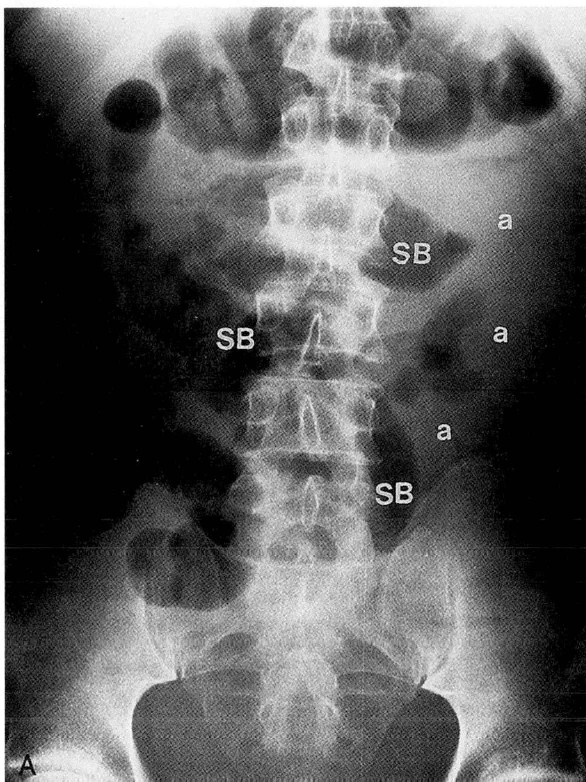

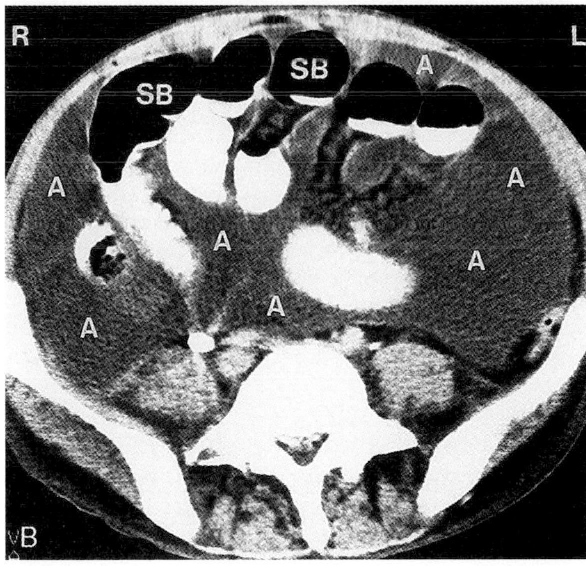

FIGURE 6-45 ■ **Ascites.** On a plain film of the abdomen *(A),* only gross amounts of ascites can be identified. This is usually seen because the ascites (a) has caused a rather gray appearance of the abdomen and pushed the gas-containing loops of small bowel (SB) toward the most nondependent and central portion of the abdomen. A transverse computed tomography (CT) scan *(B)* shows a cross-sectional view of the same appearance with the air- and contrast-filled small bowel floating in the ascitic fluid.

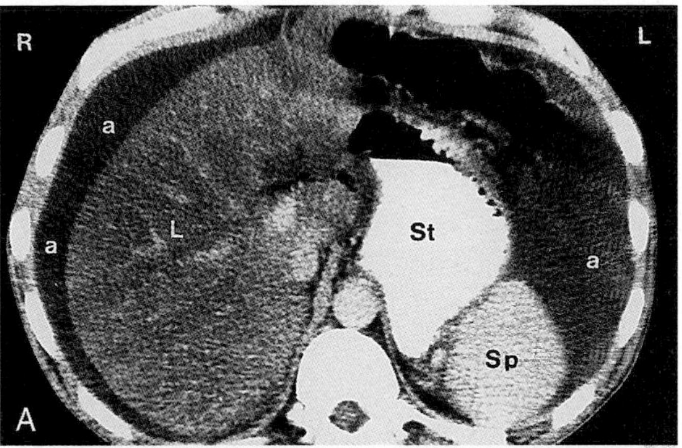

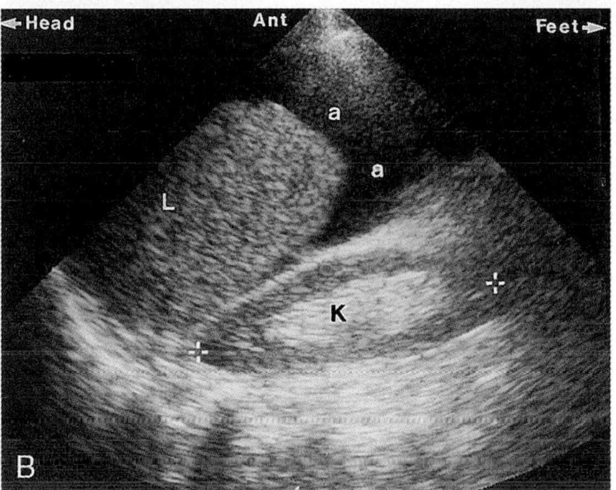

FIGURE 6-46 ■ **Ascites.** A transverse computed tomography (CT) scan of the upper abdomen *(A),* done without intravenous contrast, shows fatty infiltration of most of the liver (L). Normally, without intravenous contrast, the liver should be the same density at the spleen (Sp). Ascites (a) also can be seen around the edge of the liver (L) and in the left paracolic gutter. A longitudinal ultrasound image *(B)* shows ascitic fluid (a) along the inferior aspect of the right lobe of the liver. The kidney (K) also is seen.

risk of mortality. Intraparenchymal liver hemorrhages may ultimately be resorbed.

Hepatic Tumors

The most common benign hepatic tumor is a hemangioma. This is often discovered incidentally on ultrasound examination, where it appears as an area of increased or bright echo within the liver. Hemangiomas also are discovered incidentally on noncontrasted CT scans of the abdomen. On this type of scan, the lesion

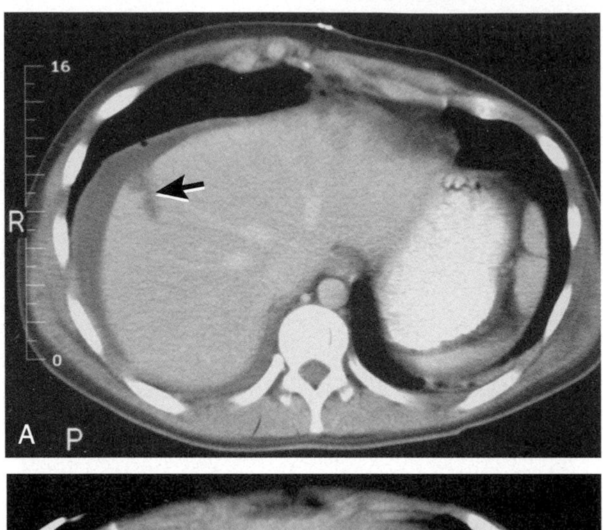

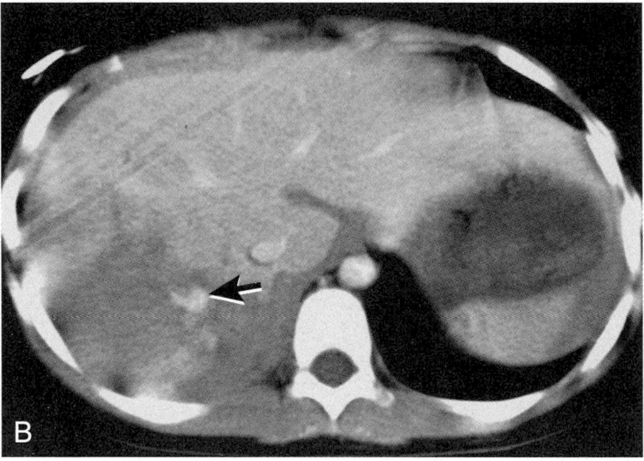

FIGURE 6-47 ■ Small and large hepatic lacerations. *A,* A computed tomography (CT) scan was obtained through the upper abdomen in this patient after a motor vehicle accident. A small area of low density *(arrow)* is seen in the lateral portion of the right lobe, and blood surrounds the liver. A CT scan in another patient *(B),* who was drunk and in a motor vehicle accident, shows a much larger area of lacerated liver in the posterior aspect of the right lobe. A central area of increased density (white) *(arrow)* indicates acute hemorrhaging at the time of the scan.

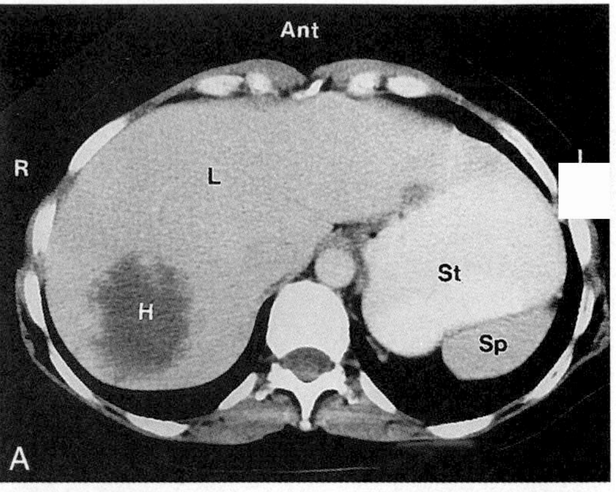

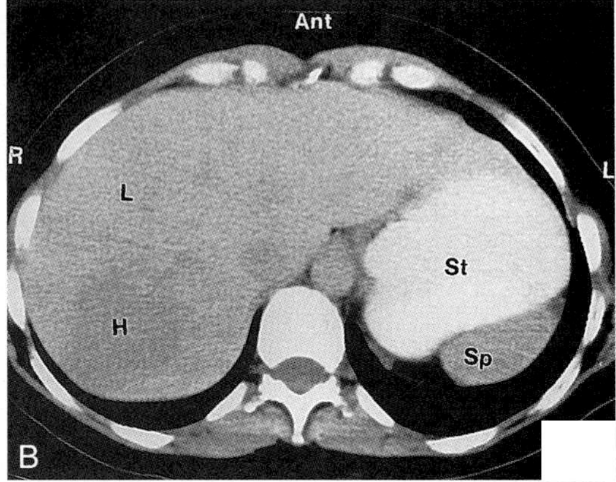

FIGURE 6-48 ■ Hepatic hemangioma. On an initial image of the contrast-enhanced computed tomography (CT) scan of the upper abdomen, hemangioma (H) appears as a low-density area with irregular margins in the posterior aspect of the liver (L). This was an unexpected and incidental finding in this young woman. A scan through exactly the same level obtained 20 minutes later shows that the lesion has almost completely disappeared. In this patient, no further workup is indicated.

appears as a rounded area of low density within the liver. A hemangioma can look like a malignant primary tumor or even a metastatic lesion. One way to differentiate a benign hemangioma from other lesions is to do serial CT scans over a period of minutes as intravenous contrast is administered. Usually, over a period of 10 to 15 minutes, the hemangioma will fill in with contrast and look like normal liver, whereas most malignancies will not do this (Fig. 6-48).

The most common primary malignant hepatic tumor is a hepatoma. On a noncontrasted CT scan, this appears as an irregular dark area within the liver, but these tumors can show pronounced vascularity on an arterial phase CT (Fig. 6-49). Remember that hepatomas can be multifocal. Five percent of patients with cirrhosis and 10% of patients with chronic hepatitis B will develop hepatocellular carcinoma. Hepatocellular carcinomas are solitary 25% of the time, multiple 25% of the time, and diffuse 50% of the time.

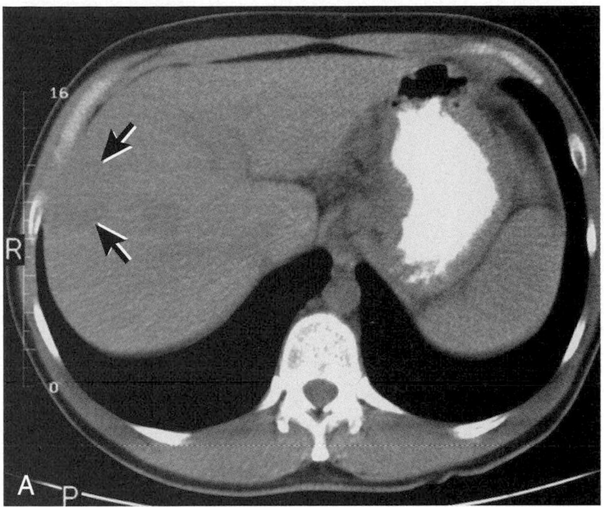

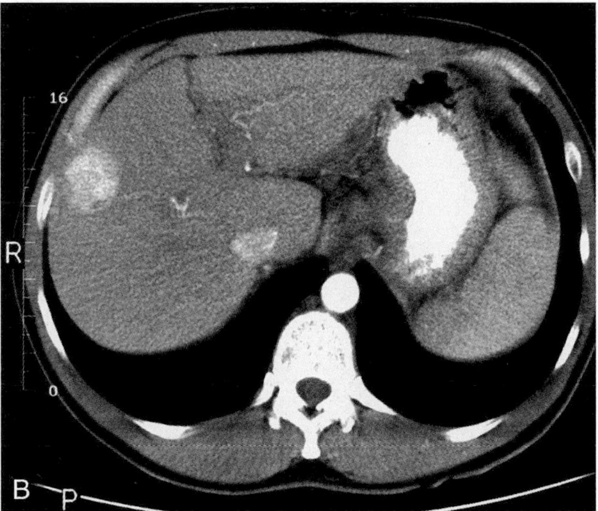

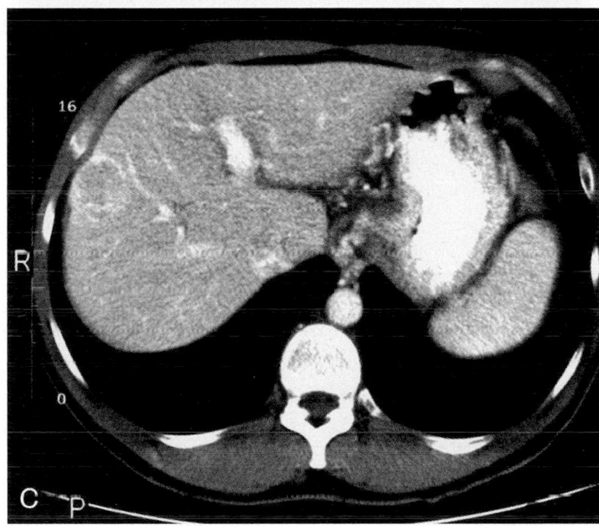

FIGURE 6-49 ■ Hepatoma on a three-phase computed tomography (CT) scan. In this patient with chronic hepatitis, on a noncontrasted CT scan *(A)* there is a low-density lesion in the lateral aspect of the right lobe that is barely visible *(arrows)*. Within seconds of administration of intravenous contrast, an arterial phase image *(B)* shows the lesion to be very vascular, and on a venous phase image *(C)*, the lesion retains some peripheral enhancement. This is characteristic of a hepatomas, but not all hepatomas show this much enhancement.

Metastatic lesions of the liver are very common. Forty percent of hepatic metastases are from cancer of the colon, 25% from stomach, 20% from pancreas, 15% from breast, and 15% from lung. Metastatic lesions may be small or large and single or multiple. Be aware that the visibility of hepatic metastases on a CT scan varies greatly, depending on the technical factors used when the filming is done from the computerized data. If a CT scan is done with very wide windows (wide-contrast scale) and without using intravenous contrast, it may be difficult to see the lesions. The best detectability is achieved by using intravenous contrast and narrow window settings (Fig. 6-50). Technologists will often produce both types of images. The less-useful images for this purpose are more pleasing to the eye. You should be sure that you are looking at those with narrow window settings. Normally these images are coarser or have more grain than those done with wide windows.

Hepatic Cysts

Hepatic cysts are quite common and are usually incidental findings on CT scans. They are lower density than the liver and are clearly defined. They may be single or multiple. Sometimes people are concerned as to whether these might be abscesses or neoplasms. The simplest way to

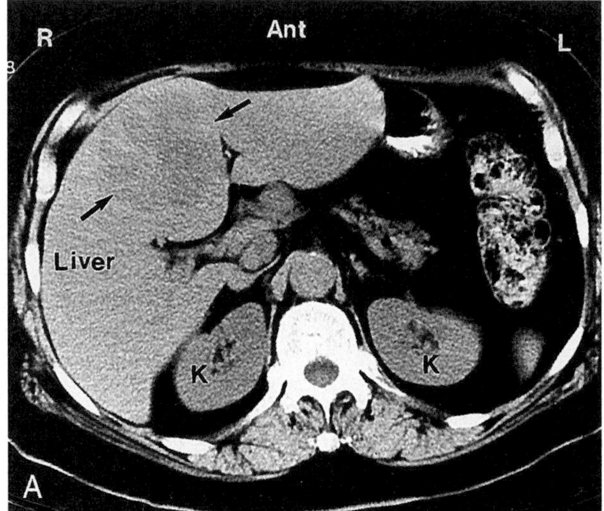

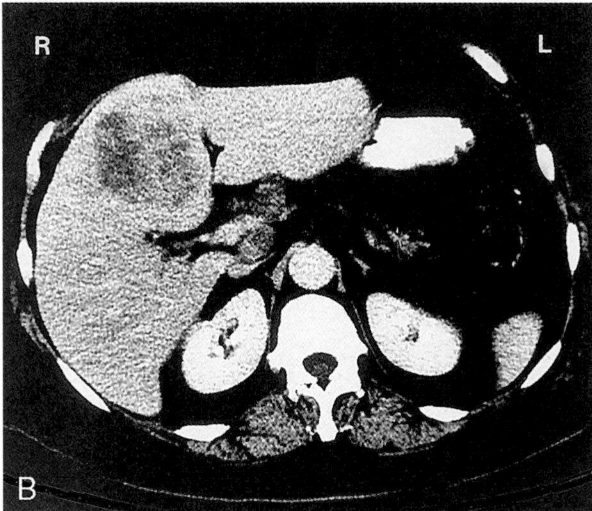

FIGURE 6-50 ■ Effect of different computed tomography (CT) techniques on detection of metastases. This patient has a fairly large metastatic deposit from colon carcinoma in the lateral segment of the left lobe of the liver. A CT scan performed without intravenous contrast *(A)* and filmed by using wide windows makes it very difficult to see the metastasis *(arrows)*. With intravenous contrast and filming the study with narrow windows *(B)*, the image looks much coarser, but the metastatic deposit is much easier to see.

determine what they are is to have the CT technologists measure the density (Hounsfield units) on the CT scan. If this measures between 0 and 20, the lesion is almost certainly a cyst and can be ignored (Fig. 6-51). If it is higher than this

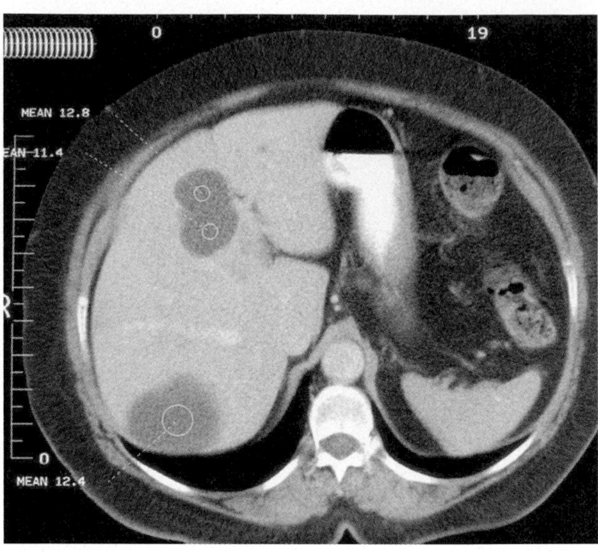

FIGURE 6-51 ■ Hepatic cysts. Low-density areas were found within the liver on this computed tomography (CT) scan done for other purposes. The mean measurements of the Hounsfield units are less than 15, indicating that these are definitely simple cysts.

value, more workup or follow-up is required. Sometimes the cysts are too small to measure accurately (<0.5 cm), and then they should be followed up in 6 months or so.

Hepatitis

Usually no need exists to image the liver in a patient with known infectious hepatitis. The diagnosis is best made by serum antibody evaluation. If hepatomegaly is seen on physical examination, the antibody tests are negative, and no history of hepatotoxins is known (e.g., alcohol, niacin, sulfa, rifampin, tetracycline, estrogens, acetaminophen), an ultrasound study is indicated to exclude biliary obstruction by occult masses. Occasionally CT or MRI scans are done to evaluate the patient for suspected secondary hepatoma.

Hepatic Abscess

Most hepatic abscesses are visualized with CT scanning. They are low density, or darker than the liver. Unless they have gas within them; their differentiation from neoplasm can be very difficult. Usually the clinical presentation of a very sick, febrile patient is enough to suggest the correct diagnosis. If not, CT scanning can be used to help in the diagnosis and also to direct a needle aspiration and place a drainage catheter. Abscesses suspected anywhere in the abdomen are best imaged by CT with both intravenous and oral contrast.

GALLBLADDER AND BILIARY SYSTEM

Anatomy and Imaging Techniques

Several ways exist of visualizing the gallbladder and biliary system, depending on the clinical presentation. Ultrasound is the least expensive and easiest method for looking for gallstones or biliary dilatation. Unfortunately, the distal common duct is difficult to see. Nuclear medicine hepatobiliary scans are more functional and generally provide physiological information and information about bile leaks. The fine architecture of both the biliary and the pancreatic ducts can be visualized by use of an endoscopic retrograde cholangiopancreatogram (ERCP). To do this, a large tube is passed down the esophagus and through the stomach to the duodenum. The ampulla of Vater is then cannulated. Contrast is injected into the pancreatic and common bile ducts (Fig. 6-52). An ERCP is a very useful way to assess the diameter of a stricture as well as its length (Fig. 6-53*A*). During an ERCP, it also is possible to do a papillotomy and remove stones from the common duct. Recently it has become possible to visualize the ductal system with MRI (Fig. 6-53*B*), but this is usually reserved for cases in which ERCP is impractical or impossible.

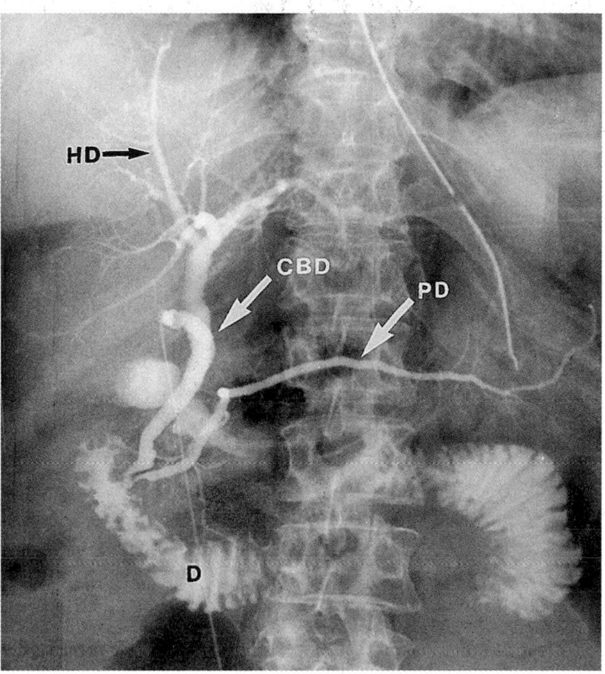

FIGURE 6-52 ■ Normal endoscopic retrograde cholangiopancreatography (ERCP). Placement of a fiberoptic gastroscope allows cannulation of the common bile duct (CBD) and pancreatic duct (PD) at the level of the ampulla of Vater. Retrograde injection of contrast also allows visualization of intrahepatic ducts (HD). Contrast is seen spilling around the cannulation site into the duodenal sweep and proximal jejunum.

Acute Cholecystitis

If acute cholecystitis is suspected, the examination of choice is a nuclear medicine hepatobiliary scan. In a normal hepatobiliary scan, the liver will clear the radioactive tracer, and it should appear in the gallbladder, common bile duct, and proximal small bowel within 1 hour (Fig. 6-54). Failure to visualize the gallbladder when imaging is carried out to 4 hours has a very high specificity for acute cholecystitis, because in acute cholecystitis, usually blockage of the cystic duct occurs, and the radioactive tracer cannot get into the gallbladder (Fig. 6-55). In chronic cholecystitis, the gallbladder fills with activity, but this occurs later than normal. Some authors advocate the use of ultrasound for acute cholecystitis and look for gallbladder wall thickening and pain when the ultrasound transducer is pressed on the right upper quadrant. You should have noted the latter finding when you examined the patient before you ordered the test. Moreover, gallbladder wall thickening is nonspecific and can occur with other entities, such as hypoproteinemia.

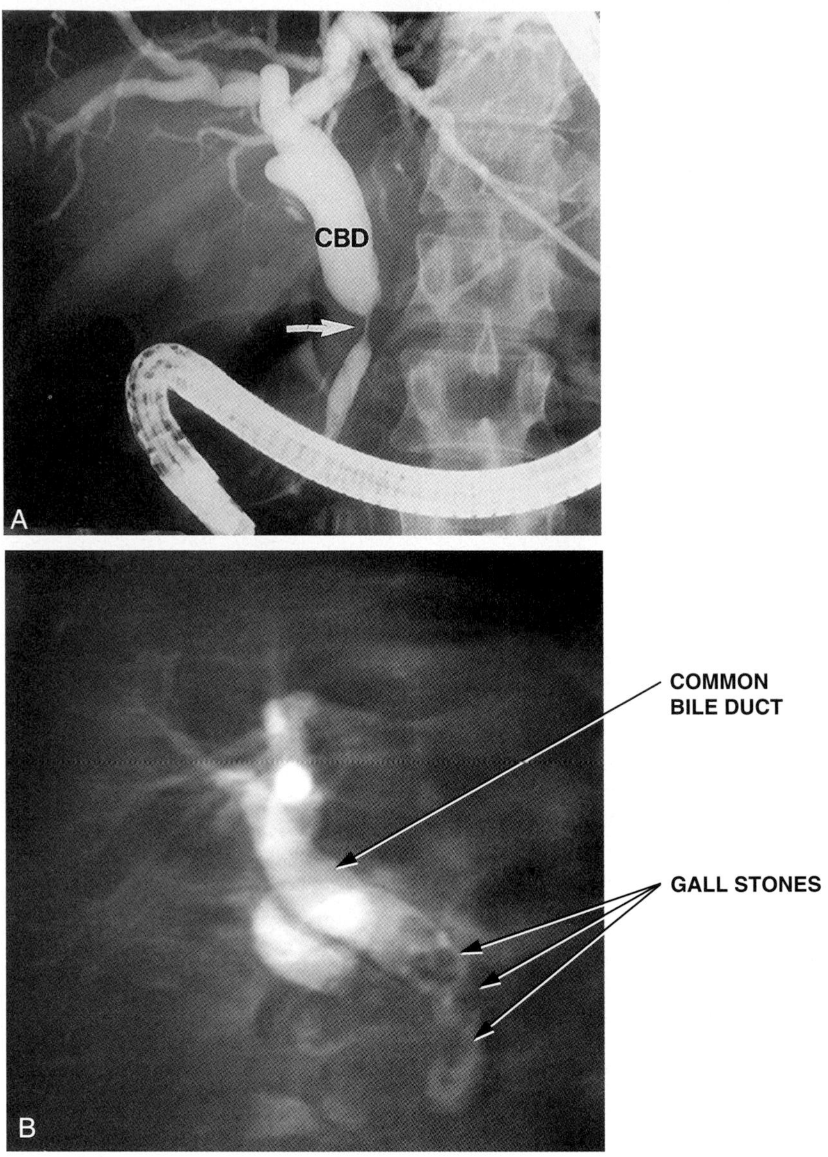

FIGURE 6-53 ■ Common bile duct pathology. *A,* With an endoscopic retrograde cholangiopancreatography (ERCP), retrograde injection of contrast shows a stricture in the midportion of the common bile duct (CBD) *(arrow)* and dilatation of the proximal and intrahepatic biliary system. In a different patient, a magnetic resonance imaging (MRI) scan *(B)* was used to visualize a dilated common bile duct (CBD) containing multiple stones *(arrows).*

Chronic Cholecystitis and Cholelithiasis

If you suspect gallstones (cholelithiasis) or biliary duct obstruction, the quickest, cheapest, and most efficient imaging test is an ultrasound examination of the right upper quadrant (see Fig. 6-10*B*). On a nuclear medicine hepatobiliary scan, chronic cholecystitis is apparent as delayed gallbladder filling (1 to 4 hours).

Biliary Obstruction and Jaundice

When jaundice is present and a question arises about whether it is due to parenchymal liver disease, such as hepatitis, or to an obstructive lesion

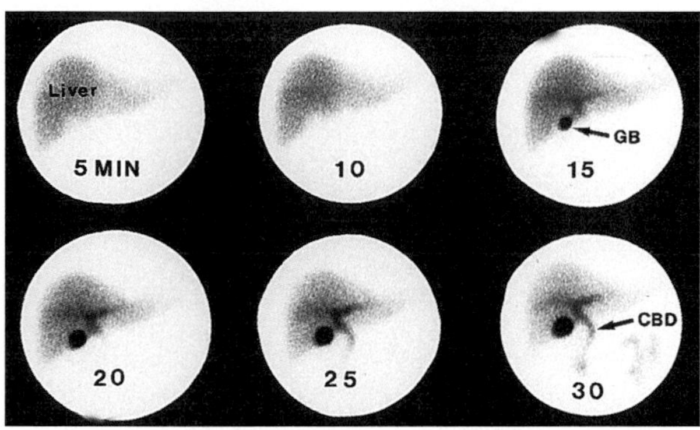

FIGURE 6-54 ■ Normal nuclear medicine hepatobiliary study. Intravenous administration of a small amount of radioactively labeled material that is cleared by the biliary system allows visualization of the liver, the gallbladder (GB) by 15 minutes, and the common bile duct (CBD) by 30 minutes.

of the common bile duct, the initial imaging examination often is ultrasound. When complete ductal obstruction has been present for more than 24 hours, dilatation of the common and intrahepatic ducts is relatively easy to see with ultrasound. The upper portion of the common duct (normally measured at ultrasound) is usually less than 4 mm in diameter. It becomes slightly dilated with age and can be up to 7 mm in some patients younger than 60 years. In normal persons who are older than 60 years, the common duct diameter should be less than 10 mm. The common duct diameter also can be larger than 4 mm (up to 6 to 7 mm) if

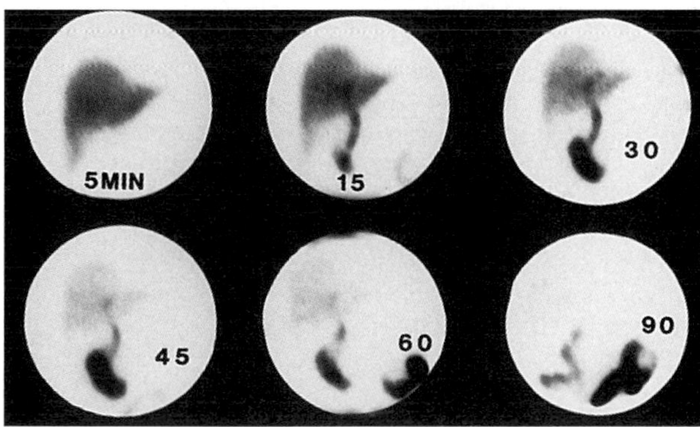

FIGURE 6-55 ■ Acute cholecystitis. A nuclear medicine hepatobiliary study shows the liver, common bile duct, and activity in the jejunum by 60 and 90 minutes. The gallbladder was never visualized, even at 4 hours after injection. This is because with acute cholecystitis, blockage of the cystic duct occurs. If the gallbladder is visualized only 1 to 4 hours after injection, chronic (rather than acute) cholecystitis is likely.

the patient has had a cholecystectomy. Because a CT scan provides information on ductal dilatation as well as other useful information (Fig. 6-56), many clinicians will order a CT scan instead of an ultrasound examination.

Intrahepatic obstruction of the common duct is usually due to cholangitis, Caroli's disease, or an intrahepatic neoplasm (hepatoma compressing the ducts or a rare biliary neoplasm). Extrahepatic biliary obstruction usually occurs distally in the intrapancreatic portion of the duct. Common causes are gallstone, pancreatic cancer, and pancreatitis.

Sometimes, after a cholecystectomy and removal of stones from the common duct, a T

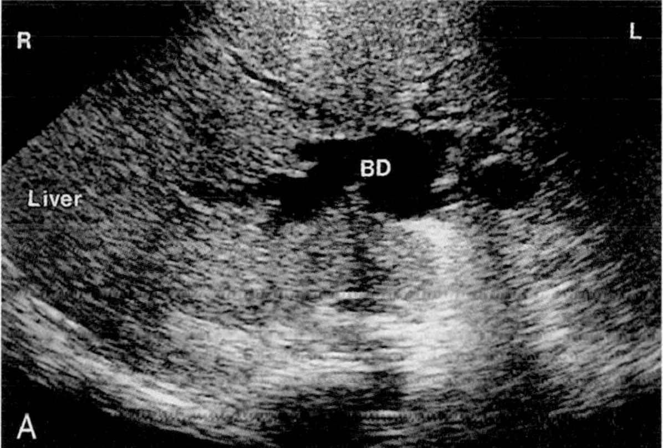

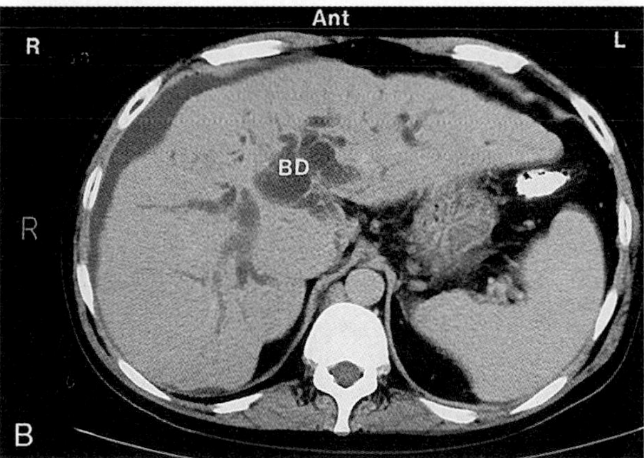

FIGURE 6-56 ■ Biliary ductal dilatation. *A,* A transverse ultrasound image through the liver shows a central branching area without echoes that represents dilated bile ducts (BD). A computed tomography (CT) scan of the same patient *(B)* also demonstrates the intrahepatic dilated biliary system. As a screening test, ultrasound is cheaper and just as effective. CT scanning is more useful to localize the cause of obstruction, such as a pancreatic carcinoma.

tube is left in place. This is done to allow bile drainage through the abdominal wall while edema related to surgery and prior stones resolves. Before the tube is pulled, contrast is injected into the T tube to look for possible retained stones.

Occasionally, as a result of surgery, air from the GI tract will reflux into the biliary system. This may be visualized on a KUB (plain film of the abdomen). Air in the biliary tract is usually centrally located in the region of the porta hepatis, and the air is prevented from going very distally into the smaller bile ducts by flow of bile toward the porta hepatis. You must be able to differentiate this relatively benign finding from that of air in the portal venous system. Air in the portal venous system is usually seen as branching air collections near the periphery of the liver (within 2 mm). The air goes peripherally because that is the direction of the flow of blood in the portal veins. Visualization of branching lucencies in the outermost 2 cm of the liver is considered presumptive evidence of portal venous air. This is seen in diabetic patients and is associated with a high mortality (Fig. 6-57).

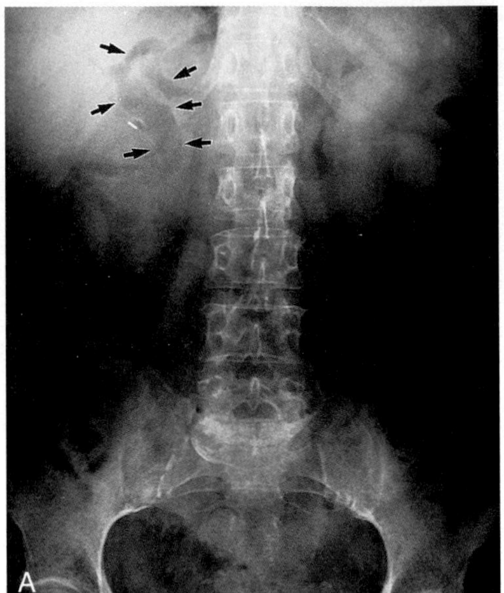

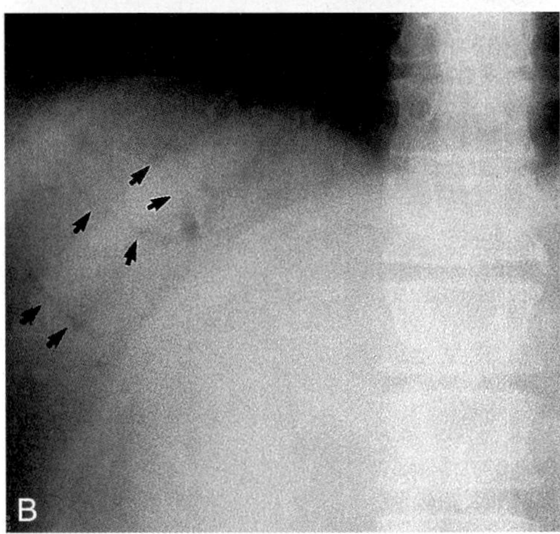

FIGURE 6-57 ■ **Air within the liver.** A branching or serpiginous collection of air is seen within the right upper quadrant on a kidneys, ureter, and bladder (KUB) examination *(A)*. This air is in the region of the porta hepatis and represents air within the biliary system. This is a common finding after gallbladder surgery and has little clinical significance. In contrast, branching collections of air seen peripherally in the liver *(B)* in a different patient represent air within the portal venous system, and this has a high associated mortality.

PANCREAS

Pancreatitis and Complications

Seventy percent of cases of pancreatitis are caused either by alcoholic pancreatitis or by obstruction due to a gallstone in the distal common duct. The diagnosis is usually made by clinical findings of epigastric or lower abdominal pain and hyperamylasemia. Unfortunately, about 30% of patients with pancreatitis have a normal serum amylase level, and about 35% of persons with hyperamylasemia have a disease other than pancreatitis. The most useful imaging method for a patient with pancreatitis is CT scanning. In rare patients who have very sudden onset pancreatitis, the pancreas may be of normal size, but the serum amylase value may be elevated. Most patients with acute pancreatitis have an enlarged pancreas with peripancreatic inflammation, thickening of the perirenal fascia, and peripancreatic fluid collections (Fig. 6-58). Occasionally, one or several dilated loops of small bowel over the central abdomen may be caused by a focal ileus from the underlying inflammation in the pancreas.

Late complications of acute pancreatitis are pancreatic duct obstruction, pseudocyst formation, and abscess (Fig. 6-59). A pseudocyst usually takes approximately 6 weeks to mature fully. At this time, a CT scan shows a well-defined cystic area (see Fig. 6-59*B*), and CT can be used

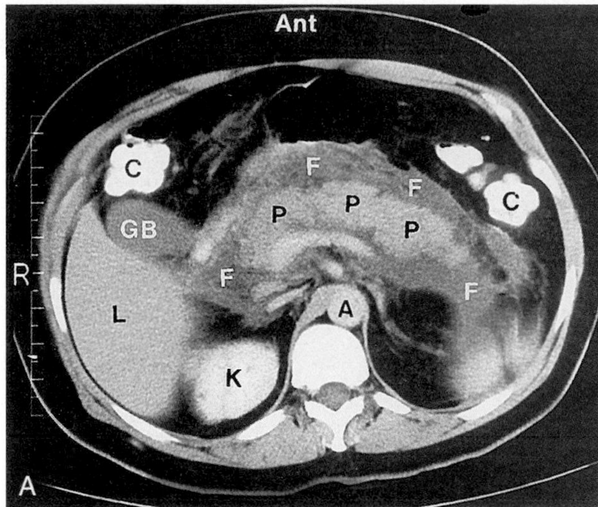

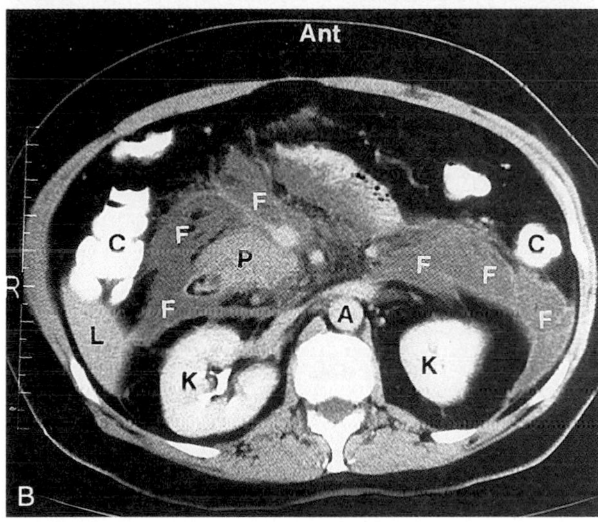

FIGURE 6-58 ■ **Acute pancreatitis.** *A,* A computed tomography (CT) scan in this young woman with hyperlipidemia shows the body of the pancreas (P) and surrounding fluid (F). The liver (L), kidney (K), gallbladder (GB), and colon (C) also are identified. Another image in the same patient obtained slightly more inferiorly *(B)* shows a marked amount of fluid (F) around the uncinate portion of the pancreas (P) and fluid extending around into the left paracolic gutter with associated thickening of Gerota's fascia.

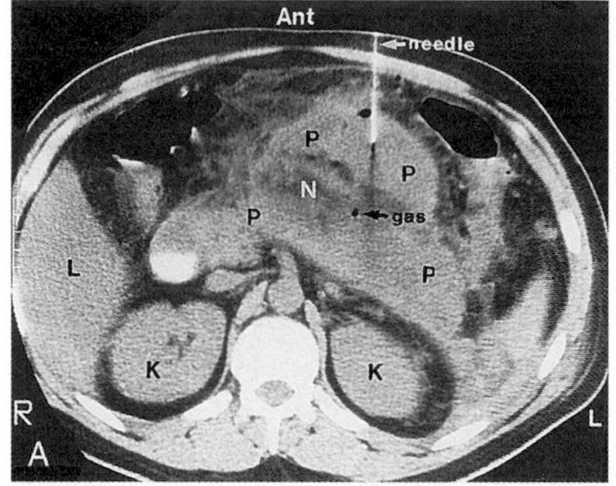

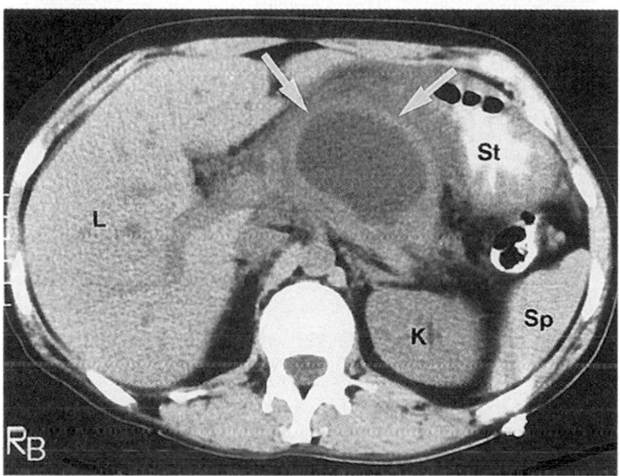

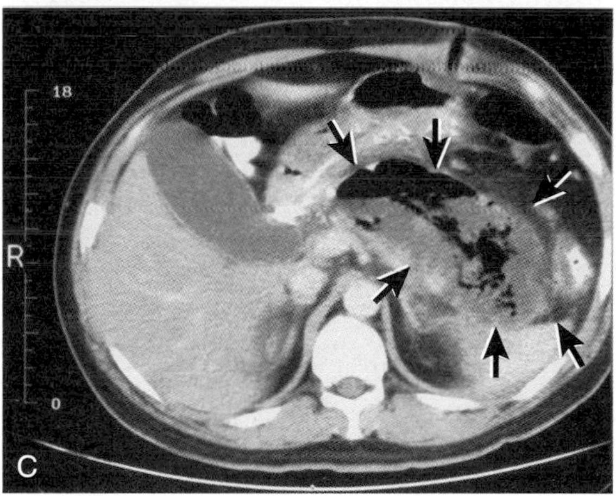

FIGURE 6-59 ■ **Complications of pancreatitis.** A transverse computed tomography (CT) scan *(A)* in a patient with pancreatitis and a persistent fever shows a very enlarged pancreas (P); a low-density area within it represents necrosis of the pancreas. Also noted is a small gas bubble due to formation of a pancreatic abscess. A needle has been inserted under CT guidance to obtain material for culture and to place a percutaneous drain. In a second patient who is a chronic alcoholic, the CT scan *(B)* demonstrates a well-defined low-density area within the pancreas *(arrows)*. This represents a pancreatic pseudocyst. In a third patient *(C)*, the CT scan demonstrates a pancreatic abscess in the body and tail *(arrows)*. The air within it *(small dark areas)* indicates an abscess.

to perform percutaneous drainage. Be aware that pseudocysts are not necessarily in the pancreas itself. They can be focal fluid collections anywhere in the abdomen and occasionally even in the pelvis or thorax.

With fulminant pancreatitis, formation of an abscess may be noted. This is seen on CT scan as a large soft tissue mass that contains air bubbles, in the region of the pancreas. This condition has a very high mortality rate, and usually a percutaneous drain will be placed to try to drain the abscess. Another complication is progressive pancreatic necrosis due to digestion of tissue (a *phlegmon*). This is seen on CT as multiple areas of lucency within the pancreas. This condition also has a high mortality rate.

Tumor

Adenocarcinoma accounts for 95% of all pancreatic cancer. It has a very poor prognosis, with a 1-year survival rate of 10% or less. Clinically, the patients initially are seen with jaundice, weight loss, and occasionally with a dilated, nontender gallbladder. CT scanning is the imaging modality of choice to assess not only the tumor size and location but also the possibility of hepatic and nodal metastases.

SPLEEN

Splenomegaly

Imaging of the spleen is sometimes done to assess splenic size, although this really should be done clinically by palpation and percussion. The spleen is usually about 10 cm in length, and up to 13 cm may be normal. Causes of splenomegaly are leukemia [especially chronic lymphocytic leukemia (CLL)], lymphoma, infection (mononucleosis), storage diseases (amyloid and Gaucher's disease), portal hypertension, and hematologic abnormalities (anemias, thalassemia, myelofibrosis).

Trauma

After blunt trauma, the spleen is the most commonly injured intra-abdominal organ, and a splenic fracture or hematomas may be found. Although surgeons usually try to manage these injuries conservatively, splenic rupture may be noted even a week to 10 days after the initial injury. If you suspect splenic trauma, a CT scan is the test of choice. Hemorrhage and hematoma usually appear as areas of lower density than the spleen (Fig. 6-60). Round or irregular dark areas represent intrasplenic hematomas or lacerations, and abnormal crescentic areas at the edge of the spleen represent subcapsular hematomas. Occasionally, with conservative management, an abscess may subsequently form and can be identified as such on a CT scan because it contains gas.

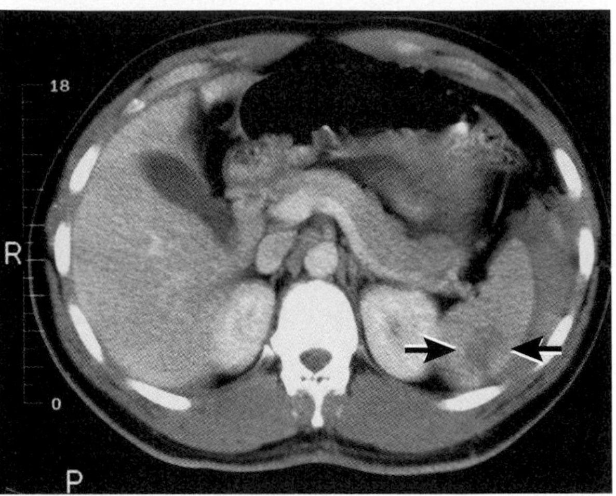

FIGURE 6-60 ■ **Splenic laceration.** The computed tomography (CT) scan done on a patient after a motor vehicle accident shows a dark area near the posterior aspect of the spleen *(arrows)*. This is the laceration. Note also the blood surrounding the spleen.

In addition to being identifiable as trauma, focal splenic lesions can easily be seen on a CT scan. These can be due to splenic abscesses, infarcts, tumors, and occasionally cysts. The sensitivity of CT for detection of these is high, but the specificity is poor, and often the clinical history is necessary to narrow the differential diagnosis.

SMALL BOWEL

You should be able to recognize some small bowel abnormalities by examining the gas pattern on plain film of the abdomen. Small bowel can be identified by its central location and by its rather thin mucosal markings that extend across the entire lumen. One of the most common remarks that you hear when a physician is examining a small bowel film is that air/fluid levels are present. The implication is that this is abnormal, but it is, in fact, quite normal, because small bowel contents are mostly fluid, and any air or carbon dioxide that is swallowed and passes through the stomach will cause an air/fluid level in the small bowel.

Obstruction versus Ileus

A standard question in reference to a patient with abdominal pain is whether he or she has either a small bowel obstruction or paralytic ileus. This question can be resolved with a stethoscope rather than an x-ray, because if bowel sounds are present and relatively frequent, a paralytic ileus is unlikely. On a plain film x-ray of the abdomen, the diameter of the small bowel should not exceed 3 cm; if it does, try to determine whether an obstruction or an ileus is present.

If the small bowel dilatation is greater than 4 cm, you are almost certainly looking at an obstruction, because in a paralytic ileus, only mild dilatation is found. The upright film is used to look at the nature of the air/fluid levels. As mentioned earlier, air/fluid levels can be normal, but if you find them in bowel and the small bowel is dilated, look on an upright film for a single loop of small bowel to see whether the air/fluid levels at either end of the loop are at the same level or at different levels. If they are at different levels in a given loop of small bowel, an obstruction is present. This is because muscle tone within the small bowel causes the different levels, and this would not be present with a paralytic ileus (Fig. 6-61).

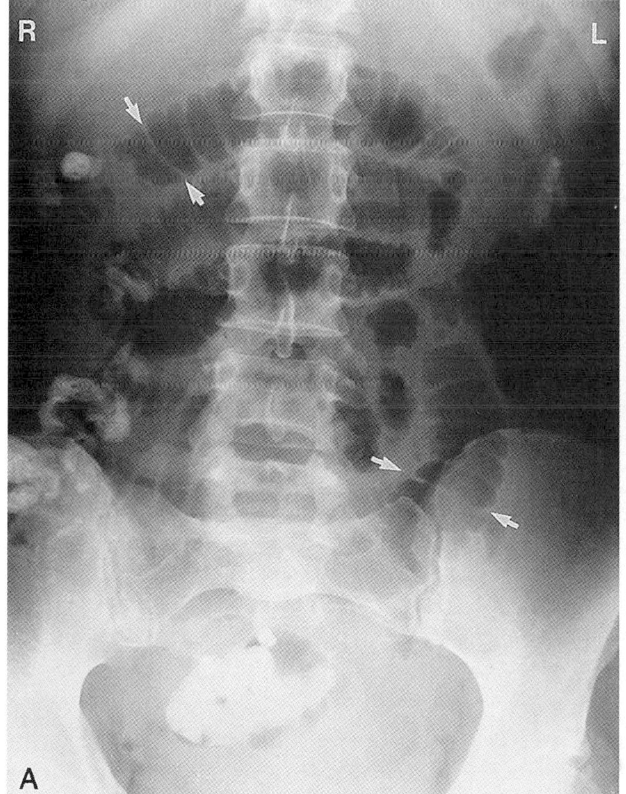

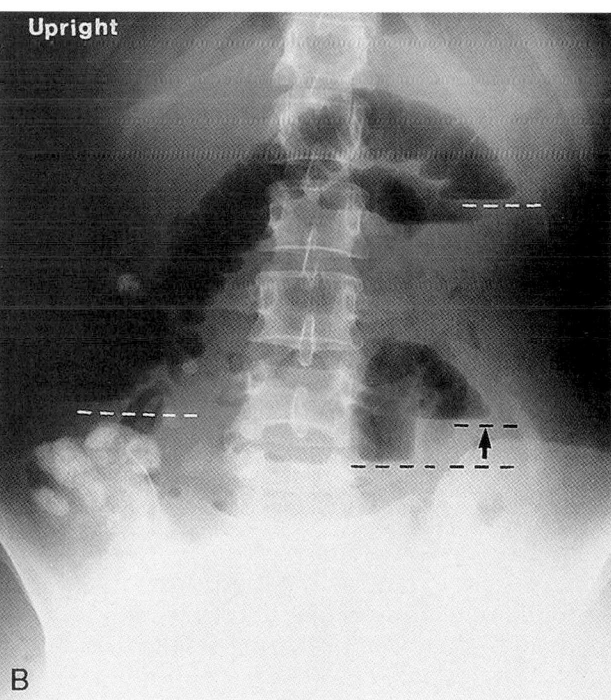

FIGURE 6-61 ■ **Small bowel obstruction.** On a supine kidneys, ureters, and bladder (KUB) scan *(A)*, a large amount of dilated small bowel is seen. This can be recognized as small bowel by the very regular mucosal pattern of the valvulae extending across the lumen and looking like a set of thick, stacked coins *(arrows)*. The small bowel normally should not exceed 3 cm in diameter. On an upright film of the abdomen *(B)*, the air/fluid levels within the same loop of bowel are at different heights. This indicates an obstruction rather than a paralytic ileus.

Continued

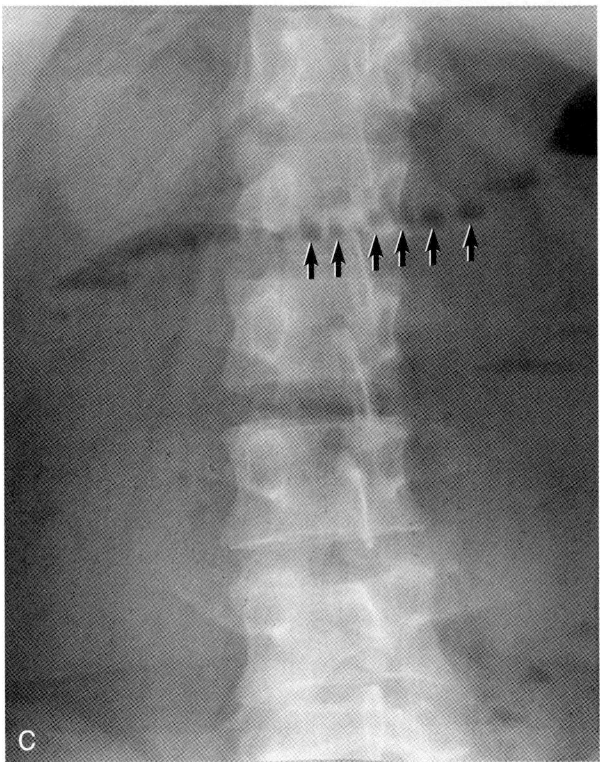

FIGURE 6-61 cont'd ■ A close-up view of the right midabdomen in another patient *(C)* shows the "string of pearls" air bubbles *(arrows)* that indicate a fluid-filled and obstructed small bowel.

Remember that a long-standing bowel obstruction can ultimately result in a paralytic ileus. The common causes of a paralytic ileus are a postoperative state, vascular ischemia, nearby inflammatory processes (such as pancreatitis and appendicitis), electrolyte imbalance, and drugs (morphine and its derivatives). Small bowel obstructions are mostly due to adhesions, tumors, hernias, and inflammatory strictures.

With a very dilated diameter of the small bowel (i.e., obstruction), look to see how far bowel gas extends. If dilated small bowel extends to the lower portion of the abdomen, you are looking at an obstruction that is at least in the distal small bowel or perhaps in the proximal colon. If you see air distally in the colon or in the rectum, you may be looking at either a partial small bowel obstruction or a very acute complete small bowel obstruction (the distal air not yet having been expelled). Sometimes, as the lumen of obstructed small bowel fills with fluid, small bubbles of air are trapped in the most superior part of the lumen between the valvulae conniventes. This leads to the appearance of a "string of pearls" (Fig. 6-61*C*).

The cause of a small bowel obstruction is often difficult to identify on a plain x-ray. Look carefully for gas in the inguinal region to exclude a strangulated hernia (Fig. 6-62). Dilatation of the small bowel in a child older than a few years should raise the suspicion of appendicitis (Fig. 6-63). When you see this, look carefully over the region of the sacrum and right ileum to see if an appendicolith may be present.

Benign Diseases

A wide variety of diseases can affect the small bowel and can be visualized on a barium study of the small bowel. The finer points of radiologic differential diagnosis of small bowel disease are

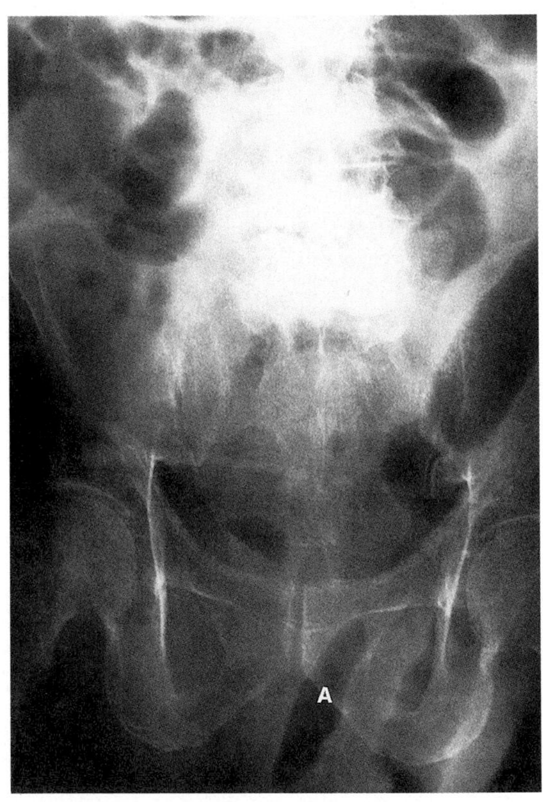

FIGURE 6-62 ■ **Strangulated inguinal hernia.** A film of the pelvis demonstrates some dilated loops of small bowel in the upper abdomen. Over the left groin, two air collections (A) represent loops of small bowel descending into the scrotum.

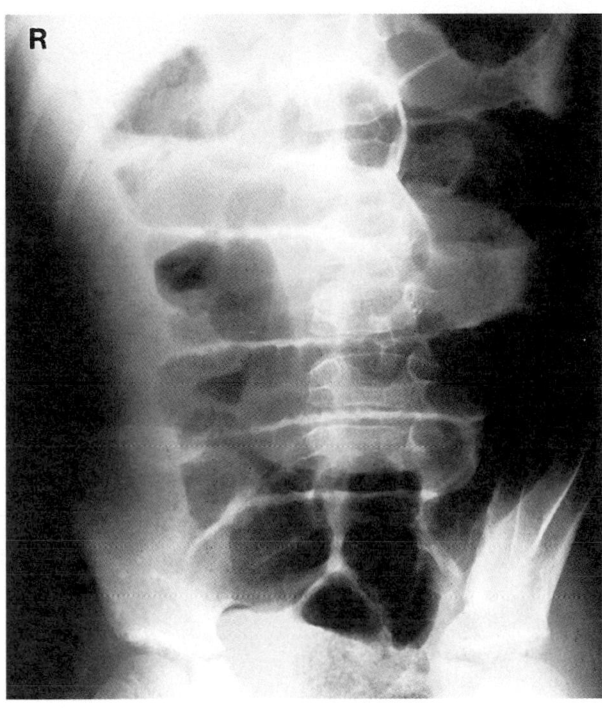

FIGURE 6-63 ■ **Acute appendicitis.** In this supine film of the abdomen of a young child, dilated small bowel loops are seen centrally. No definite gas is seen in the colon. Dilated small bowel loops in a young child should raise the consideration of appendicitis as well as intestinal obstruction.

beyond the scope of this text, but in general, you are looking for mucosal thickening, nodules, dilatation, and areas of stricturing. Fold thickening is assessed by looking at the mucosal pattern. The valvulae conniventes should not measure more than 2 to 3 mm in thickness. The mnemonic for the differential diagnosis of small bowel fold thickening is WAG CLEM, which refers to *W*hipple's disease, *a*myloid, *g*iardiasis, *c*ryptosporidiosis, *l*ymphoma, *e*osinophilic gastroenteritis, and *M*ycobacterium avium complex. The mnemonic for dilatation without fold thickening is SOSO, which stands for *s*prue, *o*bstruction (or ileus), *s*cleroderma, and *o*ther (medicines and vagotomy). I find it easier to remember the diseases than to figure out what these mnemonics stand for, but perhaps they will be useful to you.

Some diseases and conditions result in areas of stricturing. The most common are prior surgery, tumor, and Crohn's disease (regional enteritis). Lesions of regional enteritis are most common in the terminal ileum, and about half the patients also have involvement of the colon. Patients have weight loss, recurrent abdominal pain, and diarrhea. Extraintestinal manifestations include skin, eye, joint, and liver abnormalities. Characteristic features are areas of relatively fixed narrowing in the terminal ileum (the string sign) (Fig. 6-64), sinus tracts, and fistulas. In the colon, there may be areas of stricture and ulceration with skip areas that have normal mucosa in between.

Occasionally, collections of air or gas in subserosal portions of the small bowel are found (pneumatosis intestinalis) (Fig. 6-65). In adults, this is often a benign finding, whereas in children, it may be associated with necrotizing enterocolitis or ischemia. In adults, the benign form can occur in patients with chronic obstructive pulmonary disease (COPD) who have air dissecting down from the chest into the abdomen and along the mesentery of the bowel. This also may be associated with asymptomatic pneumoperitoneum. GI bleeding can occur as a result of a Meckel's diverticulum in the small bowel. Because this is most common in children, it is discussed in Chapter 9.

Tumors

Tumors of any sort in the small bowel are rare. Tumor incidence in the colon is about 40 times higher. The most common benign growths of the small bowel are leiomyomas, lipomas, adenomas, and polyps. Malignant tumors tend to be adenocarcinomas and to a lesser extent carcinoid, melanoma, and lymphoma. Symptoms of any tumor in the small bowel are obstruction and bleeding.

COLON

All of the colon can be directly visualized with an endoscope. This procedure allows biopsy of lesions, but it requires sedation and is expensive. Radiographic examination of the colon is begun by examining the plain film, but it is best performed by barium or water-soluble contrast

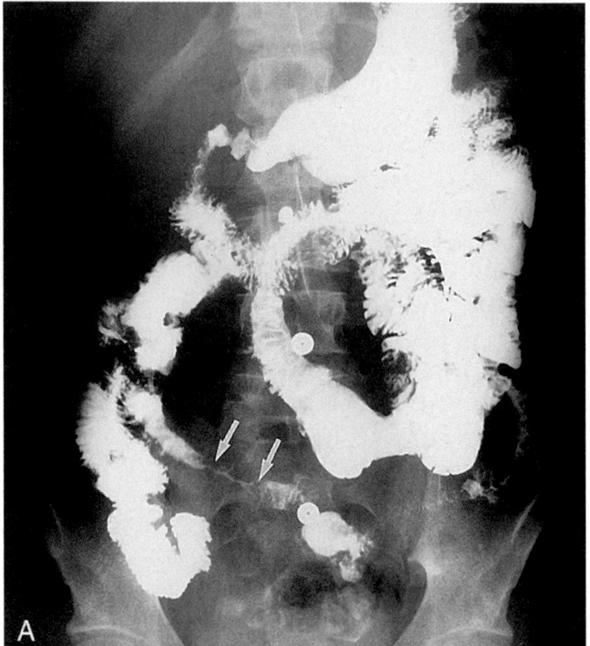

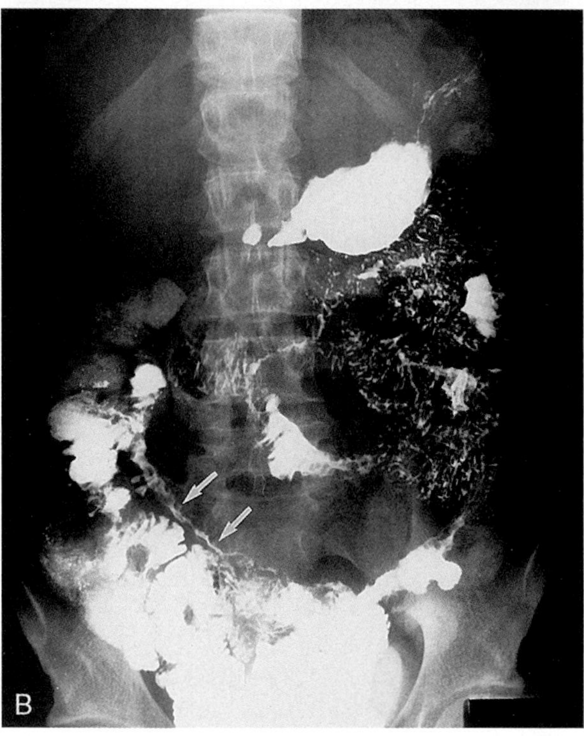

FIGURE 6-64 ■ Crohn's disease of the small bowel. A film obtained midway through a contrast study of the small bowel *(A)* demonstrates a narrowed segment of distal ileum *(arrows)*. Another film obtained at the end of the study *(B)* shows that most of the barium has passed into the colon, but the previously identified area of narrowing remains and, therefore, represents a stricture rather than peristalsis.

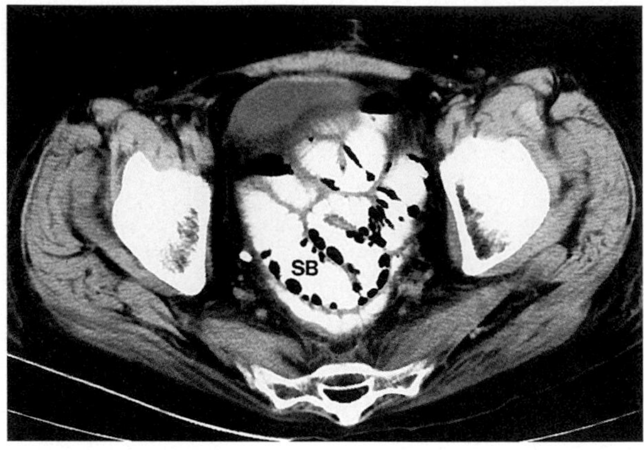

FIGURE 6-65 ■ Pneumatosis of the small bowel. A transverse computed tomography (CT) scan of the lower pelvis shows contrast-filled small bowel (SB). Small dark collections of gas in the wall of the small bowel are seen indenting the contrast-filled lumen.

enema. It is imperative that the colon be cleansed before the examination; otherwise, residual fecal material can be mistaken for polyps or malignant lesions. The diagnostic enema can be done either by filling the colon completely with barium (single-contrast examination) or by putting in a small amount of barium and then using air (double-contrast examination). The double-contrast examination has a higher sensitivity than the single-contrast examination. On a barium enema, a number of different views and projections are obtained. This is essential, because otherwise one loop of bowel would overlie another, and lesions would be obscured. The ascending, transverse, and descending colon as well as portions of the sigmoid can be appreciated on the anteroposterior (AP) or posteroanterior (PA) views of the abdomen (Fig. 6-66). Lateral views of the rectum are usually obtained (Fig. 6-67) as well as steep oblique views of the hepatic and splenic flexures (Fig. 6-68).

It is important to be sure that patients are well hydrated after a barium enema. If the barium remains in the colon for several days, water will be reabsorbed, and the patient will have difficulty in excreting the barium. Occasionally barium gets into the appendix during a barium enema. This is a normal finding. It may, however, stay there for months after the remainder

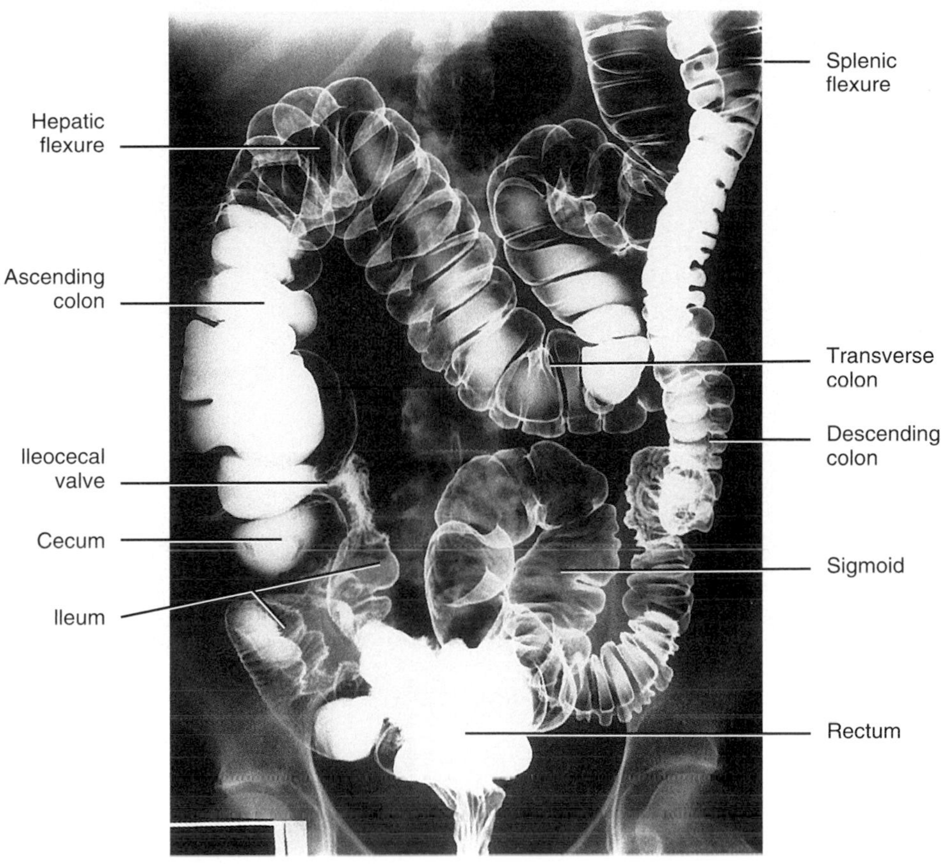

FIGURE 6-66 ■ Normal supine film on double-contrast barium enema.

of the barium is excreted. This can present a somewhat unusual and confusing appearance on a plain film of the abdomen (Fig. 6-69). It is important to understand the appearance of different lesions on a barium study. These are shown graphically in Figure 6-70. These appearances apply to all types of contrast studies.

Colonic Obstruction versus Paralytic Ileus

The key to the differentiation of colonic obstruction and paralytic ileus on a plain abdominal film is whether dilatation of the cecum is present. The cecum, compared with the rest of the colon, is most dilated in colonic obstruction. Colonic obstruction is most frequently due to a cancer (65%), but it also can be due to diverticulitis (20%) or a volvulus (5%). If the transverse colon is more dilated than the cecum, consider a diagnosis of ileus. The term for an abnormally distended transverse colon is a *megacolon*, and this refers to dilatation greater than 6 cm in diameter. A toxic megacolon can result from ulcerative colitis, Crohn's disease, or infectious causes.

When an acute colonic distention (cecum >9 cm) is found, a risk of perforation exists, and the likely causes are tumor obstruction, volvulus, and paralytic ileus. A number of patients have a chronically distended colon, and they have only a small risk of perforation. In such cases, chronic distention may be a result of chronic laxative abuse, neuromuscular disorders (including diabetes), psychogenic problems, or metabolic problems (electrolyte imbalance, hypothyroidism, use of morphine derivatives).

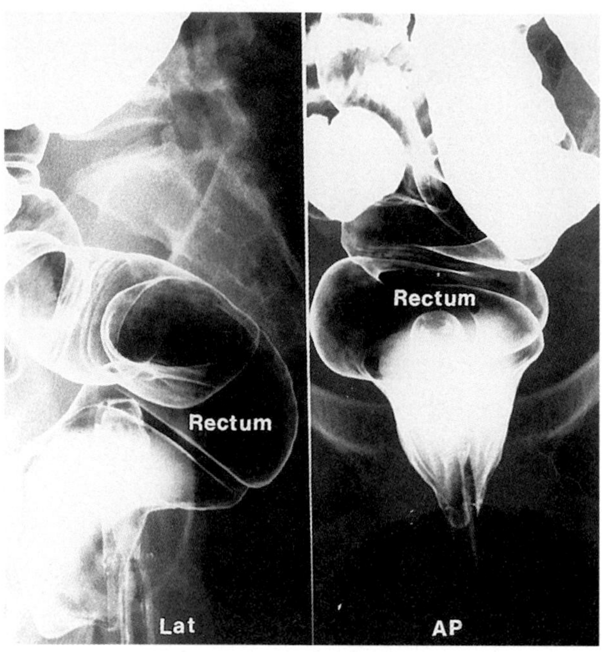

FIGURE 6-67 ■ Anteroposterior (AP) and lateral views of the normal rectum on a double-contrast barium enema.

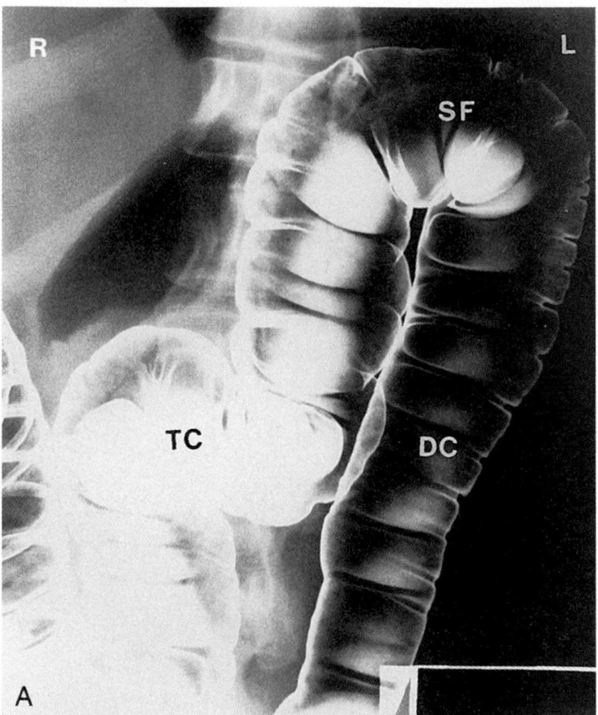

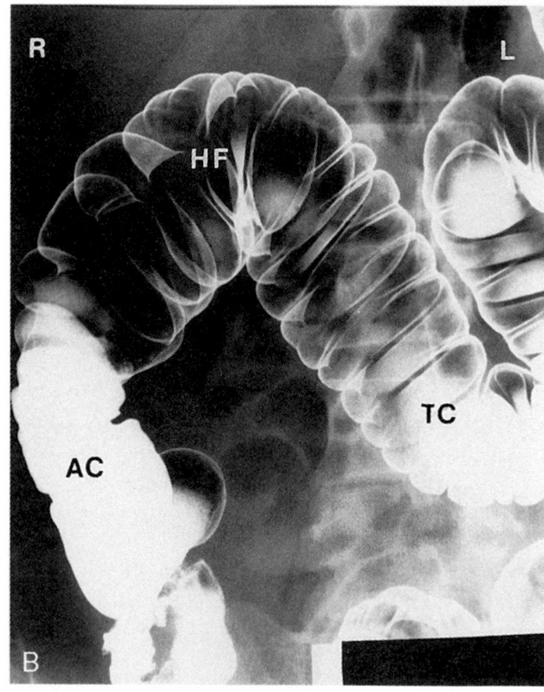

FIGURE 6-68 ■ Normal splenic and hepatic flexure of the colon. A steep oblique view of the left upper quadrant *(A)* shows the splenic flexure (SF) and the transverse (TC) and descending colon (DC), whereas an oblique view of the right upper quadrant *(B)* shows the hepatic flexure (HF) and transverse and ascending colon (AC).

Appendicitis

Acute appendicitis is usually diagnosed clinically. Because the differential diagnosis can include acute gasteroenteritis, cholecystitis, intestinal obstruction and perforation, urinary tract infection, or female pelvic pathology, and other conditions, some confusion may be apparent as to which imaging tests are indicated. Appendicitis should be suspected if there is a combination of abdominal pain; symptoms including nausea, vomiting, constipation, and diarrhea; the physical findings of guarding, rebound, rectal tenderness, and fever; or an elevated white blood cell count with a left shift.

The initial imaging test is usually of a posterior-anterior (PA) chest and supine and upright abdomen. This is useful to look for free air, dilated bowel, abnormal gas collections in an abscess, and possibly an appendicolith. Dilated central bowel in a child should suggest appendicitis. Some authors have recommended appendiceal ultrasound, but it is a difficult procedure to perform. A positive ultrasound finding

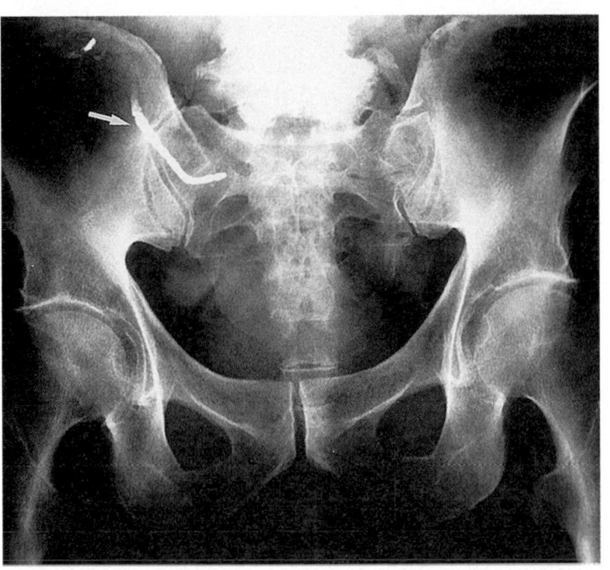

FIGURE 6-69 ■ **Residual barium in the appendix.** A view of the pelvis obtained on a patient who had a barium enema several months earlier reveals residual barium within the wormlike appendix *(arrow)*. Residual barium also can be seen in diverticula, but these appear round.

is a total outer wall to outer wall appendiceal thickness of greater than 6 mm. Unfortunately, much of the time, an overlying ileus with bowel gas makes it difficult or impossible to diagnose appendicitis by using ultrasound.

Both CT and ultrasonography can exclude other causes of pain as well as implicate the appendix. CT gives a much more comprehensive view of the abdominal structures. The normal appendix may be difficult to identify on CT (Fig. 6-71). Conversely, if is not visible and no surrounding edema is noted, appendicitis is unlikely. In appendicitis, inflammatory changes or abscesses around the cecum or appendix can easily be seen (Fig. 6-72). Ultrasonography is less commonly used because the images are harder to interpret, and if the ultrasound images are nondiagnostic, a CT scan is usually needed.

Diverticulosis and Diverticulitis

Prolonged lack of fiber in the diet causes herniation of mucosa outward through the bowel wall (diverticula). Fifty percent of individuals older than 50 years have acquired diverticula. Of this group, 15% to 30% will present with rectal

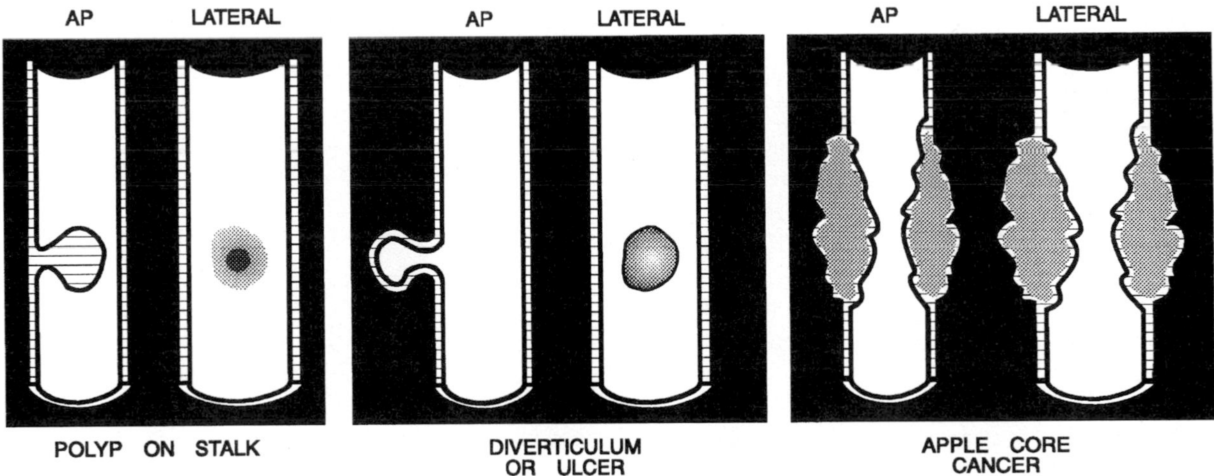

FIGURE 6-70 ■ **Schematic appearance of various gastrointestinal lesions on contrast examinations.** A polyp seen in profile will show a stalk. Seen end-on, it will be darkest in the center, with an ill-defined fading edge. A diverticulum seen in tangent will project outside the lumen, and when seen end-on, it will have very sharp edges. A cancer can be in one wall or, if circumferential, can leave contrast in the lumen that resembles an apple core.

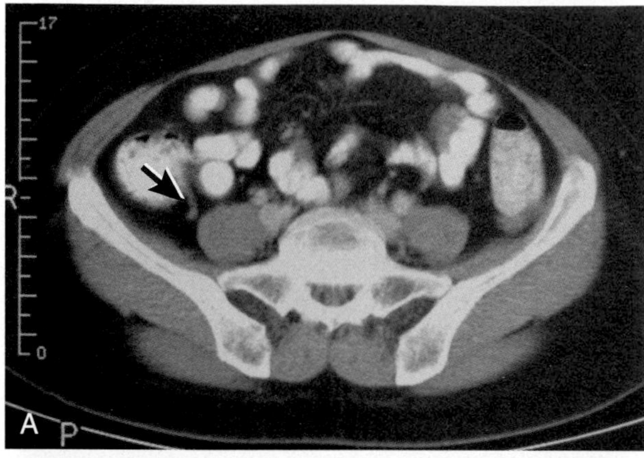

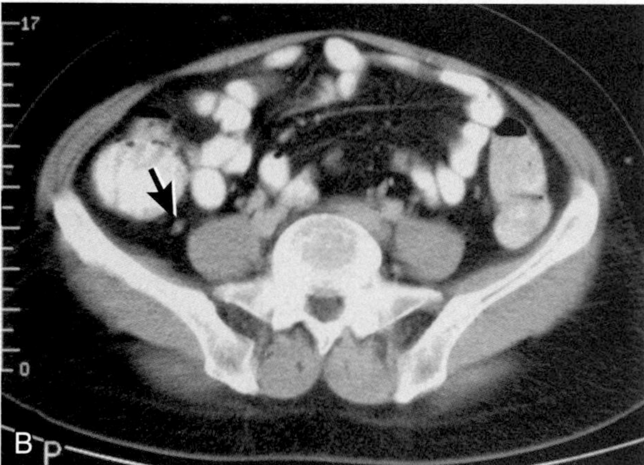

FIGURE 6-71 ■ **Normal appendix.** The appendix can be seen on these computed tomography (CT) scan slices where it joins the cecum *(A) (arrow)* and at a lower level *(B) (arrow)*. In many normal people, the appendix cannot be seen on CT.

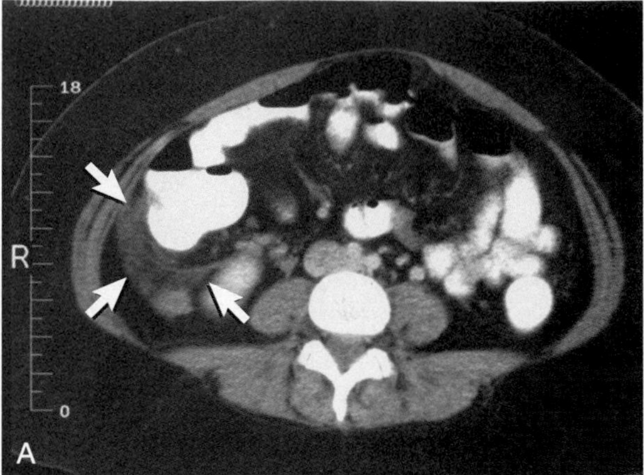

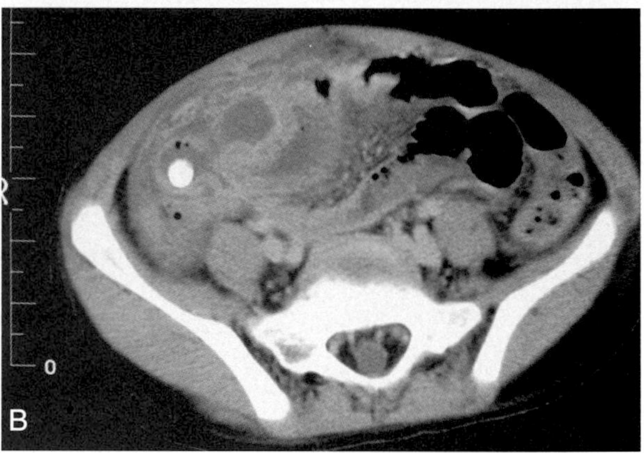

FIGURE 6-72 ■ **Appendicitis.** In a patient with mild appendicitis, the computed tomography (CT) scan *(A)* shows stranding due to edema *(arrows)* in the tissues surrounding the cecum. In the right clinical setting, this is highly suggestive of appendicitis. In a different patient, the CT scan *(B)* demonstrates more-advanced findings with an inflammatory mass around the cecum and a central calcification (an appendicolith).

bleeding and pain. Ninety-five percent of diverticula are located in the region of the sigmoid and descending colon. Diverticulosis simply refers to the presence of multiple diverticula. Diverticulosis is often seen in CT scans of older persons (Fig. 6-73).

Diverticulitis is an inflammatory process often caused by extravasation of bowel contents from the tip of the diverticulum. It is confined to the sigmoid colon in 90% of patients, and usually significant resultant bowel wall thickening or formation of intramural abscesses is found. Patients present with left lower quadrant pain 70% of the time, and they also may have diarrhea or constipation, fever, and leukocytosis. Diverticulitis can sometimes be seen on a contrast enema as a small longitudinal track of barium within the wall of the colon. If the diagnosis of diverticulitis is suspected, however, it is better to order a CT scan (Fig. 6-74), because it is possible to have diverticulitis without diverticula being identified on the barium enema.

Ulcerative Colitis

Ulcerative colitis is associated with arthritis and arthralgia, and the patients have diarrhea and rectal bleeding. The disease is confined to the mucosa and submucosa. It begins in the rectum and then spreads from the distal to the proximal

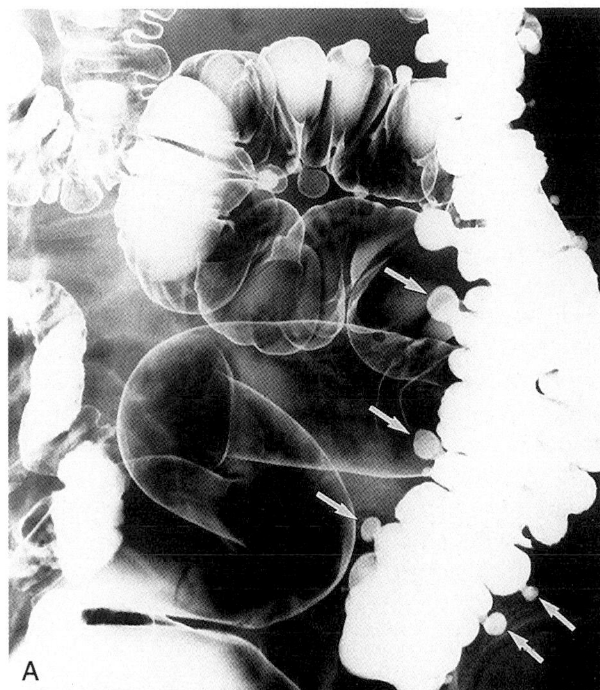

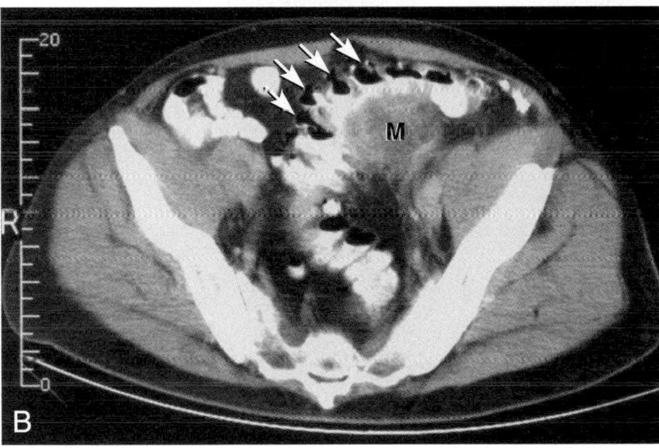

FIGURE 6-73 ■ **Diverticulosis of the colon.** An oblique view of the sigmoid colon *(A)* during a double-contrast barium enema shows multiple outpouchings *(arrows)* that represent diverticula. Diverticula also can be seen in a computed tomography (CT) scan *(B)* as outpouchings *(arrows),* but a developing focal inflammatory mass (M) also is compatible with a developing abscess.

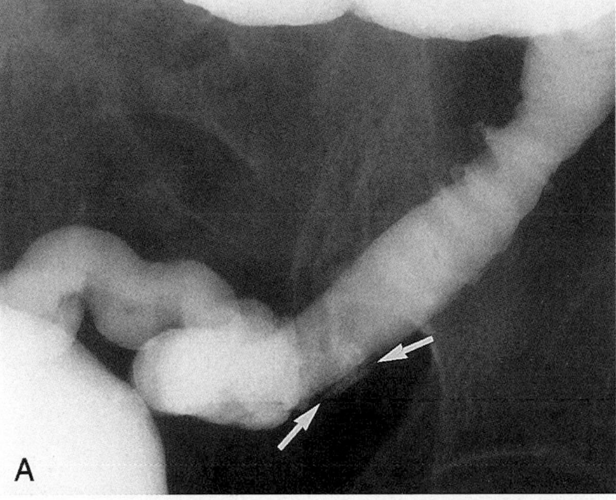

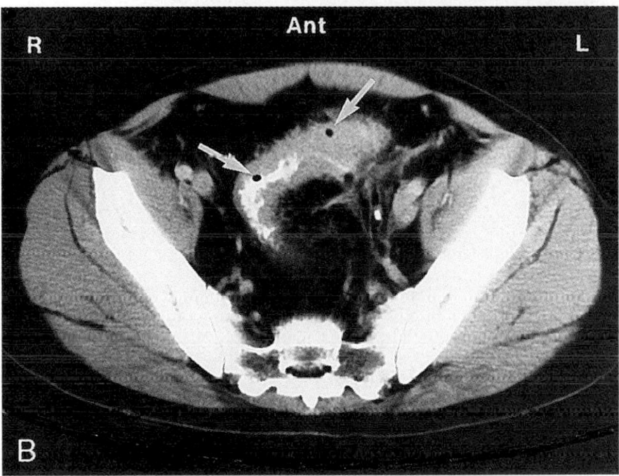

FIGURE 6-74 ■ **Diverticulitis.** *A,* A view of the sigmoid colon obtained during a single-contrast barium enema shows tracking of the barium within the wall of the colon *(arrows).* A transverse computed tomography (CT) scan *(B)* in the same patient shows the sigmoid colon with a markedly thickened wall. Several gas bubbles *(arrows)* are seen within the wall of the colon, representing abscess formation.

colon. Backwash ileitis with involvement of the terminal ileum also may occur. Patients with ulcerative colitis are at a 5- to 30-fold higher risk for malignancy than is the general population. The barium enema features of this disease are a short colon with granular mucosa and shallow, confluent ulcers (Fig. 6-75).

Crohn's Disease

Crohn's disease can affect the colon as well as the small bowel. In contrast to ulcerative colitis, it is transmural and rarely involves the rectum. On a barium enema, visualization of aphthous erosions, ulcers, cobblestone fissures, fistula, and strictures may occur. Characteristically, the disease is noncontiguous and skips areas of the

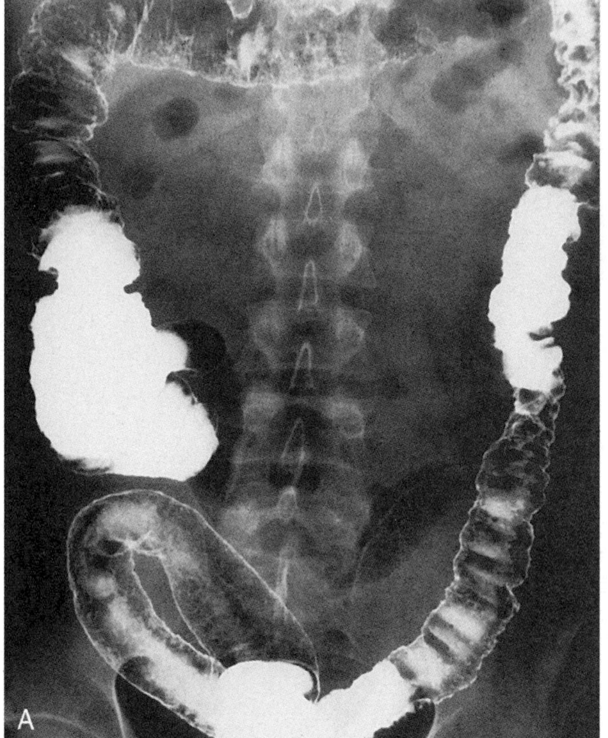

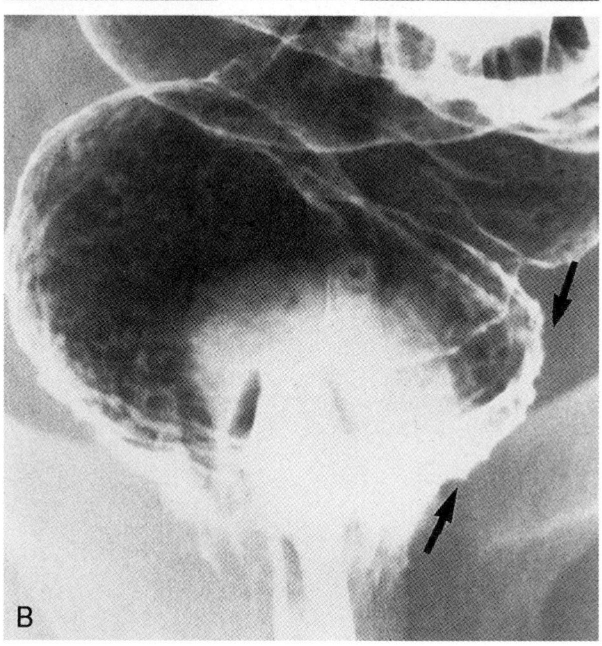

FIGURE 6-75 ■ **Ulcerative colitis.** A double-contrast barium enema *(A)* shows very small irregular ulcers extending back from the rectum to at least the hepatic flexure. A spot view of the rectum *(B)* shows the tiny ulcers in better detail. (Case courtesy of Michael Davis, M.D.)

colon, so diseased areas of the colon have segments of normal colon in between.

Ischemic Colitis

Ischemic colitis can result from thrombosis of the superior or inferior mesenteric artery, hypercoagulable states, small-vessel disease, or obstruction of the colon. Initial symptoms are usually vague and nonspecific. This is followed by abdominal pain that seems out of proportion to clinical findings, and often by rectal bleeding. The goal is to make the diagnosis without causing perforation or other complications. A plain abdominal film may reveal free air or "thumbprinting" from mucosal edema or intramural hemorrhage. A patient without signs of peritonitis and in whom the plain film findings are nonspecific may have endoscopy or a single-contrast barium enema. In either case, the distention of the colon should be kept to a minimum during the procedure.

Infectious Colitis

Pseudomembranous colitis and a number of other infections caused by *Campylobacter*, *Shigella*, and *Salmonella* sp. can produce a radiographic pattern similar to that of ulcerative colitis. Cytomegalic virus colitis usually occurs in immunocompromised persons and has variable radiographic features, including ulceration, which can be either localized or pancolonic (Fig. 6-76).

Ulcerative colitis and, less commonly, other colitises, can result in a toxic megacolon. A barium enema should not be ordered on a patient in whom a toxic megacolon is suspected, and proctoscopy should be performed. The radiographic feature of toxic megacolon is a dilated colon with a deformed bowel wall, most evident in the transverse portion of the colon. The wall may be nodular, irregular, or haustral, or even show what looks like thumbprints of soft tissue extending into the colonic lumen. This thickened-fold appearance also can be due to ischemia of the colon, but it is usually limited to the appropriate vascular distribution, that is, proximal to the splenic flexure for the superior mesenteric artery and distal to the

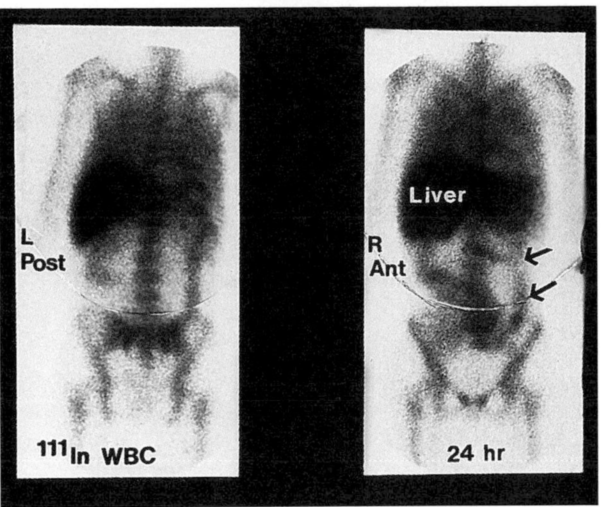

FIGURE 6-76 ■ **Infectious colitis.** A nuclear medicine abscess-localization study done with radioactively labeled white blood cells shows the front and back views of the torso of an immunosuppressed patient with a fever. Activity in the marrow and liver is normal. The abnormal activity in the lungs and colon *(arrows)* is due to infection by cytomegalic inclusion virus.

splenic flexure for the inferior mesenteric artery distribution.

Polyps

About 90% of polyps are hyperplastic and non-neoplastic. Of those that are neoplastic, adenomas are the most common. Of the adenomatous polyps, 50% are multiple, and although many are asymptomatic, they can cause diarrhea, pain, and bleeding. Seventy per cent of polyps occur in the rectum and sigmoid, and 10% each in the ascending, transverse, and descending colon.

The larger the polyp, the more likely it is to be malignant. Of polyps smaller than 1 cm, only 1% are malignant; between 1 and 2 cm, 25% are malignant; and over 2 cm, 40% are malignant. A benign polyp is usually less than 2 cm in diameter, has a thin stalk and a smooth contour, is single, and has a smooth underlying colonic wall. Malignant polyps usually are larger than 2 cm, have no definite stalk, can be multiple, and are often irregular or lobulated (Fig. 6-77*A*).

A number of syndromes include multiple polyps, including familial polyposis, Gardner's

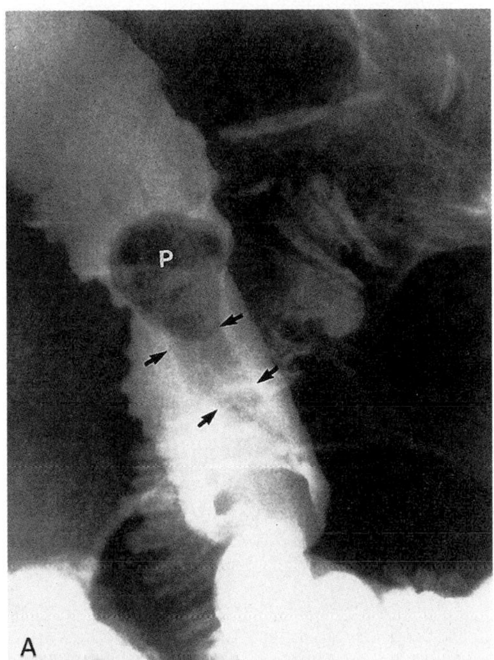

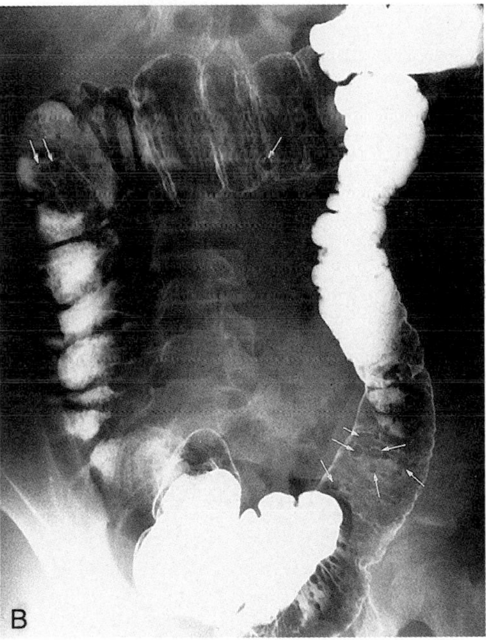

FIGURE 6-77 ■ **Colonic polyps.** A magnified spot view of the sigmoid during a barium enema *(A)* outlines a single polyp (P) as well as its stalk. In a different patient, a barium enema *(B)* reveals multiple tiny polyps *(arrows)* extending throughout the colon.

syndrome, Peutz-Jeghers syndrome, and juvenile polyposis. Most of the polyposis syndromes have adenomas as the underlying histology, but the familial type and Gardner's and Turcot's syndromes have an extremely high rate of malignancy. In familial polyposis, the rate of malignancy is so high that screening of family members begins at puberty (Fig. 6-77*B*), and treatment often involves a prophylactic total proctocolectomy.

Colon Carcinoma

Colon cancer is the second most common cancer in men and women. The most common cancer in men is lung, and in women, it is breast cancer. Fifty percent of colon cancers occur in the rectum or sigmoid, and about 10% each in the cecum, ascending colon, transverse colon, and descending colon. The clinical presentation is most commonly colonic obstruction or rectal bleeding. A debate is ongoing as to whether colonoscopy, barium enema, or CT virtual colonoscopy is the appropriate method of workup or screening. Barium enema is relatively inexpensive compared with colonoscopy, and it has about the same accuracy rate. The advantage of colonoscopy is that if a lesion is identified, a biopsy can be performed immediately. Screening for polyps and colon cancer is commonly done by a fecal occult blood test (FOBT) and sigmoidoscopy. An FOBT has a high incidence of false-positive results from a diet high in red meat or peroxide-containing vegetables (e.g., broccoli, turnips, cauliflower). Sigmoidoscopy provides only very limited visualization of the colon. After a positive FOBT, colonoscopy is usually performed. If colonoscopy is not available or if there is inadequate visualization of the entire colon, a double-contrast barium enema is usually performed.

The recommendations for colon cancer screening in asymptomatic persons vary among organizations. For persons older than 50 years, the American Cancer Society, American College of Physicians, and National Cancer Institute recommend an annual FOBT and a flexible sigmoidoscopy every 3 to 5 years. The American Cancer Society also recommends annual digital rectal examination beginning at age 40 years. The U.S. Preventive Services Task Force has concluded that insufficient evidence exists to recommend either for or against screening in asymptomatic persons. In 1994, the Canadian Task Force on the Periodic Health Examination reported that insufficient evidence exists to support inclusion or exclusion of FOBT, sigmoidoscopy, or colonoscopy for screening in persons older than 40 years.

Some asymptomatic individuals are at a higher than average risk for colorectal cancer. These include persons with ulcerative colitis; Crohn's disease; familial polyposis syndromes; a personal history of colorectal, breast, ovarian, or endometrial cancer; hereditary nonpolyposis colorectal cancer (HNPCC); and a history of adenomas or colorectal cancer in first-degree relatives. For such individuals older than 40 years, the American College of Physicians recommends a double-contrast barium enema or colonoscopy every 3 to 5 years and an annual FOBT. The American Cancer Society recommends colonoscopy or double-contrast enema every 5 years beginning at the age of 35 years. Recommendations of the U.S. Preventive Services Task Force has concluded that it is prudent to offer screening tests to such persons older than 50 years.

The barium enema appearance of a colon cancer may be a polypoid lesion extending into the lumen of the colon, or a mass on one wall of the colon; if more advanced, the lesion may be circumferential, resulting in an "apple core" (Fig. 6-78). You should not be so filled with gratification when you see a colon cancer that you stop looking. Remember that in about 5% of patients, a second colon cancer is present at the same time. The radiologist will not usually put a lot of barium retrograde past a high-grade obstructing lesion because the barium will stay there; the colon will absorb the water, and it will almost turn to concrete. At surgery, however, one must look for second tumors.

CT scanning is usually done to assess the extent of disease locally and in lymph nodes and the liver. Accuracy for detection of lymph node metastases is poor (~60%). If the nodes are enlarged, they probably have tumor within them, but nodes can be of normal size and still contain tumor. A CT scan with intravenous con-

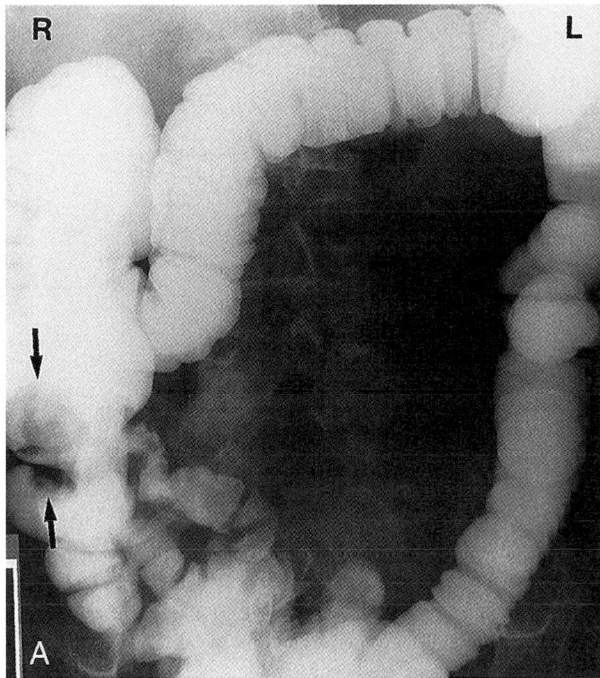

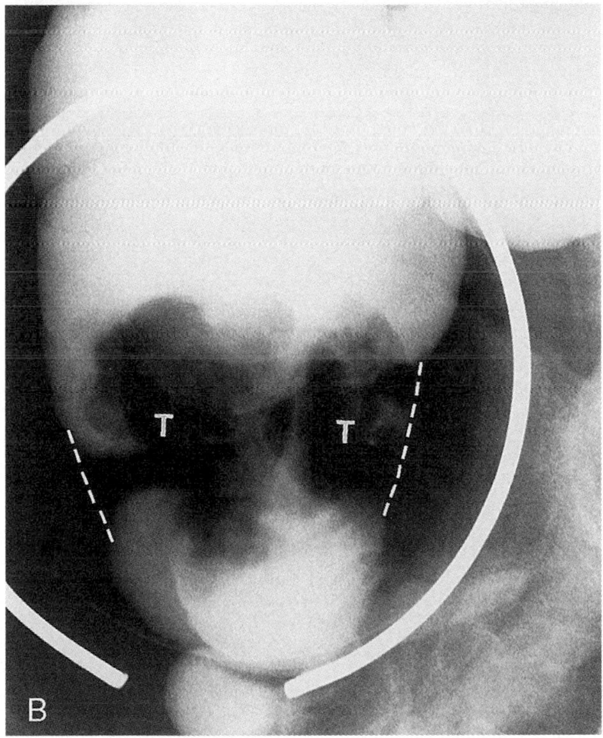

FIGURE 6-78 ■ Colon carcinoma. A single-contrast view of the colon *(A)* demonstrates a filling defect in the cecum *(arrows)*. A compression ring was applied, and a spot view *(B)* was taken of the cecum. This shows that the tumor (T) has encircled the lumen, producing a typical "apple-core" lesion with overhanging edges. This is characteristic of a cancer.

trast of the liver often will show multiple low-density metastases (see Fig. 6-50). FDG PET scans are currently being used to assess patients with suspected recurrence of cancer.

Gastrointestinal Bleeding

Bleeding is a common presentation of GI pathology. Although bright red blood from the rectum implies a rectal or colonic lesion (98% of the time), this is not necessarily the case; distal small bowel lesions are rarely seen this way. When the source of GI bleeding cannot be found by colonoscopy, it is often valuable to perform a nuclear medicine GI bleeding study. This is done by labeling the red blood cells with radioactive material and then doing sequential imaging over the abdomen to look for abnormal pooling (Fig. 6-79). This examination should be ordered before an angiogram or barium enema. A nuclear medicine study should be ordered only when the patient is having active bleeding, and it is capable of localizing the bleeding site with bleeding rates as low as 0.5 mL/min. In contrast, an angiogram needs approximately 4 mL/min for

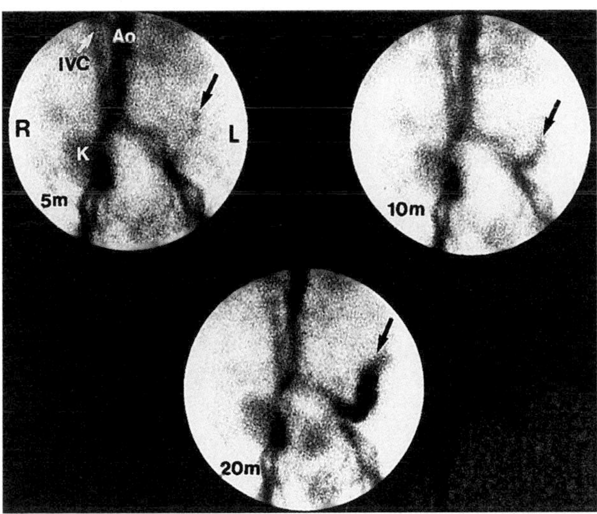

FIGURE 6-79 ■ Colonic bleeding from a diverticulum. A nuclear medicine gastrointestinal bleeding study done by tagging red cells with a small amount of radioactive material has images of the abdomen obtained at 5, 10, and 20 minutes. The aorta (Ao), inferior vena cava (IVC), and a transplanted kidney (K) are visible. In the left lower quadrant, increasing activity *(black arrow)* appears on the sequential images as a result of bleeding into the colon from a diverticulum.

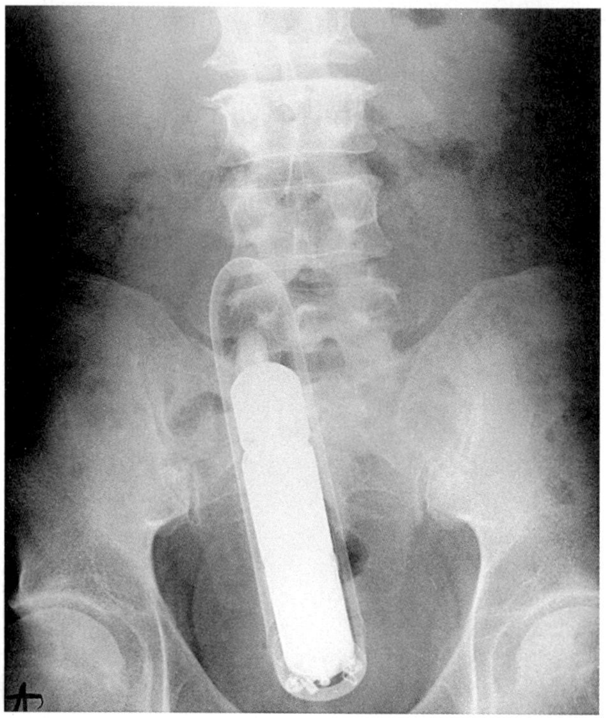

FIGURE 6-80 ■ **Vibrator in the rectum.** This plain film shows the vibrator in this patient who "accidentally fell on it while gardening in the nude."

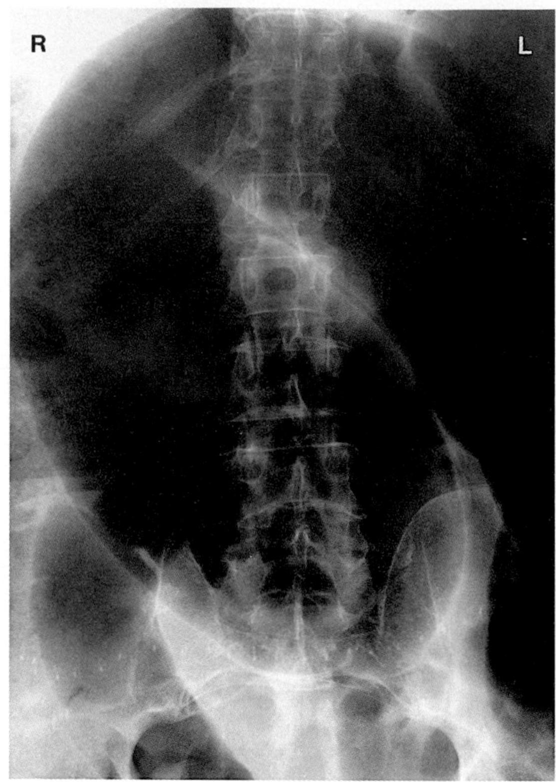

FIGURE 6-81 ■ **Sigmoid volvulus.** A plain film of the abdomen shows the massively dilated "inverted U" of colon pointing toward the right upper quadrant. (Case courtesy of Michael Davis, M.D.)

the bleeding site to be identified. A nuclear medicine scan also is helpful to direct the radiologist as to which vessels to catheterize if an angiogram is needed. Occasionally bleeding and other symptoms may be due to a foreign body (Fig. 6-80). Most patients with these have very imaginative stories.

Volvulus

Twisting of the colon can cause either a sigmoid or a cecal volvulus. This obstruction causes severe colicky pain, nausea, abdominal distention, and vomiting. A sigmoid volvulus is about 3 times more common than a cecal volvulus. A sigmoid volvulus is seen on the KUB film as a massively dilated loop of colon that looks like an inverted U projecting up out of the pelvis toward the right upper quadrant. This is also called the "omega loop" sign (Fig. 6-81). Air usually is seen in the proximal colon. With a cecal volvulus, a dilated loop of colon points toward the left upper quadrant, and usually there is associated small bowel dilatation. The diagnostic study of choice for both these entities is a barium enema.

Suggested Textbooks on the Topic

Eisenberg RL: Gastrointestinal Radiology: A Pattern Approach, 4th ed. Philadelphia, Lippincott Williams & Wilkins, 2002.

Gore RM, Levine MS: Textbook of Gastrointestinal Radiology, 2nd ed. Philadelphia, WB Saunders, 2000.

7 Genitourinary System and Retroperitoneum

ANATOMY AND IMAGING TECHNIQUES

The urinary system may be imaged in a number of ways. The initial study of choice for many suspected clinical problems is shown in Table 7-1. The most common radiographic method is by intravenous injection of an iodine-based contrast agent, which is rapidly cleared by the kidneys. This is called an intravenous pyelogram (IVP). The normal anatomy is shown in Figure 7-1. Initially, a plain x-ray image of the abdomen (KUB) is obtained. You should examine this carefully, looking for abnormalities in the skeleton; soft tissue margins of the liver, spleen, and psoas regions; and the gas pattern in the bowel; as well as for calcifications. Of particular interest are those calcifications that project or overlie the region where you expect to find kidneys, ureters, and bladder. After injection of a contrast material, a tomogram may be obtained as part of the procedure. The tomogram essentially blurs structures in front of and behind the kidneys, leaving only the kidneys and part of the spine in focus.

The kidneys should be examined for size, shape, position, and axis. The length of kidneys on a radiographic study is typically about 13 cm. On an ultrasound examination, they are smaller, only about 10 to 11 cm in length. The reason is that magnification occurs on the images, and the intravenous contrast being excreted during an IVP causes the kidneys to enlarge 1 to 2 cm in length. Normally the left kidney is somewhat higher than the right; the long axis of the kidneys should be tilted slightly inward, with the superior pole of the kidney being more medial than the lower pole. Look for uniform thickness of the cortex relative to the calyces of the collecting system. The shape of the kidneys should be relatively smooth in outline, although occasionally a slight lump is seen on the lateral margin of the kidneys. The lateral lump is sometimes referred to as a "dromedary hump," or column of Bertin. Although this is a common variant, you cannot exclude a cyst or neoplasm if a major difference is found between the thickness of the cortex between the calyces and the outer margin of the kidney or if one portion of the cortex is focally thicker than another. Often a renal ultrasound is the most cost-efficient and innocuous way of resolving this problem.

On the IVP, a dark area normally surrounds the collecting system of the kidneys, and this represents fat in the hilum of the kidney. Look carefully at the calyces to make sure that they are very sharp and pointed, not blunted, at their outer corners, and examine the renal pelvis and ureters for any intrinsic or extrinsic defects. The ureters should course inferiorly and medially from the kidneys and anterior to the psoas muscles at the L3 to L5 level. On the anteroposterior (AP) projection, the ureters typically are most medial and project over the lateral aspect of the transverse processes at L3, L4, and L5. As the ureters pass over the sacrum, they deviate laterally and then enter the bladder from the posterolateral aspect.

Renal ultrasound is a simple noninvasive examination (Fig. 7-2). Remember that all

TABLE 7-1 ■ **Initial Imaging Studies for Common Clinical Genitourinary Problems**

Clinical Problem	Imaging Study
Ureteral calculus	Noncontrasted CT
Hematuria	IVP, CT
Infection	
Recurrent in a female	Cystoscopy
First time in a male	IVP
Abscess	CT with and without intravenous contrast
Renal trauma	CT with intravenous contrast
Hydronephrosis	IVP initially, US for follow-up
Probable cyst on IVP	US
Probable mass on IVP	CT with and without intravenous contrast
Bladder rupture	Cystogram or CT cystogram
Urethral obstruction or tear	Retrograde urethrogram
Bladder cancer	Cystoscopy, CT with intravenous contrast
Suspected renovascular hypertension	Nuclear medicine captopril renogram or MR angiogram
Testicular torsion	Doppler US or nuclear medicine testicular scan
Testicular or scrotal mass or trauma	US
Pelvic mass (female)	US
Pelvic pain (female)	US
Cervical cancer	CT with intravenous, oral, and rectal contrast
Ovarian cancer	CT with intravenous, oral, and rectal contrast
Uterine cancer	CT with intravenous, oral, and rectal contrast
Uterine fibroids (initial, enlarging, painful, or bleeding)	Pelvic US
Prostate cancer	PSA measurement and biopsy (not imaging), bone scan (to exclude metastases)
Infertility	Physical examination, hormone levels, US
Vaginal bleeding	(See text)
Premenopausal, physical examination normal	US
Postmenopausal, not taking hormone currently or taking it for > 6 mo	US

CT, computed tomography; IVP, intravenous pyelogram; PSA, prostate-specific antigen; US, ultrasound.

ultrasound images are "slices" and that the easiest view of the kidney to understand is the longitudinal view. The right kidney is easily visualized by transmitting sound through the right lobe of the liver. Because bowel and stomach gas prevents ultrasound transmission, the left kidney is usually visualized from the patient's back. The kidney is bean shaped and has bright central echoes because of the fat surrounding the collecting system. Ultrasound is typically ordered to exclude hydronephrosis or to evaluate renal size or suspected renal cysts.

Computed tomography (CT) is commonly used as another major imaging mode of the urinary system. CT is often used as the initial imaging test for suspected renal cell carcinoma, complicated renal or ureteral stones, or trauma. Magnetic resonance imaging (MRI) or CT may be used in cases of renal cell carcinoma to exclude renal vein or inferior vena cava thrombus. Nuclear medicine techniques are used when function or other parameters must be quantitated. Common indications for radioisotope techniques include evaluation of renal transplants to determine whether a dilated collecting system is obstructive or nonobstructive and to detect renovascular hypertension.

Although the bladder is seen on the IVP, remember that the contrast medium is heavier than urine and layers posteriorly in the bladder. What you are really looking at when you

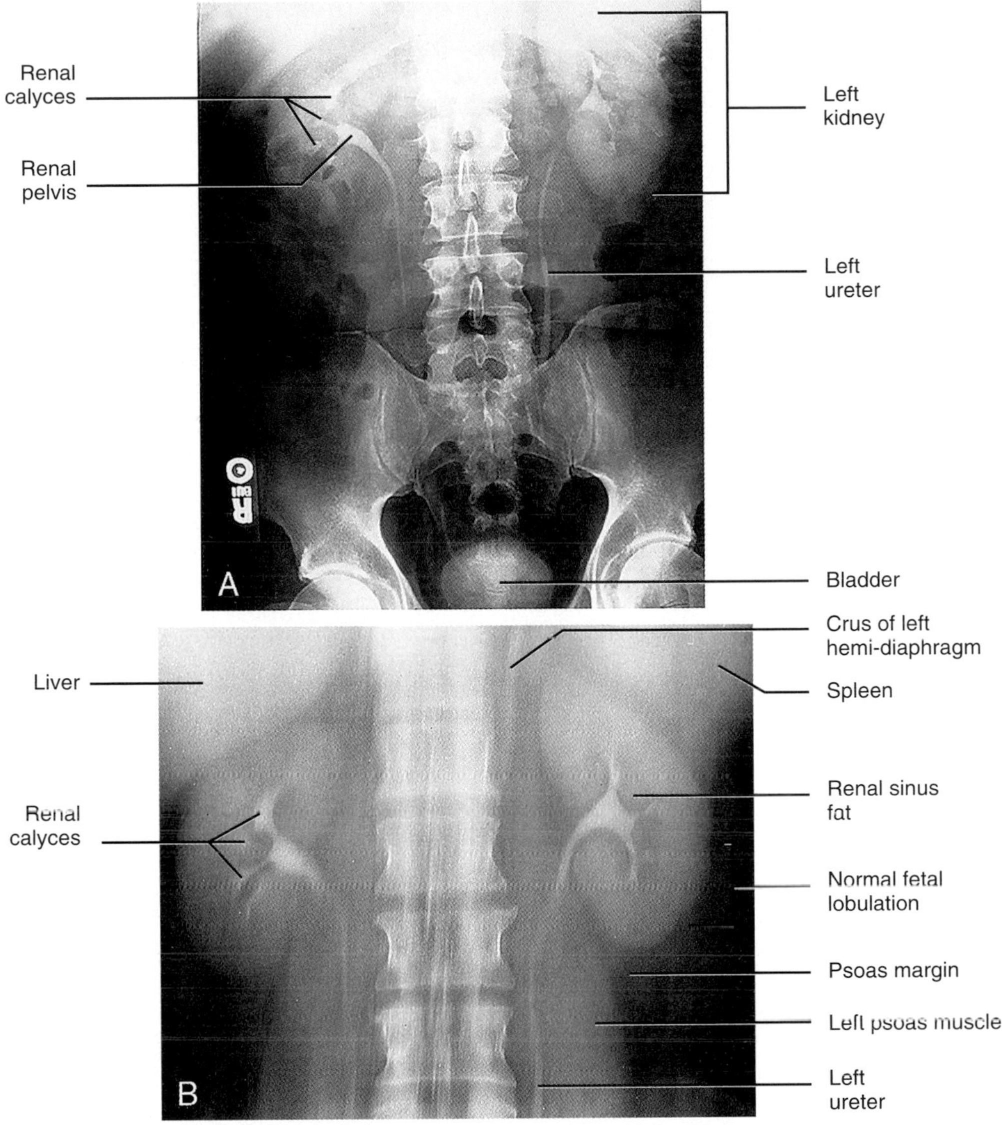

FIGURE 7-1 ■ Normal anatomy of the kidneys, ureters, and bladder on an intravenous pyelogram *(A)*. Normal anatomy also is shown on the tomographic image *(B)* taken during an intravenous pyelogram.

think you see the bladder on IVP images often is only the lateral margins of the back of the bladder (Fig. 7-3). The anterior portion of the bladder is usually not well seen. Consequently, if you wish to see the entire bladder, a Foley catheter can be placed directly into the bladder, the urine drained, and the bladder refilled with contrast material. This procedure is called a *cystogram*. On a cystogram, images of the bladder are obtained in several different projections. When the catheter is removed, the patient may be asked to void. In male patients, this gives a very good demonstration of the urethra (Fig. 7-4). The

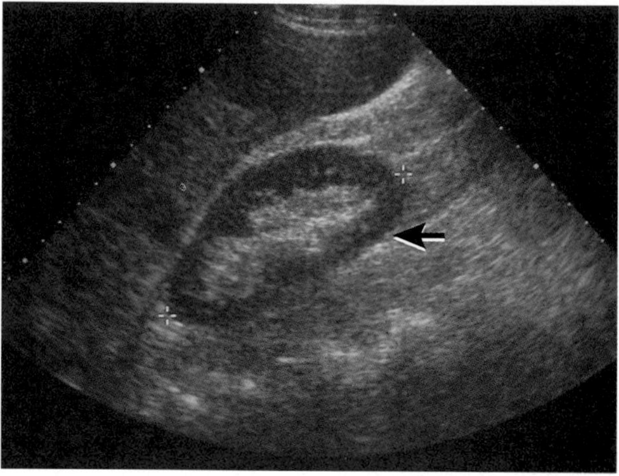

FIGURE 7-2 ■ **Normal renal ultrasound.** A longitudinal view of the right kidney was obtained by passing the sound beam through the right lobe of the liver. The kidney is seen behind this, outlined by the markers. The central bright echoes in the kidney are due to fat around the collecting system.

male urethra also can be studied in a retrograde fashion by inserting a small tube in the tip of the penis and injecting the contrast material. This is usually done only in cases of suspected urethral trauma or stricture.

KIDNEYS

Congenital Abnormalities

Congenital abnormalities of the urinary tract occur quite frequently, and you should be aware of the most common variants. Embryologically, the ureter buds and grows superiorly from the bladder to meet and connect with the renal parenchyma. The ureter can divide as it ascends, causing a person to have two, partially duplicated or completely separate, collecting systems for one kidney. If complete ureteral duplication is found, the ureter that supplies the upper half of the kidney often becomes obstructed. If the obstruction is not too bad, this can be seen filling with contrast on an IVP (Fig. 7-5). If the upper pole of the kidney is completely obstructed, all that is visualized is the normally

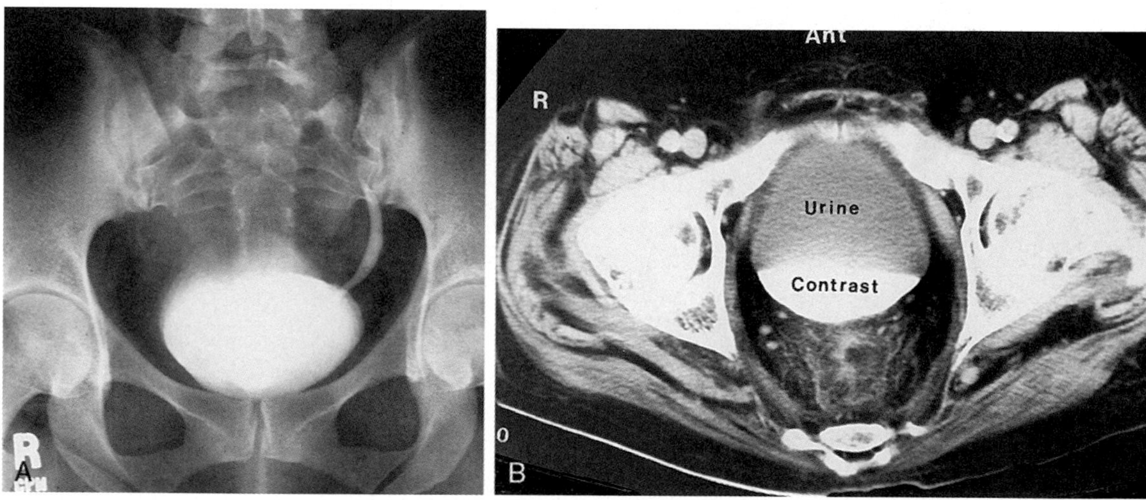

FIGURE 7-3 ■ **Distal ureters and bladder.** A single supine view of the pelvis during an intravenous pyelogram *(A)* shows the distal left ureter and what appears to be the bladder. A computed tomography (CT) scan obtained on this patient at the same time at the level of the bladder *(B)* shows that the contrast from the intravenous pyelogram is layering only in the dependent portion of the bladder. Thus on an intravenous pyelogram, when you think you are looking at the bladder, you are simply seeing a puddle of contrast in the back of the bladder.

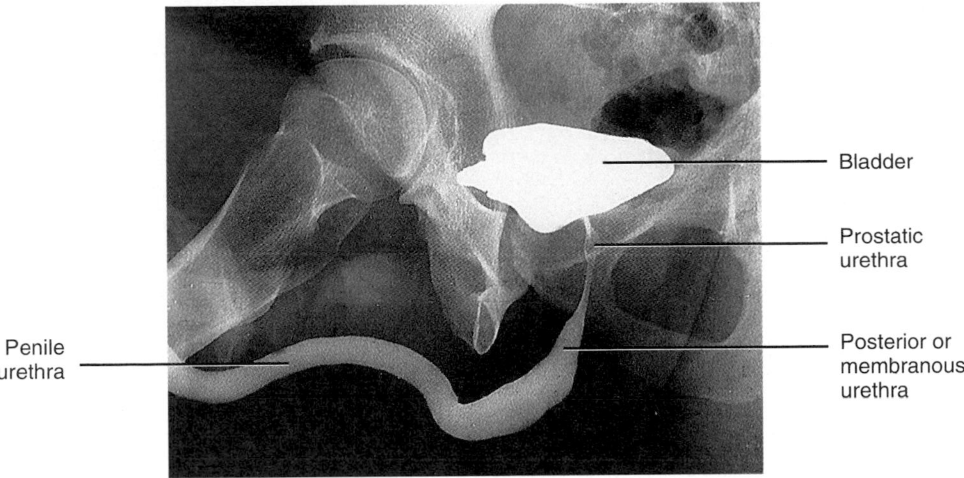

FIGURE 7-4 ■ Normal voiding urethrogram.

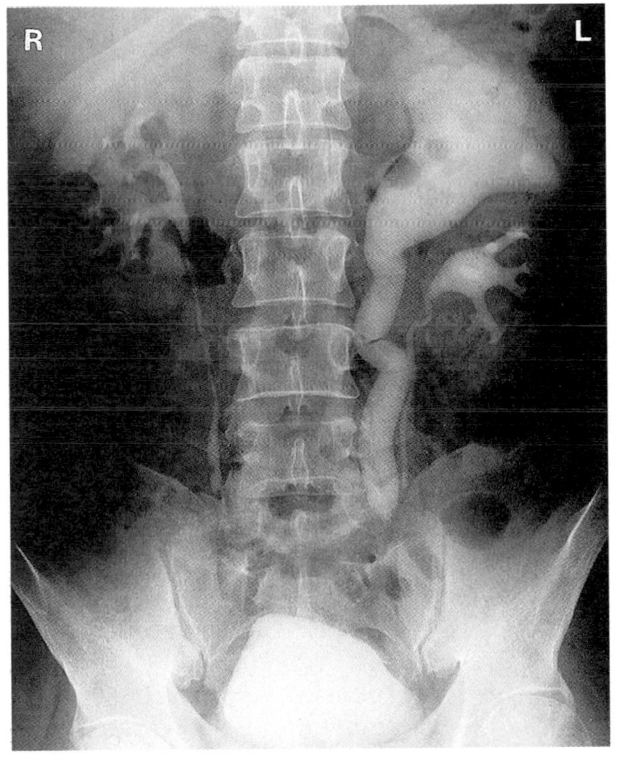

FIGURE 7-5 ■ Duplicated collecting system of left kidney. A film from an intravenous pyelogram shows a normal right collecting system and ureter. On the left is a completely duplicated collecting system. As happens frequently with duplicated systems, the collecting system to the upper pole is dilated and obstructed.

draining lower pole collecting system, and it looks like a drooping lily. You should also be aware that the duplicated ureter that supplies the upper pole may often have an ectopic insertion into the bladder, urethra, or vagina.

A number of other anomalies occur in the course of the normal embryologic ascent of the kidneys out of the bony pelvis. These anomalies include one kidney rising normally and the other kidney remaining in the pelvis. Remember that it is very rare to have a unilateral kidney, and thus if you see only one kidney in normal position, you should look elsewhere for an ectopic kidney (Fig. 7-6). Another common variant is fusion of the inferior aspect of both kidneys (a "horseshoe" kidney). This is relatively easy to identify, because the axis of the kidneys is abnormal, with the superior aspect of the kidneys tilted outward instead of inward (Fig. 7-7).

Renal Cysts

Renal cysts are quite common, and their incidence increases with age. Most persons older than 60 years have one or more simple renal cysts. These are often found incidentally on an IVP, and they are frequently seen on CT scans ordered for other reasons. Ultrasound is a good, inexpensive initial test to characterize a suspected renal cyst found on an IVP. The margins

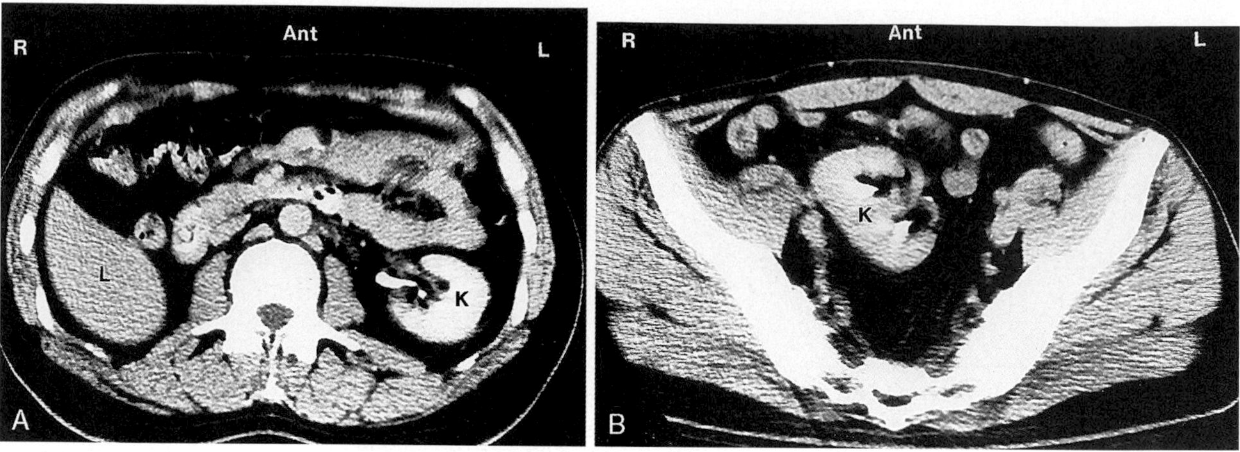

FIGURE 7-6 ■ **Pelvic kidney.** In this young woman, a questionable mass was felt in the pelvis during a routine gynecologic examination. A transverse contrast-enhanced computed tomography (CT) scan of the upper abdomen *(A)* reveals only the left kidney. The liver (L) is seen, but no right kidney is identified. Continuing the scan down into the pelvis *(B)* shows that the right kidney is ectopic.

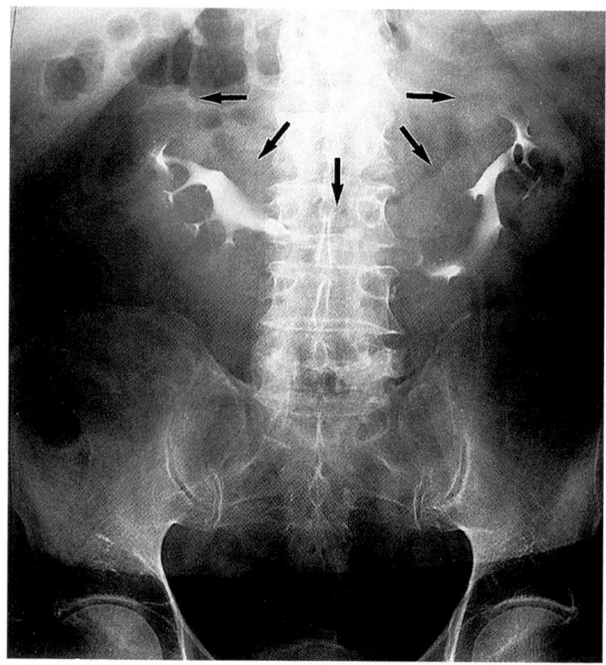

FIGURE 7-7 ■ **Horseshoe kidney.** On this intravenous pyelogram, the inferior aspects of the right and left kidneys are joined. Note the abnormal axis of both the right and the left collecting systems, with the upper portion tipping outward from the spine instead of tipping slightly inward.

of a benign simple cyst should be well defined, and increased echoes should be seen on the posterior aspect of the cyst because of good transmission of sound through the fluid in the cyst (Fig. 7-8). If a cyst has septa or internal echoes, a CT scan is ordered to evaluate further for a possible cystic neoplasm.

Currently renal cysts or cystic masses are classified according to the Bosniak criteria. Bosniak I lesions are benign cysts that are round or oval with a thin wall, no septations, Hounsfield CT units of 0 to 20, and no enhancement with intravenous contrast. Follow-up is not usually needed. Bosniak II lesions are the same but with a few septations or a few thin calcifications or both. These are often followed up in 6 to 12 months, but both Bosniak I and II lesions have a very small chance of being a malignancy. A Bosniak III lesion has any or all of the following: a thick wall, calcifications, Hounsfield density of 0 to 20, and no enhancement of nodules. These lesions have about a 60% chance of being malignant. Bosniak IV lesions have a thick wall, thick septations, coarse calcifications, Hounsfield density of more than 20, and enhancement with intravenous contrast. All of these lesions should be considered to be malignant and require further workup.

Polycystic renal disease presents a difficult imaging problem. In the adult form of this heri-

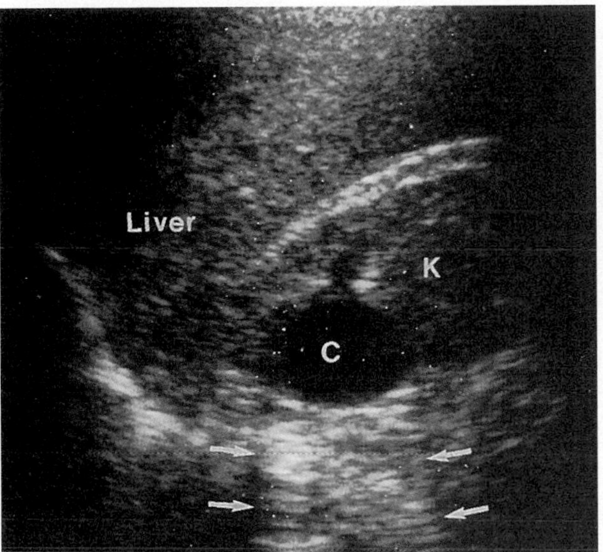

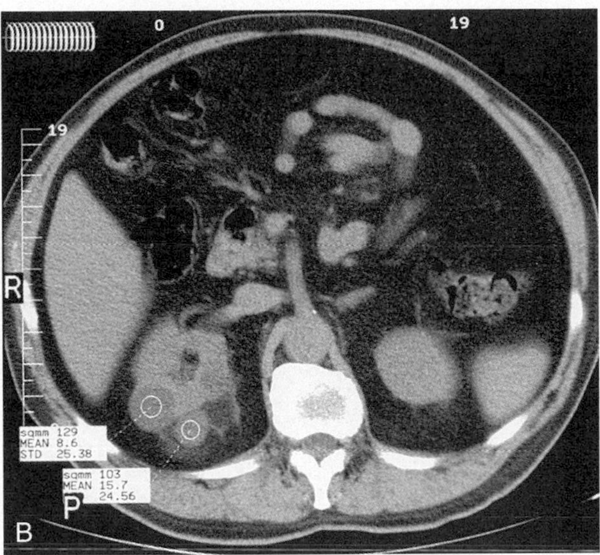

FIGURE 7-8 ■ **Simple renal cyst.** *A,* A longitudinal ultrasound image shows the normal liver and renal parenchyma with a cyst (C) in the upper and posterior aspect of the right kidney (K). Notice that no (white) echoes appear within the cyst and that increased transmission of sound occurs through the fluid of the cyst, producing a posterior enhanced echo pattern *(arrows).* Renal cysts are common incidental findings on computed tomography (CT) scans *(B).* In this case, attenuation measurements (Hounsfield units) have a mean of less than 20, clearly indicating a simple cyst. If the value were >20, it would need further workup to exclude an inflammatory process, complex cyst, or neoplasm.

table disorder, often progressive renal failure occurs. A CT scan will demonstrate very lumpy kidneys, but the cysts may not be well defined, because hemorrhage often is found within the cyst. Cysts also are usually identified in the liver and sometimes in the pancreas (Fig. 7-9).

Hematuria

Hematuria can be traumatic or nontraumatic and visible or microscopic. In cases of trauma and visible hematuria, a CT scan is indicated. In cases in which trauma, microscopic hematuria (<50 red blood cells [RBCs] per high-power field [HPF]), and little suspicion of injury to other organs are found, many physicians do not do any imaging but rather wait 48 hours to see if the hematuria clears.

Of patients with nontraumatic visible hematuria, about 25% have cancer, 25% have infection, and 15% have calculi. About 5% of patients with nontraumatic microscopic hematuria (5 RBCs/HPF) have a urologic cancer. Obviously, the presence of unilateral flank pain suggests calculi, which are discussed later. If RBC casts are seen in urine immunologic studies, renal biopsy is usually performed. Neither an IVP nor an ultrasound examination can completely exclude a urologic malignancy, because an IVP can miss small parenchymal renal tumors, and ultrasound is poor for detection of small urothelial tumors. Both are poor for evaluation of bladder tumors. The best evaluation of painless, nontraumatic hematuria often begins with cystoscopy and, possibly, retrograde pyelograms at the same time. If this is negative, a CT scan is indicated.

Renal Stone Disease

Calcification can occur within the substance of the kidney or within the collecting system. Calcification within the substance of the kidney (nephrocalcinosis) may be cortical (near the

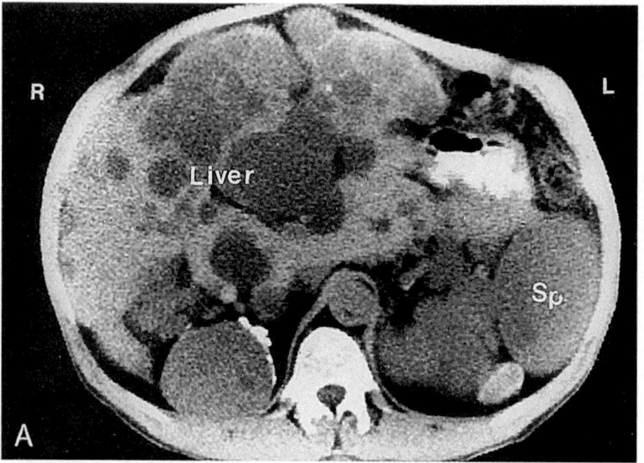

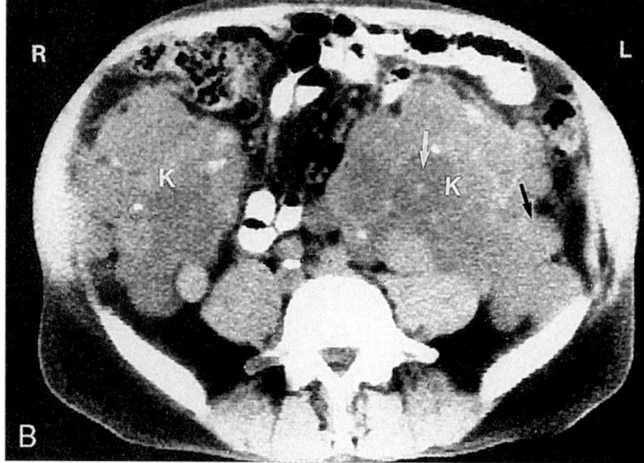

FIGURE 7-9 ■ **Adult polycystic disease of the liver and kidneys.** A computed tomography (CT) scan through the upper abdomen *(A)* shows the liver, with multiple low-density areas throughout it due to cysts within the liver. A transverse scan obtained slightly lower *(B)* shows markedly deformed kidneys bilaterally. Notice that some of the cystic areas within the left kidney are of low density *(white arrow),* and some of the cysts are of higher density *(black arrow).* This makes it very difficult to exclude a malignancy in this patient.

periphery of the kidney) or medullary (near the ends of the calyces). Cortical calcification can be due to chronic glomerulonephritis, cortical necrosis, or acquired immunodeficiency syndrome (AIDS)-related nephropathy. Medullary calcification may be idiopathic or caused by papillary necrosis, medullary sponge kidney, or other hypercalcemic states (including hyperparathyroidism and osteoporosis) (Fig. 7-10).

At least 80% (and ≤90%) of renal calculi are radiopaque and appear dense (or white) on a

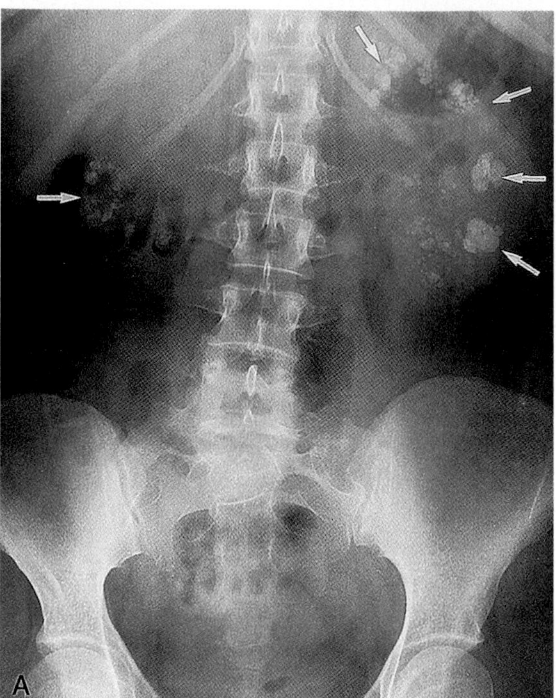

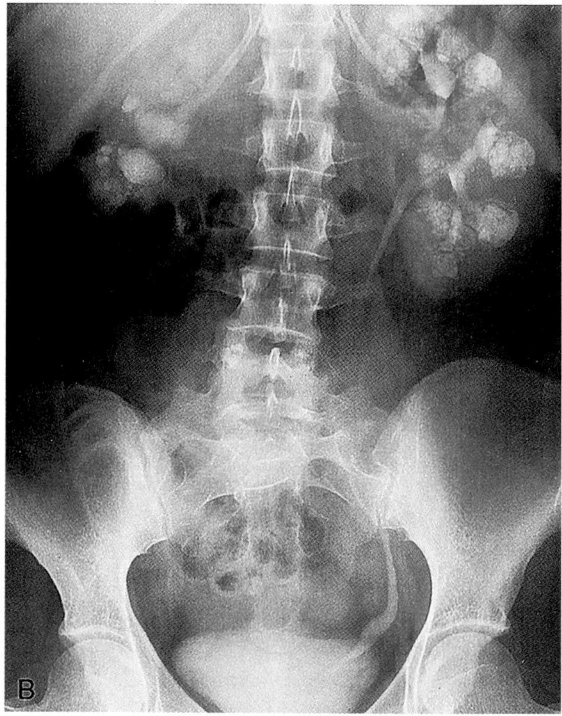

FIGURE 7-10 ■ **Nephrocalcinosis.** A plain film of the abdomen *(A)* shows multiple calcifications *(arrows)* within the left kidney. On an intravenous pyelogram *(B),* the calcifications are located near the ends of the calyces (medullary) rather than in the cortex. This patient had medullary sponge kidneys.

routine x-ray (Fig. 7-11*A*). Occasionally renal stones become very large and essentially fill the collecting system of the kidney. These are referred to as "staghorn calculi" (Fig. 7-11*B*). If calculi are radiopaque and are overlying the kidneys or are within the course of a ureter, they are usually fairly easy to see. Sometimes it can be difficult to visualize a small stone in the region where the ureter passes anterior to the sacrum. Remember that a large number of vascular calcifications occur low within the bony pelvis and to the sides of the bladder. These phleboliths typically can be recognized because they are round, have a lucent (dark) center, and are more lateral and lower in the pelvis than the normal course of the ureter.

The most common clinical presentation of stone disease is intense flank pain with hematuria. If the patient is having a first presentation of renal stone disease, a spiral noncontrasted CT scan or IVP is indicated, even if no calculus is seen on the plain film of the abdomen. If a history of renal stones is known, imaging is not always needed. Imaging may be reserved for those patients who have pain uncontrolled by medication, those with continued flank pain for more than 5 days, those who have continued hematuria 2 weeks after passing a stone, those with microscopic hematuria for more than 1 month, and those who have acute flank pain and are known to have a solitary kidney or pelvic tumor.

On an IVP, the obstruction of the ureter by a stone may cause delayed visualization of the affected kidney and ureter. When it does visualize, the ureter is usually dilated, and the renal calyces are blunted (Fig. 7-12). On delayed images, whereas the normal kidney is completely clear of contrast, the affected kidney and ureter will be seen retaining contrast. Delayed images are often necessary to determine the exact level of the ureteral obstruction.

Although renal and ureteral calculi can be identified on IVP, noncontrasted CT scanning is the test of choice. One reason is that no risk of a reaction to the intravenous contrast is present. On a noncontrasted CT scan, even tiny stones that cannot be seen on an IVP are easily visualized. Dilatation of the renal pelvis and ureter also is quite obvious. Usually a kidney with an

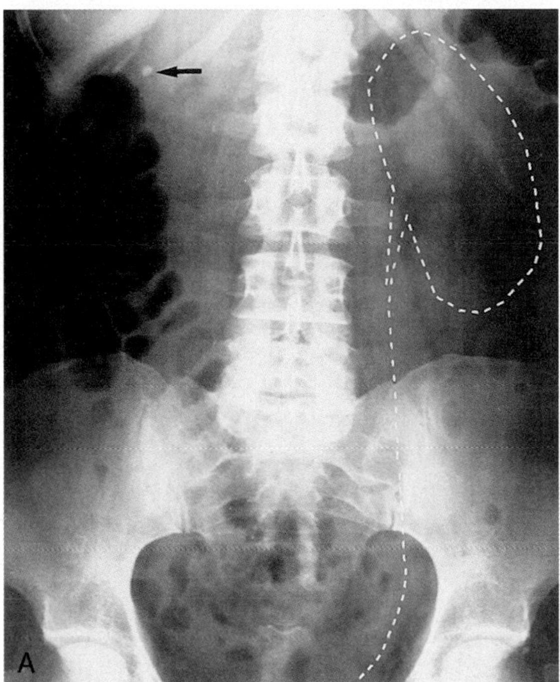

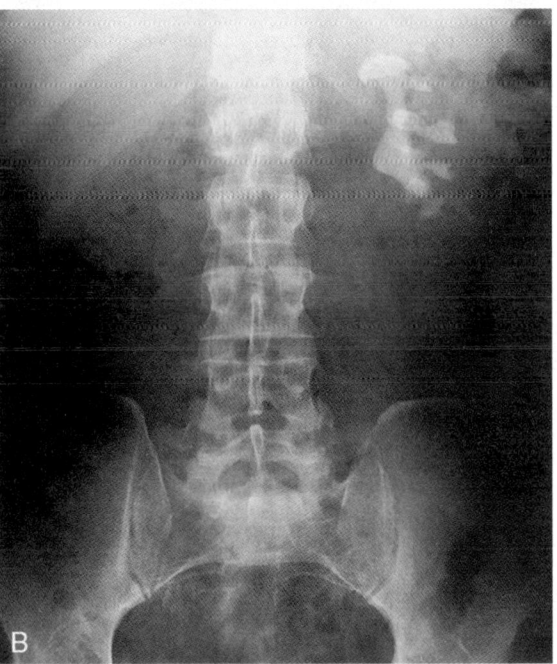

FIGURE 7-11 ■ **Renal calculi.** On a plain film of the abdomen *(A)*, a single calcification is seen in the right upper quadrant *(arrow)*. This is a right renal calculus. Renal calculi should be suspected any time a calcification is seen within the renal outline or along the expected course of the ureter *(dotted lines)*. In a different patient, a plain film of the abdomen *(B)* shows a calcification conforming perfectly to the collecting system of the left kidney. This is referred to as a "staghorn calculus."

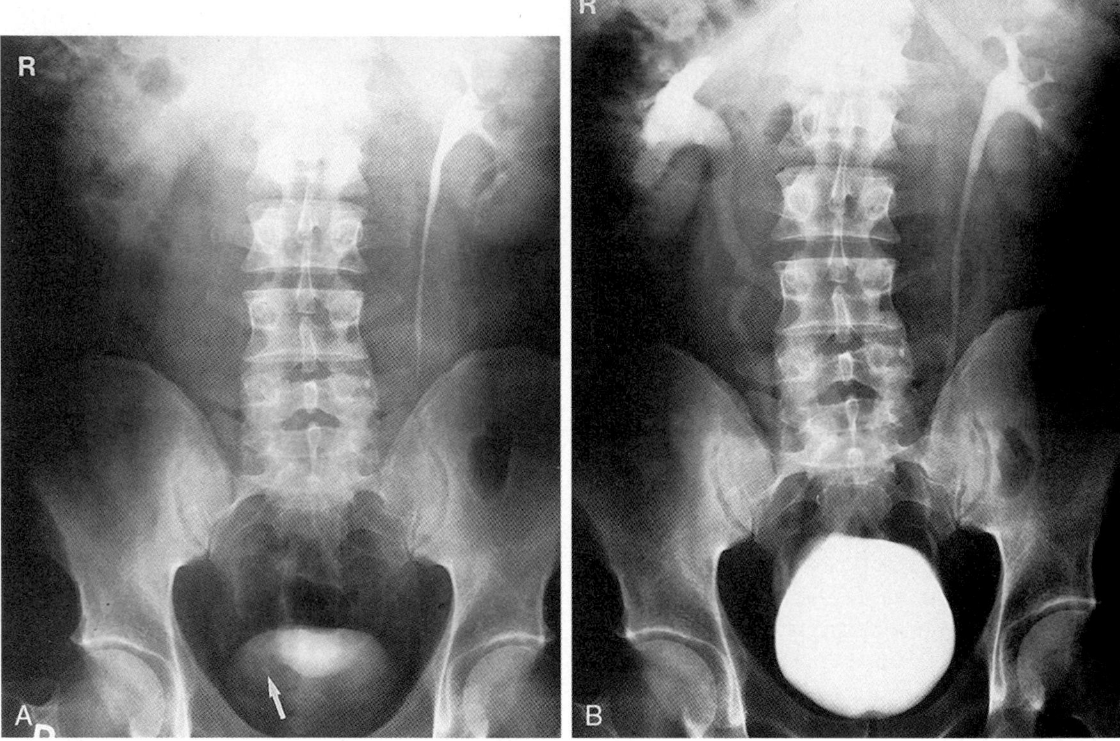

FIGURE 7-12 ■ Ureteral calculus. This young male had intense right flank pain and hematuria. An image taken at 5 min during an intravenous pyelogram shows good function of the left kidney, and the left ureter is well seen. The right kidney is faintly seen, and a small calcification is seen at the ureterovesicular junction *(arrow)*. A delayed image 20 min later *(B)* shows a dilated right renal collecting system and right ureter due to obstruction by the distal ureteral calculus.

acute problem with renal calculi will have associated perirenal edema in the adjacent soft tissues (Fig. 7-13*A*). Age-related perinephric stranding is usually bilateral and occurs mostly in persons older than 55 years. If a stone is lodged in the distal ureter, a dilated proximal ureter can often be seen (Fig. 7-13*B*). Sometimes it is difficult to differentiate ureteral calculi from atherosclerotic vascular calcification or from vascular phleboliths. One way is to look for a soft tissue rim around the calculus (Fig. 7-13*C*). Phleboliths are most common in the lower pelvis below the middle portion of the femoral heads, whereas the ureters have almost always entered the bladder at a more cephalad level.

Occasionally the back pressure caused by an obstructing ureteral stone can rupture a renal calyx or renal pelvis. When this occurs, extravasation of urine and contrast outside the kidney into the perirenal space is seen. When an obstructing lesion of the ureter is present, the urologist may perform cystoscopy and then put a little tube into the distal ureter and inject contrast (a retrograde pyelogram). The ureter, renal pelvis, and calyces are usually visualized. Because pressure is being exerted during the injection, minimal blunting of the calyces is normal under these circumstances. A retrograde pyelogram is useful for looking at small lesions within the collecting system, such as a transitional cell carcinoma. Occasionally, air bubbles will be inadvertently injected along with the contrast, and this may give the appearance of filling defects. The key to differentiation of these entities is that tumors will not move around on different views; many calculi also have sharp or geometric borders (Fig. 7-14). Air bubbles move and are completely round.

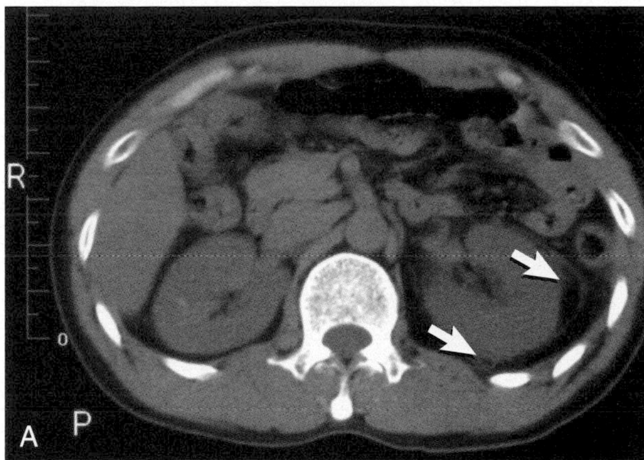

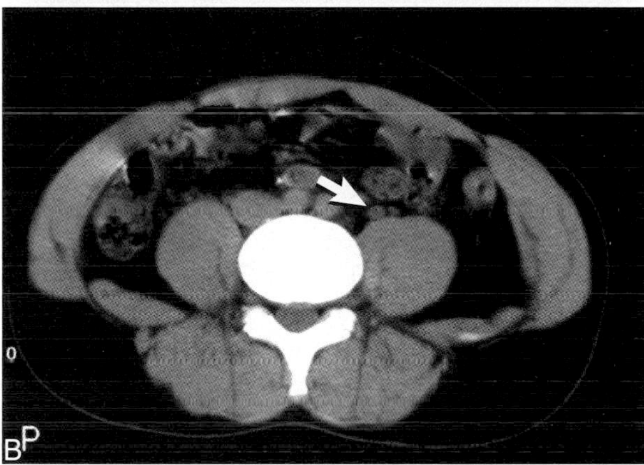

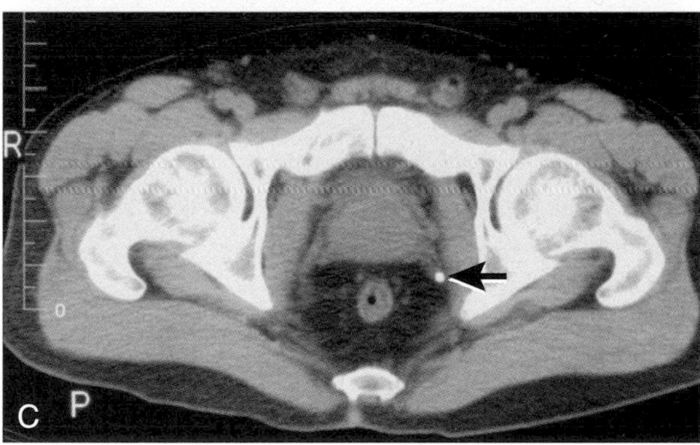

FIGURE 7-13 ■ Obstructing left ureteral calculus. On this noncontrasted computed tomography (CT) scan, at the level of the kidneys *(A)*, there is stranding *(arrows)* around the left kidney but not around the right kidney. At a lower level *(B)*, a dilated left ureter is seen *(arrow)*, and at the level of the bladder *(C)*, a calculus is seen at the left ureterovesicular junction *(arrow)*. The small rim of soft tissue around the calculus helps distinguish it from a phlebolith.

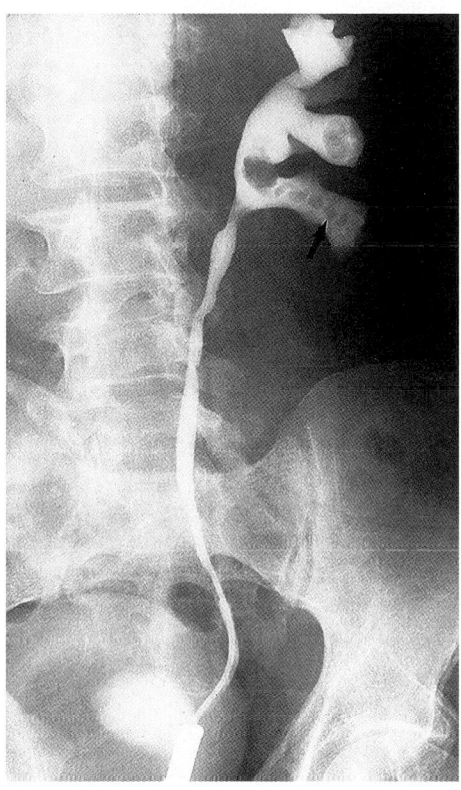

FIGURE 7-14 ■ Ureteral calculi on a retrograde pyelogram. A cystoscope has been put in the bladder, and the orifice of the left ureter catheterized. Contrast is then injected retrograde. Multiple lucencies can be seen within the collecting system of the left kidney *(arrow)*. That these defects are not round but rather have sharp corners indicates that they are calculi and not inadvertently injected air bubbles.

Renal Failure

Imaging is indicated in patients with unexplained oliguria or new onset of renal insufficiency or failure (serum creatinine level >2 mg/dL). Most imaging studies of the kidneys rely on normal function. The most common clinical question is whether renal failure is due to obstruction or to medical renal disease. Because the intravenous contrast material used for an IVP or a CT scan can reduce renal function, the imaging examination of choice in these circumstances is ultrasonography. Normally, the cortex of the kidney has the same ultrasound echo density as the liver or has fewer echoes than the substance of the liver. In cases of medical renal disease, more echoes are found within the renal cortex than within the liver. This is probably the result of fibrosis and scarring (Fig. 7-15).

Pyelonephritis and Renal Infections

The clinical findings of pyelonephritis include fever, flank pain, and pyuria. Most patients with pyelonephritis have no discernible findings on imaging studies. Imaging studies are usually not warranted in women unless repetitive episodes or persistent, worsening pain after 3 days of appropriate antibiotic therapy occur. Sometimes, in patients who have severe acute pyelonephritis, enough edema of the renal parenchyma is present that the swelling causes compression of the calyces or renal pelvis, and there is poor visualization of the collecting system on an IVP. Occasionally with acute pyelonephritis, focal areas of edema can be seen on CT scans. The real purpose of ordering CT scans in these cases should be to look for a renal parenchymal or perirenal abscess.

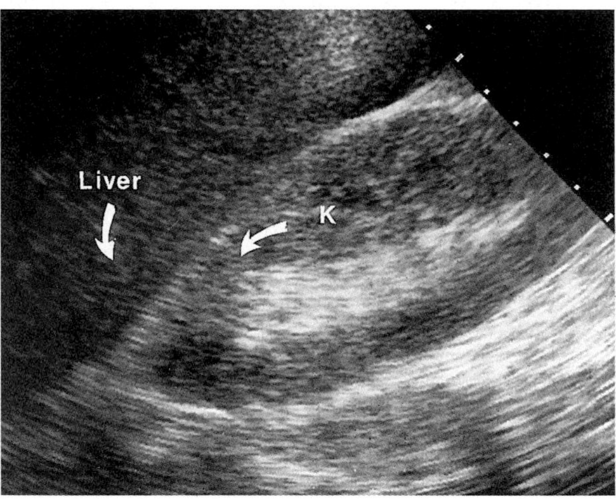

FIGURE 7-15 ■ Medical renal disease. Ultrasound is often performed in patients with renal failure to differentiate between hydronephrosis and renal parenchymal disease. Patients with renal parenchymal disease usually have smaller than normal kidneys. In this longitudinal ultrasound image of the right kidney, note that the parenchyma of the kidney has more echoes or is whiter than that of the liver at the same depth. Normal renal parenchyma will have a number of echoes equal to or lower than those of the liver (see Fig. 7-27 for an ultrasound image of hydronephrosis).

In patients with chronic pyelonephritis, the kidney is usually shrunken and has an irregular outer margin. The cortex also is typically thinned. The irregularities of the outer cortical margin are fairly characteristic, with dimpling or scarring directly over a calyx. If there is dimpling or a defect in the margin of the kidney between two calyces, it is more likely to be the result of a focal infarct.

Persons with diabetes are particularly prone to an unusual form of acute pyelonephritis, which is called *emphysematous pyelonephritis*. In these patients, gas is generated by the bacteria within the parenchyma of the kidney. Usually the kidney is nonfunctional, and a dark radiating striated gas pattern is seen where you would normally expect to find a kidney (Fig. 7-16).

Occasionally, inflammatory abnormalities can cause enlargement of both kidneys, particularly in acute glomerulonephritis. The differential diagnosis for bilaterally enlarged kidneys includes bilateral obstruction, leukemia, glycogen storage diseases, lymphoma, and polycystic disease, as well as a number of other entities (Fig. 7-17).

Infections of the kidney can progress to the stage at which the kidney is essentially nonfunctional. In an entity known as *xanthogranulomatous pyelonephritis*, a nonfunctional kidney is seen, with some calcification visible within (Fig. 7-18). The kidney is removed surgically. On the basis of any imaging study, it is difficult to differentiate xanthogranulomatous pyelonephritis from a renal tumor.

Renal tuberculosis can affect the kidneys, ureter, and bladder; the infection typically begins in the kidneys, and you should look there first. In the early stages, narrowing or amputation of the infundibulum is seen between a renal calyx and the renal pelvis. In late stages, a nonfunctional shrunken kidney with clumps of calcification is found (Fig. 7-19). A number of fungal infections can affect the kidney in diabetic and immunosuppressed patients. Fungal infections often cause large fungal clumps or balls within the collecting system that can obstruct the kidney (Fig. 7-20).

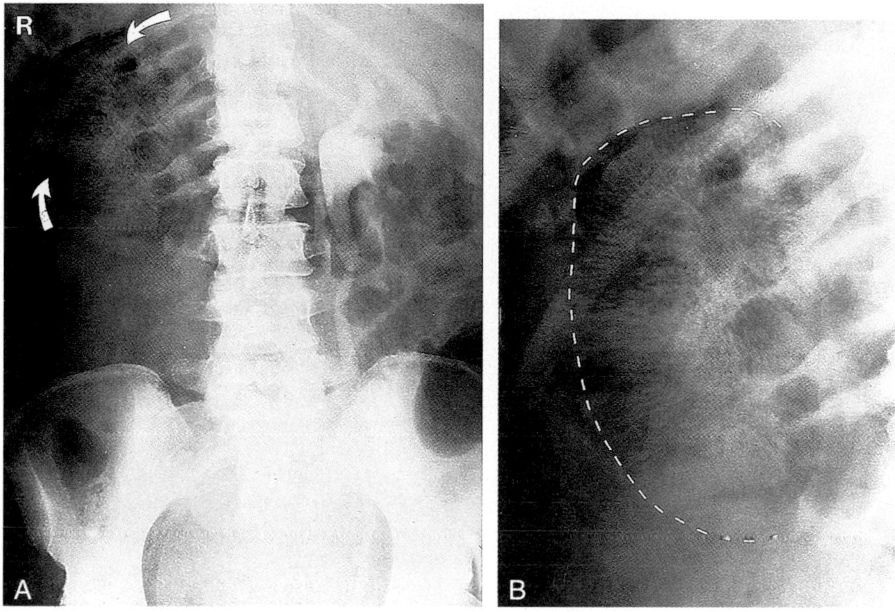

FIGURE 7-16 ■ **Emphysematous pyelonephritis.** This condition most commonly occurs in diabetics. On an intravenous pyelogram *(A)*, nonfunction of the affected kidney is seen, in this case, on the right *(arrows)*. A more detailed view of the right upper quadrant *(B)* shows radiating dark, thin lines of gas within the parenchyma of the right kidney.

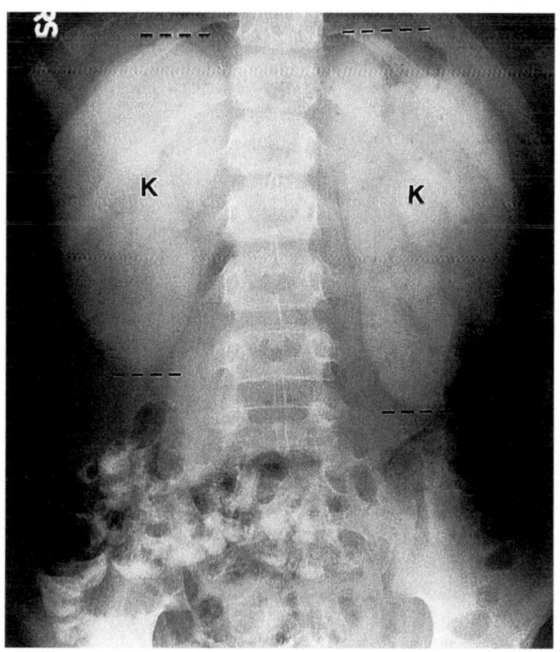

FIGURE 7-17 ■ **Acute glomerulonephritis.** An intravenous pyelogram in this child demonstrates markedly enlarged kidneys bilaterally. The injected contrast has made the kidneys visible, but the kidneys are unable to excrete the contrast.

Renal Trauma

Blunt trauma, particularly during motor vehicle accidents, can cause a number of renal abnormalities. Significant kidney trauma should be suspected when a fracture of the twelfth rib or fractures of the transverse processes of the lumbar vertebrae are found. Another useful sign on the plain film is nonvisualization of the psoas margin on one side. In a renal contusion, the kidney is intact, but interstitial edema may lead to reduced blood flow. Lacerations and intrarenal hematomas can be incomplete (not extending into the calyceal system), whereas complete lacerations are usually accompanied by a significant hemorrhage and urine extravasation (Fig. 7-21). Minor renal injuries are usually treated conservatively, and even kidneys that have large lacerations may ultimately heal. Surgical intervention may not be required unless there is major blood loss. Occasionally, avulsion of the renal vascular pedicle occurs with disruption of the blood supply (Fig. 7-22).

The advantage of CT scanning in cases of renal trauma is that you can assess other

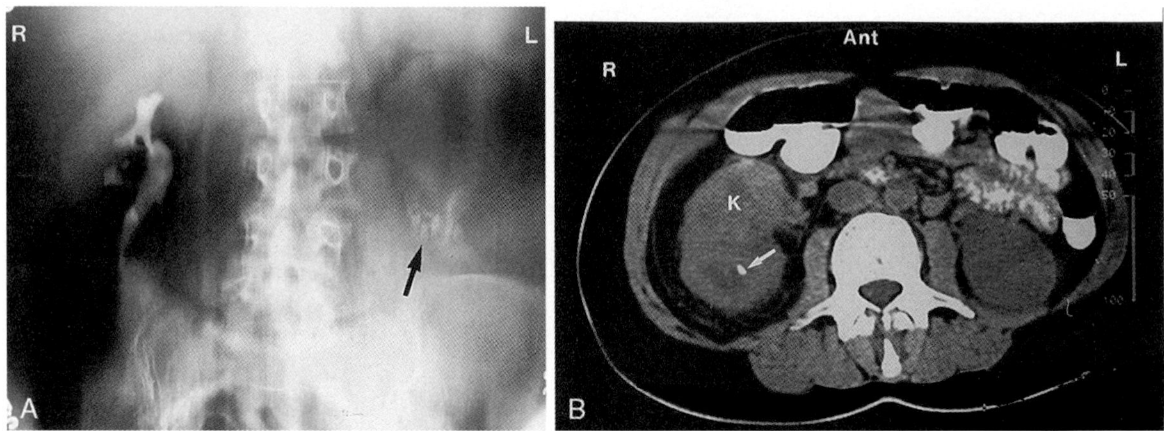

FIGURE 7-18 ■ Xanthogranulomatous pyelonephritis. On an intravenous pyelogram *(A)*, no function is seen in the left kidney, although some evidence of calcification is noted *(arrow)*. In a different patient with the same condition in the right kidney, a computed tomography (CT) scan *(B)* again shows nonfunction, with areas of low density and calcification *(arrow)*. With any imaging modality, it is very difficult to differentiate this condition from a neoplasm.

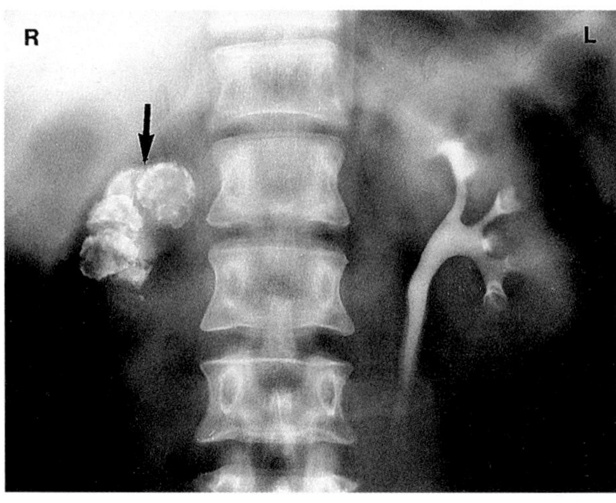

FIGURE 7-19 ■ End-stage renal tuberculosis. A tomogram obtained during an intravenous pyelogram shows a normally functioning left kidney, but a completely nonfunctional shrunken right kidney replaced by mottled calcification *(arrow)*.

organs, such as the liver and spleen, for concomitant injuries and the peritoneal and retroperitoneal areas for hematomas. Although it is not generally appreciated, lithotripsy (ultrasound used to fragment renal stones) can cause significant renal trauma. Postlithotripsy hemorrhage generally resolves without intervention, and imaging studies are not usually ordered.

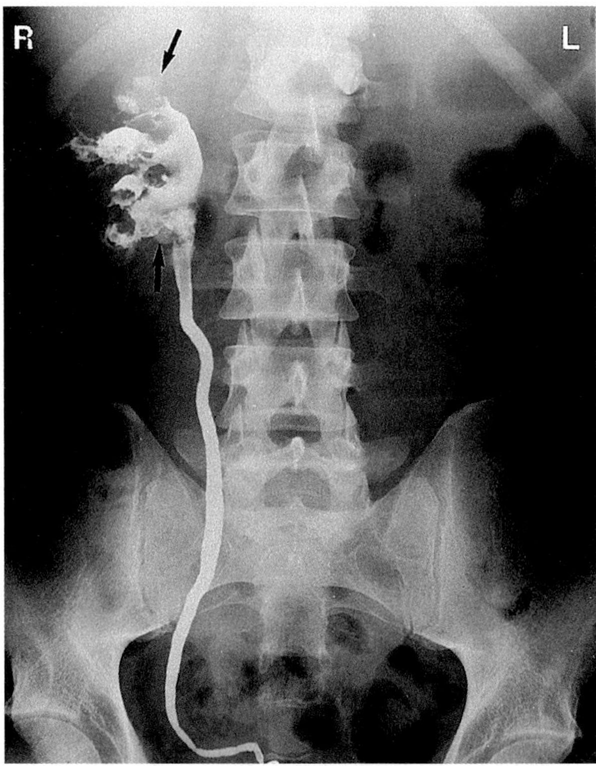

FIGURE 7-20 ■ Aspergillosis. In this immunocompromised patient, no function of the right kidney was identified on an intravenous pyelogram. Therefore a right retrograde pyelogram was performed and is shown here. Marked irregularity of the renal pelvis and collecting system is seen, with intraluminal irregular defects *(arrows)*. These are due to fungus balls and debris within the collecting system.

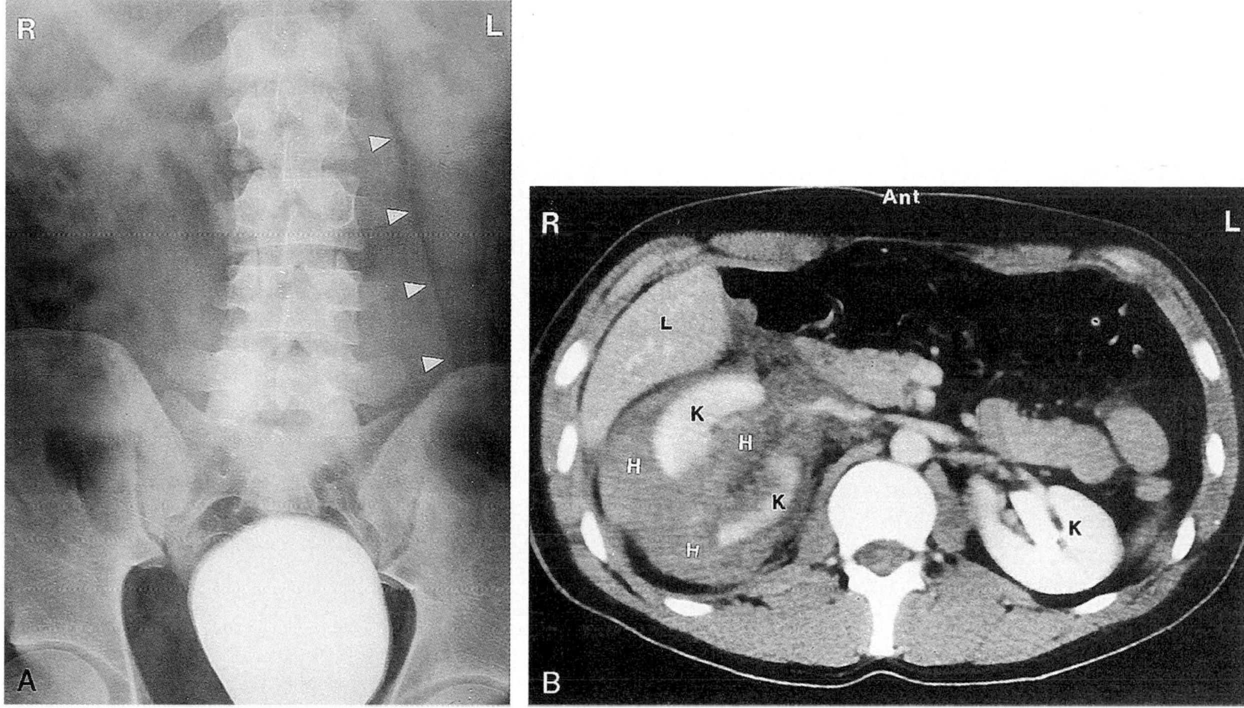

FIGURE 7-21 ■ **Renal laceration.** A plain x-ray image of the abdomen *(A)* in a young male patient involved in an automobile accident shows a well-defined left psoas margin *(arrowheads)*. The right psoas margin is not identified, and a contrast-enhanced computed tomography (CT) scan *(B)* at the level of the kidneys shows a fracture through the midportion of the right kidney. The kidney can be seen in two separate pieces with intervening and surrounding hemorrhage (H).

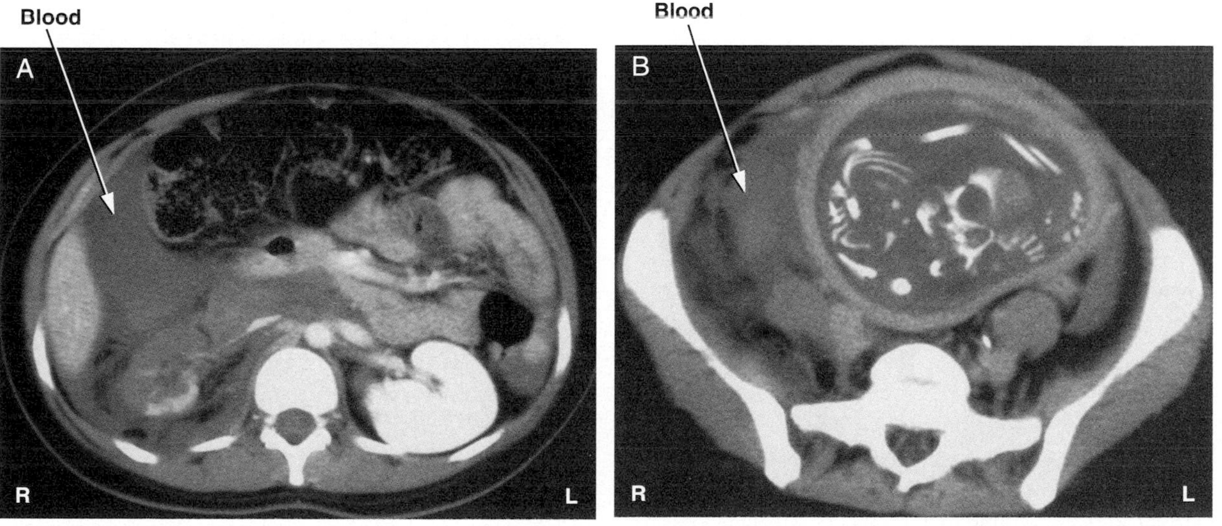

FIGURE 7-22 ■ **Disruption of the renal pedicle.** A computed tomography (CT) scan of a hypotensive pregnant woman who was in an auto accident shows that at the level of the kidneys *(A)*, intravenous contrast appears in the left kidney but not in most of the right kidney. This is because the right renal artery has been avulsed, and free blood (Bl) is present around the kidney. At a lower level *(B)*, a fetus is identified with free blood along both sides of the uterus. Mother and child survived after emergency surgery.

Renal Tumors

Among the occasional benign tumors of the kidneys is an angiomyolipoma. It is easily identified on CT scanning by the presence of fat within the mass (Fig. 7-23). Other tumors include fibromas, oncocytomas, and hamartomas.

Renal cell carcinoma constitutes about 85% of all primary renal malignancies. It usually occurs in the sixth decade, and male patients are affected twice as often as female patients. The classic clinical triad consists of gross hematuria, flank pain, and a flank mass, although this triad is seen in only approximately 10% of patients. Typically, gross or microscopic hematuria raises the suspicion of a urinary malignancy. Large mass lesions within the kidney will displace the collecting system and produce an irregular contour of the kidney on an IVP, but very small tumors or pedunculated neoplasms can be difficult to appreciate. CT scanning with and without intravenous contrast (with thin cuts through the kidneys) is now the imaging procedure of choice in an older patient with persistent painless hematuria, a normal IVP, and normal cystoscopy. MRI also can be used to evaluate renal masses (Fig. 7-24).

Most renal cell carcinomas are relatively solid, but some are very cystic, and you may have some difficulty differentiating a cystic neoplasm from a benign renal cyst. On a CT scan, the finding of a thickened wall or a mural mass within a cystic abnormality is a criterion for malignancy. On the CT scan, also look for potential extension into the renal vein and inferior vena cava, as well as into the nearby nodes (Fig. 7-25). Metastases from renal cell carcinoma tend to go either to the lung or to the bone. On the chest x-ray, the metastases are usually nodules ranging from 0.5 cm to several centimeters. When the metastases are in bone, they tend

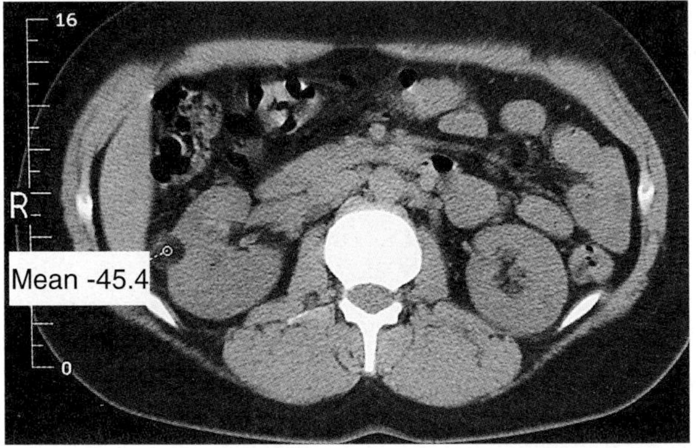

FIGURE 7-23 ■ Renal angiomyolipoma. A computed tomography (CT) scan shows a mass in the right kidney with low-density dark areas. Measurement of the attenuation values indicates that the mean Hounsfield unit is less than zero (minus 45), indicating the presence of fat. This is essentially diagnostic of an angiomyolipoma.

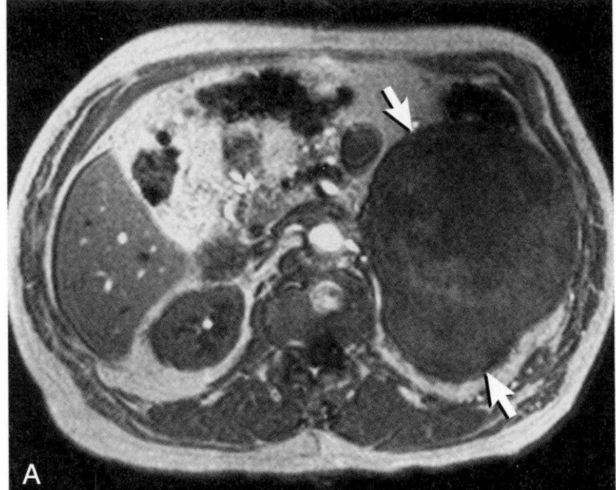

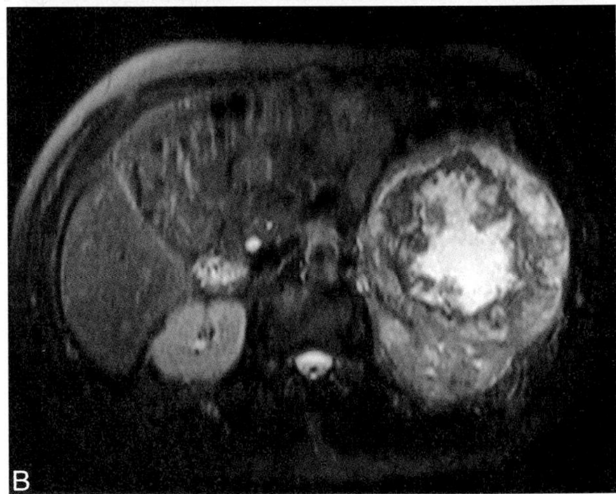

FIGURE 7-24 ■ Renal cell carcinoma. A T1-weighted magnetic resonance (MR) scan *(A)* shows a large left renal mass *(arrows)*. On a T2-weighted sequence *(B)*, the tumor has high signal and appears whiter.

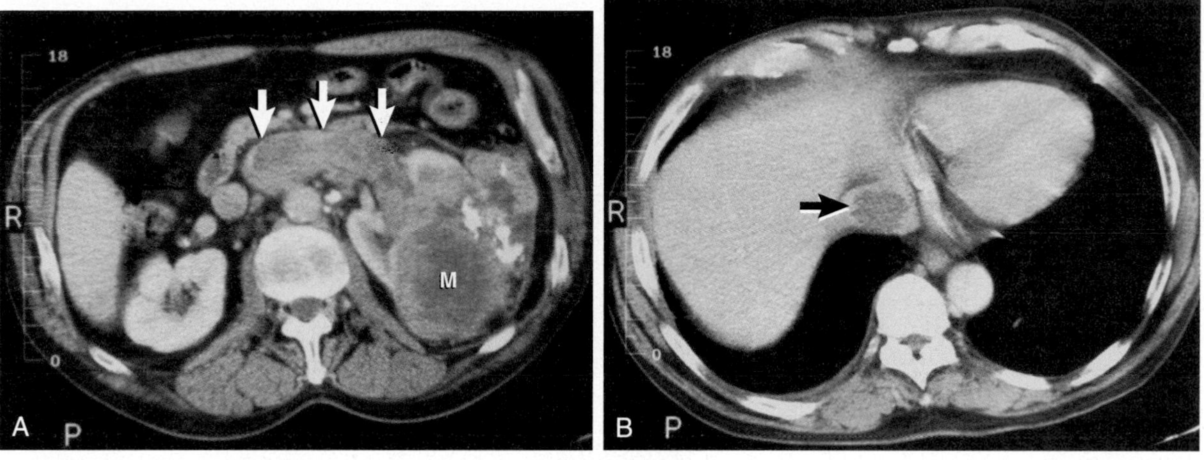

FIGURE 7-25 ■ Renal cell carcinoma. In this patient, the computed tomography (CT) scan at the mid portion of the kidneys *(A)* demonstrates a large left renal mass (M) that extends into the renal vein and into the inferior vena cava *(arrows)*. An image at the level of the base of the heart shows that the tumor thrombus *(arrow)* extends into the right atrium.

to be very aggressive, expansile, and lytic (destructive) (Fig. 7-26).

Renal Artery Stenosis

Fewer than 5% of patients with hypertension have renal artery stenosis as the cause. Imaging is usually reserved for those patients whose hypertension is uncontrolled by two medications or uncontrolled by medication and have increasing levels of serum blood urea nitrogen or creatinine. Imaging studies for suspected renal artery stenosis are discussed in Chapter 5 .

Obstruction of the Renal Collecting System

Obstruction of the ureter of the kidney is easily visualized by an IVP, which affords a detailed view of the anatomy; however, ultrasound or CT may be more useful. Although it is difficult or impossible to visualize the full length of the ureter by ultrasound, it is very easy to determine whether dilatation of the collecting system exists within the kidney itself (Fig. 7-27). This is seen as an area with relatively few echoes splaying the high-intensity echoes (caused by fat) around the renal collecting system. If you are monitoring a patient with known hydronephrosis, ultrasound is the test to order. Ultrasound also is the test of choice to differentiate hydronephrosis from medical renal disease in a patient who has renal failure. CT scans have the advantage of assessing pathology in other organs as well as being able to clearly visualize external causes of urinary tract obstruction.

Occasionally dilatation of the renal pelvis is not caused by obstruction. This may have a congenital basis or may be the result of a flaccid collecting system. A simple way of differentiating the two is to order a nuclear medicine furosemide (Lasix) renogram (Fig. 7-28). The patient is injected with a radioactive material that is rapidly cleared by glomerular filtration. This will give a picture of both kidneys that looks like a poor man's IVP. The advantage of this study, however, is that you can inject the patient with furosemide approximately 15 minutes into the study. If rapid clearance of activity from the kidney and renal pelvis is found, you know that you are dealing with a flaccid system rather than an obstructed one.

THE URETER

You should be able to recognize frequent and characteristic lesions that occur in the ureter. Duplication of the ureter and collecting system

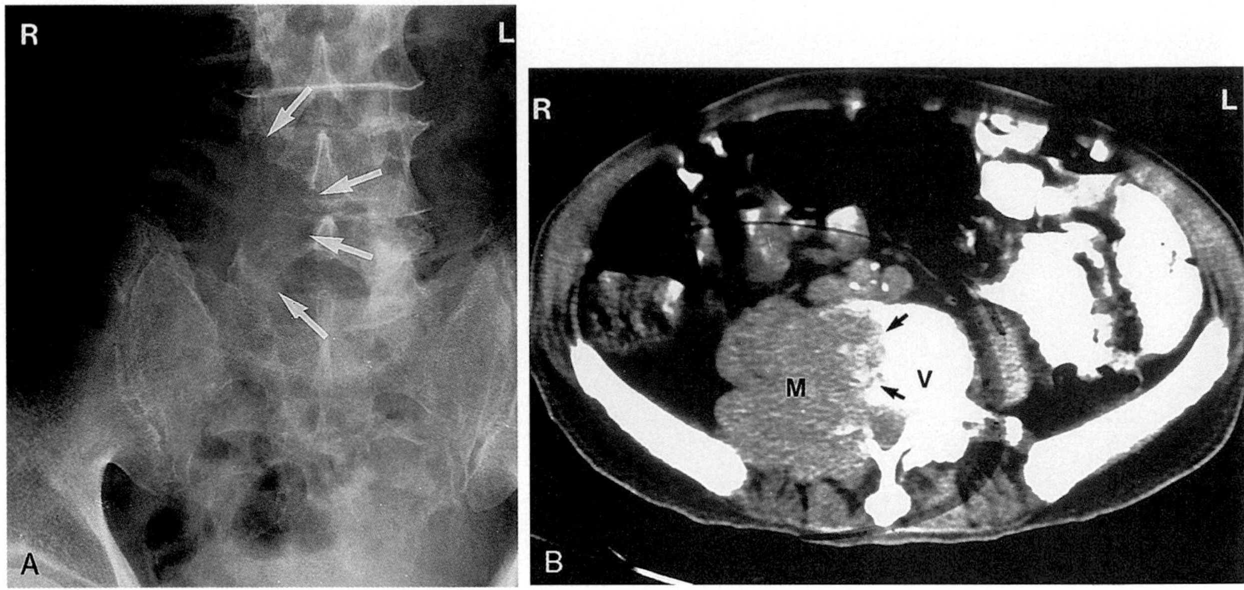

FIGURE 7-26 ■ Bone metastasis from renal cell carcinoma. An anteroposterior (AP) view of the lower lumbar spine *(A)* shows destruction of the right lateral aspects of L4 and L5 *(arrows)*. A transverse computed tomography (CT) scan at the same level *(B)* shows that not only has the vertebral body (V) been destroyed, but also a significant soft tissue tumor mass (M) extends laterally.

has already been discussed. Sometimes the ureter has an abnormal entrance into the bladder, with dilatation of the ureter as it passes through the bladder wall (ureterocele) causing a "cobra head" deformity (Fig. 7-29). Ureteroceles are not of much clinical importance and generally do not require treatment.

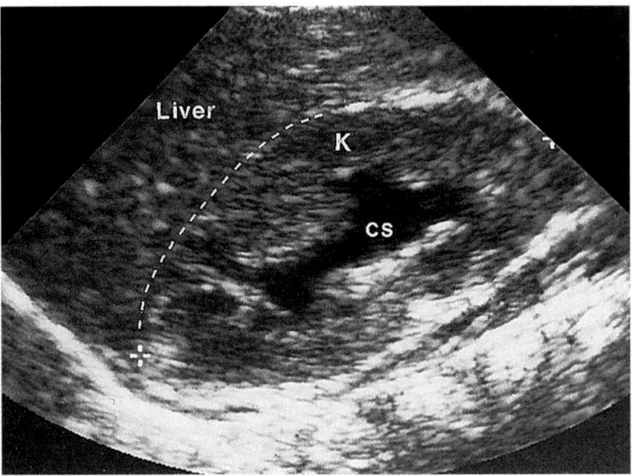

FIGURE 7-27 ■ Hydronephrosis. Ultrasound is the simplest and most cost-effective way of determining whether hydronephrosis is present. Here, a longitudinal image of the right kidney (K) demonstrates a dilated collecting system (cs). This persisted even after the patient had voided.

The ureter normally has peristaltic waves, and therefore on any single image, usually visualization will occur of some portions of the ureter and not others. Do not be fooled into diagnosing a stricture unless you see contrast above, below, and at the level of the lesion and are able to confirm it on several different films. Because an IVP is done with the patient supine and contrast is heavier than urine, the most anterior portions of the ureters (as they pass over the sacroiliac [SI] joints into the pelvis) are usually very difficult to see. Sometimes the radiologist will order a prone image to rectify this situation.

Dilatation of a ureter is diagnosed only when the ureter is seen to be greater than 8 mm in diameter and contrast is backed up in the ureter without peristaltic waves. When an acute obstruction is present, there is almost always calyceal blunting as well. Dilatation of a ureter usually elicits a reflex response from students, who immediately say "hydronephrosis" and then "obstruction." Dilatation can be due to a

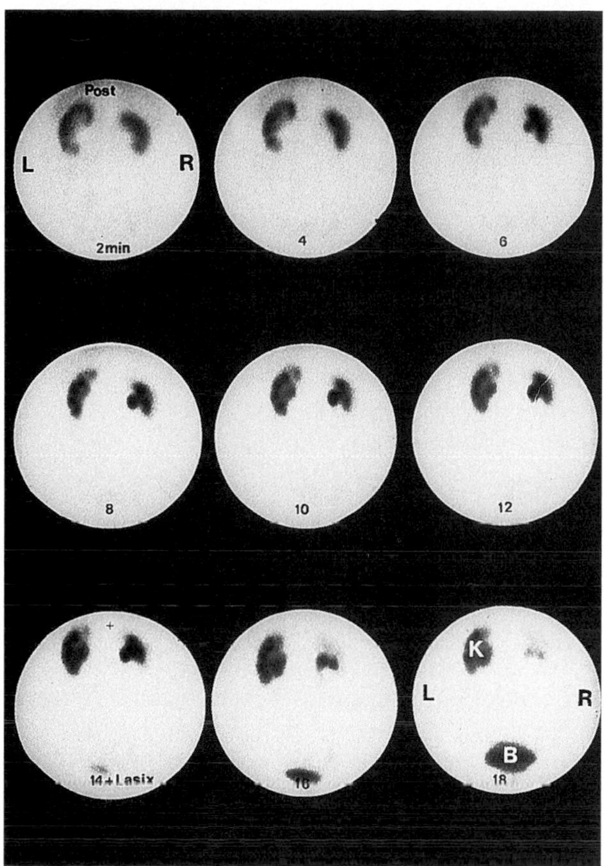

FIGURE 7-28 ■ **Differentiation of causes of a dilated collecting system.** A nuclear medicine renogram is performed by administering a small amount of radioactivity that is cleared by the kidney. Two-minute sequential images are obtained in a posterior projection. At 14 min, activity is seen in both the right and the left dilated collecting systems, and furosemide (Lasix) is given intravenously. The right kidney excretes its activity into the bladder (B), but the left kidney (K) remains essentially unchanged, indicating a flaccid dilated collecting system on the right but an obstructed left collecting system.

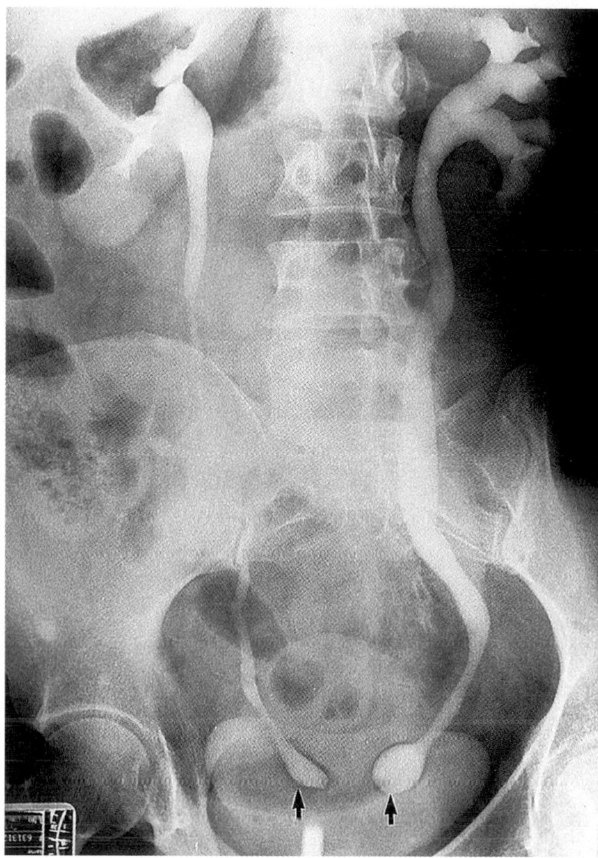

FIGURE 7-29 ■ **Bilateral ureteroceles.** This intravenous pyelogram demonstrates a congenital variant with dilatation of the distal ureter as it enters through the bladder wall. This produces a typical "cobra head" deformity *(arrows),* which is usually of little clinical significance.

number of other causes, including ureterovesicular reflux, infection, and congenital megaureter.

Common intraluminal abnormalities of the ureter are renal calculi (see earlier), blood clots, transitional cell carcinomas, and, occasionally, fungal lesions. A clot within the ureter is not visible on a plain film, and on an IVP, it will be a filling defect that can look like a nonopaque stone (Fig. 7-30). Remember that most renal calculi (80%) are radiopaque. A clot should be suspected after trauma and in patients who are taking anticoagulants.

Transitional cell carcinomas can occur either in the renal collecting system or in the bladder. In the renal collecting system, they can form a mass that spreads the renal sinus fat and can cause obstruction (Fig. 7-31*A*). In the ureter, a renal cell carcinoma may look like a lesion in the wall of the ureter, or it may cause an "apple core" deformity with encirclement of the lumen. Occasionally on an IVP, an intraluminal transitional cell carcinoma causes an appearance that looks like an upside-down goblet (Bergman's sign) (Fig. 7-31*B*).

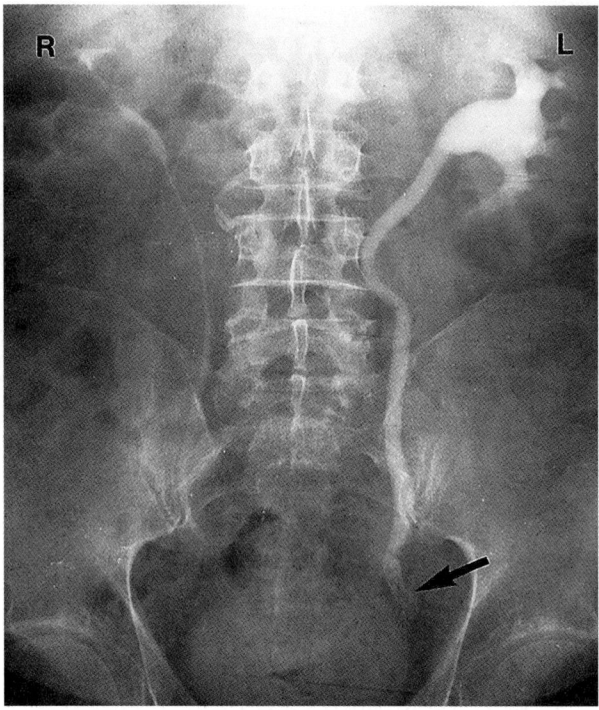

FIGURE 7-30 ■ **Ureteral clot.** In this patient, who was receiving anticoagulant therapy, hematuria and left flank pain developed. The intravenous pyelogram demonstrates a filling defect in the distal left ureter *(arrow)* caused by a clot that has partially obstructed the left collecting system, causing it to be dilated compared with the right ureter.

In addition to lesions that are entirely contained within the lumen, lesions may project into the lumen or may be the result of extrinsic pressure. In some patients, indentations seen across the upper one third of the collecting system are caused by vascular impressions of blood vessels as they cross over the ureter. Collateral vessels may cause ureteral notching (Fig. 7-32). In patients who have an infection, small fluid-filled cysts in the ureteral wall may project into the lumen (pyelitis cystica). Occasionally even metastases can indent the ureter at multiple locations. This most often is the result of metastatic melanoma. If a suspected ureteral lesion is seen on an IVP, this is almost always confirmed by the urologist, who will perform a retrograde ureterogram before surgery.

Deviation of the ureter can signal nearby pathology. In the region between the lower pole of the kidney and the sacrum, the normal course of the ureters on an anteroposterior (AP) or a posteroanterior (PA) image is over the transverse processes of the spine. Lateral deviation of a ureter can be the result of retroperitoneal adenopathy, retroperitoneal tumors, abdominal aortic aneurysms, and occasionally, large psoas muscles (in young men or horse riders). Medial deviation can be due to traction caused by fibrosis from chronic leakage of an aneurysm, by methysergide use, or, if only on the right side, by a congenital retrocaval ureter.

BLADDER

Anatomy and Imaging Techniques

As the bladder fills with urine, it has a water or soft tissue density. The bladder can often be seen on a plain x-ray, because it is frequently outlined by perivesicular fat. As the bladder enlarges with urine, it pushes the small bowel superiorly and laterally. An enlarged bladder can be very striking (Fig. 7-33), and without having contrast material in the bladder, it is often difficult to tell whether you are looking at an enlarged fluid-filled bladder or some other soft tissue mass arising from the pelvis or an abdominal mass. One of the rules I use is that it is unusual for abdominal masses or tumors to grow down into the pelvis, but it is very common for pelvic masses to grow up out of the pelvis into the lower abdomen. Thus if you see a soft tissue mass that involves both the lower abdomen and the pelvis, the mass probably arose in the pelvis. The differential diagnosis of a pelvic mass includes uterine enlargement, ovarian cysts, and tumor or pelvic sarcomas. In the female patient, if the bladder is displaced to one side, you should expect an ovarian etiology. Usually the bladder is visualized by using water-soluble contrast from an IVP, CT, or cystogram.

Trauma

Fractures of the pelvis are accompanied by hematomas. These may displace the bladder to one side if they are unilateral, but more often

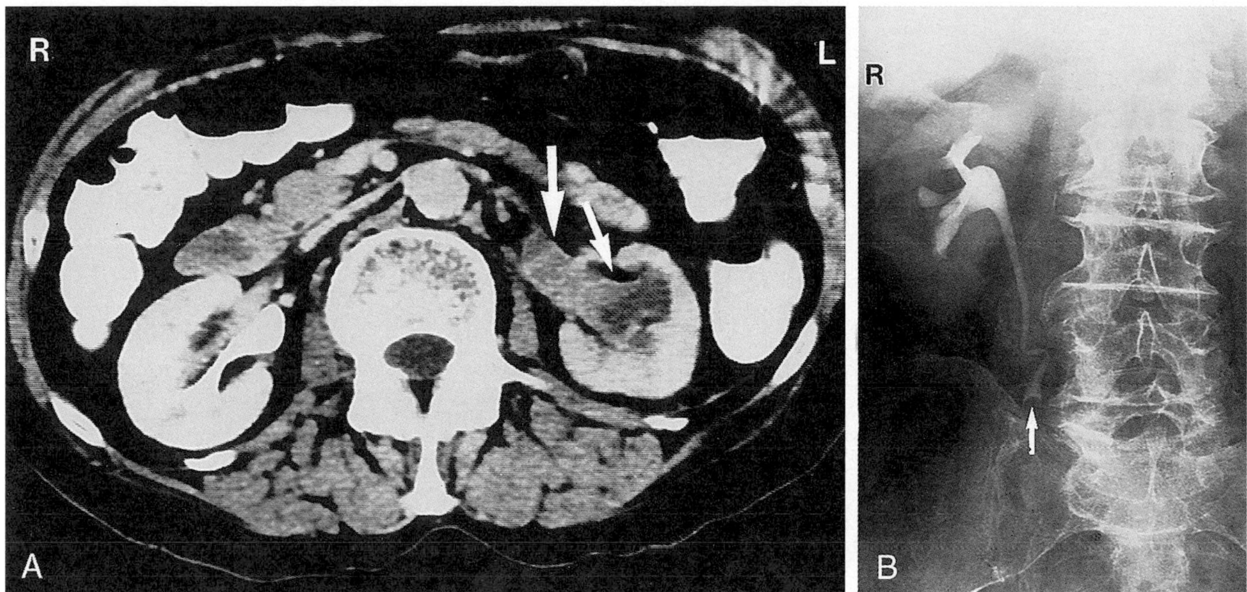

FIGURE 7-31 ■ **Transitional cell carcinoma.** A transverse contrast-enhanced computed tomography (CT) scan at the level of the kidneys *(A)* shows expansion of the left renal pelvis *(arrows)*. This is due to a transitional cell carcinoma within the renal pelvis. In a different patient, an intravenous pyelogram *(B)* demonstrates an upside-down goblet deformity (Bergman's sign) in the right midureter *(arrow)*. This is a sign of a ureteral transitional cell carcinoma.

pelvic hematomas are bilateral, and they will compress and elevate the inferior portion of the bladder (Fig. 7-34) so that it looks like an upside-down teardrop. This shape of the bladder also can be caused by pelvic adenopathy, pelvic lipomatosis (mostly in black males with hypertension), and by very prominent iliopsoas muscles.

With pelvic fractures or as a result of direct compression of a fluid-filled distended bladder, bladder rupture can occur. This is almost always accompanied by hematuria. About 10% of patients who have a pelvic fracture will have bladder rupture. The bladder can rupture either extraperitoneally (80%) or intraperitoneally (20%). Intraperitoneal rupture of the bladder is recognized on an IVP or a cystogram because contrast extravasation into the peritoneal cavity outlines loops of bowel, and the contrast also will layer in the paracolic gutters.

The vast majority of patients with an extraperitoneal bladder rupture will have associated pelvic fractures. With extraperitoneal rupture, the extravasated contrast material will be in a streaky or sunburst pattern (Fig. 7-35). About 10% of patients with ruptured bladders will have both an intraperitoneal and an extraperitoneal component.

Pelvic trauma also can result in injury to the urethra. Because the female urethra is so short, it is rarely, if ever, injured in an accident. In the male patient, urethral injuries are more common than bladder injuries. Because the urethra is fixed at the prostatomembranous junction, tears in this area are secondary to shearing. In a patient with pelvic trauma who has blood at the urethral meatus and who is unable to void or can void only with difficulty, a posterior urethral tear should be suspected. In these cases, a retrograde urethrogram should be done before any attempt is made to catheterize the bladder, because a small initial tear may be significantly enlarged by any attempt at catheterization (Fig. 7-36). Injuries to the anterior portion of the urethra are much less common. Injuries to the bulbous portion of the urethra are most commonly due to a straddle injury in which the patient falls astride a solid object, such as a beam.

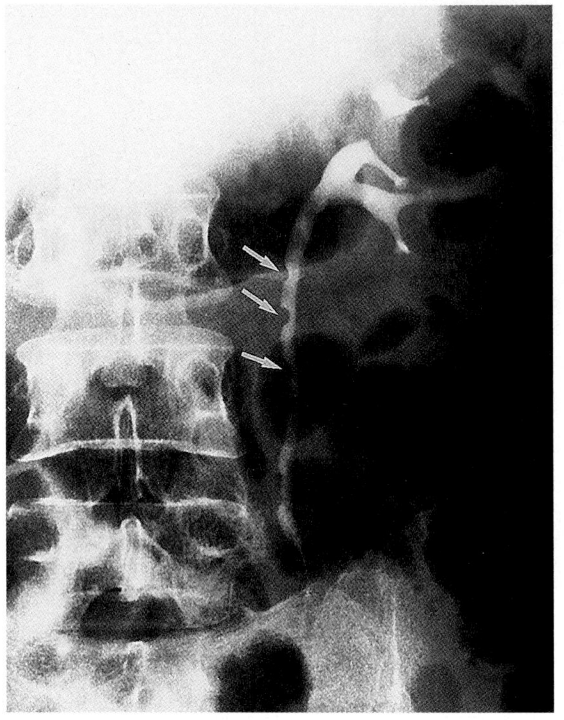

FIGURE 7-32 ■ Ureteral notching. On this intravenous pyelogram, notching along the medial aspect of the proximal left ureter is easily seen *(arrows)*. This can be due to a number of abnormalities, but in this case, it was due to impression on the lumen of the ureter by collateral vessels.

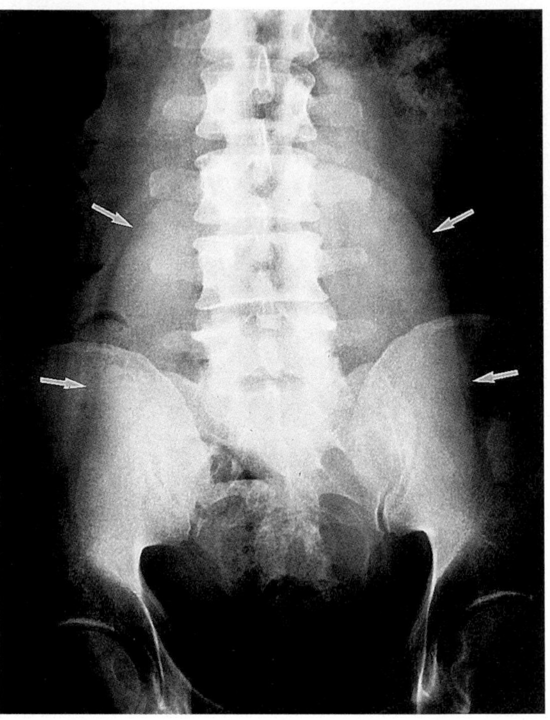

FIGURE 7-33 ■ Distended bladder. On this plain x-ray image of the abdomen, a large soft tissue mass is seen arising from the pelvis *(arrows)*. It has pushed the small bowel out of the way. The differential diagnosis includes a pelvic tumor, distended bladder, or cystic abnormality arising from the pelvis.

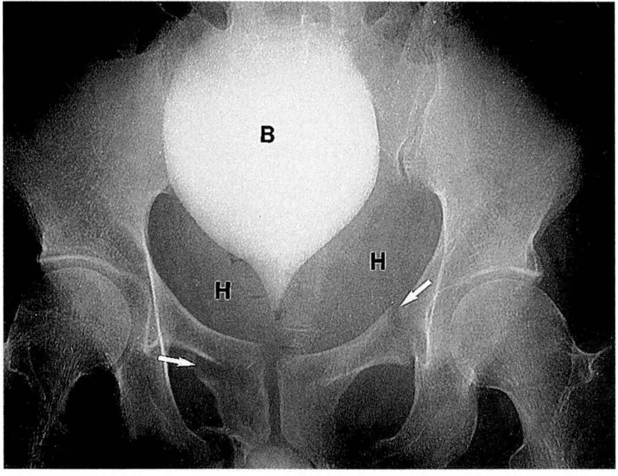

FIGURE 7-34 ■ Pelvic fractures with hematoma. This cystogram demonstrates multiple pelvic fractures *(arrows)*. The associated bilateral hematomas (H) have elevated and compressed the bladder.

Incontinence

Incontinence in some form affects about 10 million persons in the United States. Inability to hold urine results from a wide number of etiologies. The mechanism of urination involves the bladder wall, sphincters, and pelvic musculature, as well as neurologic control in the bladder, spinal cord, and brain. The workup is best begun with a thorough medical history, physical examination, urinalysis, and evaluation of postvoid residual volume. The four forms of incontinence are urge, stress, overflow, and mixed.

Urge incontinence can be due to lesions (infection, stones, or neoplasm) of the bladder near the trigone, causing uncontrolled contractions. Stress incontinence occurs with increased intra-abdominal pressure (e.g., coughing, sneezing) and is most common in parous

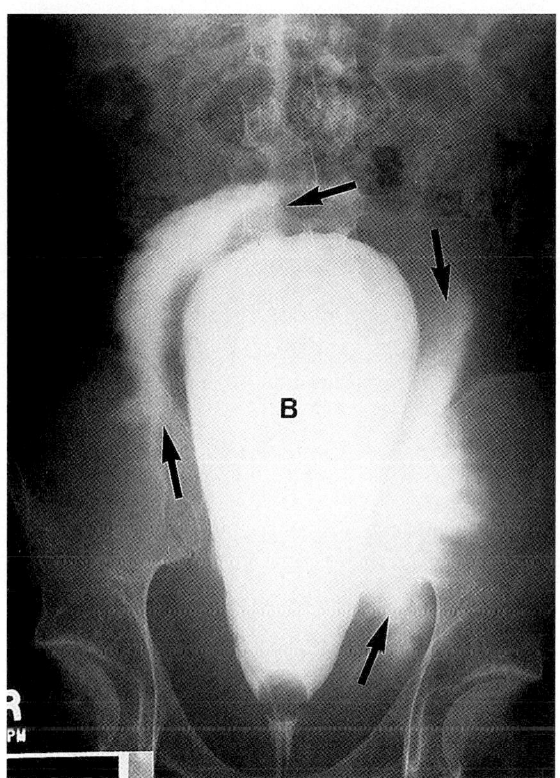

FIGURE 7-35 ■ Bladder rupture. A cystogram done in a patient after a motor vehicle accident shows extravasation of contrast *(arrows)* into the tissues surrounding the bladder, an extraperitoneal bladder rupture. With an intraperitoneal bladder rupture, contrast would be seen outlining loops of bowel.

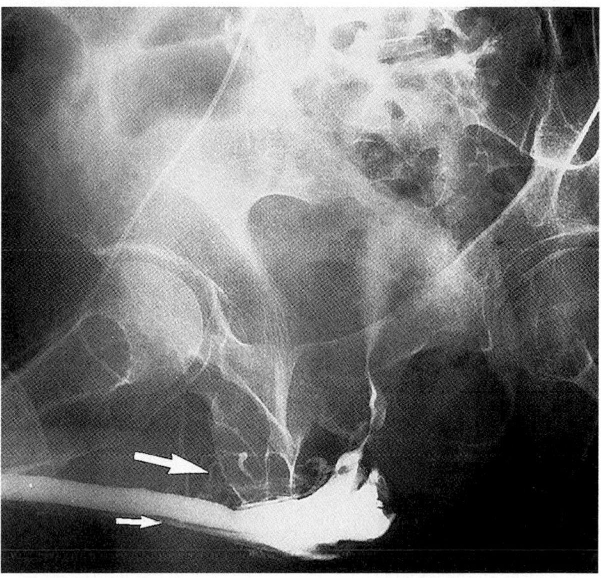

FIGURE 7-36 ■ Urethral rupture. After a straddle-type injury, this young male patient had hematuria and was unable to void. A retrograde urethrogram was performed, and there was extravasation of contrast into the soft tissues *(small arrow)* as well as into nearby venous structures *(large arrow).*

postmenopausal women; this is a result of estrogen deprivation and relaxation of the pelvic musculature with loss of the normal ureterovesicular angle. Imaging is not usually indicated, and most women are treated conservatively with exercise of the pelvic muscles. In men, stress incontinence is usually secondary to prostatic surgery. Other causes that should be considered include multiple sclerosis or other neurologic abnormalities. Overflow incontinence is due to large volumes in an atonic bladder secondary to spinal cord injury, diabetes, hypothyroidism, chronic alcoholism, or collagen vascular disease. In patients with incontinence and suspected urologic abnormality, urodynamic studies should be conducted before imaging procedures.

Neurologic Abnormalities

If trauma compromises the spinal cord, the bladder may become either flaccid or spastic. On a contrasted study, a spastic bladder has the shape of a Christmas tree, with little outpouchings along the lateral margins (Fig. 7-37). These areas of outpouching of contrast or urine are pseudodiverticula caused by hypertrophy of the bladder musculature. A hyper-reflexive bladder usually occurs when the spinal cord lesion is at the level of T5 or higher. These patients are prime candidates for urinary infection, calculi, and bilateral collecting system dilatation. Hyporeflexive bladders are usually the result of a herniated disk, multiple sclerosis, diabetic neuropathy, or lower spinal cord tumor. Although these patients may demonstrate a large bladder, the upper urinary collecting systems are usually within normal limits, and vesicoureteral reflux is rare.

Infections

There is little reason to do imaging studies in female patients with uncomplicated cystitis. If

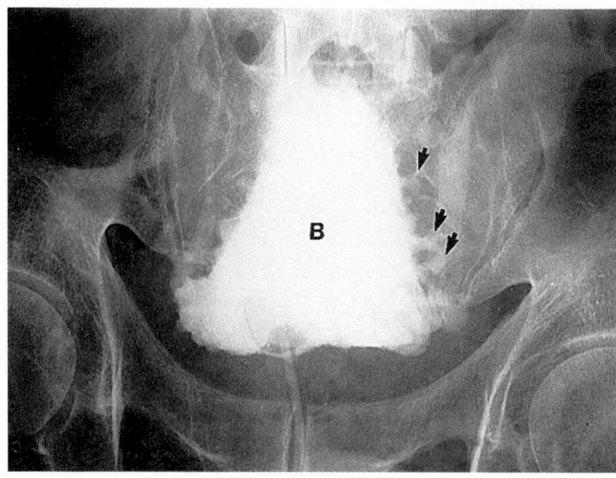

FIGURE 7-37 ■ Spastic bladder. In this patient with a spinal cord injury, the typical "Christmas tree" deformity of the bladder with lateral diverticula is seen *(arrows)*.

repeated bouts of infection have occurred, an IVP may be indicated to exclude anatomic abnormalities. Because cystitis is rare in male patients, an IVP may be indicated after an initial infection. With severe cystitis, mucosal thickening may be noted; however, this should not be evaluated on a study that has a nondistended bladder. Once the bladder is fully distended, it may be possible to image thickened mucosa, although this finding rarely changes treatment.

In a number of unusual bladder infections, imaging findings are fairly characteristic. In diabetic patients, emphysematous cystitis may develop, in which gas is present in either the wall or the lumen of the bladder (Fig. 7-38*A*). In contrast to emphysematous pyelonephritis, morbidity is not increased with emphysematous cystitis. This condition usually responds well to antibiotic therapy. Air within the bladder itself is more likely due to instrumentation or a bladder/bowel fistula.

Tuberculosis can affect the bladder, but this is extremely rare without strictures and stenosis of the ureters and stenosis of the calyces of the renal collecting system. Schistosomiasis, although very rare, can produce characteristic bladder wall calcification (Fig. 7-38*B*). A number of inflammatory conditions can cause a small bladder, including interstitial cystitis, cyclophosphamide cystitis, and radiation therapy. These also can cause calcification within the bladder wall. With the exception of the small capacity, very little is characteristic or disease specific about the imaging findings.

Tumors

Ninety-five percent of bladder tumors are transitional cell carcinomas. Transitional cell carcinoma is 4 times more common in men than

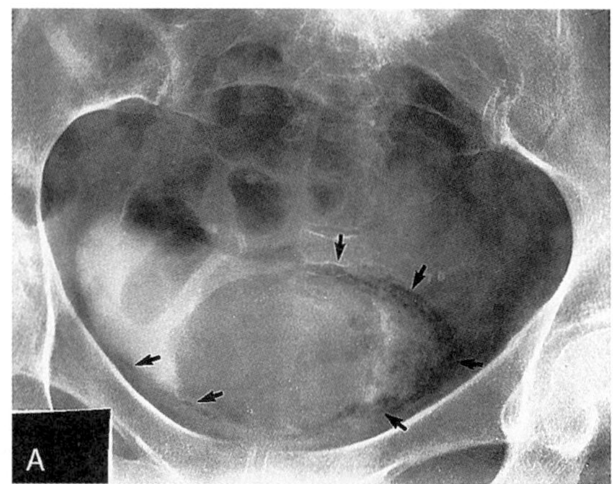

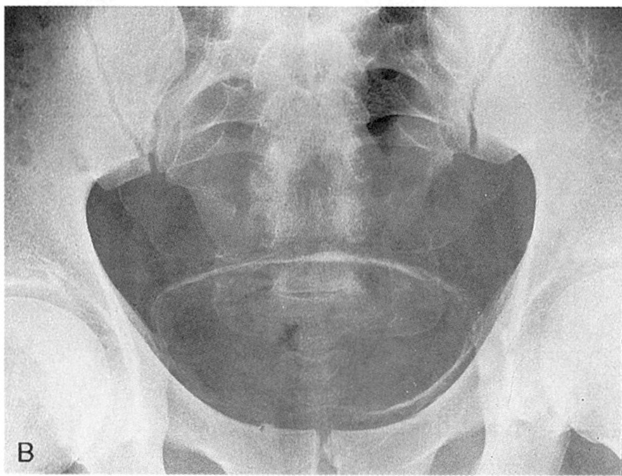

FIGURE 7-38 ■ Unusual forms of cystitis. A view of the pelvis obtained during an intravenous pyelogram *(A)* in a diabetic patient shows air within the wall of the bladder as well as within the bladder *(arrows)*. This is called emphysematous cystitis. In a different patient, calcification of the bladder wall is seen on a plain x-ray image of the pelvis *(B)*. This is due to schistosomiasis.

in women, and a significantly increased incidence has been associated with cigarette smoking. Patients frequently are initially seen with hematuria and occasionally with urinary frequency and dysuria. Pelvic lymph node extension is relatively common. Hematogenous metastases tend to go to liver and lungs and, to a much lesser extent, to bone. When bone lesions are seen, they are typically lytic. Transitional cell carcinoma of the bladder is associated with upper tract transitional cell tumors, and close follow-up of these patients is essential.

Tumors of the bladder rarely calcify, and the diagnosis of tumors is not obvious on plain x-ray images. An IVP may show a filling defect within the lumen of the bladder (Fig. 7-39). Be very cautious about saying that no cancer is present on the basis of an IVP. As pointed out earlier, intravenously administered contrast is heavier than urine and layers dependently in the bladder. A tumor will not be visualized unless it is located in the dependent portion of the bladder. CT scanning is useful only to evaluate invasion of adjacent organs and pelvic lymphadenopathy. If a bladder carcinoma is suspected, the initial study of choice should be direct visualization using cystoscopy.

PROSTATE AND SCROTUM

Anatomy and Imaging Techniques

Enlargement of the prostate causes elevation of the base of the bladder (Fig. 7-40). Prostate enlargement is most often the result of benign prostatic hypertrophy rather than prostatic car-

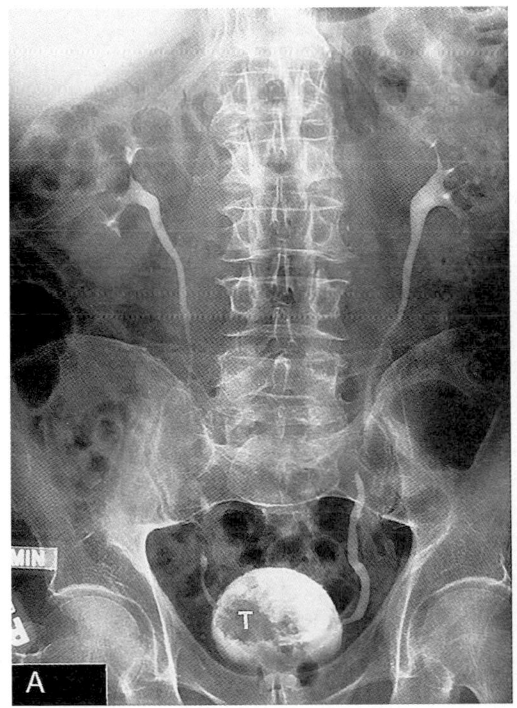

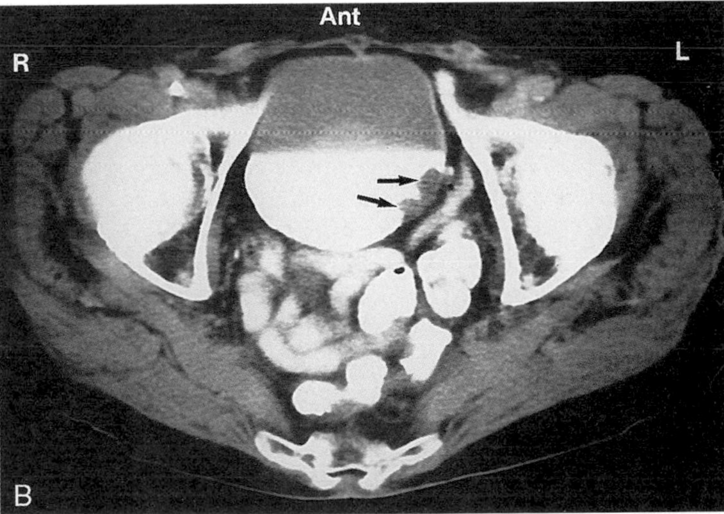

FIGURE 7-39 ■ **Bladder carcinoma.** An intravenous pyelogram *(A)* in a patient with hematuria clearly shows a large, irregular filling defect within the bladder caused by a tumor (T). A computed tomography (CT) scan *(B)* in a different patient shows a small bladder carcinoma *(arrows)*. This is visible only because the tumor happens to be in the dependent portion of the bladder with the contrast. Had this lesion been on the anterior surface of the bladder, it probably would not have been visualized on either a CT scan or an intravenous pyelogram.

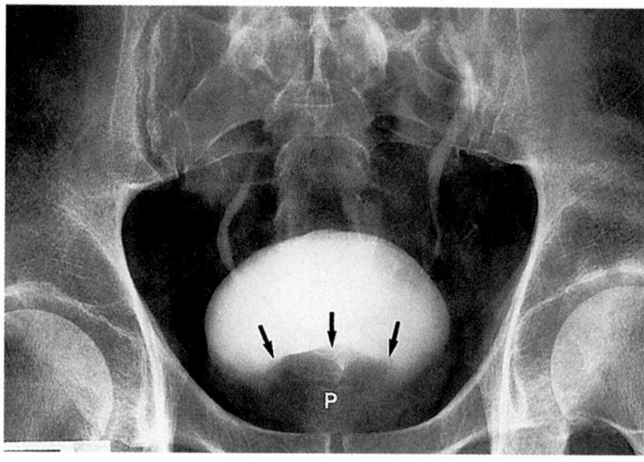

FIGURE 7-40 ■ Benign prostatic hyperplasia. A view of the bladder obtained during an intravenous pyelogram shows a smooth defect impressing on the inferior aspect of the bladder *(arrows)* caused by a benign enlargement of the prostate (P).

cinoma. If the prostate is big enough, outlet obstruction of the bladder may occur. Prostate cancer is common. Much interest has been expressed in the transrectal ultrasound examination of the prostate as a screening test for prostate cancer. This is not a useful test by itself, and no screening modality has been shown to reduce mortality. The initial investigation for suspected prostate carcinoma should be by digital rectal examination and evaluation of the serum level of prostate-specific antigen (PSA). Unfortunately, PSA is neither sensitive nor specific for prostate cancer. If the serum PSA value is elevated, ultrasonography may be helpful in locating a suspicious area in which a transrectal biopsy may be performed. A number of other indices besides total PSA levels are being used, including age-specific PSA and PSA velocity. In general, the level of PSA in men between the ages of 40 years and 50 years should not exceed 2.5 ng/mL, and in men older than 50 years, it should not exceed 3.5 to 4.0 ng/mL. Note that patients taking finasteride have a PSA level about 50% lower than the true value. Ultrasonography, CT, and MRI are not extremely accurate in determining local extension of a tumor. CT or MRI can show metastatic lesions in the rest of the abdomen; however, in a patient with a known prostate carcinoma and an increasing PSA level, radionuclide bone scan is the initial test of choice.

Testicular Pain and Masses

The most common lesions of the scrotum that may require imaging are epididymitis, testicular torsion, and hydrocele, in addition to evaluation for testicular tumors. In cases in which testicular torsion must be differentiated from epididymitis, Doppler ultrasound or less commonly a radionuclide testicular scan is used. Epididymitis will be seen as a lesion with hyperemia on the affected side. In acute torsion, an area of decreased blood flow will appear on the side in which pain occurs. In a torsion that has been present for a day or more (missed torsion), a lesion without much blood flow centrally, but with a hypervascular rim, may be seen. Imaging evaluation of the testicle for either a hydrocele or a tumor should be done with ultrasound. In general, any mass within the testicle itself should be considered malignant, whereas those lesions outside the testicle but within the scrotum are usually benign. Ninety-five percent of solid testicular masses are germ cell tumors (seminoma, embryonal carcinoma, choriocarcinoma, and teratoma).

FEMALE PELVIS

Anatomy and Imaging Techniques

The most common and fruitful imaging methods are pelvic ultrasound and CT. Ultrasound is undoubtedly the most widely used method, because it can easily image the uterus and adnexal regions. Because it does not use ionizing radiation, it can even be used during pregnancy. Imaging of the female pelvis with a plain x-ray is usually of low yield, because most significant pathology associated with female pelvic organs is not calcified. Sometimes a large soft tissue mass can be seen displacing bowel.

Female pelvic ultrasound is done either transabdominally (by having the transducer on the lower anterior abdominal wall and using the bladder as a window) or transvaginally.

Transvaginal ultrasound has a much smaller field of view, and it is often very difficult to orient yourself with respect to the images unless you were actually there when they were taken. With transabdominal ultrasound, orientation is much easier. Remember that ultrasound imaging gives you a "slice" picture. The slices are typically either longitudinal or transverse. In the longitudinal plane, you can easily see the vagina, cervix, uterus, and bladder (Fig. 7-41). Areas of high-intensity echoes can be seen in the vagina and sometimes in the center of the uterus as a result of mucus production, hemorrhage, or decidual reaction. Fluid in the bladder, uterus, or cul-de-sac appears as an area without echoes. A small amount of fluid within the cul-de-sac can be a normal finding in the middle of the menstrual period, but in patients in whom an ectopic pregnancy is suspected, this may represent hemorrhage (Fig. 7-42).

Evaluation of the uterus by ultrasound does not allow determination of patency of the fallopian tubes. A hysterosalpingogram is typically done to assess tubal patency. This is done by putting a cannula in the cervical os and injecting a water-based contrast material. After the uterus is filled, the contrast goes out the fallopian tubes and spills into the peritoneal cavity. In cases in which obstruction of the fallopian tubes (hydrosalpinx) is present, the contrast proceeds to the point of obstruction and then collects in a dilated portion of the fallopian tube without free spill into the pelvis (Fig. 7-43).

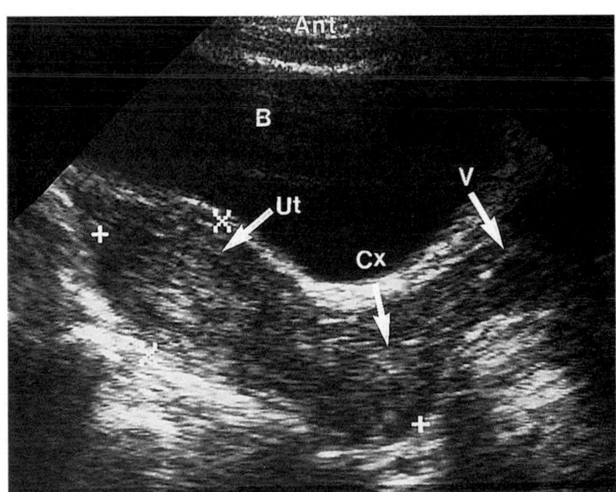

FIGURE 7-41 ■ Normal female pelvic transabdominal ultrasound. On this longitudinal image obtained in the midportion of the pelvis, the bladder (B), uterus (Ut), cervix (Cx), and vagina (V) are easily visualized.

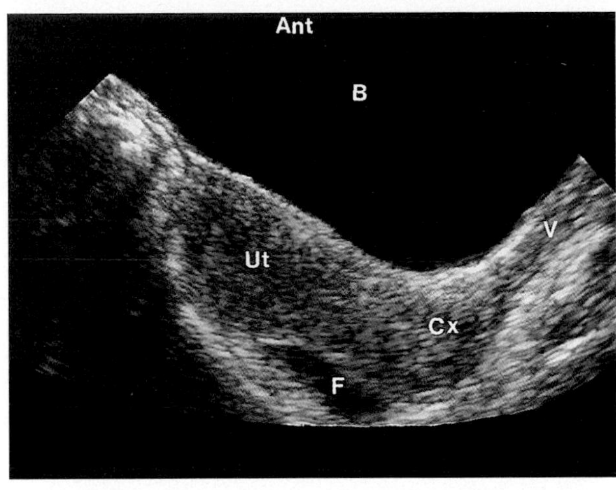

FIGURE 7-42 ■ Free fluid in the cul-de-sac. This longitudinal image of the pelvis demonstrates a collection of fluid (F) behind the uterus (Ut). This can be a normal finding during the middle of the menstrual cycle or may represent bleeding from entities such as an ectopic pregnancy. Cx, cervix; V, vagina.

Infertility

Infertility is the inability to become pregnant in 12 months if younger than 30 years or in 6 months if older than 30 years. It may be due to abnormalities of the man or woman. In the woman, it can be due to absent ovulation from any cause and anatomic factors such as tubal scarring, fibroids, congenital uterine abnormalities, or adenomyomatosis. Initial evaluation includes a complete physical examination, a pelvic examination, and a measurement of serum hormone levels. An ultrasound image can be used to assess follicle development. If ovulation is confirmed and physical examination, complete blood cell count, basal body temperature, thyroid function, and pituitary function are normal, and if the male partner is normal, a hysterosalpingogram to assess tubal patency is indicated. It also is indicated to assess tubal

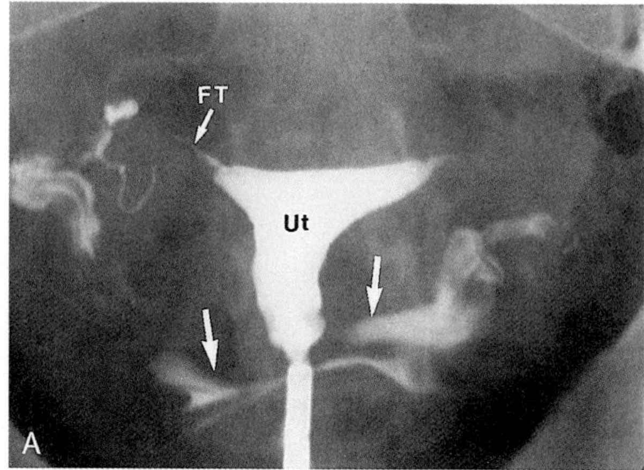

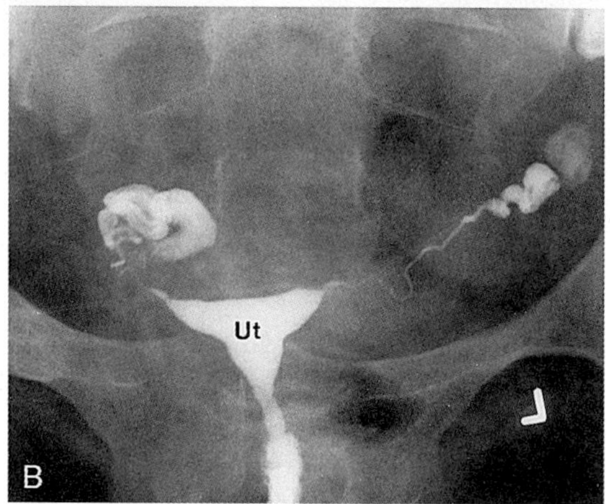

FIGURE 7-43 ■ Normal and abnormal hysterosalpingogram. In a normal patient *(A)*, the uterine cervix is cannulated, and contrast is injected to visualize the uterus (Ut). Contrast then goes out the fallopian tubes (FT) and has free spill into the pelvis *(arrows)*. In a different patient complaining of infertility, a hysterosalpingogram *(B)* demonstrates the uterus and dilated fallopian tubes with no spill into the pelvis. This is known as hydrosalpinx.

patency after surgery or in cases of repeated spontaneous abortion.

Vaginal Bleeding

Dysfunctional uterine bleeding is due to a number of causes including hormonal imbalance and tumors. Imaging procedures are not in the initial workup. An ultrasound examination is indicated in a premenopausal woman who has a normal cervix and vagina by physical examination and who has bleeding continuing after three cycles of hormone therapy. Ultrasonography also is indicated in postmenopausal women with bleeding who are not taking hormonal replacement therapy or who have been taking daily or cyclical hormonal therapy for more than 6 months.

Ectopic and Intrauterine Pregnancy

Ultrasound is the imaging method of choice to evaluate the status of a pregnancy. Indications for use of ultrasound during pregnancy are shown in Table 7-2. In very early pregnancy, transvaginal, rather than transabdominal, ultrasound is the most sensitive. By measuring the fetal crown/rump length as well as a number of other parameters, the gestational age of the fetus can be determined (Tables 7-3 and 7-4). The age that is usually quoted refers to menstrual age rather than to the conceptual age. Thus a report that indicates a 5-week pregnancy (gestational age) really corresponds to a 3-week pregnancy (conception dates).

The first ultrasound sign of pregnancy is the appearance of the gestational sac at 28 to 30 days. A yolk sac can be seen at 5 to 6 weeks, and this is the first reliable sign of an intrauterine pregnancy. A heartbeat also is typically seen at approximately 5 weeks (gestational age) (Fig. 7-44). As the fetus becomes more advanced, it is possible to see decidual thickening and formation of the placenta. A low-lying placenta early in pregnancy will not necessarily result in a placenta previa, because significant growth of the lower uterine segment occurs later in pregnancy.

A very common clinical question is whether a patient with pelvic pain and a missed menstrual period has an intrauterine pregnancy, an ectopic pregnancy, or an incomplete or missed abortion. An imaging study is not appropriate until the results of a pregnancy test are available. As mentioned earlier, if suspected gestational age is greater than 5 weeks, an intrauterine gestational sac should be identified. In addition, fetal components should be seen within this ges-

TABLE 7-2 ■ **Common Indications for Use of Ultrasound during Pregnancy***

Size/dates discrepancy ≥2 wk
Multiple gestation
Uterine growth less than expected between prenatal visits
Vaginal bleeding
Suspected placental abruption
Suspected congenital anomaly with abnormal estradiol, human chorionic gonadotropin, or α-fetoprotein
First-degree relative with congenital anomaly
Assistance in obtaining amniotic fluid
Obstetric history of congenital anomaly, microsomia (<10th percentile body weight), macrosomia (>90th percentile body weight), or placental structural abnormality
Maternal disease including hypertension, congenital heart disease, diabetes mellitus, renal disease, connective tissue disease, parvovirus, cytomegalovirus, rubella, toxoplasmosis, pre-eclampsia, eclampsia, or human immunodeficiency virus
Follow-up of prior identified abnormalities including oligo- or polyhydramnios, intrauterine growth retardation, placental previa
Suspected fetal demise (no movement or unable to locate heartbeat with Doppler)
Estimate fetal size before elective pregnancy termination
Preterm labor or rupture of membranes <36 wk

* "Routine" ultrasound or ultrasound for the sole purpose of identifying sex of the fetus is not necessary.

TABLE 7-3 ■ **Measurements versus Gestational Age in Early Pregnancy**

Gestational Sac Size* (mm)	Crown-rump Length (mm)	Gestational Age (wk)
10	—	5.0
13	2.0	5.5
17	3.7	6.0
20	5.5	6.5
24	7.4	7.0
27	11.3	7.5
31	14.7	8.0
34	18.2	8.5
—	21.9	9.0
—	30.5	10
—	40.4	11
—	51.7	12

* If sac is not round, use the average diameter.

tational sac, particularly if transvaginal ultrasound is used.

Patients with an ectopic pregnancy almost always have pain and bleeding, but only 40% will have a palpable adnexal mass. On ultrasound, a normal-looking uterus and normal

TABLE 7-4 ■ **Fetal Measurements versus Gestational Age**

Gestational Age (wk)	Biparietal Diameter (mm)	Abdominal Circumference (mm) (5th and 95th %)	Femur Length (mm) (50th %)
12	19	—	13.3
14	26	—	14
16	33	105 (85, 126)	17
18	40	129 (108, 150)	26
20	47	152 (132, 173)	32
22	52	175 (154, 196)	37
24	58	197 (176, 218)	42
26	64	219 (198, 239)	47
28	69	240 (219, 260)	53
30	74	260 (239, 281)	57
32	79	280 (259, 300)	62
34	83	299 (279, 320)	67
36	88	318 (297, 339)	71
38	92	336 (316, 357)	76
40	96	354 (333, 374)	80

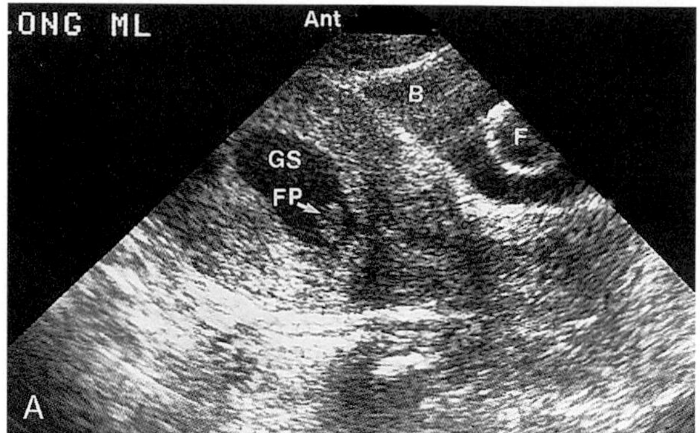

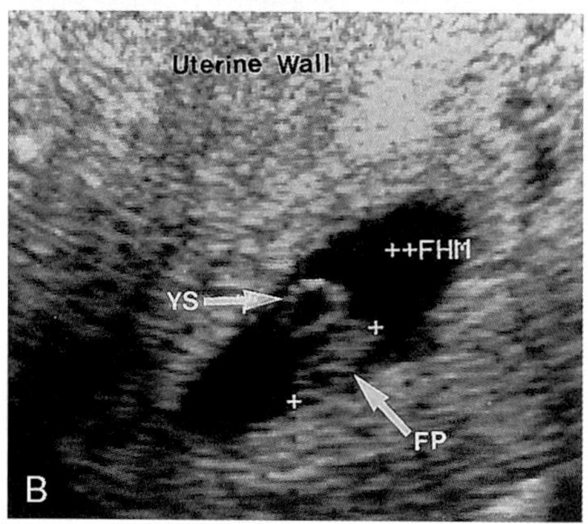

FIGURE 7-44 ■ **Early normal obstetric ultrasound.** A longitudinal transabdominal ultrasound image *(A)* demonstrates the bladder (B) and a Foley catheter (F) within it. Superior to and behind the bladder is the uterus with a gestational sac (GS) centrally and a fetal pole (FP) within it. More detail can be obtained by using transvaginal ultrasound *(B)*. In this case, the fetal pole can be measured; a yolk sac (YS) also is seen; and the technician has indicated that fetal heart motion was seen. (FHM).

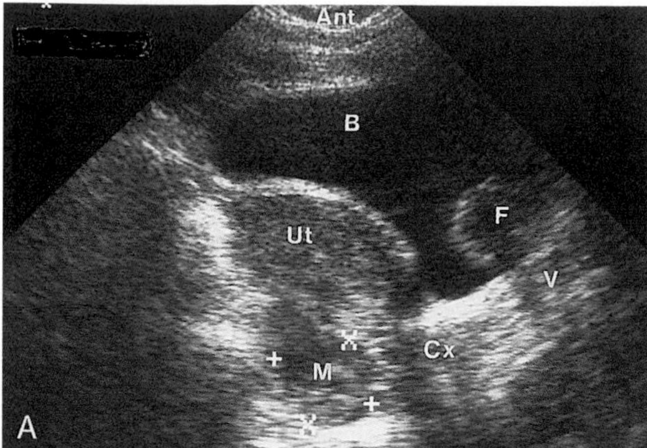

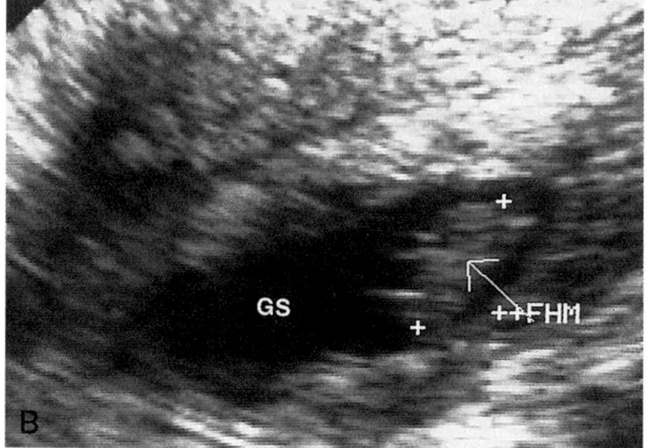

FIGURE 7-45 ■ **Ectopic pregnancy.** A longitudinal transabdominal image *(A)* clearly shows the bladder (B), uterus (Ut), and cervix (Cx). A Foley catheter (F) is within the bladder. A mass (M) is noted and marked behind the uterus. A transvaginal ultrasound *(B)* was performed to achieve better detail of this abnormality. A gestational sac (GS), a fetal pole, and fetal heart motion (FHM) were identified in this ectopic pregnancy.

adnexal areas do not exclude an ectopic pregnancy. Under these circumstances, a repeated examination in 7 to 10 days may be necessary. If the uterus appears normal and a complex adnexal mass is present, the likelihood of an ectopic pregnancy should be considered high. Sometimes a gestational sac and fetal heart motion can be seen outside the uterus. In these circumstances, the diagnosis of an ectopic pregnancy is certain (Fig. 7-45).

If an empty gestational sac is seen within the uterus, it may represent a very early intrauterine pregnancy, particularly if the diameter of the sac is 10 to 20 mm. It also may represent a blighted ovum or a pseudogestational sac in a patient with an ectopic pregnancy. A pseudogestational sac is seen in approximately 20% of patients with ectopic pregnancies.

In the second and third trimesters of pregnancy, quite complete ultrasonic evaluation of the fetus is possible. The most common reason for an ultrasound at this stage is to determine placental location, fetal growth, and gestational age. The earlier in pregnancy that gestational age is determined, the more accurate it will be. Dating is done by measuring the biparietal diameter of the head (Fig. 7-46) as well as the length of the femur and other structures. At the same time, an evaluation should be made of the intracranial structures, the heart (to see that it has four chambers), and the abdominal organs to look for abnormalities such as duodenal atresia, obstructed kidneys, and defects in the spine and anterior abdominal wall.

Radiation during Pregnancy

X-ray examinations may be done during pregnancy but only after careful consideration. Little, if any, reason exists to use x-ray images in the management of labor. Occasionally x-rays may be needed during pregnancy; for example, they may be taken to assess potential injuries of the spine, pelvis, or hips after an automobile accident. Under these circumstances, it must be ensured that the same information cannot be obtained by using ultrasonography. If x-ray examinations are necessary, it is prudent to first determine the information that is needed and whether the examination can be tailored or done with fewer than the normal number of views (Fig. 7-47). If the uterus is not in the direct beam (e.g., a chest x-ray) and the dose is quite low, little potential risk occurs to the fetus. If the fetus is in the direct beam and the examination is needed, it should be done, although a somewhat increased risk of neoplasm is present in the child and possibly later in life. Informed consent is usually obtained. A physicist usually calculates the fetal dose, and it is placed in the medical record. The fetal radiation dose from a ventilation/perfusion lung scan is low and should not be cause for concern. Fluoroscopy gives relatively high doses, and pelvic or lower abdominal fluoroscopy should be avoided during pregnancy unless no alternative is available.

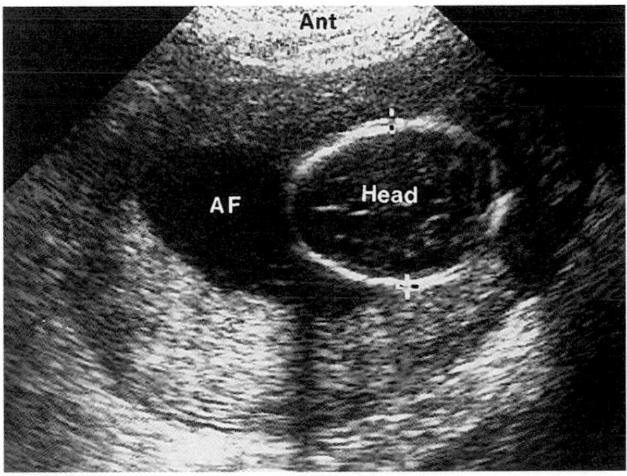

FIGURE 7-46 ■ Measurement of biparietal diameter. A transabdominal ultrasound image is done to find and measure the greatest biparietal diameter. This is one of the measurements used for estimating fetal age. Amniotic fluid (AF) is clearly seen.

Pelvic Inflammatory Disease

Pelvic inflammatory disease is an inflammatory syndrome of the upper genital tract in women and is most commonly associated with *Neisseria gonorrhoeae* and *Chlamydia trachomatis*. The diagnosis is made clinically with the combination of lower abdominal tenderness, bilateral adnexal tenderness, and cervical motion tenderness. Associated inflammatory bowel symptoms may be present. Imaging plays a small role in simple pelvic inflammatory disease, but about 15% of patients with acute pelvic inflammatory disease have a tubo-ovarian abscess. This is best detected with ultrasonography, although CT and laparoscopy also can be used.

Pelvic Pain and Masses

Pelvic pain should be classified as acute or chronic. In most cases, patient age, medical history, physical examination, complete blood cell count, pregnancy test, and urinalysis help assign priorities for the differential diagnosis. An ultrasound examination with Doppler is the imaging test of choice for suspected ectopic pregnancy, tubo-ovarian abscess, and ovarian torsion. It identifies any free fluid in the cul-de-sac. No good imaging test exists for endometriosis;

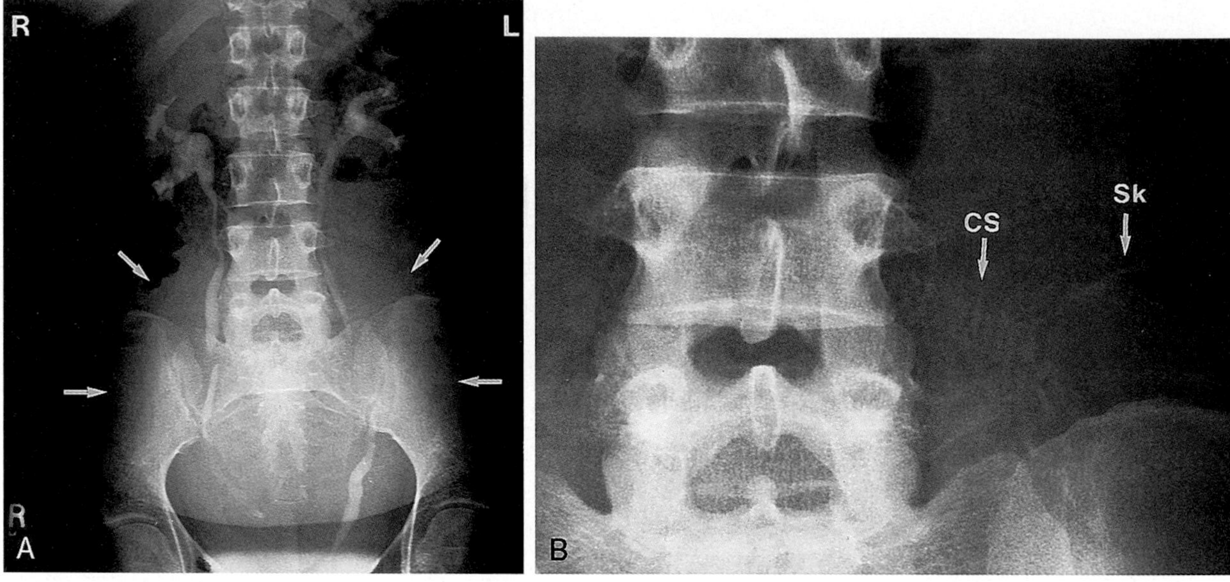

FIGURE 7-47 ■ Tailored intravenous pyelogram during pregnancy. This young pregnant woman was in a motor vehicle accident and had hematuria. Clinicians wished an assessment of bony structures as well as an assessment of renal function. Rather than do all the routine images of an intravenous pyelogram, only a single image was taken at 10 min after injection *(A)*. This showed the enlarged uterus *(arrows)* and bony structures, as well as both kidneys and ureters. A close-up view *(B)* clearly shows the fetal skull (Sk) as well as the fetal cervical spine (CS). This procedure has about one-tenth the fetal radiation dose of a computed tomography (CT) scan.

therefore that diagnosis is usually made laparoscopically.

An ovarian lesion is the most common pelvic mass in women, but other etiologies such as uterine, bladder, and intestinal lesions also must be considered. Most masses are found during routine pelvic examination, and the size, shape, and location are determined. Associated symptoms such as fever, pain, or menstrual abnormalities can provide valuable clues. Laboratory tests such as a complete blood cell count, a urinalysis, and a CA-125 assay also are potentially helpful. In terms of imaging, although an IVP, CT scan, or barium enema can provide some information, the initial imaging test should be a pelvic ultrasound. It provides information about the internal structure and vascularity of the mass. Although no imaging test is quite accurate in differentiating benign from malignant pelvic

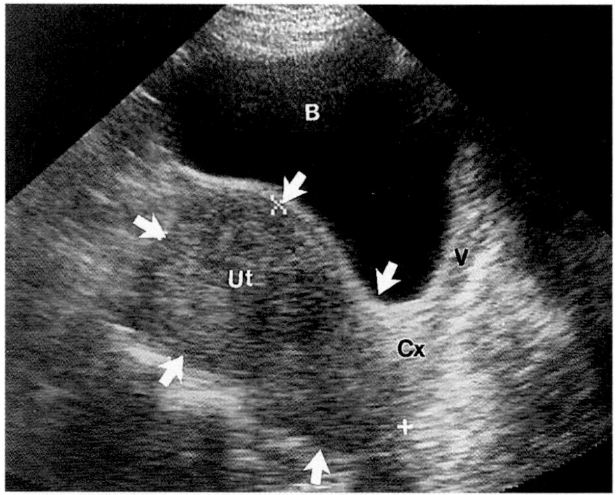

FIGURE 7-48 ■ Ultrasound of uterine fibroids. A longitudinal transabdominal view of the pelvis shows that the uterus (Ut) is enlarged and lumpy *(arrows)*. The echo pattern within the uterus is inhomogeneous; this is the most common appearance of uterine fibroids.

masses, if septations, irregular solid portions, or ascites is present, malignancy should be considered, and surgery or laparoscopy may be performed.

Tumors

The most common benign uterine tumor is a fibroid. These are often calcified and are seen on x-rays in the central portion of the pelvis. The calcification is typically somewhat popcorn shaped (see Fig. 6-17). This finding is usually incidental, because x-rays should not be ordered to look for uterine fibroids. The most common method used to image uterine fibroids and other pelvic masses, as mentioned earlier, is ultrasound. Fibroids will enlarge the uterus in a lumpy fashion and make the internal echo pattern very inhomogeneous (Fig. 7-48). Although it is difficult to differentiate fibroids from endometrial carcinoma on ultrasound, this is easily done on clinical grounds, because most endometrial carcinomas are associated with bleeding. Dermoid tumors typically contain hair, teeth, and sebaceous secretions. Often a molar-type tooth can be seen on an x-ray of the pelvis (Fig. 7-49).

Most ovarian tumors are cystadenomas or cystadenocarcinomas. Both benign and malignant tumors are bilateral in a fair number of cases. When an ovarian tumor is suspected, ultrasound imaging should optimally be done in the first 10 days of the menstrual cycle to minimize the presence of benign ovarian cysts. Cystadenomas and cystadenocarcinomas are usually large cystic adnexal lesions.

One of the most frequent clinical presentations of ovarian carcinoma is increasing weight and abdominal girth due to the presence of ascites. Pleural effusions also are common. CT scanning is often done for suspected pelvic malignancies to determine the size of the mass, possible involvement of pelvic side walls, and ureteral obstruction, as well as to look for metastatic disease. The finding of a pelvic mass on CT or ultrasound is usually somewhat nonspecific, although if the mass can be traced down into the pelvis and into the adnexa, it is most likely of ovarian origin. Ovarian carcinoma may involve the bowel, particularly the serosa (Fig. 7-50).

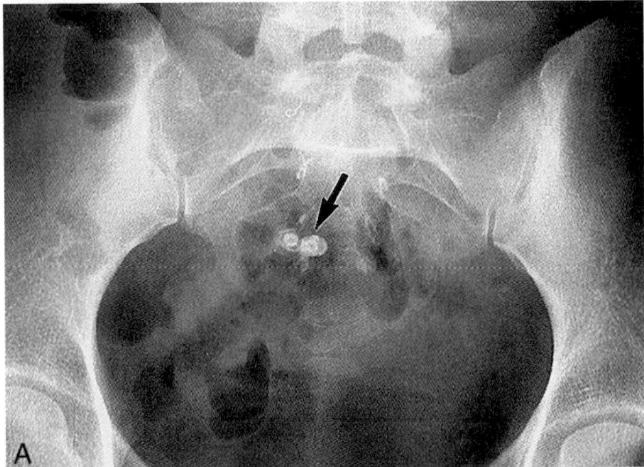

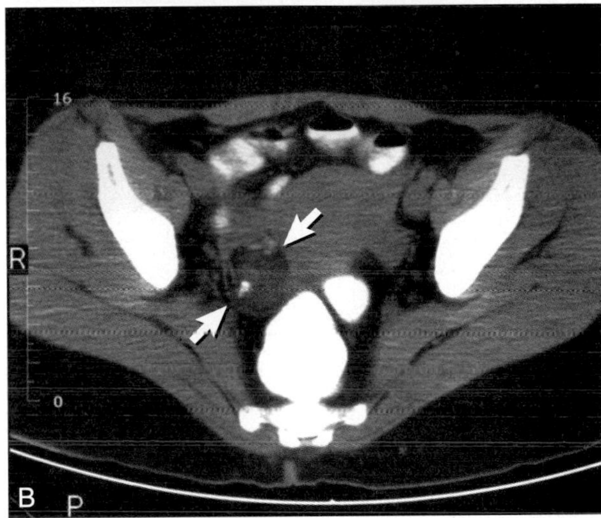

FIGURE 7-49 ■ **Ovarian teratoma.** A plain film of the pelvis *(A)* shows a relatively classic molar tooth calcification *(arrow)*. A computed tomography (CT) scan of the pelvis in a different patient shows a right adenexal mass *(arrow)* also containing a central calcification *(B)*.

Carcinoma of the cervix is usually found during annual examination and with a Papanicolaou (Pap) smear. Once a cervical carcinoma has been found, CT or MR scanning can assess the overall size of the tumor and the potential presence of metastases. Often this cancer will obstruct the cervical canal and cause buildup of fluid within the uterus. Cervical carcinomas tend to obstruct the distal ureters, and renal obstruction is the most frequent cause of death from this tumor. Evaluation can initially be done by using an intravenous pyelogram (IVP) (Fig. 7-51); however, in follow-up of these patients, it is probably cheaper and safer to look for potentially obstructed kidneys by means of ultrasound. In contrast to ovarian carcinoma, cervical carcinomas often spread locally and involve lymph nodes (Fig. 7-52). Even though CT can detect metastases if the lymph nodes are enlarged, its accuracy for detection of metastases from cervical carcinoma is only 65%, because the nodes may have small metastatic deposits and not be enlarged.

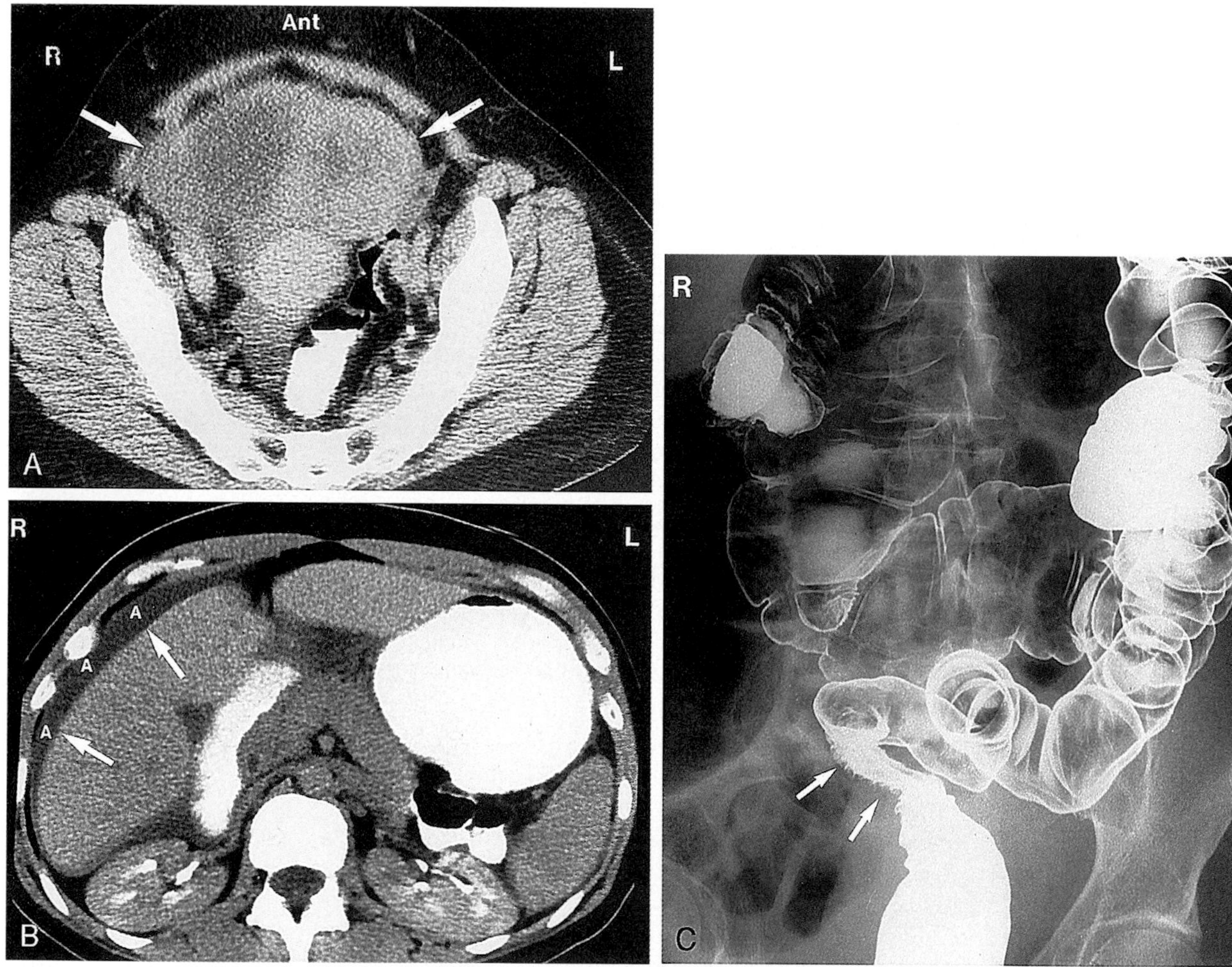

FIGURE 7-50 ■ **Ovarian carcinoma.** A transverse computed tomography (CT) scan through the pelvis *(A)* shows a large soft tissue mass *(arrows)*. Some low-density areas lie within this, suggesting necrosis. A CT scan performed higher in the abdomen *(B)* shows a small amount of ascites over the lateral aspect of the liver. A barium enema performed on the same patient *(C)* shows narrowing of the rectosigmoid with fine toothlike serrations (arrows), indicating serosal involvement by the tumor.

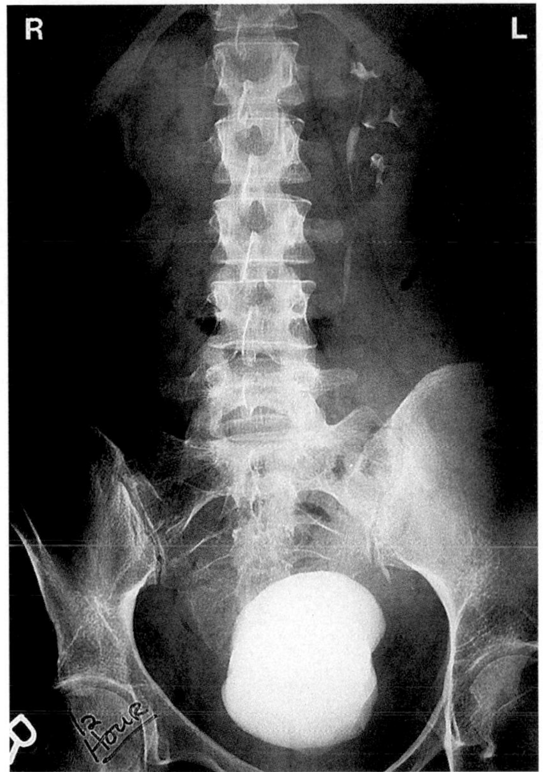

FIGURE 7-51 ■ **Carcinoma of the cervix.** On this intravenous pyelogram, the left kidney is clearly identified and is functional. No contrast is seen in the collecting system of the right kidney due to obstruction of the distal right ureter by the cervical carcinoma.

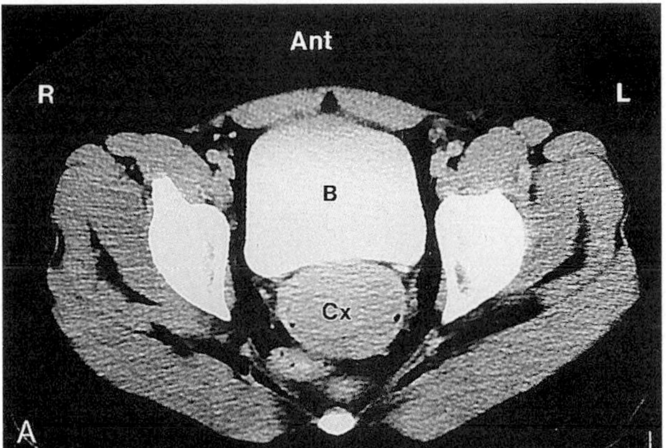

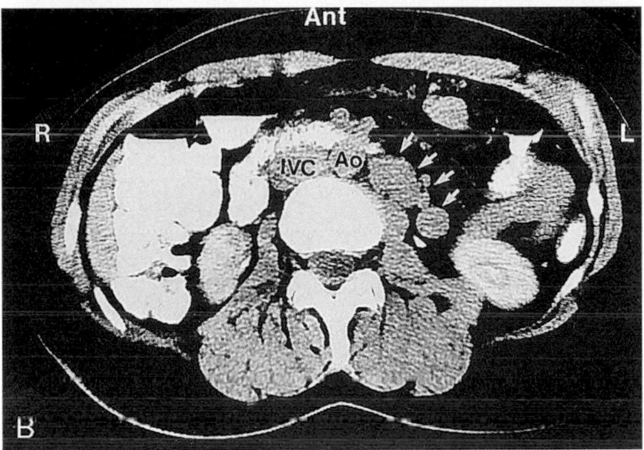

FIGURE 7-52 ■ **Cervical carcinoma.** The soft tissue extent of cervical carcinoma (Cx) is seen on a transverse computed tomography (CT) scan of the lower pelvis *(A)*. An image obtained higher in the abdomen *(B)* shows the inferior vena cava (IVC) and the aorta (Ao), but lateral to the aorta are multiple soft tissue structures representing nodes *(arrows)* enlarged with metastatic disease.

ADRENAL GLANDS AND RETROPERITONEUM

Adrenal Glands

The adrenal glands are not normally visualized on a plain x-ray image of the abdomen. They can be seen if prior hemorrhage or infection has produced calcification or if a tumor or mass large enough to displace the kidney is present in the adrenal. Most anatomy texts would have you believe that the adrenal gland sits on top of the kidney like a little cap. This is not true. The right adrenal gland is located above and slightly anterior to the right kidney, and it is between the right lobe of the liver and the crus of the diaphragm. Often it can be seen on a CT scan as just a small line. The left adrenal gland likewise does not sit on top of the left kidney but actually sits just anterior and slightly medial to the upper pole of the left kidney. The left adrenal gland typically has an upside-down "Y" shape. If you suspect adrenal pathology, the imaging study of choice is a CT scan (Fig. 7-53).

The width of the adrenal gland should be less than 1 cm, and the limbs of the Y should be 3 to 6 mm thick. Masses in the adrenal glands are the result of adenomas (50%) (Fig. 7-54),

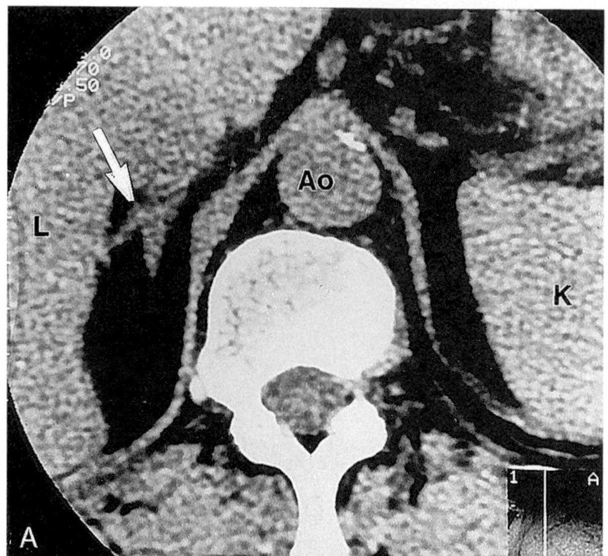

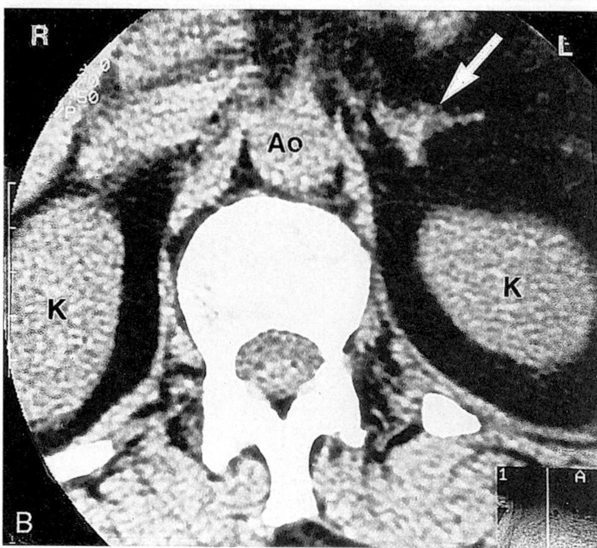

FIGURE 7-53 ■ **Normal adrenal anatomy.** A coned-down computed tomography (CT) scan of the upper abdomen above the level of the right kidney *(A)* shows the right adrenal gland *(arrow)*. It is usually shaped like an upside-down V or a thin line. The left adrenal gland is seen on a slightly lower CT cut *(B)* and is a triangular structure anterior and slightly medial to the upper pole of the left kidney.

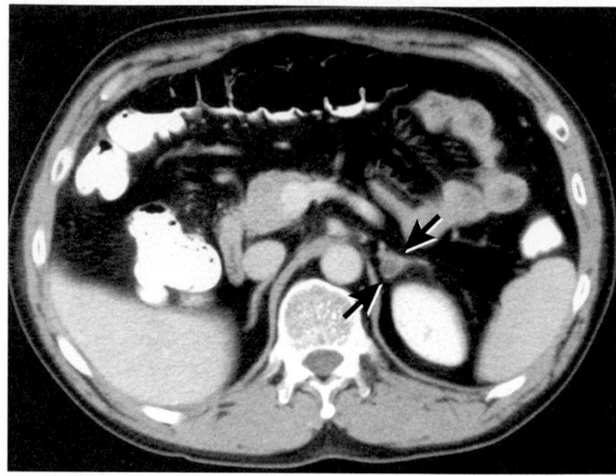

FIGURE 7-54 ■ **Adrenal adenoma.** On a computed tomography (CT) scan, incidental note was observed of a small (about 1 cm) left adrenal mass *(arrow)*. This small size combined with a relatively low-density (dark) center is consistent with a benign adrenal adenoma. Note that any adrenal mass larger than several centimeters should be suggestive of malignancy

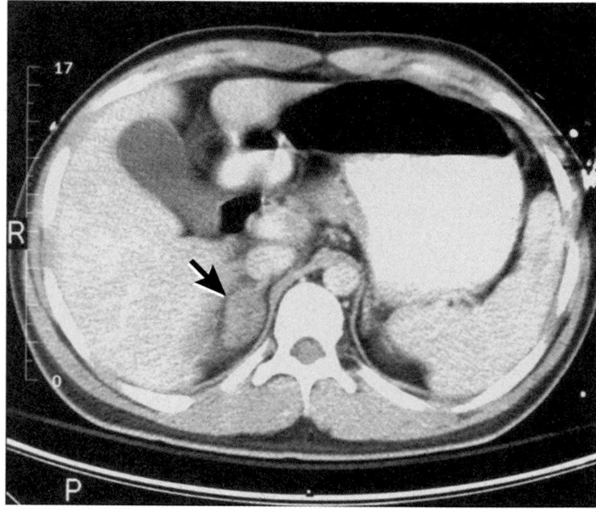

FIGURE 7-55 ■ **Adrenal hematoma.** A computed tomography (CT) scan obtained immediately after an auto accident shows a soft tissue–density mass in the right adrenal *(arrow)*.

metastases (35%), pheochromocytoma (10%), lymphoma, and neuroblastoma (in children younger than 2 years). An adrenal adenoma usually is low density (dark) on CT and occurs in about 3% of persons. It is most often found as an incidental finding on CT. After trauma, enlargement of an adrenal gland is usually due to a hematoma (Fig. 7-55).

An adrenal lesion in excess of 2 cm to 3 cm in diameter that is not low density on CT should be considered a malignancy. Bilateral adrenal masses are usually the result of metastases, bilateral pheochromocytoma, lymphoma, and granulomatous diseases. At autopsy, about 25% of individuals who died of cancer have adrenal metastases. Lung, breast, stomach, colon, and kidney are the most common primary lesions to metastasize to the adrenal gland. In a patient with cancer and an adrenal mass, a high probability exists that the latter is metastatic (Fig. 7-56).

Adrenal hyperplasia may be nodular, as in Cushing's syndrome, or smooth, as in 25% of patients with Conn's syndrome. Both these diseases are related to hormone overproduction (adrenocorticotropic hormone [ACTH], cortisol, or aldosterone), which may be caused by an adenoma, tumor, or hyperplasia. The primary diagnosis for most of these lesions is made by evaluation of serum or urine hormone levels. Tumors and clinically significant functional adenomas can usually be localized by CT, but hyperplasia can be difficult to differentiate from normal glands. Most pheochromocytomas (90%) occur in the adrenal medulla, and 10% are bilateral. Occasionally they occur elsewhere in the abdomen. Localization should be done by using a nuclear medicine scan with a substance called *meta*-iodobenzylguanidine (MIBG) or by MRI.

Retroperitoneal Adenopathy and Neoplasms

CT scanning is the only convenient and practical way to assess patients for retroperitoneal adenopathy. As mentioned earlier in this chapter, patients can have normal-sized lymph nodes that have microscopic metastases. Therefore you should not automatically assume that if adenopathy is absent, no spread of tumor exists. When nodal enlargement occurs in a patient with a known neoplasm, the chances of malignant involvement are high, although not certain, because some patients have hyperplastic lymph nodes without actual tumor involvement.

CT scanning not only can identify adenopathy but also can be used on a serial basis to assess the results of therapy. Unless intravenous contrast is given, it can be difficult to differentiate a large mass of lymphadenopathy about the aorta from an abdominal aortic aneurysm. Another major advantage of CT is that you can look at the abdominal organs and mesenteric regions for metastatic disease while you are searching for adenopathy (Fig. 7-57).

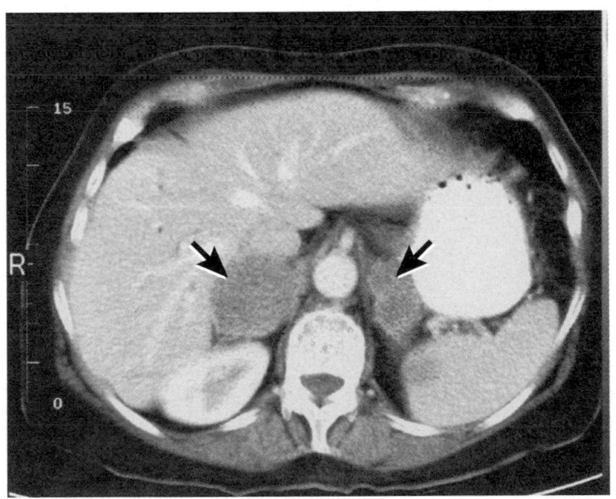

FIGURE 7-56 ■ **Bilateral adrenal metastases.** A contrast-enhanced computed tomography (CT) scan of the upper abdomen shows bilateral adrenal masses *(arrows)* due to metastases from lung carcinoma.

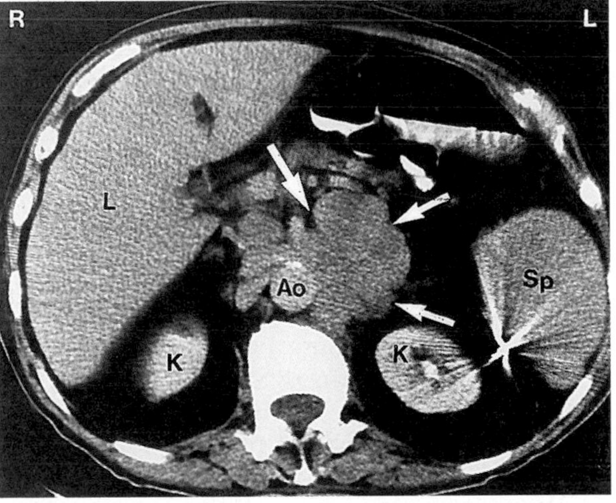

FIGURE 7-57 ■ **Retroperitoneal lymphoma.** In this young patient with suspected Hodgkin's disease, a contrast-enhanced computed tomography (CT) scan clearly shows the kidneys (K) and the aorta (Ao). The aorta is surrounded by a lobular soft tissue mass *(arrows)* due to lymphoma.

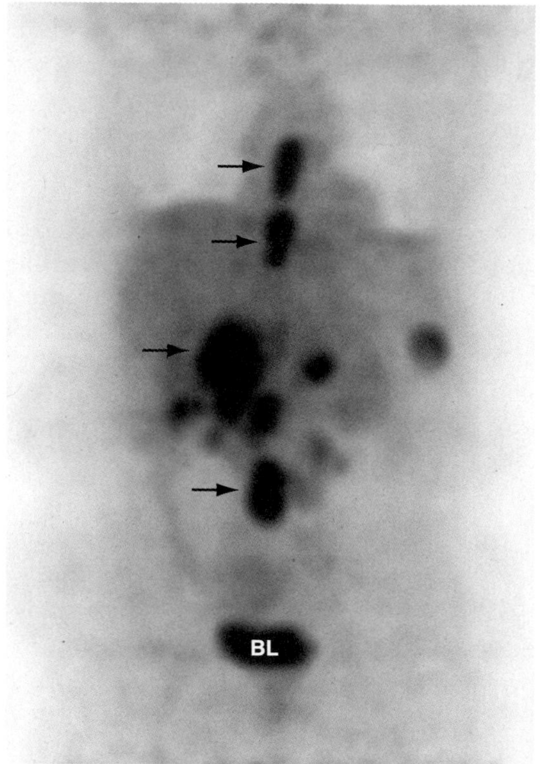

FIGURE 7-58 ■ **Staging of lymphoma.** An anterior nuclear medicine positron emission tomography (PET) scan of the chest and abdomen done with fluorine 18 fluorodeoxyglucose demonstrates multiple areas of increased activity throughout the abdomen and lower chest (some shown with *arrows*). Activity in the kidneys and bladder (Bl) is normal.

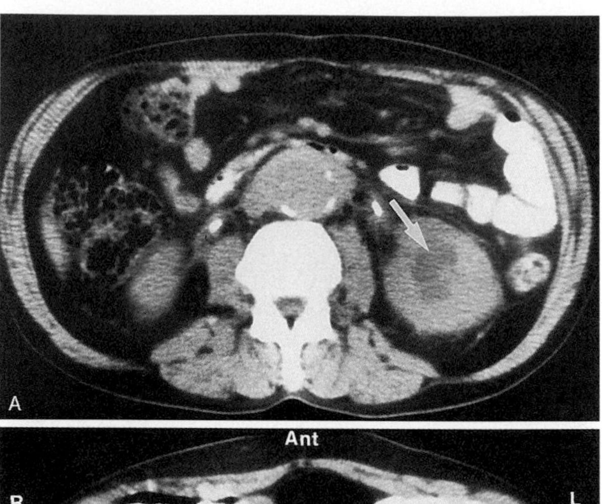

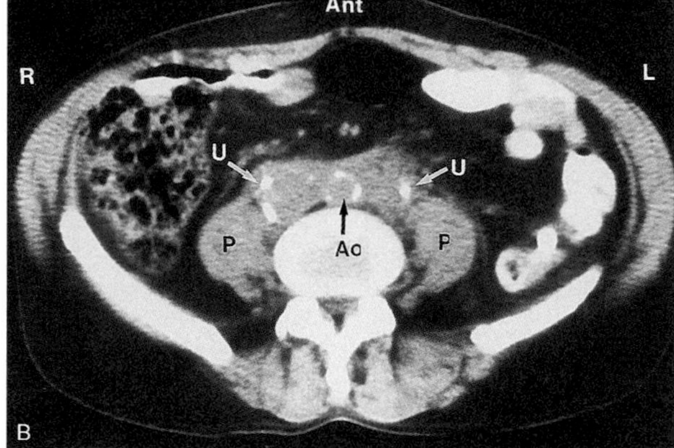

FIGURE 7-59 ■ **Retroperitoneal fibrosis.** A computed tomography (CT) scan at the lower level of the kidneys *(A)* shows dilation of the left renal pelvis *(arrow)* and, incidentally, a slightly dilated aorta. A scan obtained just below the iliac crest in the same patient *(B)* again shows the aortic wall outlined by calcium. The right and left ureters (U) are pulled medially and encased by a soft tissue mass caused by retroperitoneal fibrosis. The white densities in the ureters are from stents or tubes placed in the ureters to relieve obstruction. The psoas muscles (P) also are easily seen.

Lymphoma can involve multiple portions of the body, but adenopathy is common in the mediastinum, mesentery, and retroperitoneal areas. CT scans can identify enlarged nodes but cannot tell whether the disease is active. In the past, staging for lymphoma was often done by using whole-body nuclear medicine scans with gallium 67. This has largely been replaced with nuclear medicine positron emission tomography (PET) scans, which give a good indication not only of location of disease but also of activity (Fig. 7-58).

Retroperitoneal fibrosis can be confused with an aneurysm or retroperitoneal adenopathy. The distinction is not always easy to make on CT. One differentiating factor is that with retroperitoneal fibrosis, usually medial deviation of the ureters appears because of traction by the fibrotic process (Fig. 7-59). With adenopathy and aneurysms, there is usually lateral deviation of the ureters by a soft tissue mass.

General Textbooks on the Topic

Davidson AJ, Hartman DS, Choyke PL, Wagner BJ: Davidson's Radiology of the Kidney and Genitourinary Tract, 3rd ed. Philadelphia, WB Saunders, 1999.

Dunnick NR, Sandler CM, Newhouse JH, Amis S Jr: Textbook of Uroradiology, 3rd ed. Philadelphia, Lippincott Williams & Wilkins, 2000.

8 Skeletal System

INTRODUCTION

Fractures and other abnormalities involving the skull and face were covered in Chapter 2. Initial imaging studies for a number of clinical problems are presented in Table 8-1. A few general comments should be made about the structure of bone. Most bones consist of a densely calcified cortex, or shell, that surrounds the medullary space. The medullary space contains either active (red) marrow or fatty replaced (yellow) marrow. In the adult, red marrow is found in the skull, ribs, spine, pelvis, and proximal portions of the femurs and humeri. Because this red marrow acts as a filter, most bone metastases begin in these locations and chew outward until they involve the cortex.

TABLE 8–1 ■ **Initial Imaging Studies of Choice for Various Musculoskeletal Problems**

Clinical Problem	Imaging Study
Fracture	Plain x-ray
Occult hip fracture	MRI or bone scan
Occult knee fracture	MRI
Stress fracture	Nuclear medicine bone scan
Metastases	Nuclear medicine bone scan, plain x-ray in area of pain
Osteomyelitis	Plain x-ray; if negative, then nuclear medicine three-phase bone scan or MRI
Low back pain	Bed rest (for several weeks).
Without radiculopathy	Imaging not indicated
With radiculopathy	Noncontrasted CT or MRI
Arthritis (nonseptic)	Plain x-ray
Suspected septic arthritis	Joint aspiration, plain x-ray
Monoarticular joint pain	Plain x-ray, if conservative therapy fails, then MRI
Infection or loosening of prosthetic joint	Plain x-ray, if negative nuclear medicine bone scan
Reflex sympathetic dystrophy	Plain x-ray, if negative three-phase nuclear medicine bone scan

CT, computed tomography; MRI, magnetic resonance imaging.

The midportion of the long bones is referred to as the *diaphysis*. Toward the ends of long bones is the *metaphysis*, which extends up to the *epiphyseal plate*. Beyond the epiphyseal plate is the *epiphysis*. An epiphysis by definition involves a joint space. Occasionally growth centers are found on portions of long bones where the joint space is not involved (for example, along the greater trochanter of the femur). These centers are referred to as *apophyses*.

Growth of long bones occurs primarily at the epiphyseal plate, when new bone is added to the lengthening metaphysis, and the epiphyseal plate moves farther along. Some growth occurs along the lateral periosteum as well, to allow the bones to become thicker with age. Some epiphyses are present at birth, and most are closed by age 20 years. The different parts of long bones are important, because some lesions will preferentially affect only certain parts of the bone. For example, it is common for a Ewing's sarcoma to affect the diaphysis of a long bone, but it will rarely, if ever, affect the epiphysis.

The cortex of bone has fine white lines, which are the *trabeculae*. These are located predominantly along the lines of stress in the bone, and they provide little pillars of support. Occasional cross-linking trabeculae occur. With disuse, old age, or states of increased blood flow, calcium is carried away from bone. This does not occur in a random fashion but preferentially removes the cross-linking trabeculae first. As the process becomes more advanced, the trabeculae along the lines of stress are removed, and the bone becomes weakened and may be subject to compression fractures. This process is seen in older women. Often in a woman with osteoporosis, on the lateral chest x-ray, you will see only the outline of the thoracic vertebral bodies (because the trabeculae have been resorbed), and many mid- and upper thoracic wedge compression fractures are found. As is shown later, with disuse of an extremity or in hyperemic states, initial resorption of calcium occurs in a periarticular distribution because more blood flow is found here than along the shaft of bones.

A final word of caution before we begin: Most bone lesions will be relatively obvious to you as a result of the clinical history. More than 95% of bone films are obtained for evaluation of trauma, arthritis, degenerative conditions, or metastases. A number of classic fractures must be recognized; a few, if missed, can have dire consequences (especially cervical spine fractures). It is crucial that you spend time on these. Although some details of the various arthritic conditions are presented, these are relatively nonspecific and certainly not emergencies or life threatening. Primary bone tumors are very rare, and you should not expect to develop competence regarding these. In clinical practice (other than orthopedics or oncology), you probably will see a primary bone tumor once every 5 or 10 years. Most radiologists are lucky if they see three or four bone tumors per year. The main point is to be able to discern the lesions and refer them to a radiologist for a reasonable differential diagnosis.

CERVICAL SPINE

Normal Anatomy

The lateral view of the cervical spine is the initial view obtained, particularly in trauma cases. Table 8-2 provides a summary of how to evaluate a cervical spine examination done for trauma. Initial inspection should be directed toward the various contour lines of the cervical spine, which are shown in Figure 8-1. These include the anterior soft tissues, the anterior and posterior spinal line, the spinal laminal line, and the posterior spinous process line. On the lateral view, the cervical spine should be bowed forward and have a relatively smooth curve. No sharp angulation should be found at any level. If the patient was lying on a stretcher when the lateral view was taken, the neck is often somewhat flexed, and the cervical spine is straight rather than curved. When you see this, you cannot be sure whether the straightening is due simply to the supine positioning of the patient or to muscular spasm. If the trauma was relatively minor, an upright lateral x-ray of the cervical spine usually will solve the problem. If major trauma is suspected, a computed tomography (CT) or magnetic resonance imaging (MRI) scan may be needed.

Examination of the anterior soft tissues and spaces should be done at several vertebral levels. Evaluation of soft tissue width is typically not a problem unless the patient has an endotracheal tube in place, in which case, the normal air and soft tissue interface is obscured, and you will have to rely on other findings. Actual width of

TABLE 8–2 ■ **Items to Look for on a Trauma Anteroposterior and Lateral Cervical Spine Examination**

Lateral View
Count vertebral bodies to assure that all seven are seen (if not, consider swimmer's view or shallow oblique view)
Alignment
- Anterior vertebral body margins
- Posterior vertebral body margins
- Posterior spinal canal

Cervical curvature, straightening, or sudden angulation
Prevertebral soft tissue thickness (see text)
Widening of vertical distance between posterior processes
Common fractures
- C1 arch
- C2 odontoid
  - Arch (hangman's)
  - Widening between anterior arch of C1 and odontoid
- C3–C7 anterior avulsion
  - Wedge compression
- C6–C7 posterior process (clay-shoveler's)

Facets (to exclude unilateral locked facet)

Anterior View
Odontoid view
- Widening of the lateral portion of C1 relative to C2 (Jefferson's fracture)
- General alignment of lateral margins and spinous processes
- Lucent fracture lines

Oblique View (If No Major Trauma Is Suspected)
Neural foraminal narrowing
Alignment of facet joints

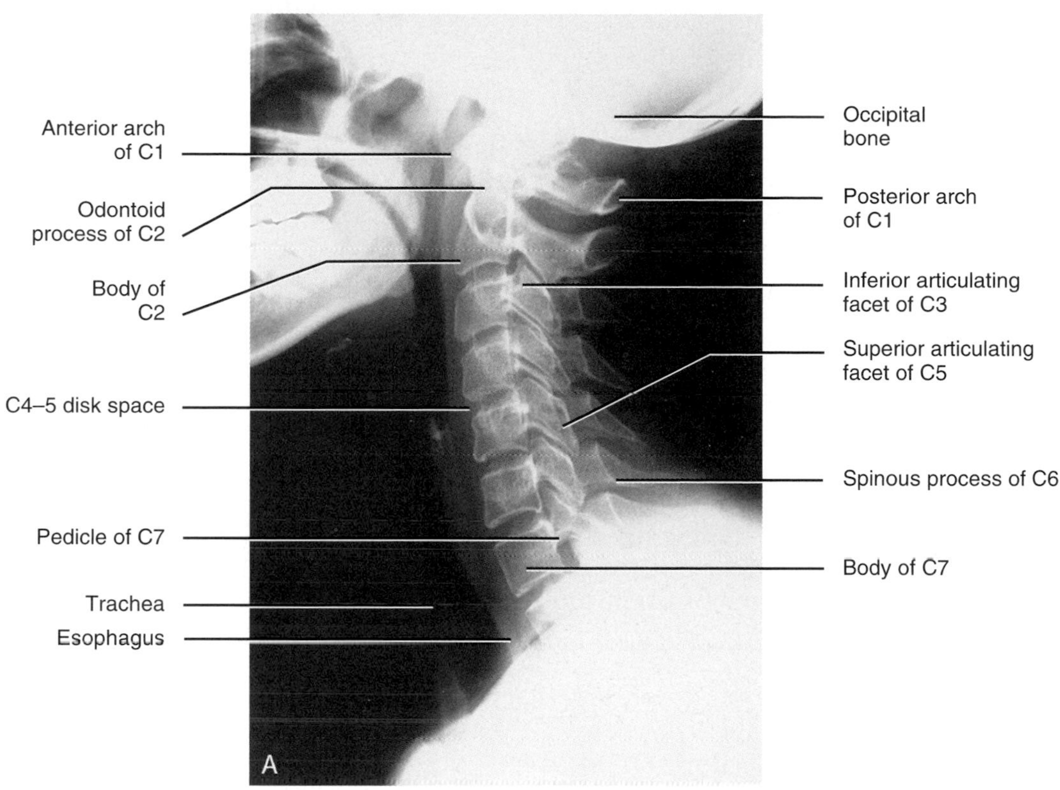

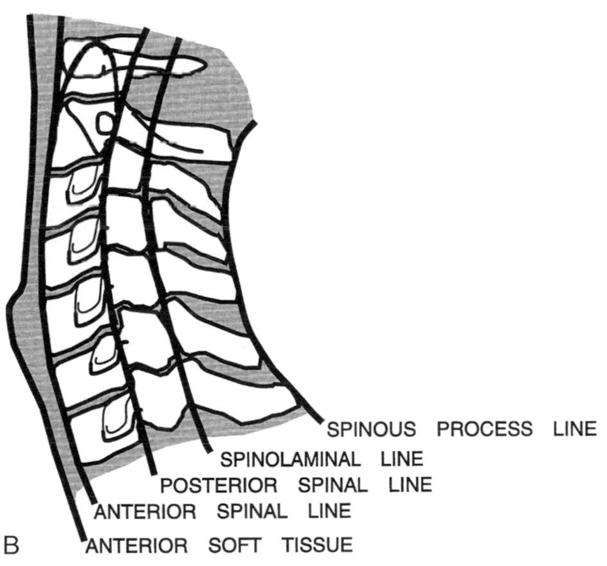

FIGURE 8-1 ■ Normal anatomy of the cervical spine in the lateral projection *(A)* and diagrammatically *(B)*.

the prevertebral soft tissues as measured on an image, of course, is dependent on the magnification that occurred as the x-ray was taken. On a portable trauma series (with the patient supine), the x-ray tube is often only 40 inches from the film cassette. As a result, significant magnification is seen, and a measurement of up to 7 mm may be normal in the prevertebral soft tissues at the C3 level. However, if the examination was done with the tube 72 inches, or 6 feet, from the film, the soft tissue normally should not exceed 4 to 5 mm.

Below the level of C4, the air column moves anteriorly in the region of the larynx; thickened soft tissue between the larynx and the vertebral bodies is due to the esophagus. Soft tissue anterior to the lower cervical bodies averages about 15 mm, with a range of 10 mm to 20 mm. If the soft tissue in this region equals or exceeds the width of the vertebra at or below the level of C4, pathology should be suspected.

Another measurement to note on the lateral view is the distance from the posterior aspect of the anterior arch of C1 to the most anterior portion of the odontoid. In an adult, this should not exceed 3 mm; in a child, it should not exceed 5 mm.

Examination of the bony contour lines is done to exclude subluxations. Remember that on the lateral view, you should be able to see down to at least the bottom of the C7 or the top of the T1 vertebral body. If difficulty is found in seeing this far down, because of the patient's shoulders being in the way, a swimmer's view can be ordered. For this view, one of the patient's arms is raised next to the head and the other arm placed down alongside the waist. This essentially raises one shoulder and lowers the other, allowing the x-ray beam to penetrate the area of the cervicothoracic junction more easily (Fig. 8-2).

Typically, two anterior views are done after the lateral cervical spine view has been examined by a physician and found to be free of fracture or subluxation. These are, first, the anterior view of the lower cervical spine with the mouth closed; this view is used to examine alignment and to exclude oblique fractures. Additionally, an open-mouth view of the odontoid is obtained (Fig. 8-3). This view

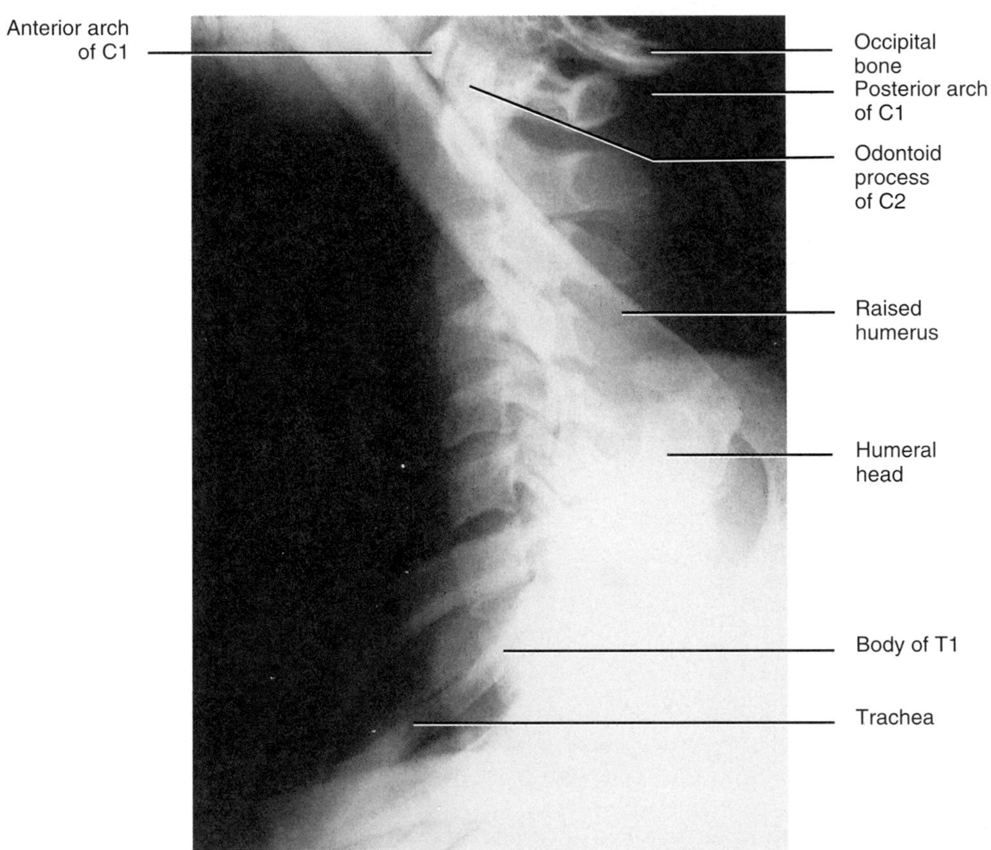

FIGURE 8-2 ■ Normal anatomy of the cervical spine on the lateral swimmer's view.

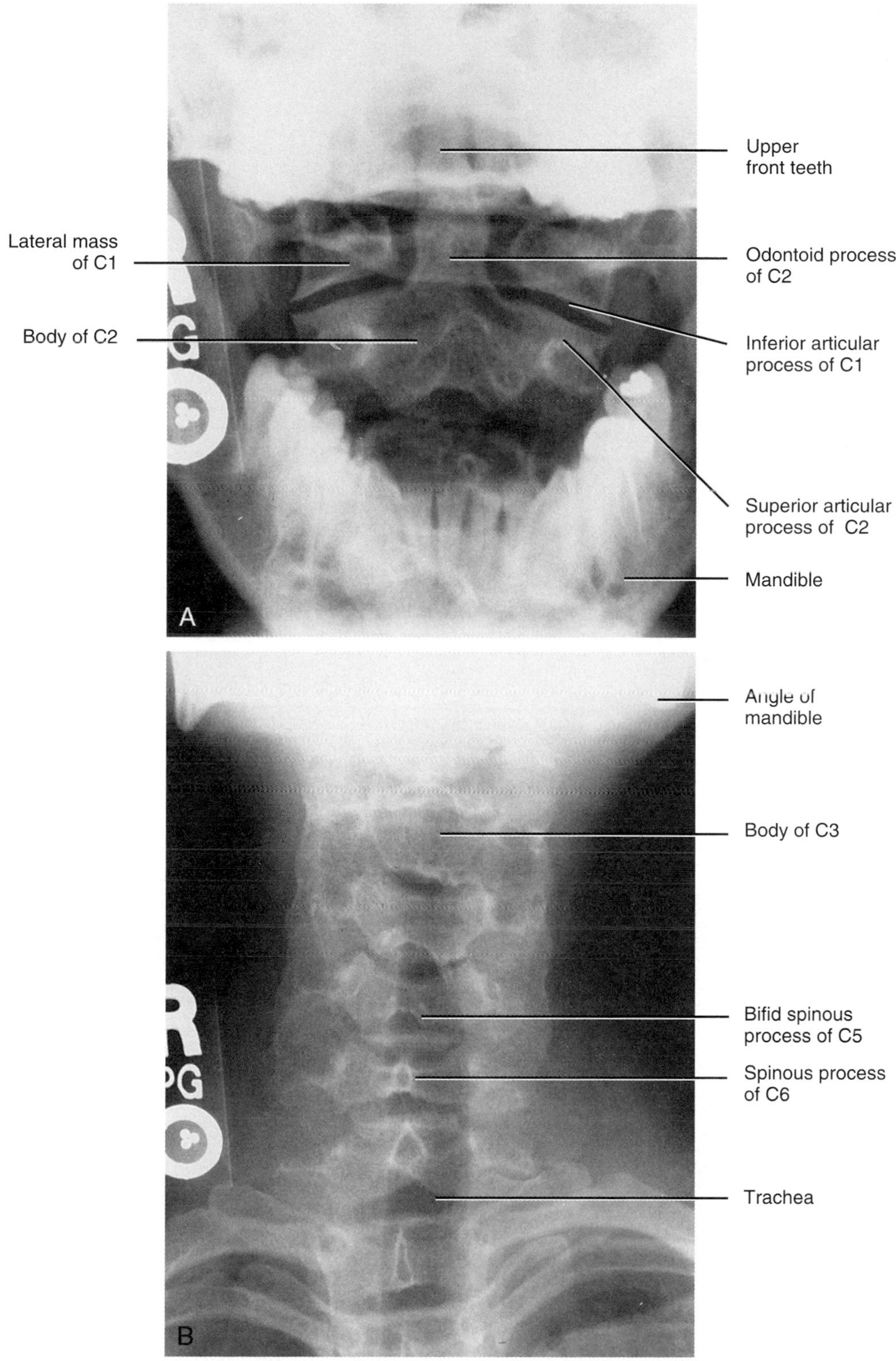

FIGURE 8-3 ■ Normal anatomy of the cervical spine on the anteroposterior (AP) odontoid view *(A)* and the standard AP cervical view *(B)*.

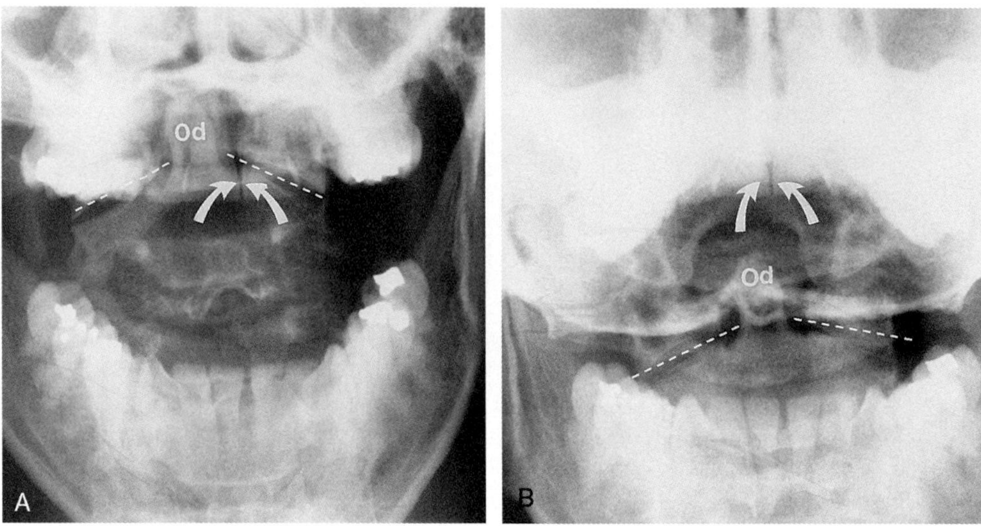

FIGURE 8-4 ■ Pseudofracture of C2. On the odontoid view *(A),* if the teeth project over the vertebral bodies, an air gap between the front teeth *(arrows)* can cause what appears to be a vertical fracture through either the odontoid process or the body of C2. The junction between the articular surfaces of lateral masses of C1 and C2 is indicated by the *dotted lines.* If a question remains, the pseudofracture artifact can be corrected by raising the maxilla and repeating the view *(B).*

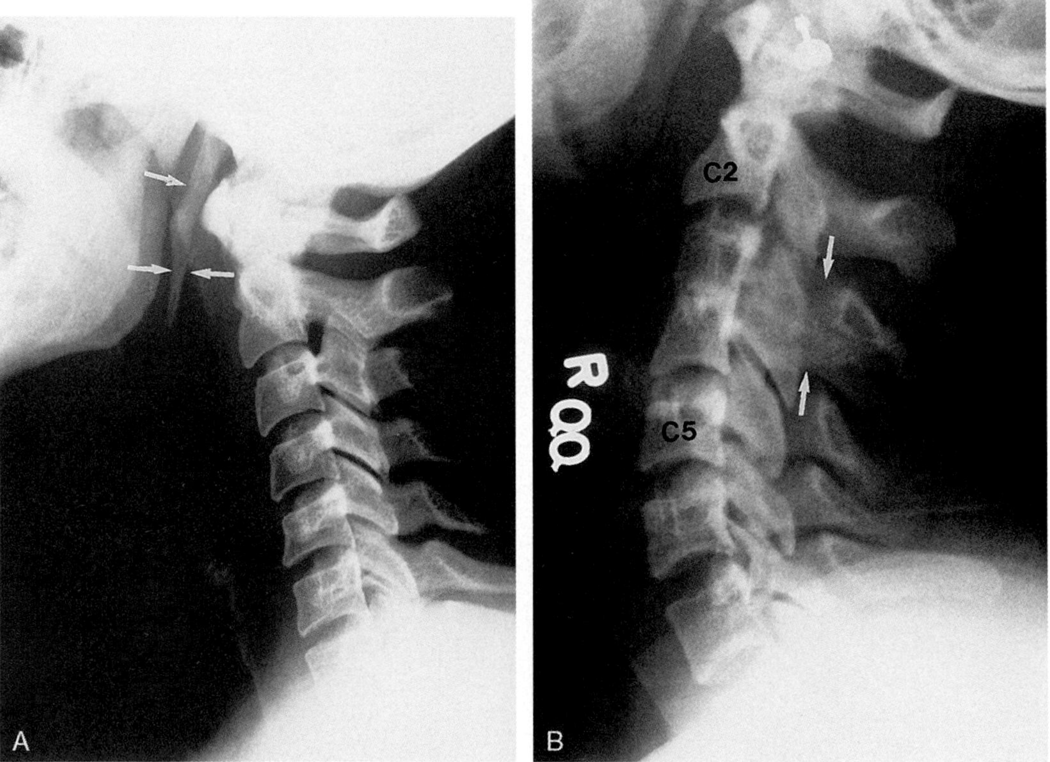

FIGURE 8-5 ■ Normal variants of the cervical spine. On the lateral view *(A),* often prominent calcification of the stylohyoid ligament appears, causing what looks like a long, calcified icicle. In a different patient, the lateral view demonstrates congenital fusion *(B)* of the bodies of C3 and C4. Note also that the posterior elements are fused.

shows the relation of the inferior aspect and lateral margins of C1 to the superior aspect and lateral margins of C2, and it also shows the odontoid very well. It is important to have the mouth open wide enough that the front teeth do not overlie the odontoid. If this happens, you can see the air gap between the two front teeth and mistakenly call this a fracture (Fig. 8-4).

Two relatively common normal variants appear on the lateral view. The first of these looks like a calcified spike or nail and represents calcification of the stylohyoid ligament. It is actually quite lateral, but on the lateral cervical spine view, it projects posterior to the mandible and anterior to C1 and C2 (Fig. 8-5). Another common variant is embryologic fusion of two or more vertebral bodies to create a "block" vertebra; this may be a complete or an incomplete fusion. Often a block vertebral body will cause abnormal motion, with associated early degenerative changes.

Oblique views of the cervical spine are obtained only when you are quite sure that no major trauma, fracture, or dislocation is present. The value of the oblique views is mostly to see whether impingement and narrowing of the neural foramina by bony degenerative spurs are present. On a good oblique view, you should be able to see the neural foramina very well from C2 down through T1 (Fig. 8-6). Additionally, look to see that the articular facets are lined up like shingles on a roof. This view may be helpful to see a unilateral perched, subluxed, or locked facet if CT is not available. Both CT and MRI are useful for imaging the cervical spine. CT is best suited to detecting subtle bony fractures, whereas MRI

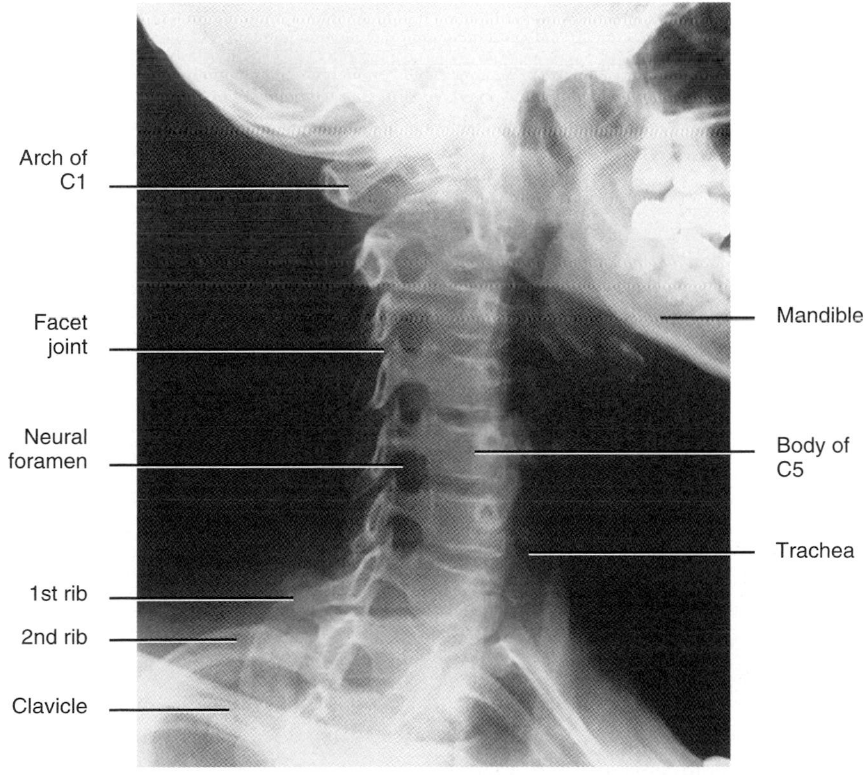

FIGURE 8-6 ■ Normal anatomy of the cervical spine on the oblique view.

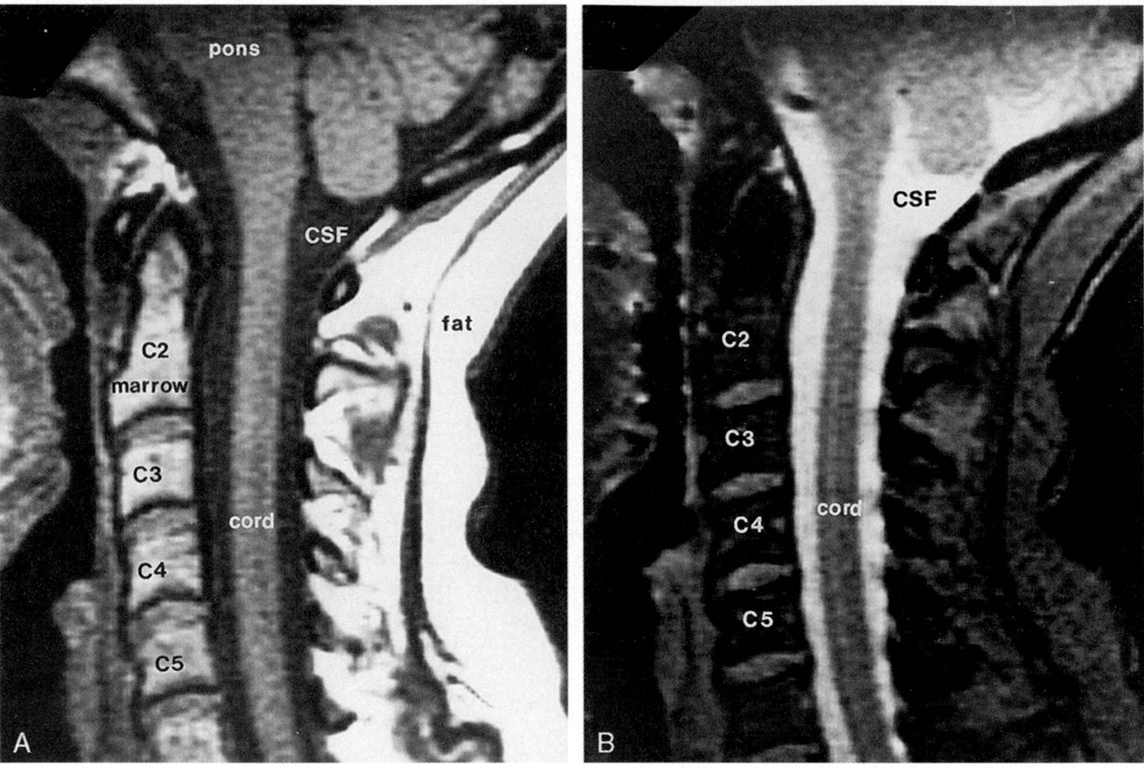

FIGURE 8-7 ■ Normal appearance of the cervical spine and spinal cord on magnetic resonance imaging. A sagittal (lateral) view with a T1-weighted sequence *(A)* shows that the subcutaneous fat and marrow within the vertebral bodies have a high signal and appear white. The cerebrospinal fluid (CSF) appears almost black, and the cerebellum, pons, and spinal cord appear gray. On the T2-weighted sequence *(B)*, the contrast is somewhat reversed, with fluid or CSF appearing white, and the fat becoming dark. The spinal cord remains gray.

provides exquisite detail of soft tissues, such as the spinal cord, and cerebral spinal fluid (CSF) (Fig. 8-7).

Trauma

Of acute traumatic spinal fractures, 50% are due to motor vehicle accidents, about 25% to falls, and about 10% to sports injuries. The most common sites are the upper (C1 to C2) and lower (C5 to C7) cervical spine and the thoracolumbar junction (T9 to L2). Twenty percent of spinal fractures are multiple, and about 5% occur at discontinuous levels.

Not all patients require imaging studies to exclude spinal injury. If a patient is fully conscious and has neurologic deficit, no pain in the spinal region, no other injuries likely to obscure the injury, and the mechanism of injury is unlikely to have produced spinal injury, further evaluation is unnecessary.

Plain anteroposterior (AP) and lateral x-rays are the primary screening tools for spinal trauma but are usually indicated in the following situations:

- Recent trauma
- Pain greater than 4 weeks' duration with conservative therapy
- Known osteoporosis or metabolic bone disease
- Infection suspected as a result of fever, increased sedimentation rate, or an elevated white blood cell count
- Known cancer
- Radicular findings including paresthesia or weakness

- Before chiropractic spinal manipulation (to find pathology that may preclude the procedure)

If a patient has severe head trauma requiring CT evaluation, most physicians simply continue the scan into the cervical spine to exclude occult fractures. About 5% of the time, fractures are found that cannot be seen on plain x-rays. In addition, about 50% of the time, plain x-rays are unable to distinguish a vertebral body compression fracture from the more serious burst fracture. MRI is better than CT for detection of the soft tissue and spinal cord components of the injury. Table 8-3 shows the indications for MRI of the spine.

Dislocation of the skull from the cervical spine (atlanto-occipital dislocation) is rare and usually fatal. Approximately 5% of cervical spine fractures involve C1. Fractures of the atlas can involve any portion of the bony ring. Combination fractures, or burst fractures of the ring of C1, are called "Jefferson fractures." This bursting is usually secondary to axial loading as a result of the skull being smashed down onto the cervical spine (as in diving into a shallow pool) (Fig. 8-8*A*).

Approximately 10% of all cervical spine fractures involve the odontoid process of C2. The most common type of odontoid fracture occurs at the very base of the odontoid process. You can identify the fracture on the lateral view by being very careful to trace the anterior and posterior cortex of the odontoid process. Often associated soft tissue swelling is found (Fig. 8-8*B*). Note should be made that in young children the odontoid may not be completely fused to the body of C2, and this should not be mistaken for a fracture (see Fig. 8-170*A*).

Occasionally, C1 to C2 injury of the transverse ligament may occur, causing traumatic atlantoaxial subluxation. Although this may occur with an associated odontoid fracture, it can also occur without it. If no fracture is present, the subluxation is often fatal, because the odontoid process pushes posteriorly into the spinal cord contained within the arch of C1. On the lateral view, the only sign of ligament injury may be some soft tissue swelling anterior to the vertebral bodies. Flexion views will sometimes demonstrate increased widening not only of the atlantoaxial space but also of the space between the posterior spinous processes. This type of subluxation also occurs as a complication of rheumatoid arthritis (Fig. 8-9).

A relatively classic fracture of C2 is the so called "hangman's fracture." This involves fracture of the posterior elements of C2, often with associated spinal cord compromise. This fracture typically occurs secondary to hyperextension and compression of the upper cervical spine, and usually anterior subluxation of the body of C2 relative to C3 is found (Fig. 8-10). In spite of the name, this is not the usual fracture that occurs as a result of judicial hangings.

Two rather characteristic fractures of the midcervical spine vertebral bodies occur. The first of these is caused by hyperextension, which typically tears off either a superior or an inferior anterior portion of the cortex from a vertebral body (Fig. 8-11). A second type of fracture that commonly occurs in the middle cervical spine is a hyperflexion injury. In this, compression of the vertebral body is found, usually with anterior wedging and sometimes with a posteriorly displaced disk fragment, and usually with associated soft tissue swelling due to the hemorrhage.

TABLE 8–3 ■ **Indications for a Magnetic Resonance Imaging Scan* of the Spine**

Radiculopathy: unchanged after 4 to 6 wk of limited activity and medications; worsening or extension after 2 wk of limited activity and medications
High-impact trauma
New or progressive neurologic deficit
Neurologic deficit inconsistent with radiographic findings
Suspected spinal tumor
Suspected spinal infection
Acute myelopathy (hyper-reflexia, gait disturbance, clonus, numbness or paresthesia in legs)
Acute urinary retention or stool incontinence
Neurogenic claudication (differentiated from vascular claudication by partial relief with back flexion, onset with prolonged standing)
Cancer elsewhere with new spine pain, new spinal bone lesion on radiographic examination, new neurologic findings

*A computed tomography scan also can be used if a magnetic resonance imaging scan is not available.

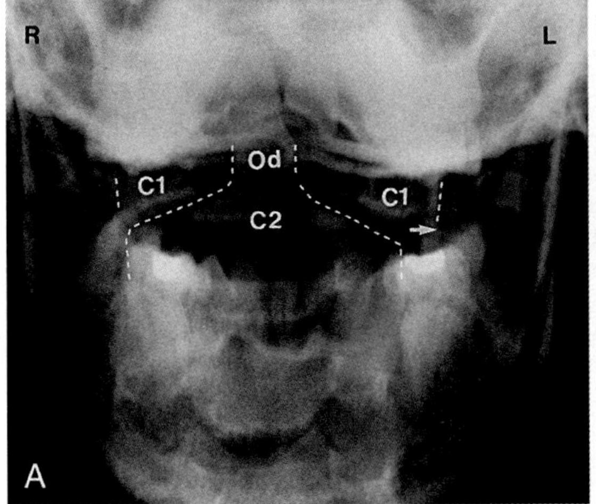

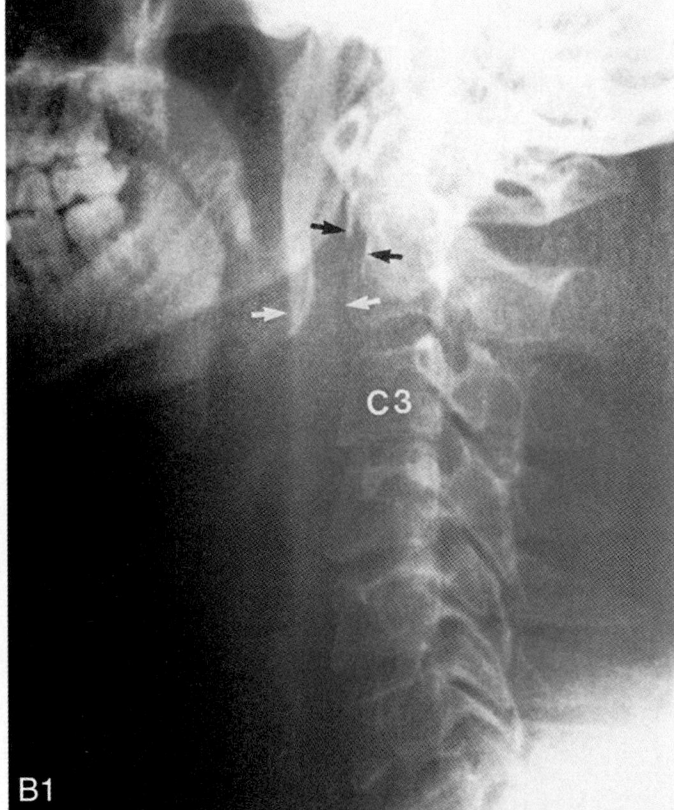

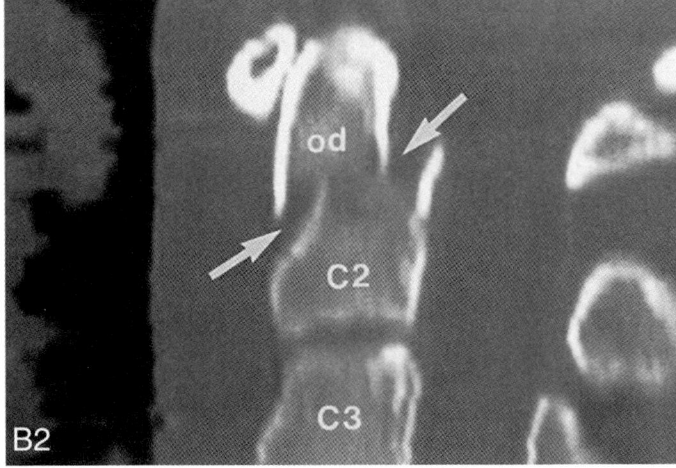

FIGURE 8-8 ■ *A,* Jefferson burst fracture of C1. On this open-mouth anteroposterior view, widening of the space between the odontoid and the left lateral mass of C1 is apparent. The lateral aspect also projects past the lateral margin of C2 *(arrow). B,* Fracture of the odontoid. In a different patient, the lateral view of the cervical spine *(B1)* shows marked soft tissue swelling in front of the body of C2 *(white arrows).* Discontinuity of the cortex along the anterior surface of C2 *(black arrows)* is seen, indicating an odontoid fracture. A sagittal reconstruction on a computed tomography scan *(B2)* shows the fracture much more clearly.

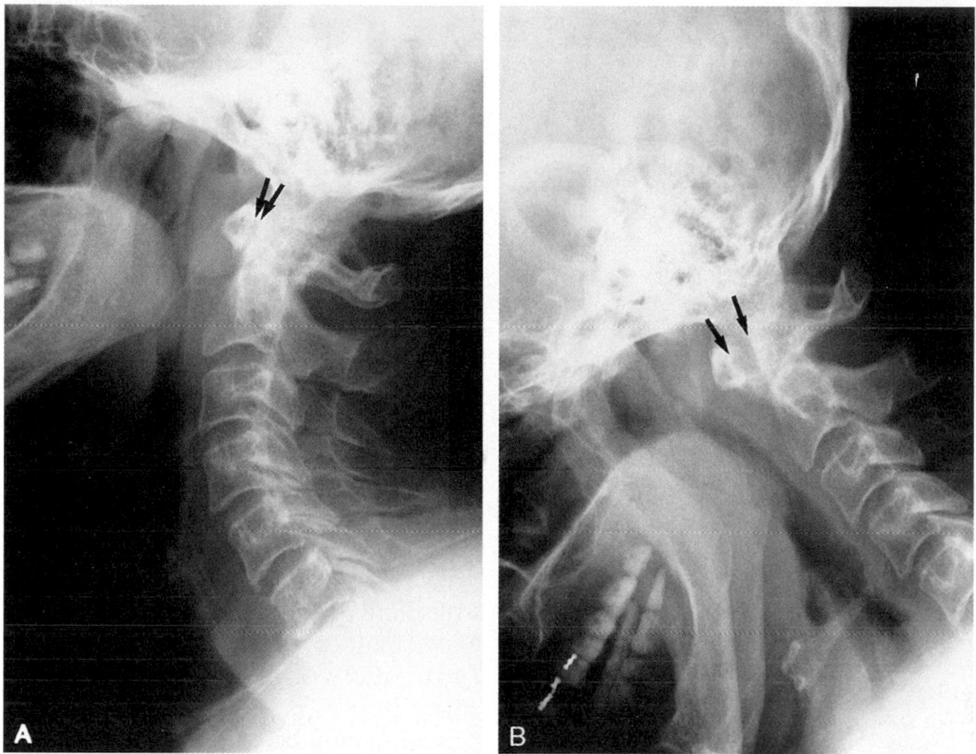

FIGURE 8-9 ■ Instability of the transverse ligament of C1. In this patient with rheumatoid arthritis, a lateral view of the cervical spine with the neck extended *(A)* shows very little space (which is normal) between the posterior aspect of the arch of C1 and the anterior portion of the odontoid *(arrows)*. With flexion *(B)*, this space markedly widens, and the odontoid is free to compress the spinal cord, which is posterior to it.

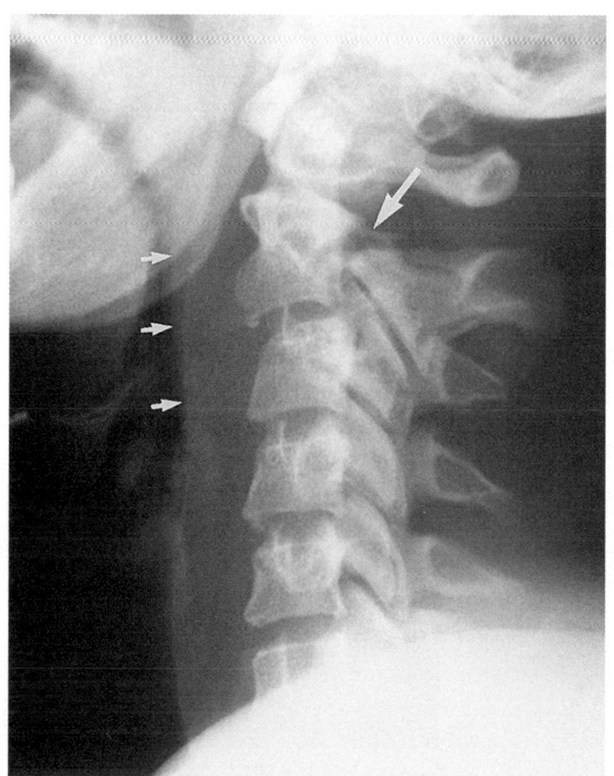

FIGURE 8-10 ■ Hangman's fracture. The lateral view of the cervical spine demonstrates marked soft tissue swelling anterior to C1, C2, and C3 *(small white arrows)*. A fracture line is seen just posterior to the body of C2 *(large arrow)*.

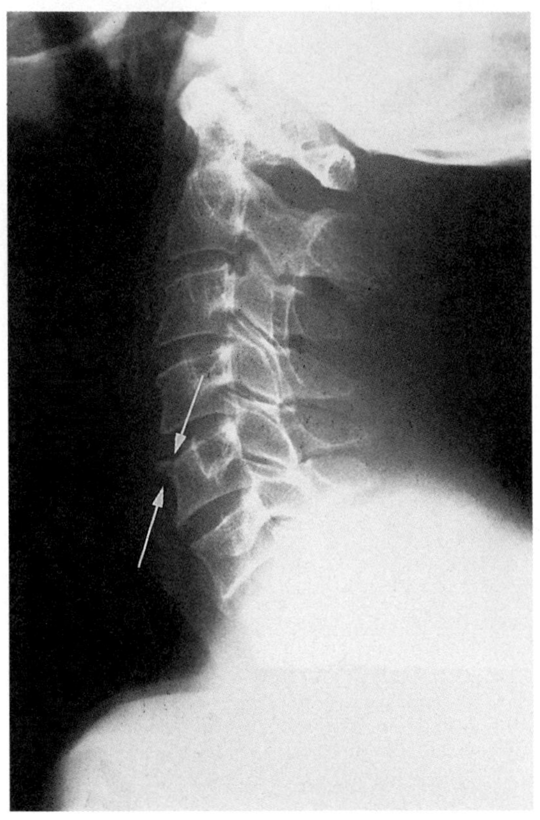

FIGURE 8-11 ■ Anterior avulsion fracture. A small avulsed fragment is seen along the superior and anterior aspect of C5 *(arrows)*.

Evaluation with MRI may show compromise of the neural canal at the level of the fracture (Fig. 8-12).

In addition to fractures associated with subluxation, ligamentous injury may allow the facets of one vertebral body to become slightly subluxated, perched, or locked. These represent a more anterior subluxation of a superior vertebral body on a lower one. Generally these injuries occur in the lower half of the cervical spine and are caused by extreme flexion of the head and neck without axial compression. Occasionally a fracture or ligamentous injury cannot be identified with plain x-rays. If a high suspicion of clinical injury exists in spite of negative plain x-rays, CT scanning (Fig. 8-13) or MRI may be useful. CT scanning is able to identify small cortical breaks, whereas the MRI scan can show areas of increased signal with hematoma or edema, suggesting at least ligamentous injury.

Three fractures of the lower portion of the cervical spine are easily missed. Occasionally oblique fractures of the lower cervical spine are seen only on the AP view (Fig. 8-14). The second fracture involves the posterior spinous process at the C6, C7, T1, or T2 level. This is called the "clay-shoveler's fracture," and it is due predominantly to hyperflexion injury (Fig. 8-15). A third

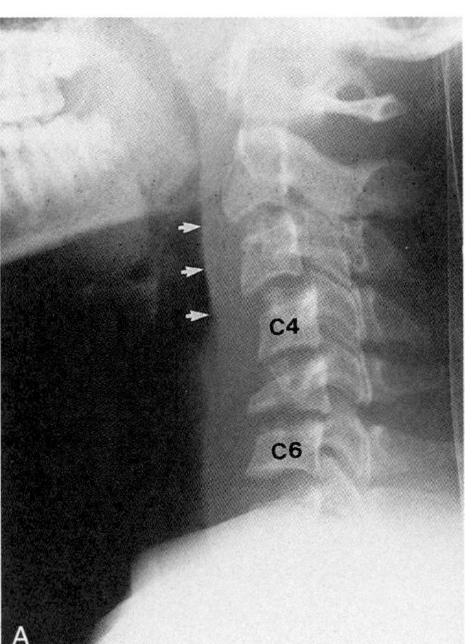

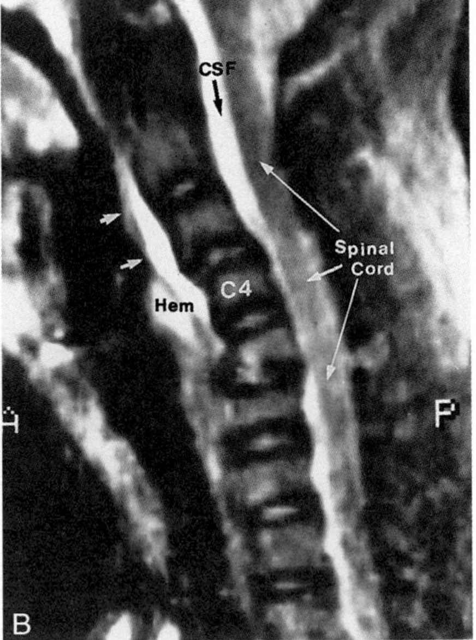

FIGURE 8-12 ■ Wedge fracture of C5. A lateral cervical spine view *(A)* demonstrates a reversed normal cervical curvature, anterior soft tissue swelling *(arrows)*, and a wedge fracture of the body of C5. A magnetic resonance imaging scan *(B)*, presented in the same projection, shows hemorrhage (Hem) as an area of high signal anterior to the body of C4. The spinal cord also is identified, and the spinal canal is clearly narrowed at the level of the fracture.

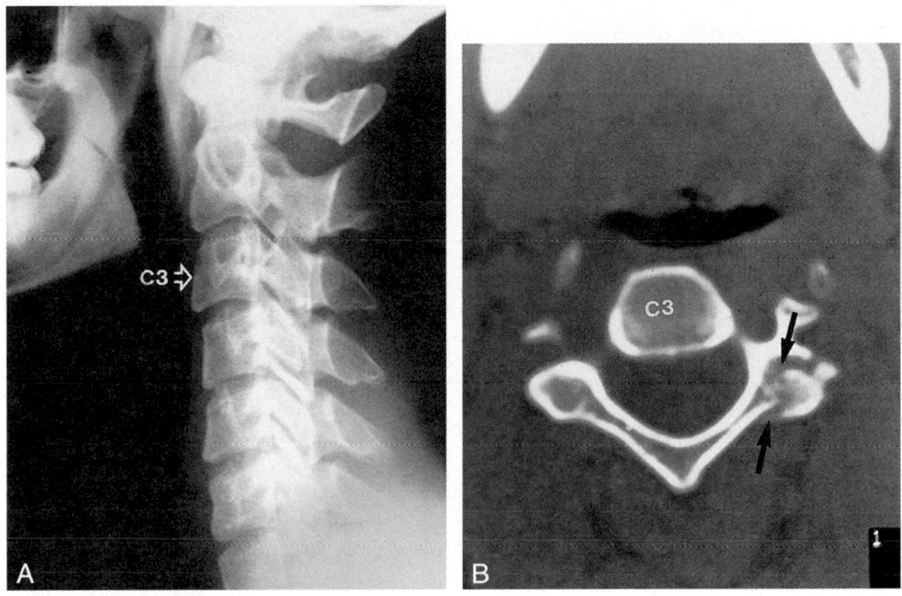

FIGURE 8-13 ■ Occult cervical spine fracture. A lateral view of the cervical spine *(A)* shows normal-appearing structures at C3. No anterior soft tissue swelling is seen. The anteroposterior view also was normal. Because the patient was complaining of severe pain and had been ejected during a motor vehicle accident, a computed tomography scan was obtained *(B)*, and a transverse image showed a fracture through the lateral mass of C3 *(arrows)*.

and most significant problem, relative to the lower cervical spine, is accepting a trauma lateral cervical spine image that does not include adequate evaluation of C6 and C7. Failure to visualize this region can result in missing significant subluxations and fractures, and for purposes of complete evaluation, either a swimmer's view or shallow oblique views through the cervicothoracic junction are necessary (Fig. 8-16).

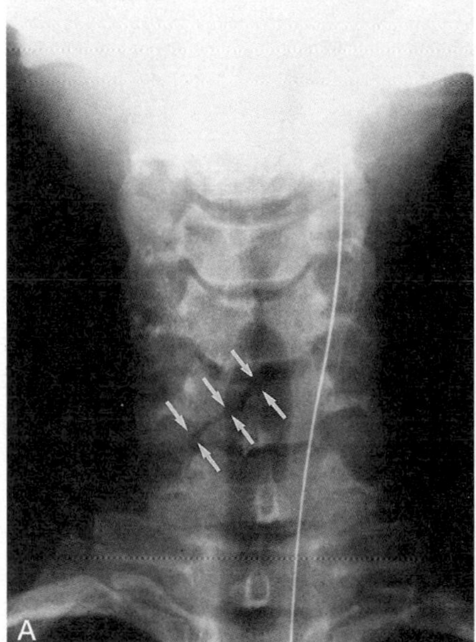

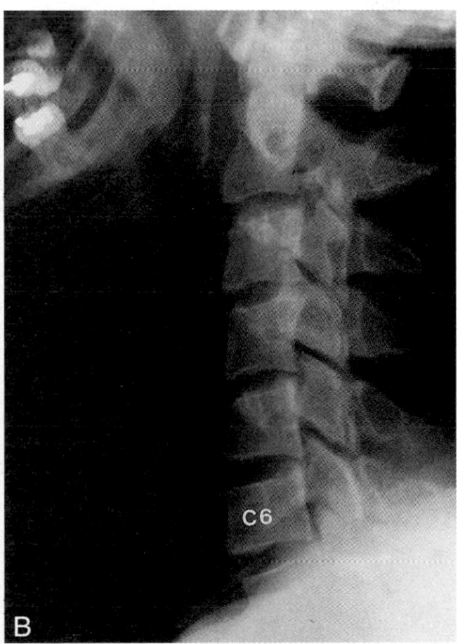

FIGURE 8-14 ■ Oblique fracture of C6. The anteroposterior view of the lower cervical spine *(A)* shows an oblique lucent line, representing a fracture, through the body of C6. This is the only view on which this fracture was seen. The lateral view in the same patient *(B)* was completely normal.

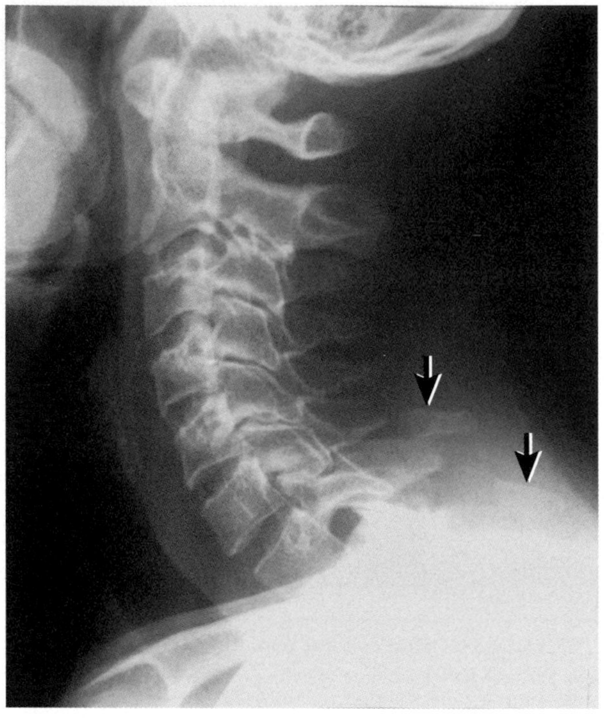

FIGURE 8-15 ■ Fracture of the posterior spinous process of C6 and C7. This fracture is identified only on the lateral view *(arrows)* and is referred to as a clay shoveler's fracture.

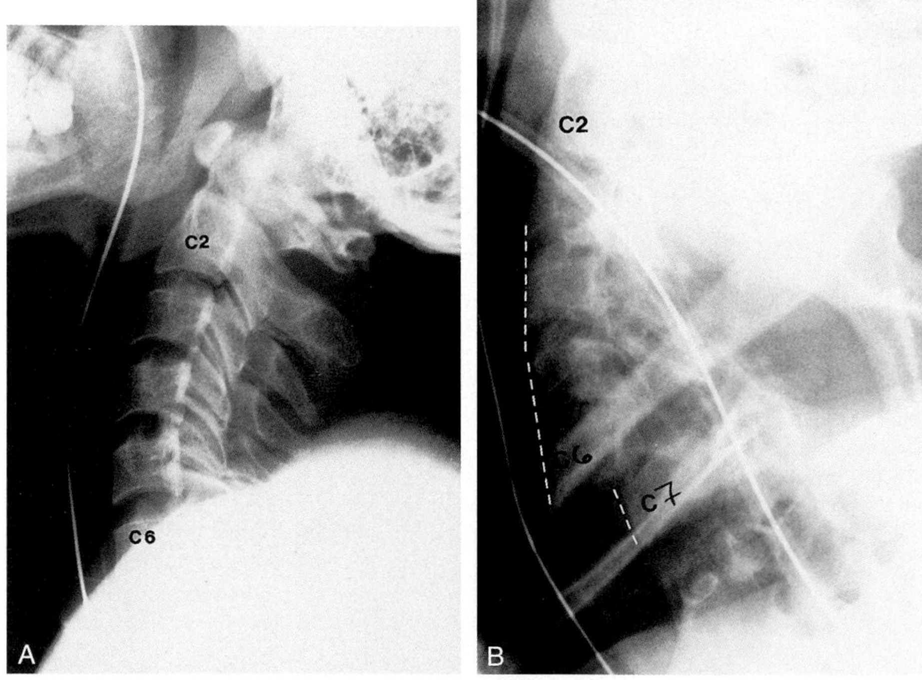

FIGURE 8-16 ■ C6-C7 subluxation. The initial lateral view of the cervical spine *(A)* in this patient with paraplegia looked normal; however, C7 was not visualized. When a swimmer's lateral view *(B)* was obtained, a complete subluxation of C6 forward on the body of C7 was noted.

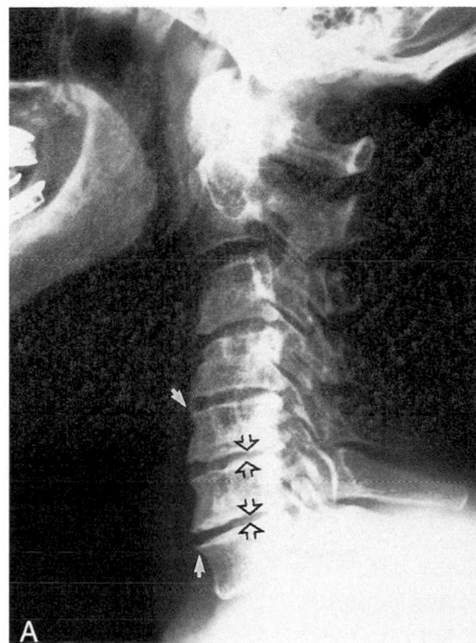

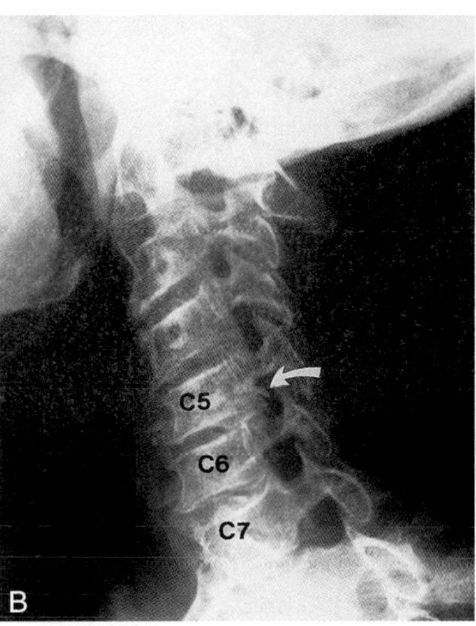

FIGURE 8-17 ■ Degenerative changes of the cervical spine. The lateral view *(A)* shows decreased disk spaces *(open arrows)* and hypertrophic spurring along the anterior aspects of the vertebral bodies. These changes are most common at the C4-C7 level. An oblique view *(B)* in the same patient shows that bony spurs are projecting into the neural foramen *(arrow)*. This can cause pain down the arms.

Degenerative Changes

In terms of anatomic and mechanical design, the lower aspect of the cervical spine is less than optimal, and by the third or fourth decade of life, degenerative changes involving C4 through C7 almost always are found. Degenerative changes are visualized as decreased disk spaces, sclerosis (increased density) of the vertebral body end plates, and beaking or spurring of the anterior, lateral, and posterior margins of the vertebral bodies. Often, patients are initially seen with arm pain, and an oblique cervical spine view can easily visualize hypertrophic osteophytes or spurs projecting into the neural foramen (Fig. 8-17). If a herniated cervical disk is suspected, the procedure of choice is an MRI scan. Metastatic disease also can involve the cervical spine with posterior or lateral extension and impingement on the spinal cord or nerve roots (Fig. 8-18).

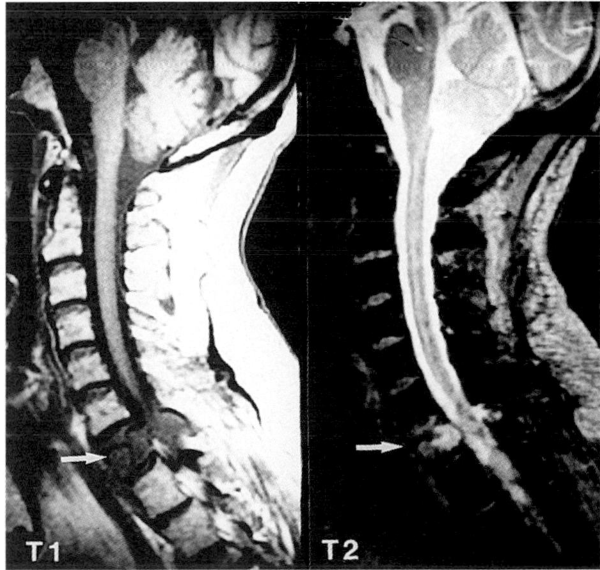

FIGURE 8-18 ■ Tumor involvement of the cervical spine. In this patient with lymphoma and neurologic deficit, a sagittal magnetic resonance image of the cervical spine demonstrates complete replacement of the marrow of C7, seen as a dark area on the T1 image *(arrow)*. The T2 image also shows the tumor as a white area *(arrow)* narrowing the spinal canal and compressing the spinal cord.

THORACIC SPINE

Anatomy

Plain x-rays of the thoracic spine are taken in AP and lateral projections. The AP projection is useful for examining spinal alignment, the paraspinous soft tissues (to exclude hematomas or other masses), and the pedicles (Fig. 8-19). The lateral thoracic spine is usually a difficult film to assess. In the upper portion, the vertebral bodies are obscured by the shoulders; as men-

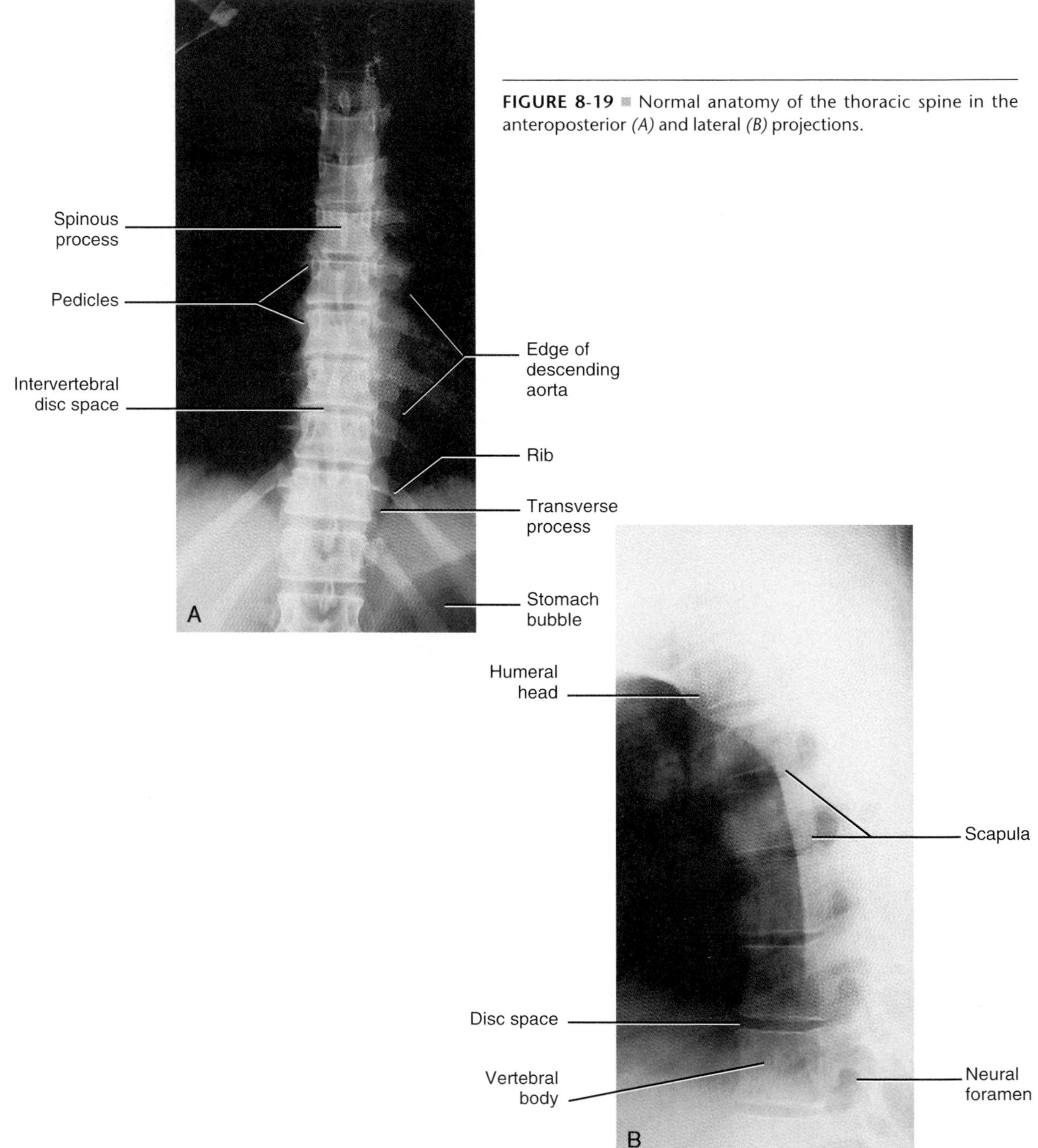

FIGURE 8-19 ■ Normal anatomy of the thoracic spine in the anteroposterior *(A)* and lateral *(B)* projections.

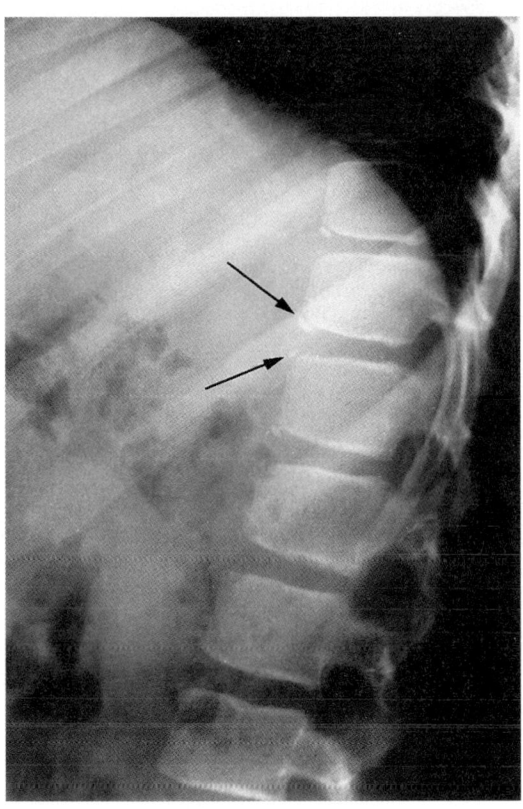

FIGURE 8-20 ■ Normal spinal apophyses. In children, a normal apophysis can occasionally be seen on the lateral projection along the anterior superior and inferior margins of the vertebral bodies. These are normal, will be seen on multiple vertebral bodies, and should not be mistaken for avulsion fractures.

tioned in the discussion of the cervical spine, if you suspect pathology in the T1 to T5 region, often a swimmer's view or shallow oblique views are necessary. The mid- and lower thoracic spine is usually well seen on the lateral view. When pathology is identified on the lateral view, it is often not easy to tell exactly the level of the vertebral body involved. Once you have identified pathology on the lateral view, you can usually go back to the AP view, look at the ribs, and then count up from T12. A common normal variant is seen on the lateral thoracic spine views in children. This apophysis that occurs along the superior and inferior anterior margins of the vertebral bodies should not be mistaken for a fracture (Fig. 8-20).

Trauma

Fractures of the thoracic spine typically are the result of motor vehicle accidents or of the normal aging process, with osteoporosis and resultant anterior wedging of vertebral bodies. Fractures due to significant acute trauma are sometimes seen well only on either the AP or the lateral view. On the AP view, you should examine the spine for malalignment of the posterior spinous processes (Fig. 8-21) as well as for paraspinous soft tissue swelling. These are both signs that a fracture may be present. If you suspect

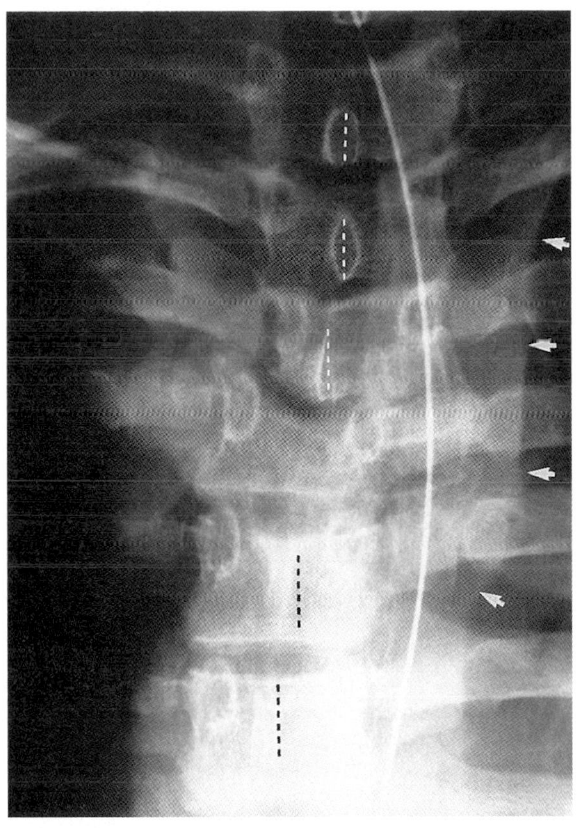

FIGURE 8-21 ■ Laterally displaced thoracic spine fracture. An anteroposterior view of the upper thoracic spine in a paraplegic patient who was hit in the driver's-side door during a motor vehicle accident shows lateral displacement of the upper thoracic vertebral bodies relative to the lower bodies. This can be assessed by looking at the line formed by the posterior spinous processes *(dotted lines)*. Also note the lateral soft tissue swelling *(arrows)* due to the paraspinous hemorrhage resulting from the fracture. This type of fracture is difficult or impossible to visualize on the lateral view.

a spinal fracture, both AP and lateral views should be examined. Sometimes significant subluxation of one vertebral body forward on another will be difficult to see on the AP view (Fig. 8-22). This usually occurs when a hyperflexion injury results in a compression burst fracture. Often retropulsed fragments of both disk and bony material project into the spinal canal and can cause significant compromise of the spinal cord.

In older persons, compression fractures of the mid- and lower thoracic spine are common (Fig. 8-23*A*). These are noted as loss of height of the anterior portion of the vertebral bodies. It is almost impossible to tell whether any one of these fractures is new or old, but it usually does not make any difference clinically. If you suspect metastatic disease as a cause of back pain in an older patient, a plain x-ray and a nuclear medicine bone scan are usually satisfactory.

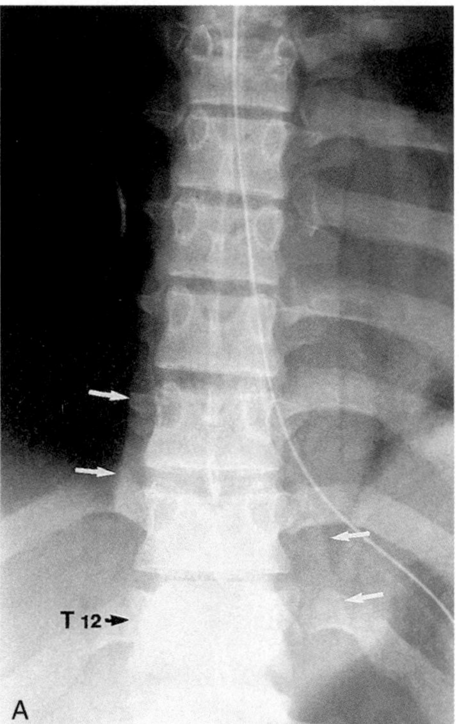

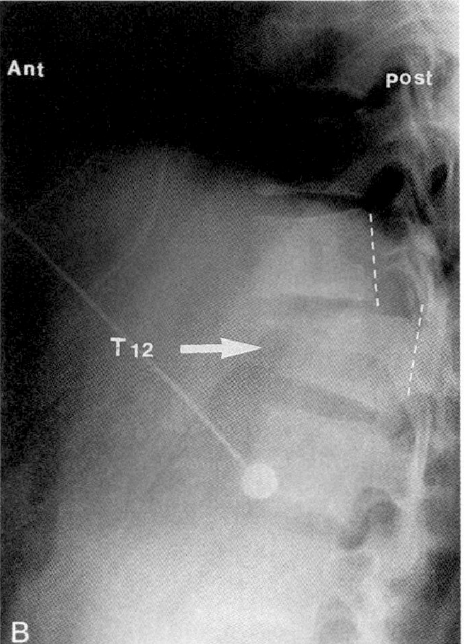

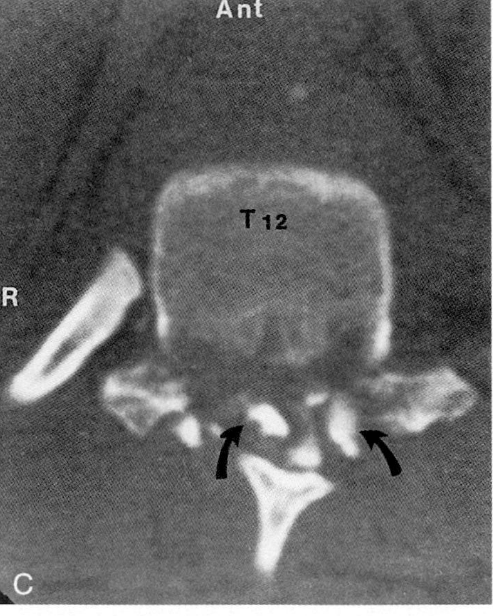

FIGURE 8-22 ■ Anterior subluxation and fracture. On the anteroposterior view of the lower thoracic spine *(A),* paraspinous soft tissue swelling due to hemorrhage is identified, although the vertebral bodies, including T12, look grossly normal. The lateral view *(B)* demonstrates a wedge compression of T12 and marked anterior subluxation of T11 on T12, causing the patient to be paraplegic. A transverse computed tomography scan *(C)* through the level of T12 shows multiple bony fragments *(arrows)* within the neural canal that have compromised the spinal cord.

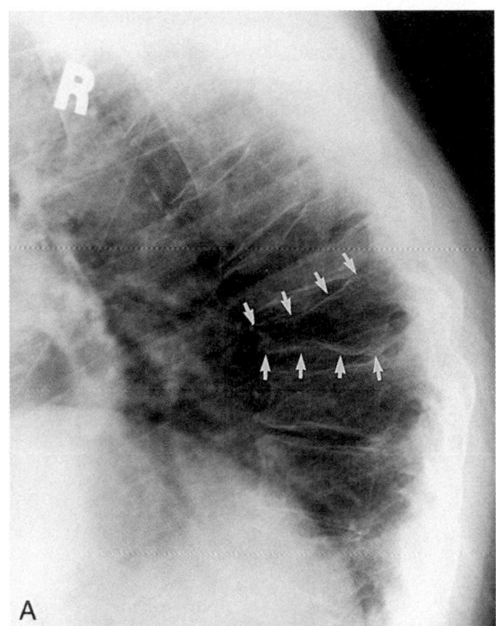

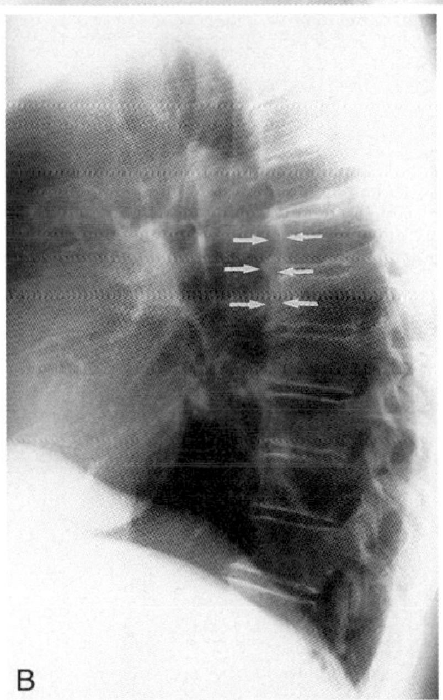

FIGURE 8-23 ■ Degenerative changes of the thoracic spine. *A,* With aging and osteoporosis, there can be wedge-compression fractures of the mid- to upper thoracic spine may occur. *B,* In a different patient, development of calcification of the anterior ligament is noted *(arrows).*

Degenerative Changes

Three relatively common degenerative findings are seen in the thoracic spine. The first are spurs or hypertrophic osteophytes, similar to those that are seen in the lower cervical spine. These are almost never a clinical issue and are not an interpretative problem unless they are very large, at which point they can cause confusing shadows on the anteroposterior (AP) or posteroanterior (PA) chest radiograph. These are pointed areas that project out to the side of the spine and are usually seen right over the proximal end of a rib. On the lateral view, these can look like lung nodules, but they always are seen to be projecting over the disk spaces (see Fig. 3-17).

A second relatively common degenerative change is calcification along the anterior ligament. This can cross over the length of several vertebral bodies (Fig. 8-23*B*) and is sometimes referred to by radiologists as DISH (diffuse idiopathic skeletal hyperostosis). It is of no clinical significance to the patient. The third, relatively common, degenerative change is

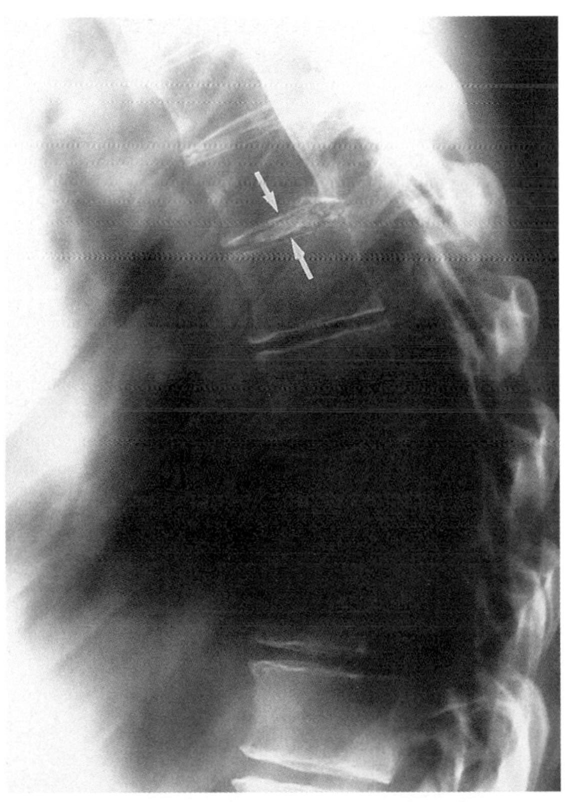

FIGURE 8-24 ■ Calcified intervertebral disk. Calcification of a single disk can be identified on this lateral view *(arrows).* This is most commonly due to trauma and is of little clinical significance. Calcification at multiple levels has a differential diagnosis, which includes hypercalcemic states as well as ochronosis.

calcification of an intervertebral disk (Fig. 8-24). This can occur at almost any level in the spine but is seen most frequently in the midthoracic region. A single calcified disk is usually the result of degenerative change or trauma. If calcification is seen at multiple disk levels, consider diseases that cause hypercalcemia or rare entities such as ochronosis.

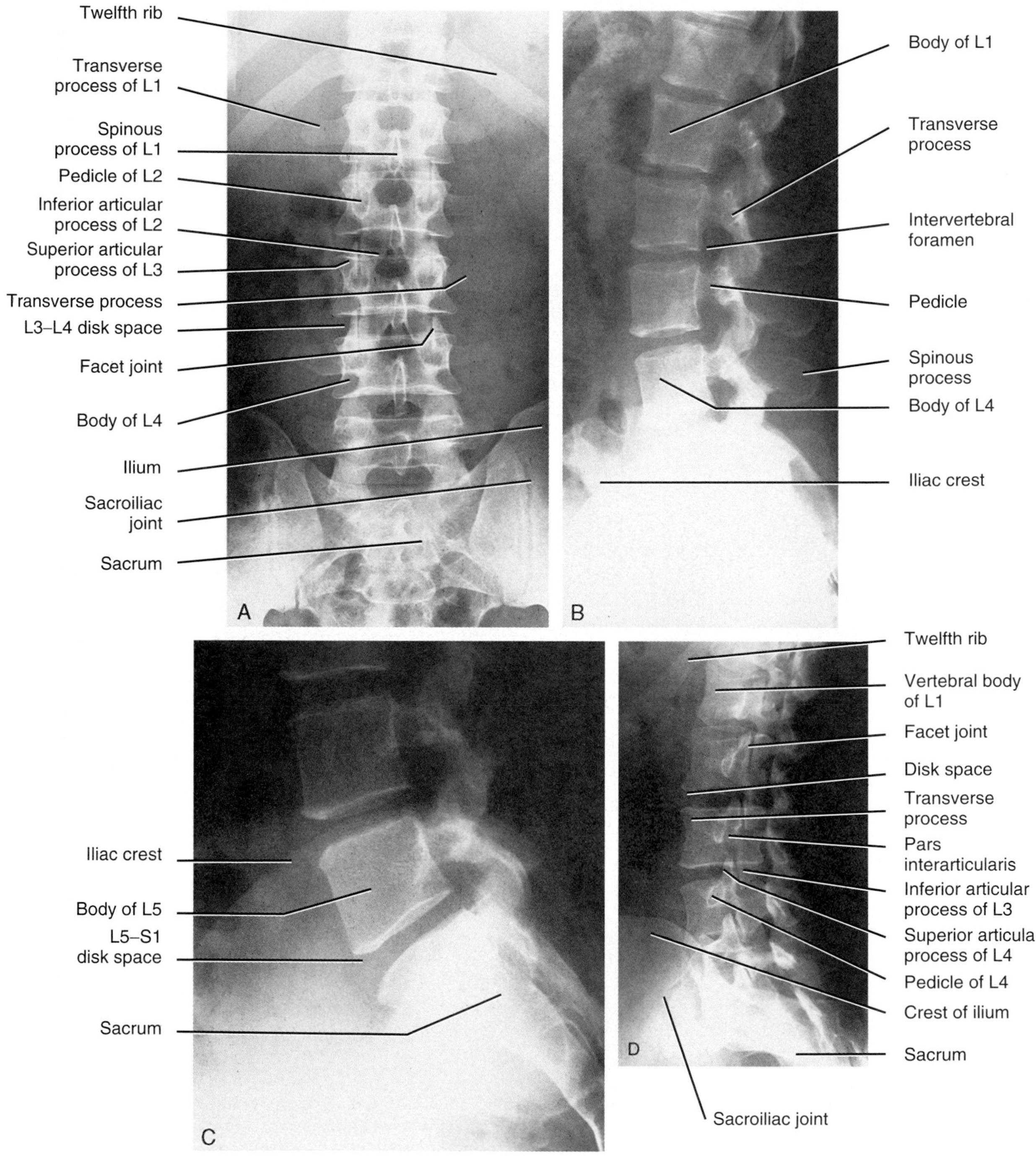

FIGURE 8-25 ■ Normal anatomy of the lumbar spine in the anteroposterior *(A)*, lateral *(B)*, lateral sacral *(C)*, and oblique *(D)* views.

LUMBAR SPINE

Normal Anatomy and Imaging Techniques

The standard views obtained of the lumbar spine are AP, lateral, and a lateral spot view of the L5 to S1 area (Fig. 8-25). The spot view is necessary because, on the lateral view, both iliac wings and a significant amount of additional soft tissue mean that more radiation exposure is necessary to penetrate and visualize the L5 to S1 area adequately.

On the AP view, examine the alignment of the spine as well as the visibility of the psoas margins bilaterally. It is often useful to count the number of vertebral bodies, because commonly six, rather than five, non–rib-bearing vertebrae may be found. The transverse processes should be examined to exclude fracture, and the pedicles at each level should be examined to make sure that they have not been eroded by a pathologic process. Additionally, the sacrum and sacroiliac joints should be examined. The sacroiliac joints can become fused in various arthritic processes (such as ankylosing spondylitis) or can be widened by a pelvic fracture.

On the lateral view of the lumbar spine, a search is made for subluxation of the vertebral bodies; this is done by looking down the contour lines formed by the anterior and posterior margins of the vertebral bodies. The height and shape of vertebral bodies and the disk spaces should be uniform. The posterior spinous processes also can be visualized.

Oblique views of the lumbar spine are useful for examining the facet joints. The typical anatomy on the oblique view is seen in the outline of a "Scottie dog" (see Figs. 8-25*D* and 8-30*B*). In this oblique projection, the pedicle is the eye of the Scottie dog, and the transverse process represents the nose. The superior articular process forms the ears, and the inferior articular process forms the front legs.

A common normal variant of the lumbar spine is incomplete fusion of the posterior aspect of L5 or S1 (so-called spina bifida occulta), which is seen on the AP view (Fig. 8-26*A*). It is of no clinical significance and

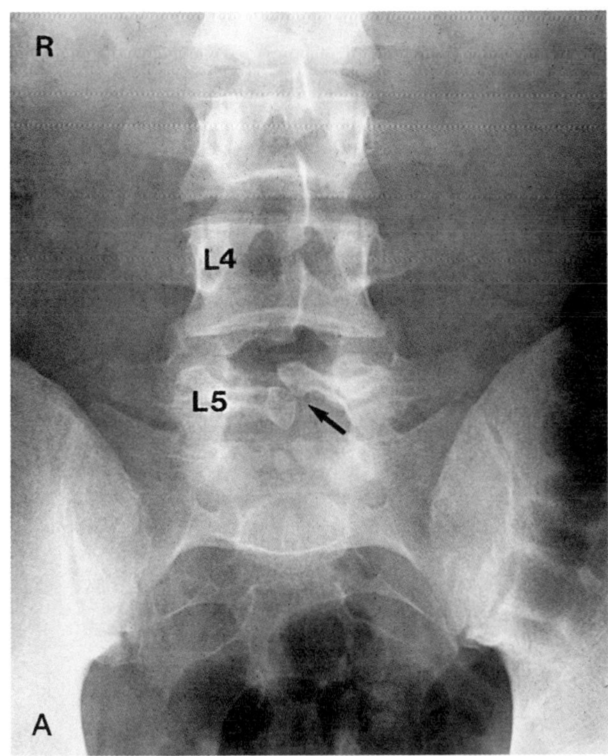

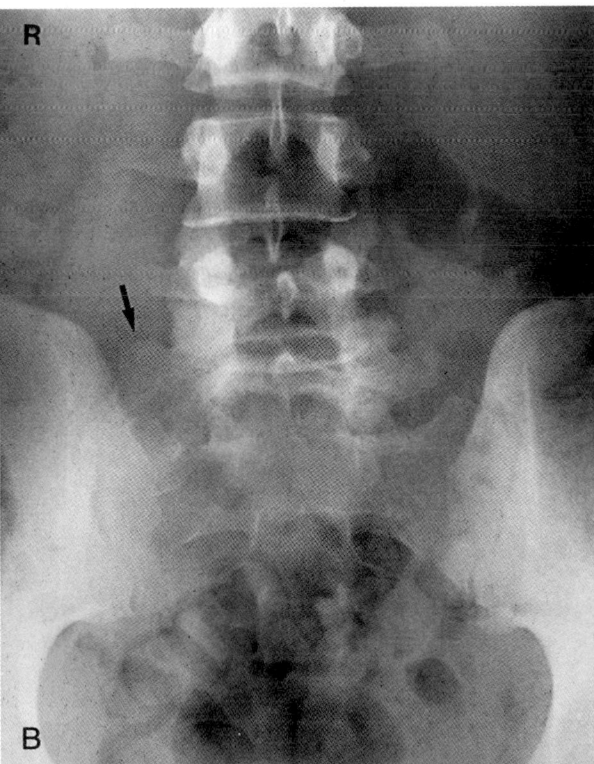

FIGURE 8-26 ■ Normal variants of the lumbar spine. *A,* Incomplete fusion of the posterior arch (spina bifida occulta) is seen on the anteroposterior view as a defect at L5 *(arrow). B,* Sacralization of the right side of L5 *(arrow).*

should be disregarded. A second common anomaly is sacralization, or partial fusion, of L5 with the sacrum (Fig. 8-26*B*). This can occur just on one side, or it can be bilateral.

On any given view of the lumbar spine or pelvis, you can see normal bowel gas projecting over bone. This looks dark and can easily mimic a destructive bone lesion. I have seen several instances in which physicians told patients that they had "cancer of the spine," which in reality was overlying bowel gas. Make sure that any bone lesion that you suspect is confined to the bone and stays within that bone on AP, lateral, and oblique views.

Postsurgical Changes

The most common postsurgical change involves either lower lumbar fusion or laminectomy. It is often not easy to appreciate laminectomy on the lateral film; however, on the frontal views, it is much easier to see that one or more posterior spinous processes are gone (Fig. 8-27). Noticing things that are missing is always harder than seeing abnormal objects that are present.

Fractures

The most common fractures of the lumbar spine are wedge-compression fractures and compression-burst fractures. These are very similar to those already described in the thoracic spine. Progression of compression fractions can be arrested and pain sometimes can be relieved by a procedure known as vertebroplasty. In this procedure, a cement or glue is injected into the vertebral body (Fig. 8-28). Note should be made, again, that the compression-burst fractures frequently have fragments that are retropulsed,

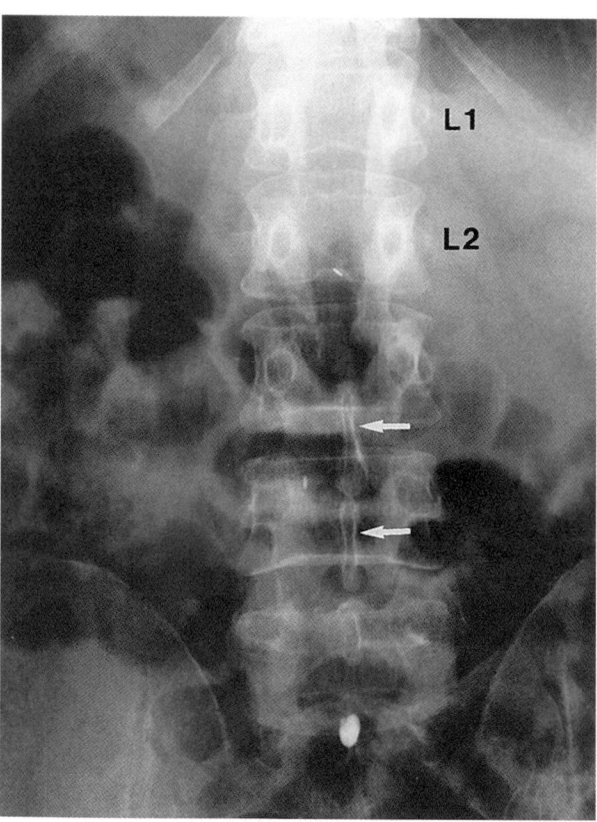

FIGURE 8-27 ■ **Postsurgical laminectomy.** On the anteroposterior view of the lumbar spine, the posterior spinous processes of L3 and L4 are clearly seen *(arrows)*. Spinous processes are absent on L1 and L2 owing to a laminectomy.

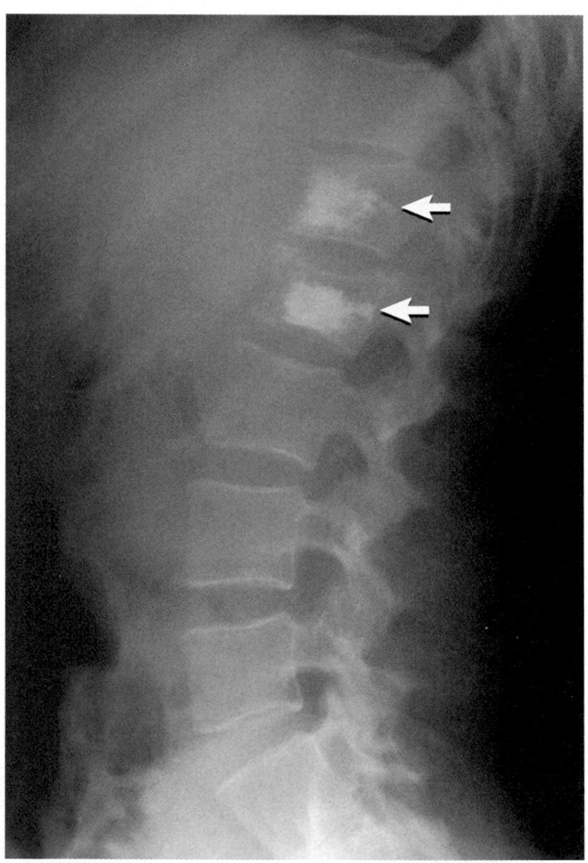

FIGURE 8-28 ■ **Vertebroplasty.** At two levels, insertion via needle of radio-opaque cement *(arrows)* has been used to arrest compression fractures.

and CT or MRI is often necessary to evaluate compromise of the spinal canal.

A somewhat unusual fracture occurs in the lumbar spine, typically at L1, L2, or L3, called a Chance fracture. In the past, this most commonly was the result of a motor vehicle accident when a lap seat belt is worn without the shoulder harness. Under these circumstances, rotation of the trunk of the body occurs about the horizontal axis of the seat belt, resulting in a vertical distraction force along the lumbar spine. This essentially tears a vertebral body (horizontally) in half. On the AP view, this fracture is recognized by discontinuity of the outline of the pedicles, and on the lateral view, by a lucency extending through the posterior spinous process and lamina (Fig. 8-29).

The pars interarticularis of the vertebral body also can be fractured. This injury typically occurs at the L4 or L5 level. It can sometimes

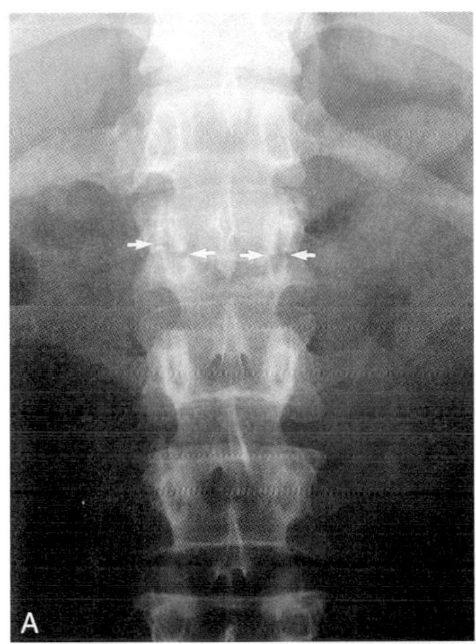

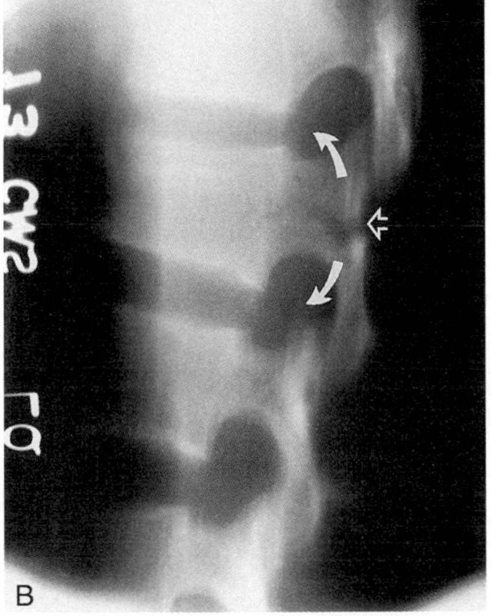

FIGURE 8-29 ■ Chance fracture. This distraction fracture usually occurs between L1 and L3. On the anteroposterior view of the lumbar spine *(A)*, all that can be identified is a discontinuity *(arrows)* in the normal white oval ring of the pedicles. On the lateral view *(B)*, a lucent dark line in the posterior elements extends toward the vertebral body *(arrowhead)*, caused by tearing of the bone due to seatbelt injury.

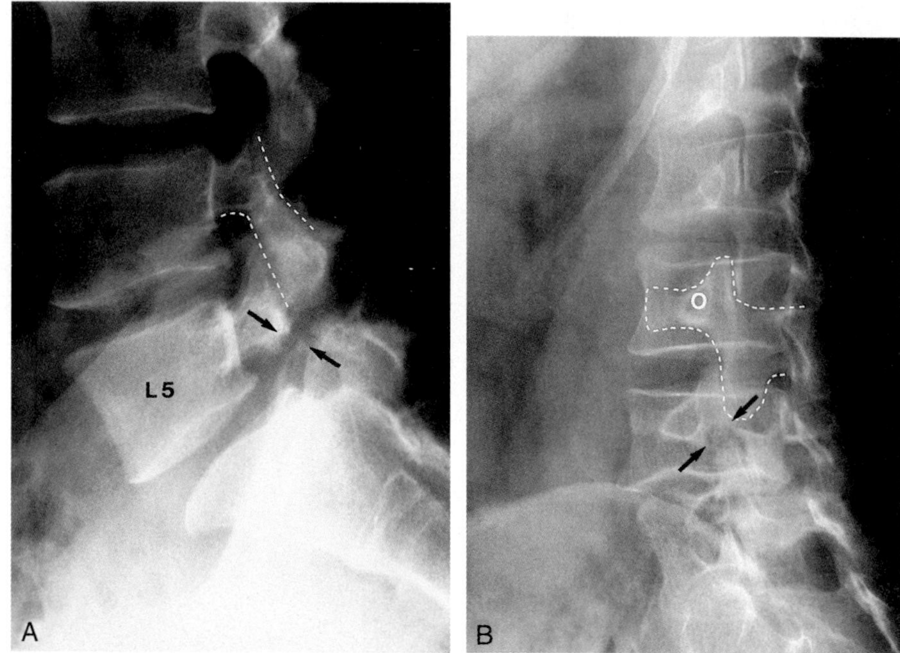

FIGURE 8-30 ■ Spondylolysis. On the lateral view of the lower lumbar spine *(A),* the normal contour of the posterior elements of L4 is outlined by the *white dotted lines.* At L5, lysis *(fracture)* of the posterior elements has occurred *(arrows).* On the oblique view *(B),* this is seen as a fracture through the neck of the "Scottie dog" *(arrows).* The normal outline for the L4 level is shown.

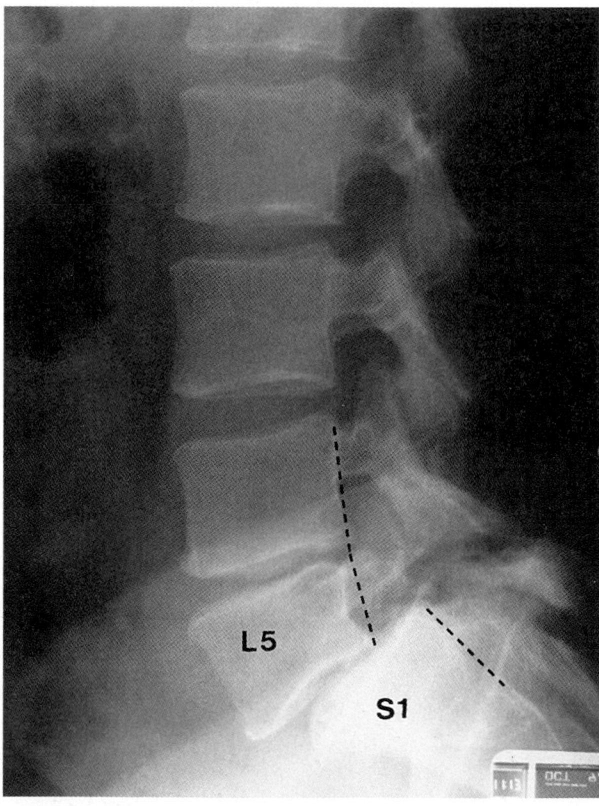

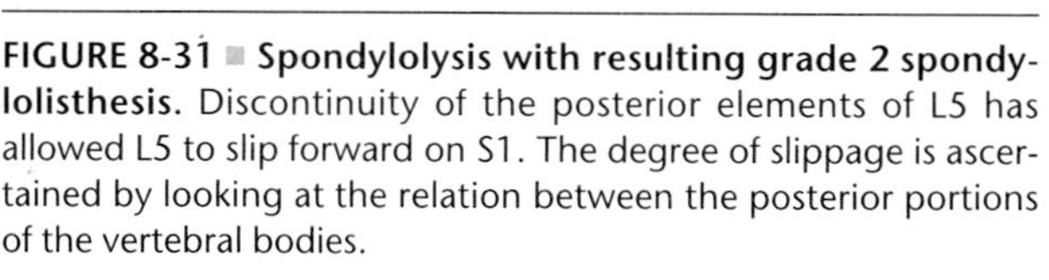
FIGURE 8-31 ■ Spondylolysis with resulting grade 2 spondylolisthesis. Discontinuity of the posterior elements of L5 has allowed L5 to slip forward on S1. The degree of slippage is ascertained by looking at the relation between the posterior portions of the vertebral bodies.

be seen on the lateral view as a lucency, but more commonly is clearly identified as a break in the neck of the "Scottie dog" on the oblique view (Fig. 8-30). This finding was originally thought to be congenital, but most of the time, it probably is the result of trauma in the early years of life. The term applied to a break in the pars interarticularis is spondylolysis. If bilateral spondylolysis is present, the vertebral body can slip forward on the vertebral body immediately below. When this happens, it is termed spondylolisthesis. The amount of offset caused by the slippage is used to grade the spondylolisthesis. If up to one fourth of the vertebral body is offset, this is called grade 1; between one fourth and one half, it is called grade 2, and so on (Fig. 8-31). In a young patient or athlete with low back pain and normal plain x-rays, a nuclear medicine bone scan with "slice" or single-photon emission CT (SPECT) technology may identify otherwise occult lesions (Fig. 8-32).

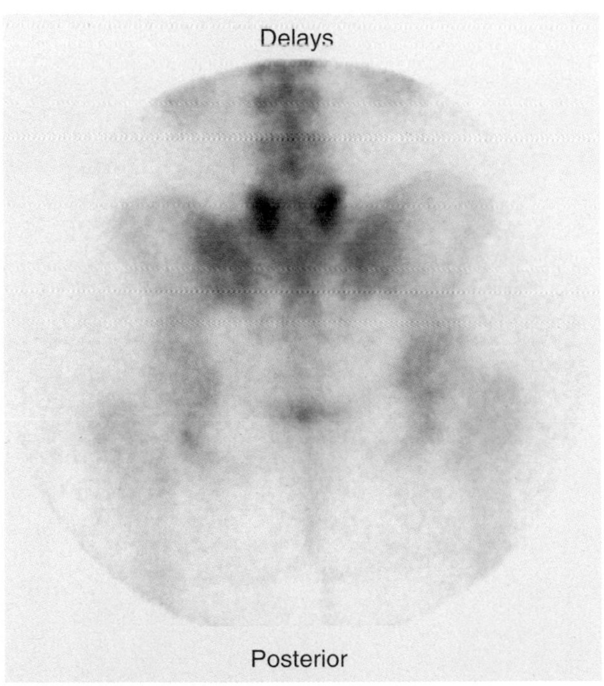

FIGURE 8-32 ■ Occult spondylolysis. In this teenage athlete with back pain, plain x-rays were normal. A nuclear medicine tomographic bone scan with a coronal image shows markedly increased activity on the both sides of L5 due to traumatic fractures of the pars interarticularis.

Degenerative Changes

As mentioned earlier, degenerative change can result in disk-space narrowing, hypertrophic spurs (osteophytes) (Fig. 8-33), or calcification of a disk. In the lumbar spine, loss of the disk space is quite common, as is hypertrophic spurring. Occasionally you can see a thin dark line in a narrowed disk space (Fig. 8-34), referred to as a vacuum disk phenomenon. Actually, it is not a vacuum; nitrogen is in the joint space. This can appear or be accentuated as a result of hyperextension of the spine, but it is a finding of no special clinical significance.

A very common degenerative change that occurs in the lower lumbar spine is a herniated disk or a protruded disk. A herniated disk often has a fragment that is asymmetrical or loose in

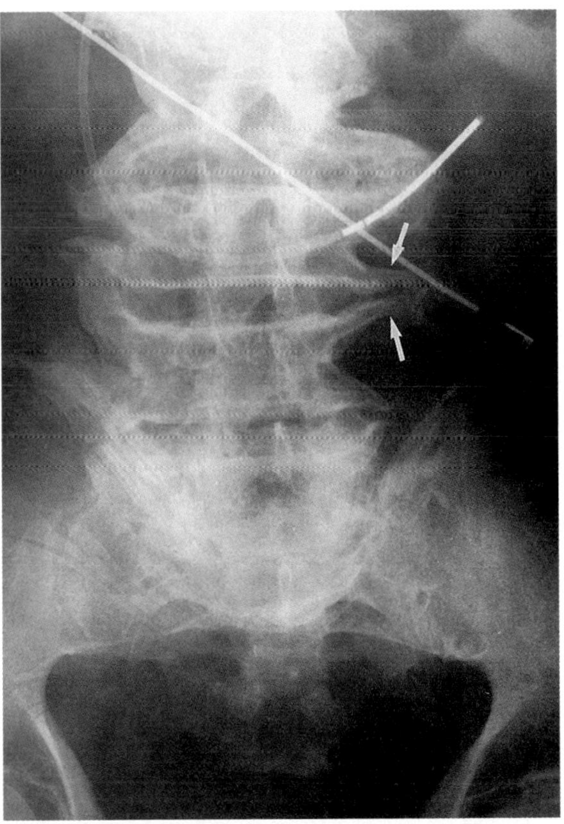

FIGURE 8-33 ■ Degenerative changes of the lumbar spine. An anteroposterior view of the lower lumbar spine shows extensive and florid bone spur formation as a result of degenerative change. The extent of these changes does not correlate very well with the presence of back pain.

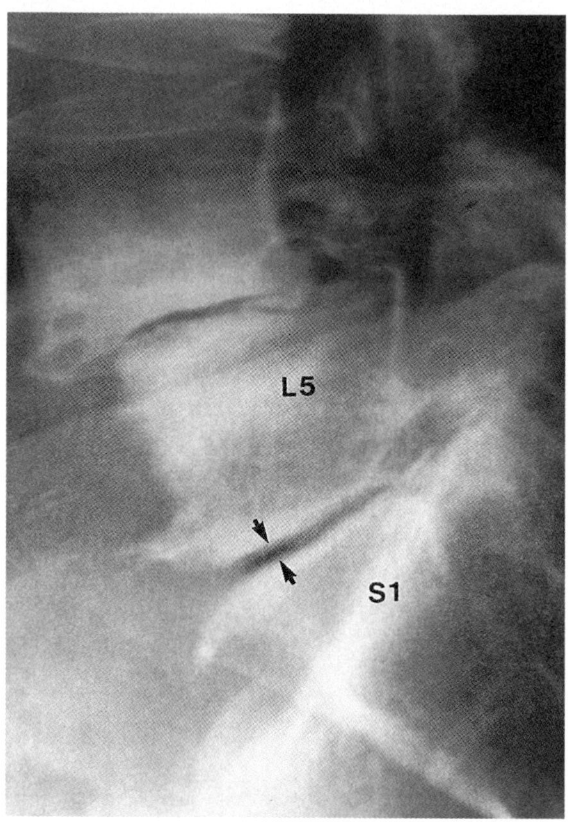

FIGURE 8-34 ■ Degenerative disk disease of the lumbar spine. A lateral view of the lower lumbar spine shows spondylolisthesis and subluxation of L4 on L5. The degenerative changes noted are almost complete loss of the disk spaces at L4-L5 and L5-S1. The small dark area within the disk space *(arrows)* is nitrogen; this is referred to as a vacuum disk.

FIGURE 8-35 ■ Disk herniation and protrusion. A transverse computed tomography scan *(A)* obtained at the L5-S1 disk space shows posterior protrusion of disk material *(arrows)* into the spinal canal. In a different patient, the sagittal or lateral magnetic resonance imaging view *(B)* of the lumbar spine shows a posterior L5-S1 disk *(arrows)* protruding into the spinal canal.

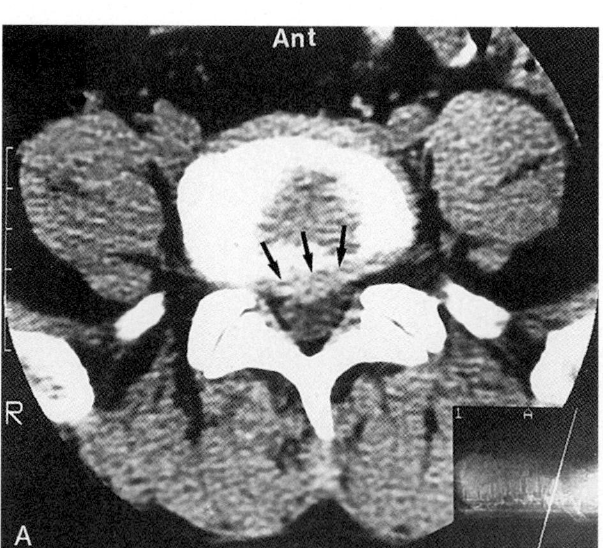

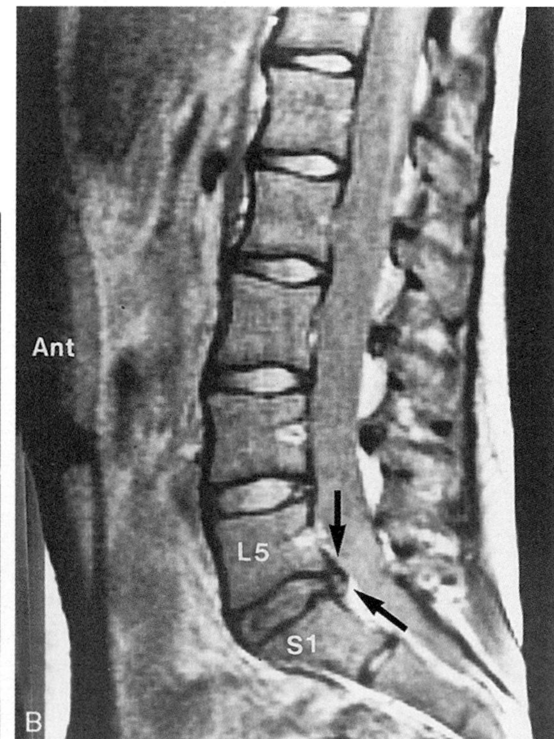

the neural canal, whereas a disk protrusion is a posterior central bulge of the disk. Both can be imaged with either CT or MR (Fig. 8-35). Currently, MRI is commonly used to make this diagnosis.

Management of Low Back Pain

This is probably one of the areas of greatest controversy in medical imaging. Low back pain affects 60% to 80% of the population at some time in their lives. The most common cause of low back pain is a herniated or bulging disk. Surprisingly, MRI and CT studies reveal a bulging disk in 25% to 50% of asymptomatic adults. Ninety percent of cases of lower back pain resolve within 4 to 6 weeks as a result of conservative therapy. Unless major acute trauma is present, plain x-rays of the lumbar spine are not of much use, because a patient can have a herniated disk and totally normal plain x-rays. Conversely, many people who have severe-looking degenerative changes are totally asymptomatic. A herniated disk is usually diagnosed by pain that extends past the knee in a dermatomal pattern. Foot drop or loss of gastrocnemius strength deserves careful monitoring rather than urgent surgery.

In the absence of serious or progressive neurologic deficit, neoplasm, spinal infection, or significant trauma, CT or MRI should not be part of the initial examination. Absence of a reflex or isolated sensory loss is not considered to be a progressive neurologic deficit. If the CT or MRI is nonspecific, a SPECT nuclear medicine bone scan may exclude occult fractures, osteoid osteomas, and spondylolysis. Indications for imaging cancer patients with back pain are given in a following section on neoplasms.

Infections

Most infections in the spine involve a disk space and will cause destruction of the vertebral body above and below (Fig. 8-36). It is very rare for a tumor to involve or cross a disk space. Tumors typically will destroy a single vertebral body and then may extend above and below. Thus if you see a destructive process centered about a disk space, an infection should be your first choice.

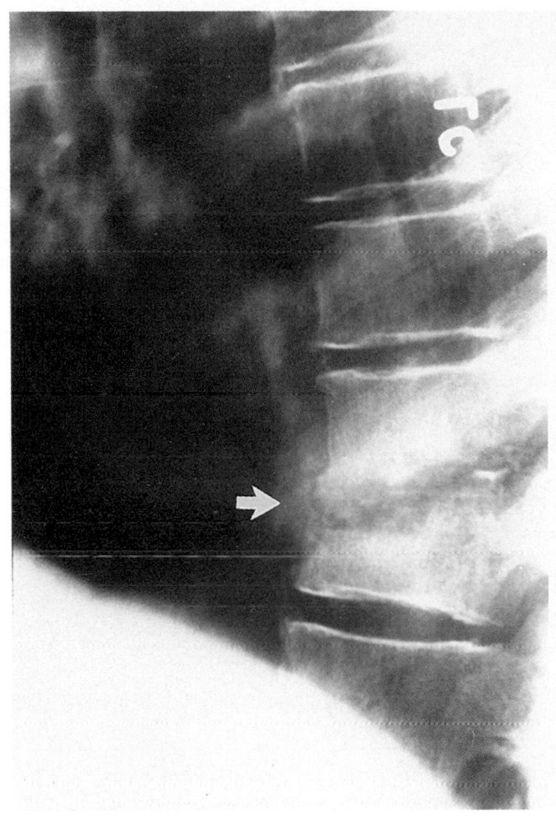

FIGURE 8-36 ■ **Osteomyelitis of the spine** A lateral view of the lower thoracic spine demonstrates destruction of the disk space *(arrow)* as well as destruction of the adjoining vertebral bodies.

Evaluation of the bony destruction of a vertebral body is best visualized by CT scan, but if a neurologic deficit is present, MRI is more appropriate.

Spinal Neoplasms and Metastases

Although primary bony neoplasms of the spine occur, they are very rare. The most common neoplastic involvement is from metastatic disease. The metastases may be destructive and cause holes (lytic lesions) in the bone, or they may be dense white (sclerotic lesions). Most neoplasms, including lung, renal, and breast cancer as well as multiple myeloma, will cause lytic lesions in bones. Most sclerotic metastases in men are due to prostate cancer, and in women, to breast cancer (Fig. 8-37).

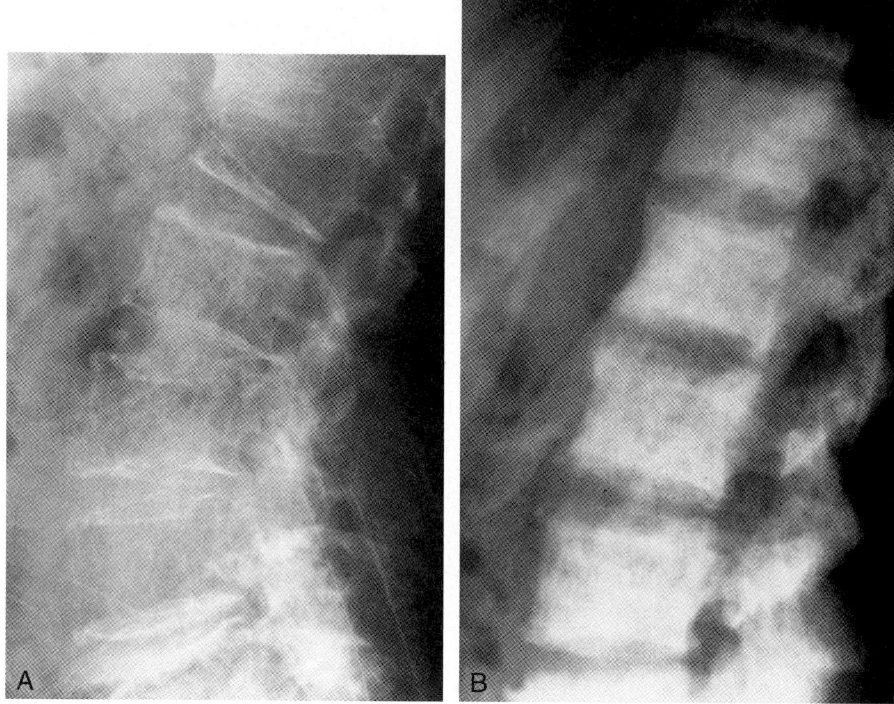

FIGURE 8-37 ■ Diffuse neoplastic involvement of the lumbar spine. In a patient with multiple myeloma, a lateral view of the lumbar spine *(A)* demonstrates vertebral bodies that are difficult to see owing to diffuse loss of calcium. Also note a vertebral body compression fracture. A lateral view of the spine *(B)* in a different patient with diffuse metastatic prostate cancer shows blastic or dense white metastases in most of the bones visualized.

Metastases do not begin in the bone cortex but rather in the red marrow, which has filtered the tumor cells out of the blood. After growing within the marrow space, the lesion becomes large enough to erode the bony cortex. The most sensitive method of finding metastatic disease in the spine is through use of MRI (Fig. 8-38). Unfortunately, MRI can focus only at limited portions of the body at one time. Therefore if you are thinking about metastatic disease to the skeleton, the most cost-effective imaging study is a nuclear medicine bone scan. If a patient has pain in a specific area, and you expect a very aggressive, destructive lesion (such as from renal cell carcinoma), order a plain x-ray of the area. Multiple myeloma not only can produce focal lytic lesions but also can diffusely involve the bones, removing enough of the calcium so that all the bones become very difficult to see.

If a patient has a known cancer of the central nervous system, head and neck, lymphoma, ovary, uterus, pancreas, colon, or rectum, and if the serum alkaline phosphatase level is normal and no bone pain is present, a nuclear medicine bone scan is not needed for initial workup. Nuclear medicine bone scans on patients with neoplasms are indicated in the following situations:

Initial staging
Non–small cell cancer of the lung, breast, or prostate cancer
Bone pain by history
Increased serum alkaline phosphatase, calcium, or prostate-specific antigen levels
Follow-up if initial bone scan was positive

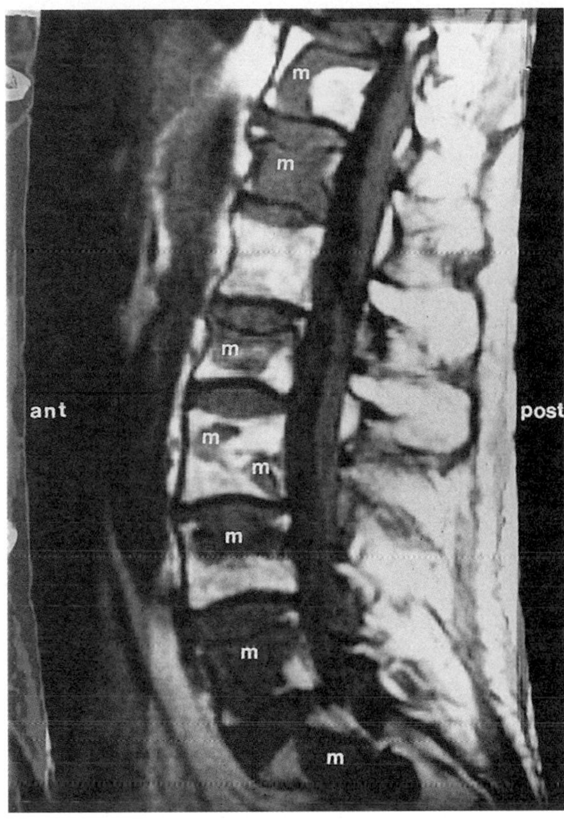

FIGURE 8-38 ■ **Focal spine metastases.** A sagittal or lateral T1-weighted magnetic resonance image of the lumbar spine shows the normal white or high signal in fat within the bone marrow. In many of the vertebral bodies, the high signal of normal marrow has been replaced by dark areas of metastatic deposits (m).

New or worsening pain
Completion of at least two cycles of chemotherapy
Six weeks after completion of chemotherapy or radiotherapy, negative initial bone scan follow-up and new pain

Unusual Lesions

A very characteristic, but unusual, lesion of the lumbar spine is ankylosing spondylitis. It occurs primarily in young male patients (onset at about age 20 years) and sometimes is associated with ulcerative colitis. Ninety-five percent of patients are positive for human leukocyte antigen (HLA)-B27. In this disease, calcification bridges the disk spaces. This is easily seen on the lateral plain x-ray and is referred to as a "bamboo spine." On the AP view, you will notice fusion of the sacroiliac joints (Fig. 8-39), and sometimes you can see "whiskering" (also called enthesopathy) of the ischial tuberosities and along the lateral ilium. About 30% of the patients will have a peripheral arthritis that spares the hands but involves the feet.

Osteoporosis and Bone Mineral Measurements

The accurate measurement of bone mineral density (BMD) with noninvasive methods can be of value in the detection and evaluation of primary and secondary causes of decreased mass. This includes primary osteoporosis and secondary disorders such as hyperparathyroidism, osteomalacia, malabsorption, multiple myeloma, diffuse metastases, and glucocorticoid therapy or intrinsic glucocorticoid excess.

By far the largest patient population is affected by primary osteoporosis. Osteoporosis is an age-related disorder characterized by decreased mass and by increased susceptibility to fractures in the absence of other recognizable

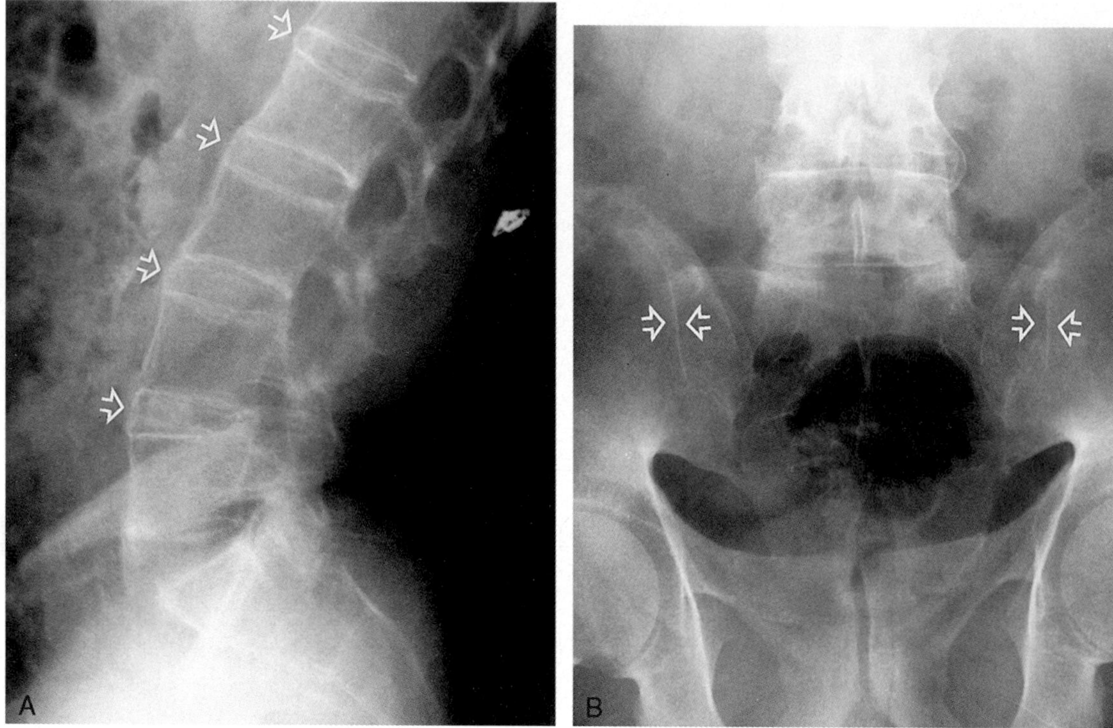

FIGURE 8-39 ■ **Ankylosing spondylitis.** A lateral view of the lumbar spine *(A)* demonstrates calcific bridging across the disk spaces *(arrows),* causing the typical "bamboo spine" appearance. *B,* Anteroposterior view of the pelvis shows that the region of the sacroiliac joints *(arrows)* is not easily visualized owing to fusion of both sacroiliac joints.

causes of loss. Primary osteoporosis is generally subdivided into type 1, or postmenopausal osteoporosis, which is related to estrogen deprivation, and type 2, or senile osteoporosis, which occurs as a result of aging.

Primary osteoporosis is a common clinical disorder and a major public health problem because of the significant number of related fractures occurring annually. Because the risk of vertebral and femoral neck fractures increases dramatically as BMD levels decrease to less than 1 g/cm^2, fracture risk in individual patients may be estimated. Furthermore, in estrogen-deficient women, BMD values may be used to make rational decisions about hormone replacement therapy and as follow-up in assessing the success of hormone replacement or specific bone-enhancing therapies.

A number of methods have been devised to permit the accurate and reproducible determination of bone mineral content. Plain x-rays generally require a loss of 30% or more of bone mineral for a change in density to be appreciated and are thus insensitive for the detection of the disease. Bone mineral measurements now are made by using dual energy x-ray absorptiometry (DEXA) or nuclear medicine techniques. Both are accurate and reliable. Results are usually presented in terms of absolute BMD (g/cm^2) as well as percentiles of reference in normal young adult and age-matched populations. Normal BMD is defined as being within 1 standard deviation of the young adult mean. Osteopenia is BMD 1 to 2.5 standard deviations less than the young adult mean. Osteoporosis is a BMD more than 2.5 standard deviations below the young adult mean.

The use of bone mineral measurement has been controversial, partly because of the wide variation of measurements in the normal population. The criteria for selecting the optimal skeletal site for evaluation have not been well

TABLE 8-4 ■ **Indications for Using DEXA to Measure Bone Mineral Density**

Intention to use hormone replacement or other medical therapy if osteoporosis is present
Suspect low bone mineral density based on osteopenia on plain radiographs
Low-impact or nontraumatic vertebral fractures by x-ray examination in a postmenopausal female (see text for additional factors) or premenopausal female or a male with normal serum thyroid-stimulating hormone, serum calcium, alkaline phosphatase, and serum protein electrophoresis levels
Loss of height >2.5 inches
Risk factors for low bone mineral density include estrogen-deficient state, chronic liver or renal disease, thyroxine therapy, steroid therapy for >6 mo (baseline and 12-mo follow-up), hyperparathyroidism, hypogonadism in a male, and nutritional disorder
Follow-up hormone therapy (only if a change in management is being contemplated)

DEXA, dual-energy x-ray absorptiometry.

defined, because bone mineral loss does not progress at the same rate at different body sites. In any case, the method can be used to determine the presence of osteopenia and to evaluate effectiveness of a therapeutic maneuver by using serial scans in which the patient acts as his or her own control. Normal results, or bone mineral content in the upper portion of the normal range, define patients in whom therapy may not be needed. Indications to use DEXA are given in Table 8-4.

SHOULDER AND HUMERUS

Normal Anatomy and Imaging

The standard view of the shoulder is obtained in an AP or a PA projection with the arm rotated internally and then externally. When the arm is in internal rotation, the humeral head looks generally smooth and spherical over the upper portion. In external rotation, a concavity of the bicipital groove is seen in the lateral aspect of the humeral head. In children, the proximal humeral epiphysis and an epiphyseal plate are visualized. This can sometimes be confused with a fracture. If the epiphyseal plate is not parallel to the x-ray beam, several lucent lines traversing

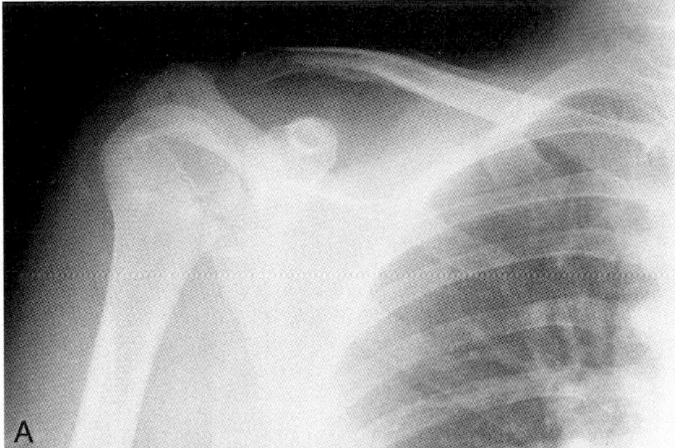

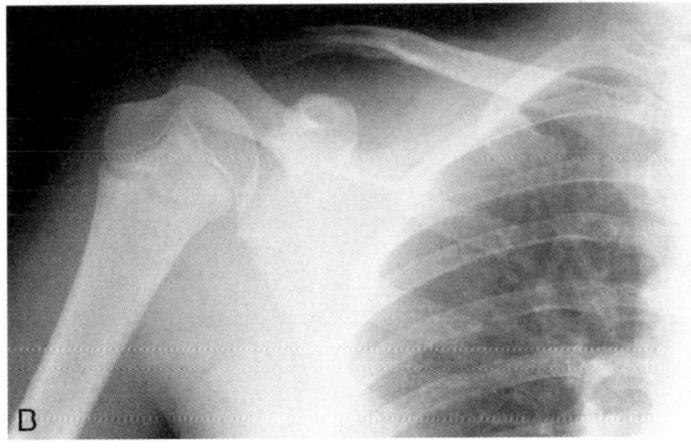

FIGURE 8-40 ■ **Normal shoulder of an 11-year-old patient in internal rotation *(A)* and in external rotation *(B)*.** The epiphyseal plate of the proximal humerus should not be mistaken for a fracture.

the proximal portion of the humerus can be seen, because the epiphyseal plate is tilted off axis relative to the x-ray beam (Fig. 8-40).

On a plain AP x-ray of the adult shoulder, the medial portion of the humeral head overlaps with the lateral aspect of the glenoid (Fig. 8-41). Sometimes the humeral head may project slightly lower or slightly higher than the center of the glenoid. Because the humerus is somewhat anterior to the glenoid, if the patient is tilted back when the image is taken, the humeral head will project high relative to the glenoid; if the patient is tilted somewhat forward, it will appear slightly low. Examine the relation of the distal clavicle to the acromion to see whether an acromioclavicular (AC) separation has occurred. In teenagers, an apophysis on the end of the coracoid process and on the

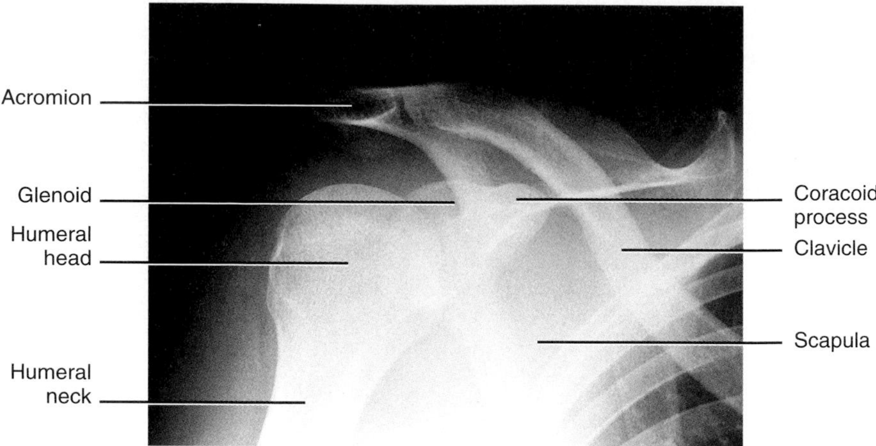

FIGURE 8-41 ■ Normal anatomy of the adult shoulder in the posteroanterior projection with the humerus in internal rotation.

acromion is seen as a thin crescentic white line and should not be mistaken for an avulsion fracture (Fig. 8-42). The clavicle, scapula, and ribs should be examined for fractures and other lesions. Also look to see whether any pathology exists in the visualized portions of the lung.

There are two other commonly ordered views of the shoulder. The first is called the "Y" view. This is done with the patient rotated somewhat so that the scapular blade is seen on end and projects off the chest wall. The acromion, spine of the scapula, and blade of the scapula form a "Y" (Fig. 8-43). The humeral head should normally project at or near the intersection of the three lines. This view is usually obtained if a shoulder dislocation is suspected and also is useful to look for fractures of the scapular blade.

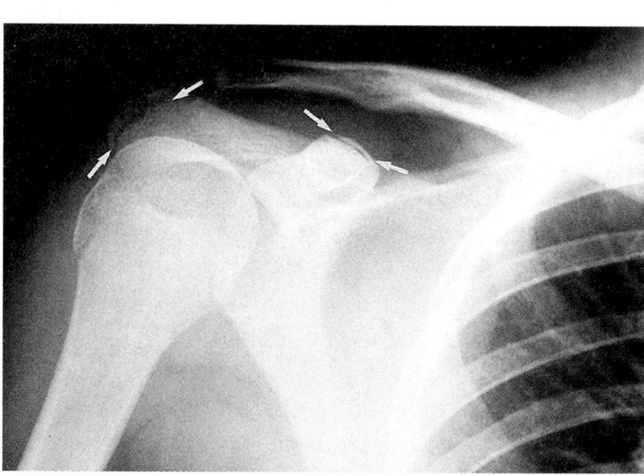

FIGURE 8-42 ■ **Normal apophysis in the shoulder of a teenager.** An apophysis with a lucent line can be seen in the distal acromion as well as the coracoid process. This should not be mistaken for an avulsion fracture.

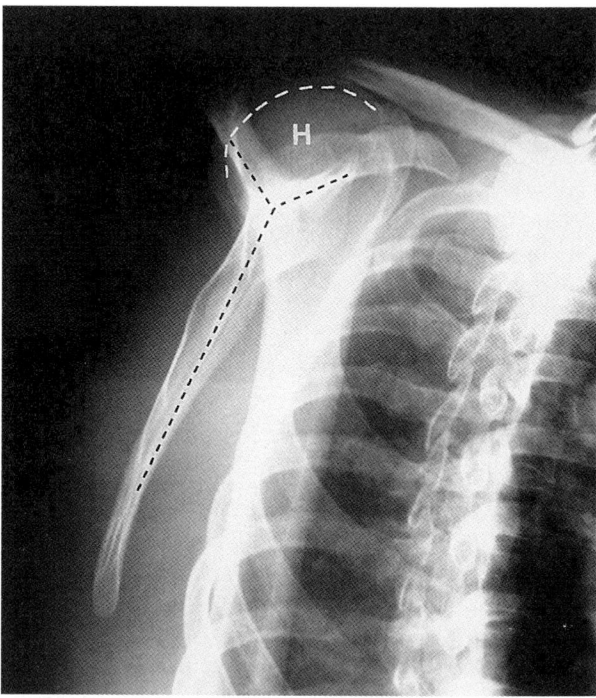

FIGURE 8-43 ■ **Normal oblique or "Y," view of the shoulder.** On this view, the elements of the scapula form a Y, and the humeral head should overlap the intersecting arms of the Y.

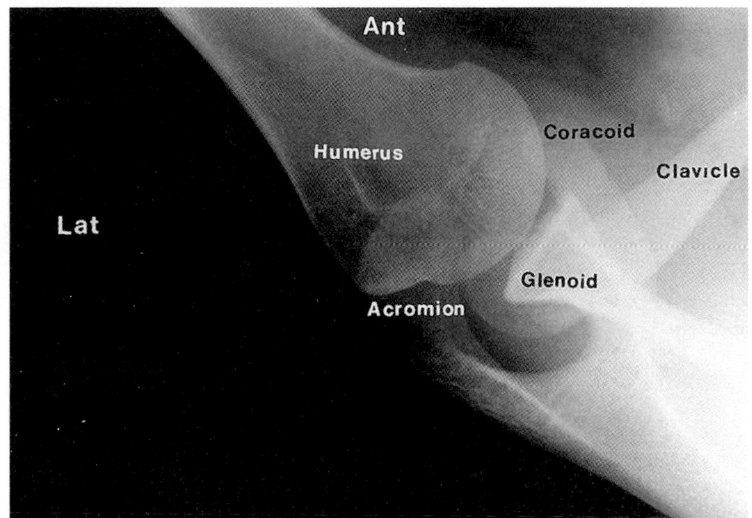

FIGURE 8-44 ■ Normal axillary view of the shoulder.

The second view often obtained is the axillary view, in which the elbow is elevated and the beam projection is directly down through the shoulder. This allows clear visualization of the relation of the glenoid to the humeral head (Fig. 8-44). Unfortunately, this view is difficult to obtain on patients who have a true dislocation. Be careful about ordering this projection if you suspect a humeral head or humeral shaft fracture, because the technologists may make the situation worse by elevating the patient's elbow in an attempt to obtain the axillary view.

Plain x-rays of the shoulder are really useful only to define bony anatomy. Many shoulder injuries involve soft tissues, and for evaluation of these, the most useful imaging test is an MRI scan. The joint and soft tissues also can be visualized by injecting contrast directly into the joint and imaging with MRI or CT. MRI allows excellent visualization not only of the muscle but also of the joint space as well as the tendons (Fig. 8-45). Remember that what appears to be a white bone on an MR image is really fat within the marrow space, and the cortex of the bone is seen as a black line around the edge. Fat in the subcutaneous areas also is seen as white, and muscle is usually gray.

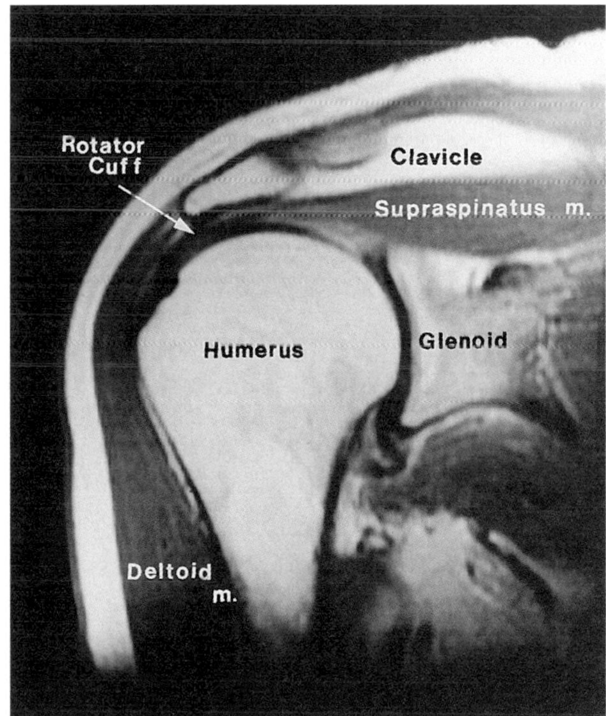

FIGURE 8-45 ■ **Normal coronal view of the shoulder with a T1-weighted magnetic resonance scan.** The osseous structures, including the humeral head, glenoid, acromion, and clavicle, are well seen. The muscular structures of the deltoid and supraspinatus also are seen, and the rotator cuff can be identified.

Trauma

Table 8-5 shows the high-yield areas to examine for upper extremity trauma. Probably the three most common acute shoulder injuries are fracture, shoulder separation [acromioclavicular (AC)] separation, and dislocation of the humeral head.

TABLE 8–5 ■ **Examination of an X-ray of the Upper Extremity Done for Trauma**

Shoulder
AP view
- Anterior dislocation, humeral head inferior and medial
- Posterior dislocation, humeral head not round and slightly lateral
- Acromioclavicular separation
- Clavicular fracture
- Scapular fracture
- Rib fracture

Y view
- Dislocation
- Scapular fracture

Elbow
AP view
- Radial head fracture
- Supracondylar fracture

Lateral view
- Posterior fat pad (always abnormal)
- Bulging anterior fat pad
- Olecranon fracture
- Coronoid fracture
- Radial head alignment

Wrist
PA view
- Distal radius
- Ulnar styloid
- Navicular
- Widening between navicular and lunate
- Two distinct rows of carpals present
- Base of thumb

Lateral view
- Alignment of radius, ulna, lunate, and distal carpals
- Dorsum (for triquetral fracture)

Hand
AP view
- Fifth metacarpal (boxer's fracture)
- Base of first metacarpal (Bennett's or Rolando's fracture if intra-articular)
- Base of first proximal phalanx (gamekeeper's thumb)
- Proximal interphalangeal joints, dislocations
- Distal phalanx, tuft fracture

Lateral view
- Base of phalanges (volar plate fracture)

AP, anteroposterior; PA, posteroanterior.

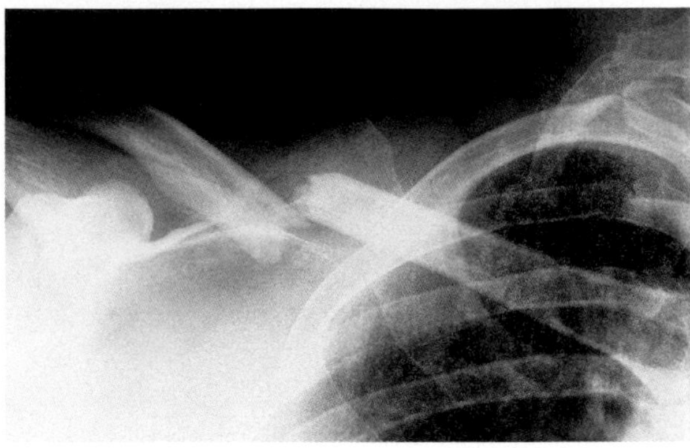

FIGURE 8-46 ■ Midclavicular fracture.

Fractures. Most clavicular fractures occur either in the midportion or the distal third of the clavicle. Usually the fractures are clinically obvious (Fig. 8-46). Rarely dislocation of the proximal head of the clavicle from the sternoclavicular joint occurs; however, this also is clinically obvious. Fractures of the scapula are

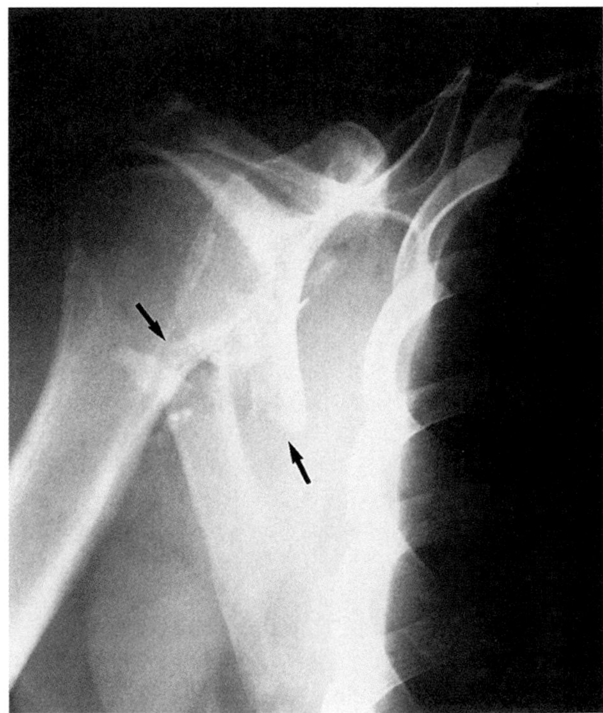

FIGURE 8-47 ■ **Scapular fracture.** A "Y" view of the shoulder clearly shows a fracture through the blade of the scapula *(arrows)*.

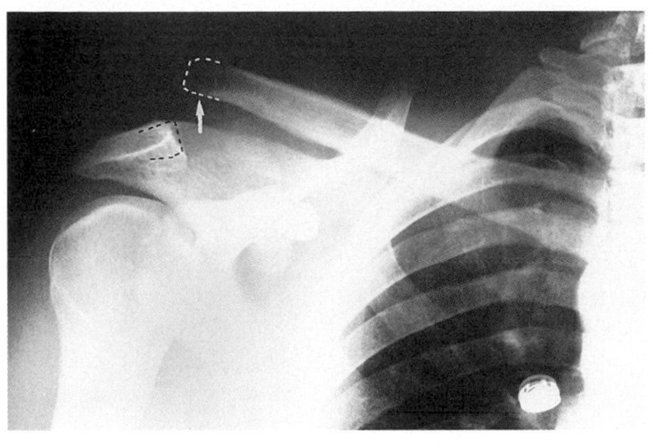

FIGURE 8-48 ■ **Acromioclavicular separation.** The distal end of the clavicle is superiorly dislocated relative to the acromion.

reasonably rare, although they can occur as the result of a direct blow. Often this is apparent on a routine shoulder film and from the clinical history (Fig. 8-47). In many cases, the fracture cannot be seen in its entirety as it traverses the blade of the scapula, and, with any additional question, a Y-view x-ray or a CT scan may be useful.

Fractures of the mid- or proximal humerus present few problems in radiographic interpretation and thus are not considered further.

Acromioclavicular Separation. In this injury, superior dislocation of the distal clavicle occurs relative to the acromion (Fig. 8-48). Because the clavicle is slightly anterior relative to the acromion, if the patient is leaning back when the film is taken, it sometimes looks as though a separation exists when none is present. If you have any question, a single view that includes both shoulders often is useful. Sometimes AP x-rays of the shoulders with the patient holding weights in both hands are ordered to see if this will accentuate a separation, but in practice this is rarely necessary.

Dislocations. More than 95% of shoulder dislocations occur with anterior dislocation of the humeral head relative to the glenoid. This is in contrast to the hip, in which the vast majority of femoral head dislocations are posterior. In an anterior shoulder dislocation, the humeral head usually is seen to be inferior to the glenoid on the AP projection with medial displacement of the humeral head from its normal position

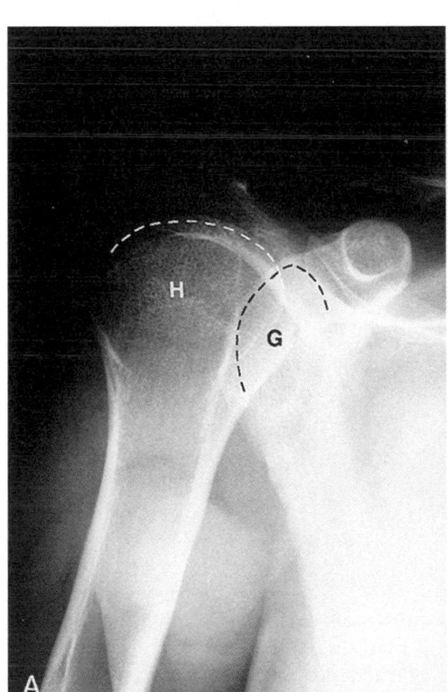

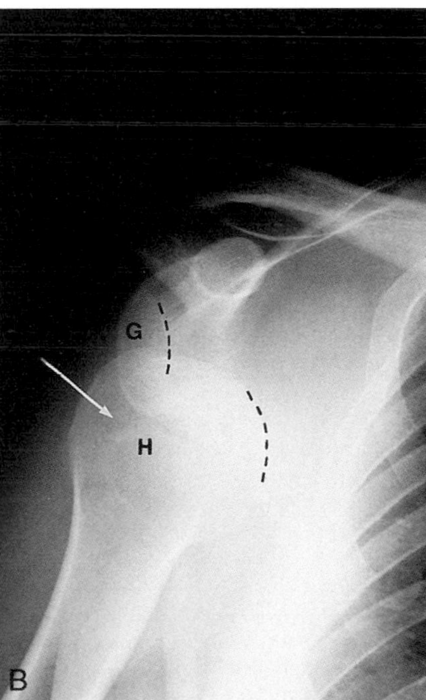

FIGURE 8-49 ■ **Anterior dislocation of the shoulder.** *A,* In the normal anterioposterior view of the shoulder, the humeral head is located lateral to the glenoid, but a small amount of overlap is seen. *B,* In the same patient with an anterior dislocation, the humeral head goes inferiorly and medially with respect to the glenoid.

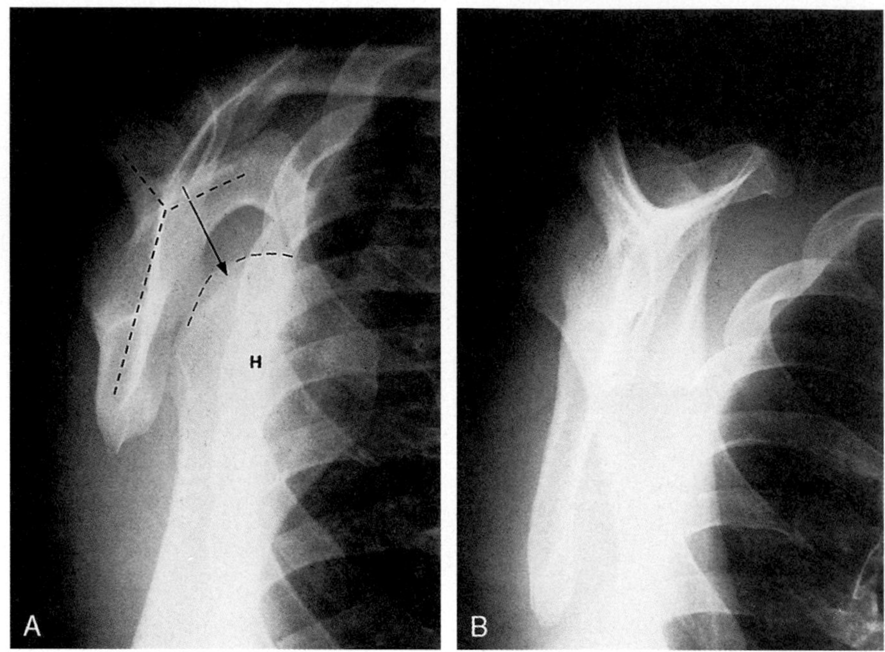

FIGURE 8-50 ■ **Anterior dislocation on the Y view.** *A,* On the Y view, the humeral head is clearly anterior and inferior to the intersection of the Y of the scapula. *B,* After relocation, the humeral head overlaps the Y formed by the scapula.

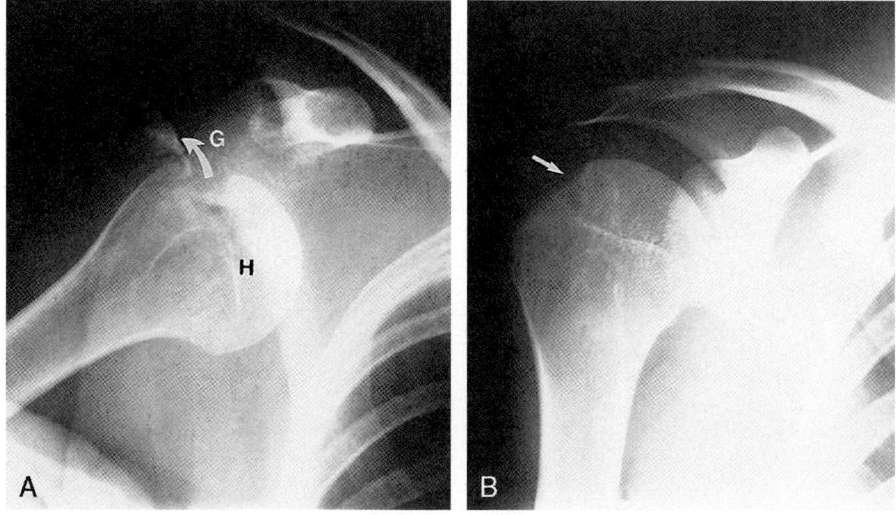

FIGURE 8-51 ■ **Complications of shoulder dislocation.** *A,* In a patient with an anterior dislocation of the humeral head, a fracture fragment arising from the humerus *(arrow)* can be identified. *B,* In a different patient, chronic anterior dislocations caused a Hill-Sachs deformity, seen as a groove in the upper outer portion of the humeral head *(arrow).*

relative to the glenoid (Fig. 8-49). As mentioned earlier, on the oblique view of the shoulder (the Y view), the humeral head should sit over the central portion of the Y. A Y view will clearly show the anterior and inferior dislocation of the humeral head (Fig. 8-50).

Two specific abnormalities may be found in addition to the dislocation. As a dislocation occurs, there is sometimes a fracture of a portion of the humeral head or of the glenoid. Some physicians relocate a dislocated shoulder without obtaining a prereduction image. If you do this, and the postreduction image demonstrates a fracture, the patient may accuse you of having been responsible for the fracture during the reduction. The second major abnormality occurs in patients who have had repeated dislocations. Chronic trauma caused by interaction of the inferior edge of the glenoid with the humeral head produces a deformity or groove in the superolateral portion of the humeral head, known as a Hill-Sachs deformity (Fig. 8-51).

Posterior shoulder dislocations are rare, and they are quite tricky to identify on a standard AP view of the shoulder. Remember that with internal rotation the humeral head on the AP projection is typically like the top half of a sphere. In a posterior shoulder dislocation, the humeral head simply does not appear to be rounded (Fig. 8-52), and a slightly increased space is seen between the humeral head and the glenoid. The Y view will clearly show you the posterior dislocation.

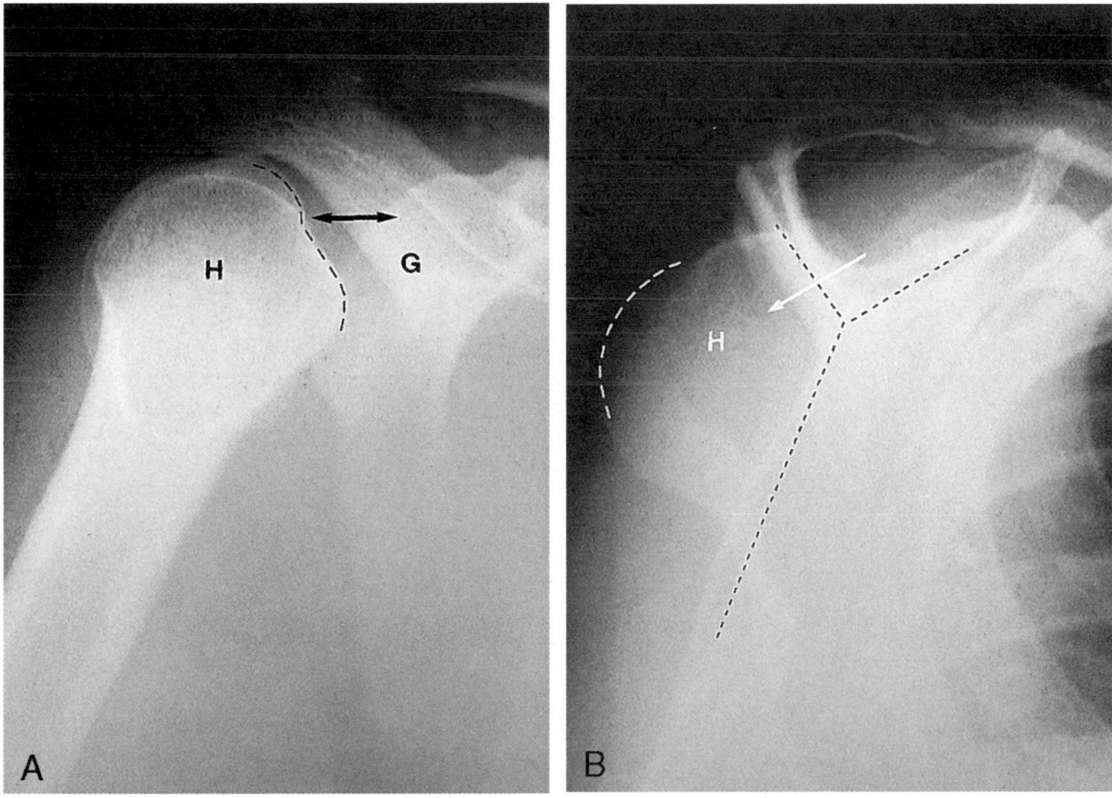

FIGURE 8-52 ■ Posterior dislocation of the humeral head. *A,* An anteroposterior view of the shoulder initially looks fairly normal. However, an increased space (double-ended arrow) is present between the humeral head and the glenoid; the fact that the humeral head is not spherical *(dotted line)* is another clue. *B,* On the Y view of the shoulder, the humeral head can clearly be seen to be displaced posteriorly relative to the central portion of the Y formed by the scapula.

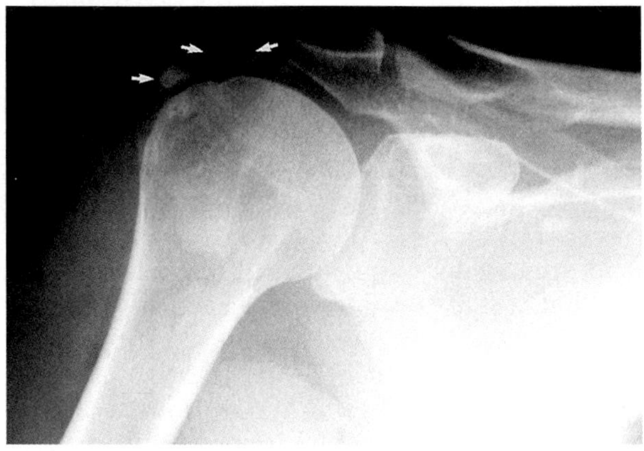

FIGURE 8-53 ■ Calcific tendinitis. Small clumps of amorphous calcification can be identified over the superior and lateral portion of the humeral head *(arrows)*.

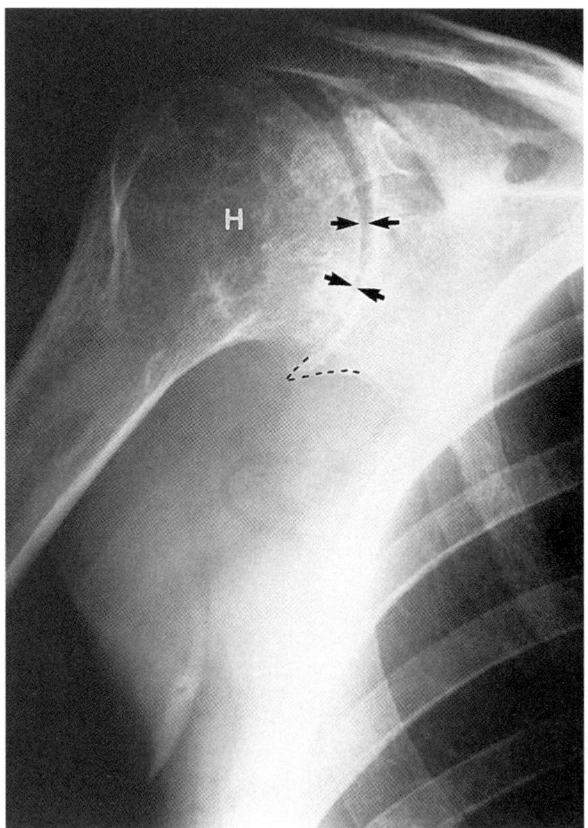

FIGURE 8-54 ■ Degenerative arthritis of the shoulder. Marked narrowing of the normal joint space *(arrows)* is seen, with flattening of the humeral head and spurring deformity of the inferior portion of the glenoid.

Shoulder Pain and Degenerative Changes

Most shoulder pain is due to degenerative change or degenerative arthritis. A degenerative change that can be seen on the plain x-ray is calcification of tendons. This usually appears as amorphous white densities over the superolateral aspect of the humeral head (Fig. 8-53). The major form of degenerative change is post-traumatic or degenerative arthritis. Because the glenohumeral joint is off axis relative to an AP x-ray beam, minimal joint-space narrowing is not easily evaluated. However, if the changes are severe enough (Fig. 8-54), it is easy to see that the joint is narrowed. Typically, associated sclerosis and often spurring and deformity of the humeral head and the inferior aspect of the glenoid are found. Degenerative change also includes rotator cuff tears. This is suspected when pain occurs with abduction and weakness at more than 60 degrees. If pain persists after 6 weeks of nonsteroidal anti-inflammatory drug (NSAID) therapy and supervised physical therapy, and if surgery is contemplated, MRI is indicated. Rotator cuff tears are best visualized by using MR scanning. With the tear, there may be a narrowing of the acromiohumeral space to less than 6 mm, an eroded inferior aspect of the acromion, and abnormal communication of the joint space with the subdeltoid bursa.

Tumors

Of the number of lesions that can be found in the shoulder, one of the most common benign tumors is the unicameral bone cyst (Fig. 8-55). This expansile, lytic, well-demarcated lesion almost always occurs in the proximal portion of the humerus in children or young teenagers. It probably is not a true cyst but may be the sequela of trauma or an intraosseous hematoma. It is usually discovered incidentally or when a fracture occurs through the weakened bone. As the child grows, the cyst usually becomes smaller and appears to progress down the shaft of the bone. Actually, it stays in the same place but appears to move with time because of the longitudinal bone growth that occurs at the epiphyseal plate.

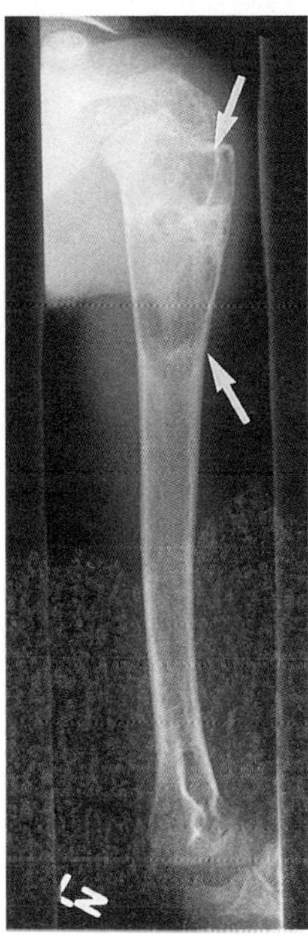

FIGURE 8-55 ■ Unicameral bone cyst. The proximal portion of the humerus is a common location for this lesion *(arrows)*. The lesion is lucent, is quite well defined, and can be slightly expansile. A fracture can occur through this area owing to the weakened bone.

Malignant lesions also develop in the shoulder. Because the scapula is a flat bone, Ewing's sarcoma can occur here. Remember that the proximal humerus is the third most frequent site of osteogenic sarcoma in children. This lesion is discussed further in the section on the knee, because the knee is a more common location.

Infection

Septic arthritis of the shoulder is seen initially as swelling of the shoulder joint with an effusion, followed by cartilage destruction and then bony destruction of both the glenoid and the humeral head. Early changes may be only widening of the joint space due to fluid or pus in the joint space. If there is a question, the joint is usually aspirated. The later changes are easily visible on a standard x-ray.

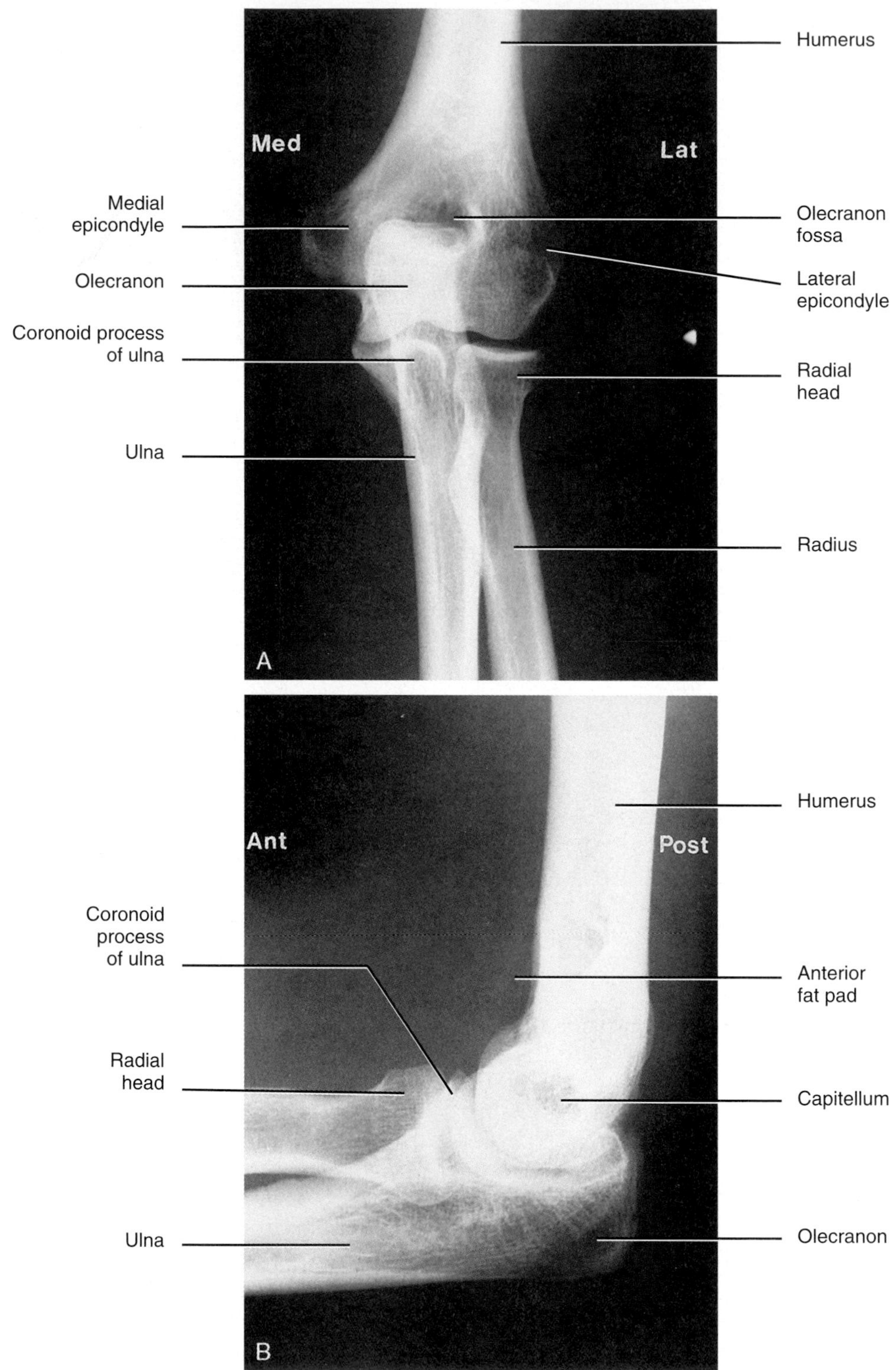

FIGURE 8-56 ■ Normal anatomy of the elbow in the anteroposterior projection *(A)* and in the lateral projection *(B)*.

ELBOW

Normal Anatomy and Imaging

Most x-ray examinations of the elbow relate to trauma. The normal images obtained include an AP and oblique view with the elbow extended and a lateral view with the elbow flexed at 90 degrees (Fig. 8-56). The lateral view is the most promising to look for pathology in the elbow. A small dark area is seen just anterior to the distal humerus. This is the anterior fat pad, and, although it is normal to see this, it should be right up against the bone. A posterior fat pad is never seen normally. In a teenager, lack of fusion of the normal epiphyses and presence of apophyses can cause confusion. The last areas of fusion include the radial head and the coronoid apophysis, which are located on the medial aspect of the elbow. In addition, an olecranon apophysis can be seen on the lateral view (Fig. 8-57). Normally these apophyses are not mistaken for fractures if you realize that they have well-defined margins without sharp edges and that the anterior fat pad is in normal position and a posterior fat pad is not seen.

Trauma

As mentioned earlier, the place to begin looking for traumatic injuries in an adult is on the lateral view. Immediately look for the anterior fat pad, which should lie against the anterior portion of the distal humerus. Anterior displacement of the fat pad is often referred to as the "sail sign." This is because, when it is pushed forward by an effusion or hemorrhage, it resembles the spinnaker on a sailboat. When you see either anterior displacement of the anterior fat pad or any visualization whatever of the

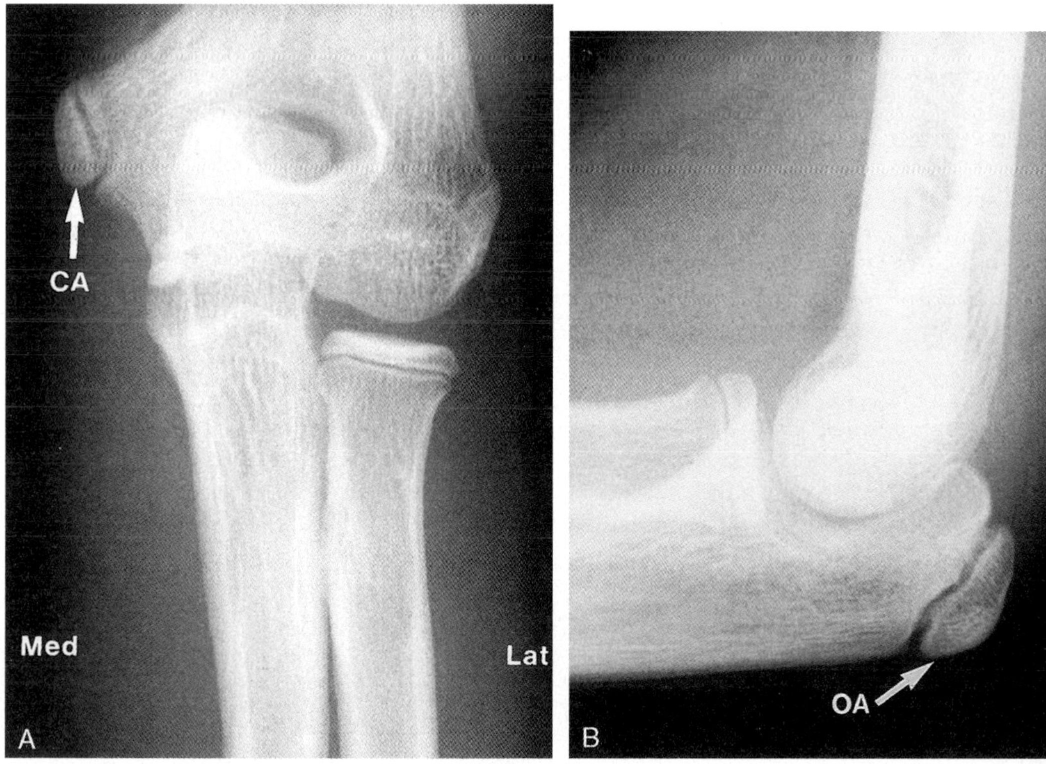

FIGURE 8-57 ■ Normal apophyses. On the anteroposterior projection *(A)*, a coronoid apophysis (CA) can be seen along the medial aspect of the distal humerus. On the lateral view *(B)*, an olecranon apophysis (OA) is often visualized in older children. The radial epiphysis has not yet fused.

FIGURE 8-58 ■ Radial head fracture. The lateral view of the elbow *(A)* shows anterior displacement of the dark stripe of the anterior fat pad *(posterior arrows)*; a posterior fat pad also is seen *(arrows)*. On the anteroposterior view *(B)*, a lucent fracture line is seen going obliquely across the humeral head.

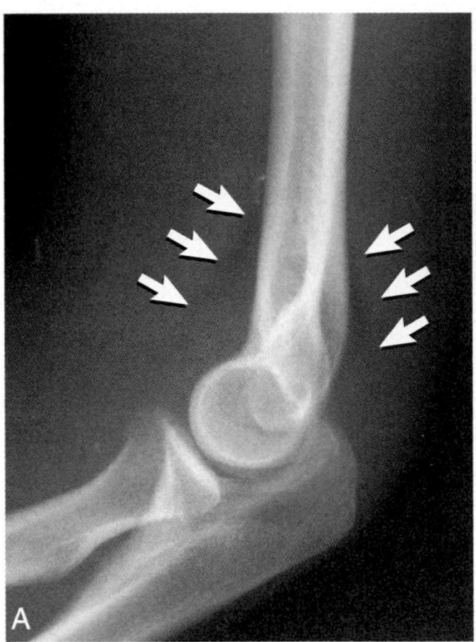

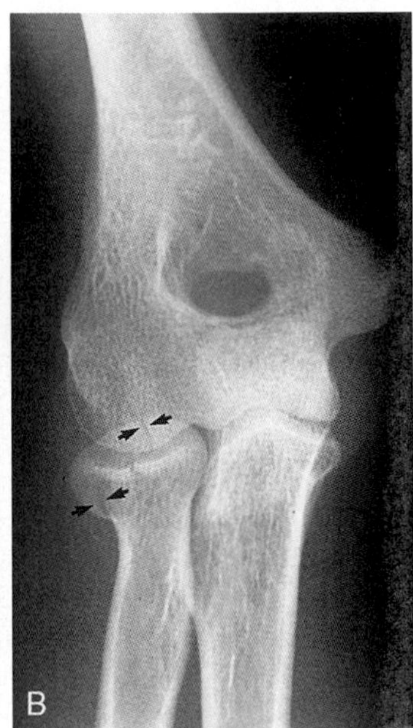

posterior fat pad, you should indicate that a fracture is likely to be present, even if you do not see it on any of the views. Sometimes repeating the examination 7 to 10 days later will allow decalcification of the fracture to occur so that it will be more easily seen.

The most common fracture of the elbow seen in the adult is a radial head fracture (Fig. 8-58). Less common are fractures of the coronoid process of the ulna (Fig. 8-59) and fractures of the olecranon. Olecranon fractures are typically caused by falling directly on the elbow when it is flexed. Orthopedic hardware used to fix elbow injuries includes screws, wire, and fixation pins (Fig. 8-60). In evaluation of postreduction and postfixation images, look at alignment and residual angulation to see that healing occurs across the fracture, that the wires and screws have not migrated, and, finally, that no increasing lucency or dark areas are present around either the screws or the pins to suggest osteomyelitis or loosening.

FOREARM

Typical normal views of the forearm are obtained in AP and lateral projections. If you suspect trauma or abnormalities of either the elbow or the wrist, a forearm view alone is not satisfactory. You should order forearm views only when you think that the abnormality is in the middle portion of either the radius or the ulna.

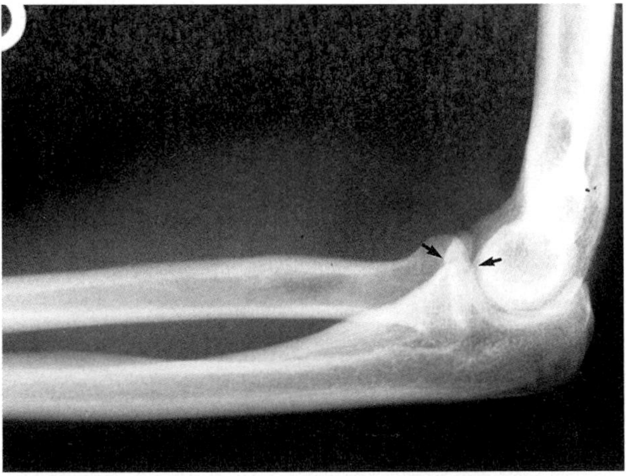

FIGURE 8-59 ■ Coronoid fracture. The anteroposterior view in this patient looked normal; however, on the lateral view, the coronoid process of the ulna has a lucent (dark) fracture line extending through it *(arrows)*.

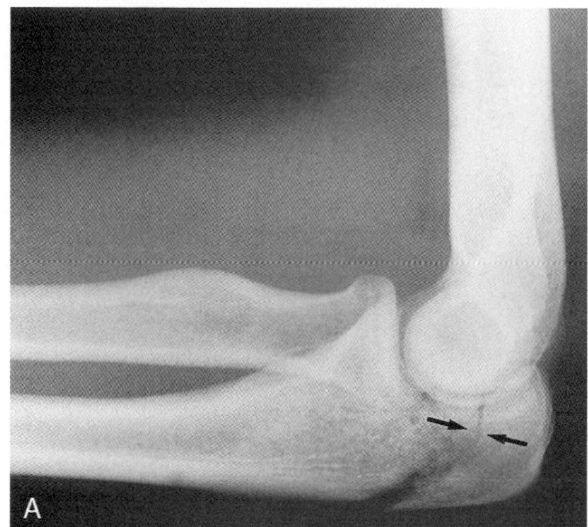

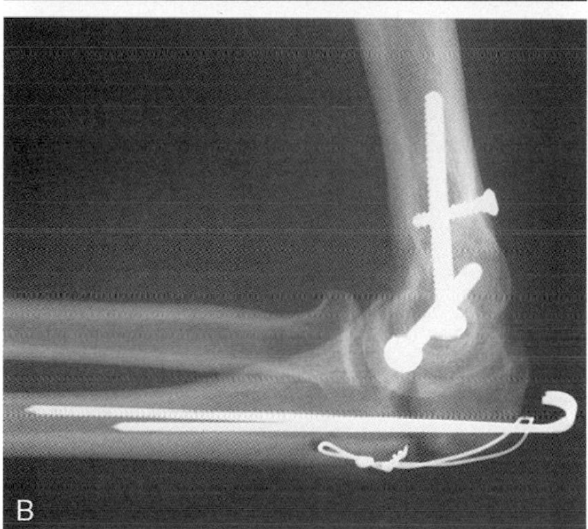

FIGURE 8-60 ■ **Olecranon fracture.** *A,* The initial lateral view of this patient who fell directly on the elbow demonstrates a fracture line extending into the joint space *(arrows)*. *B,* In a different patient, an olecranon fracture has been repaired by using two fixation pins and a tension wire. This patient also had a supracondylar fracture, accounting for the screws in the distal humerus.

Trauma

Traumatic injuries are, by far, the most common reason for ordering forearm x-rays. Of the three classic fractures that you should be aware of, the first is the "nightstick" fracture, a single fracture through the midportion of the ulna (Fig. 8-61). It is called the nightstick fracture because it usually occurs when an individual raises his or her arm to protect against being hit with a stick. A direct blow to the upraised and slightly flexed forearm means that the impact of the stick will be directly on the midportion of the ulna, causing a fracture. Fractures of the forearm often heal by a simple reduction and casting, although occasionally a compression plate and fixation screws are used. In a compression plate, the holes for the screws are somewhat elliptical, and this allows placement of the screws in such a manner that the ends of the fracture will be compressed together.

The two other classic (although uncommon) fractures of the forearm include the Monteggia fracture of the proximal ulna with dislocation of

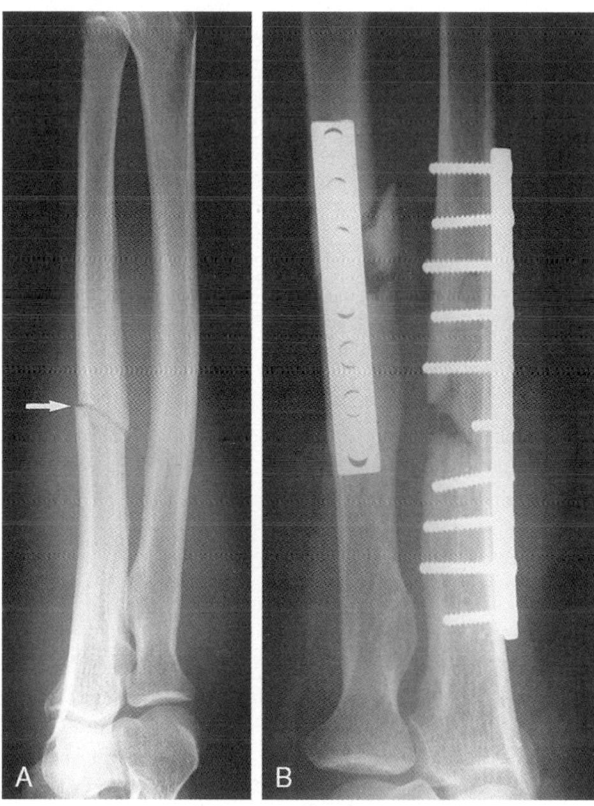

FIGURE 8-61 ■ **Nightstick fracture.** *A,* An anteroposterior view of the forearm demonstrates a single fracture across the midportion of the ulna. This is called a nightstick fracture because it occurs when the person lifts the forearm to protect against being hit with a stick. *B,* In a different patient with a much more severe fracture of the radius and ulna, the fracture has been fixed by using a plate and screws. Notice the asymmetrical holes in the plate, which allow compression of the fracture fragments.

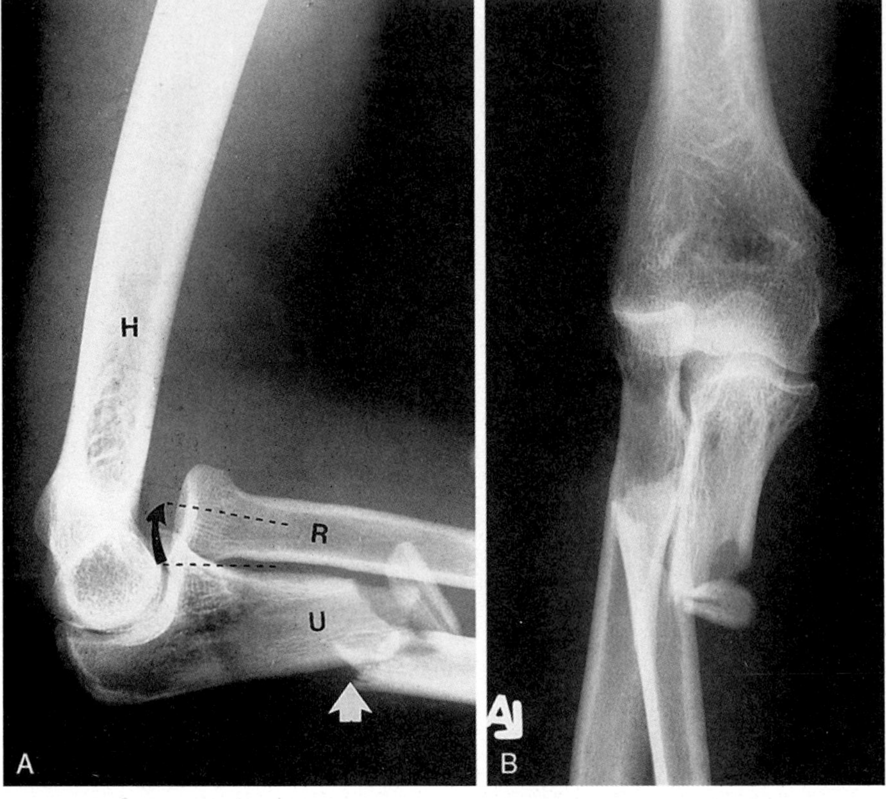

FIGURE 8-62 ■ Monteggia fracture/dislocation. *A,* The lateral view of the elbow shows a fracture of the ulna that occurs at the direct point of impact *(large white arrow)* and dislocation of the radial head from its normal position *(curved black arrow)*. *B,* On the anteroposterior projection, the ulnar fracture is clearly identified, but the radial head dislocation is impossible to see.

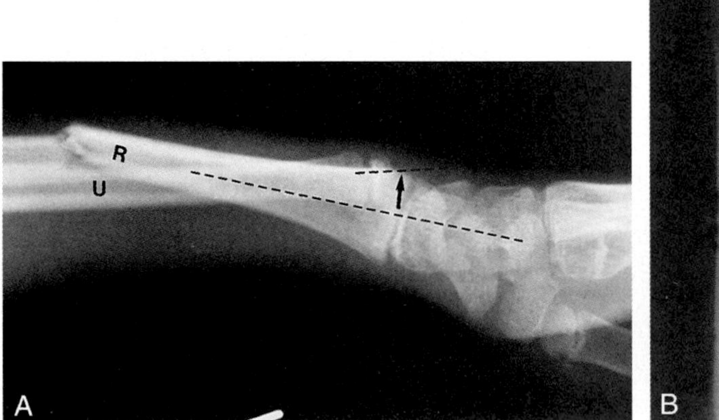

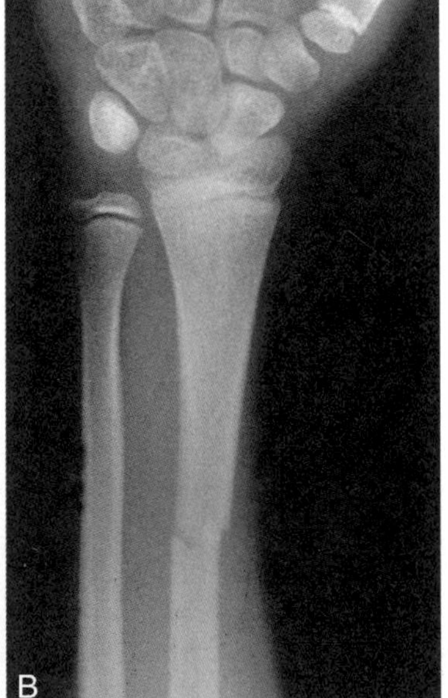

FIGURE 8-63 ■ Galeazzi fracture. *A,* A lateral view of the distal aspect of the forearm shows a fracture of the distal radius and ulnar dislocation from the normal axis of the wrist. *B,* On the anteroposterior projection, only the radial fracture is seen.

the radial head (Fig. 8-62). The dislocation of the radial head can be missed unless you realize that the radius and radial head should point toward the capitellum. The usual mechanism of this fracture is falling forward while carrying weight in the hands, such as a load of books. During the fall, a direct blow is delivered to the ulna by a sharp object, such as the corner of a stair. The weight of the body is transmitted down the humerus to the elbow while the weight of the books is in the hands, and the corner of the stair is a fulcrum located at the proximal portion of the forearm between the two weights. The Galeazzi fracture is a fracture of the distal radius with dislocation of the ulnar head from the wrist joint (Fig. 8-63). The mechanism is somewhat similar to that of a Monteggia fracture, but with the fulcrum located more distally.

HAND AND WRIST

Normal Anatomy and Imaging

The typical views obtained when either hand or wrist x-rays are ordered are AP, oblique, and lateral (Fig. 8-64). Usually these are done for assessment of trauma or degenerative changes. The wrist has many little bones that have unusual shapes and that overlap. Examination of the wrist on the AP view begins with examination of the distal radius and ulna, particularly the styloid processes of each. Next, examine the two rows of carpals (the proximal row is crescentic). The carpal joint spaces are usually quite uniform, and you should look across the carpal/metacarpal and interphalangeal joints in a sequential process.

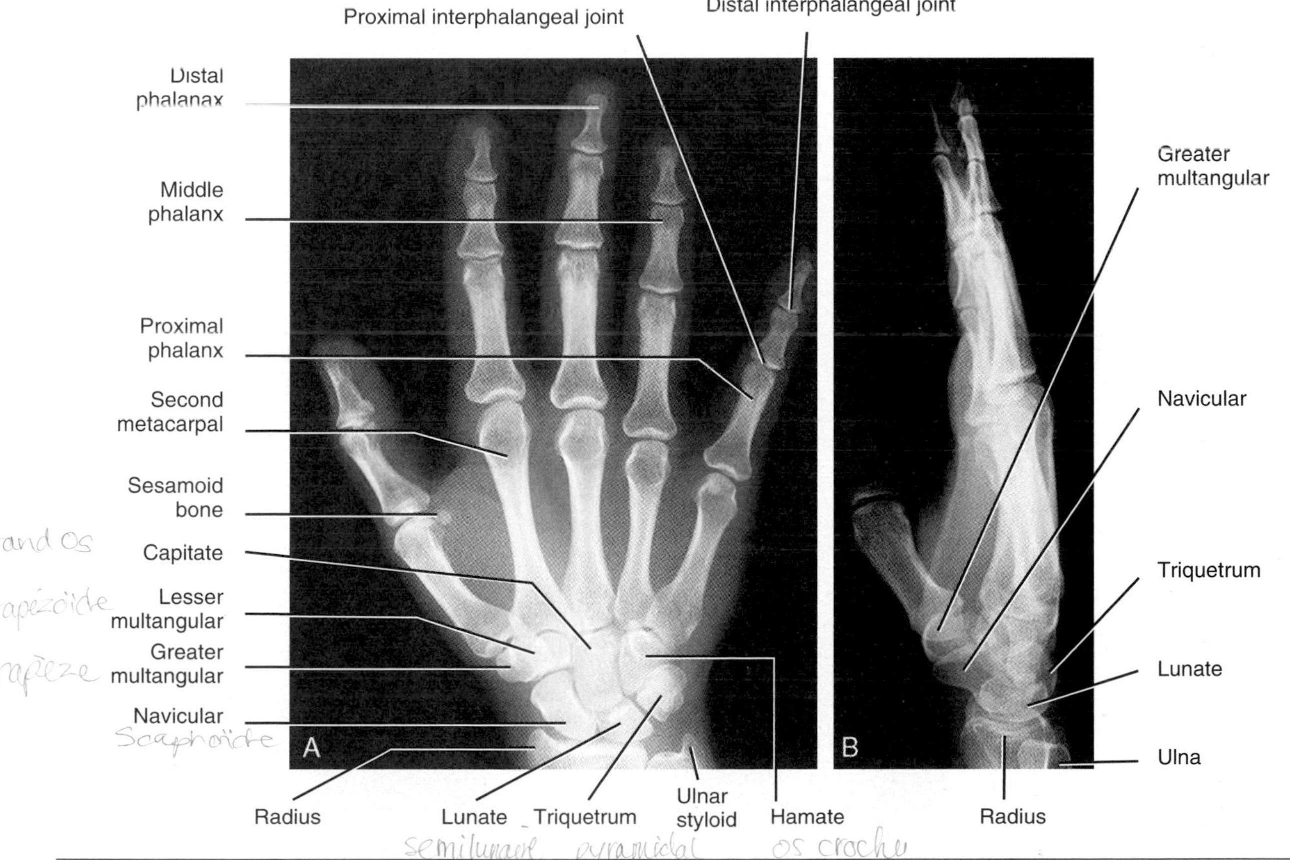

FIGURE 8-64 ■ Normal anatomy of the hand and wrist in the posteroanterior *(A)* and lateral *(B)* projections.

Wrist Pain

Carpometacarpal osteoarthritis usually occurs at the base of the thumb, and patients have pain and swelling or enlargement at the affected joint. Plain x-rays are indicated, and symptomatic patients have abnormal images with sclerosis, joint-space narrowing, and spur formation. Wrist pain also may be due to chronic ligamentous injury, usually involving the fibrocartilaginous complex. Tenderness, dorsal and volar subluxation at rest, and pain with stress are found. If pain persists after 6 weeks of NSAID therapy and a wrist splint, MRI may be indicated. Carpal tunnel syndrome is a compression neuropathy with loss of sensation in the tips of the first three digits and forearm and wrist pain. Physical examination and medical history are often diagnostic. Nerve-conduction velocity tests are indicated but not imaging. Similarly, imaging is not needed for evaluation or treatment of an uncomplicated dorsal ganglion.

Trauma

A fracture often becomes more apparent a week or so after the initial injury (Fig. 8-65). The reason is that, in the early stages of a fracture, hyperemia occurs, which is accompanied by resorption of calcium along the fracture line. This is why radiologists will sometimes indicate that, although they do not see a fracture on a particular examination, if pain persists, a repeated view in 7 to 10 days may be useful. A second phenomenon is a more general loss of calcium and coarsening of the trabecular pattern in bones around a joint that has a fracture. This process may occur over several weeks and is the result of disuse osteoporosis (Fig. 8-66). Sometimes, even with minor trauma, joint pain can persist for months with associated vasodilatation. This is termed reflex sympathetic dystrophy (RSD). The radiographic manifestations are focal osteoporosis and a coarse trabecular pattern, in an articular and periarticular distribution (Fig. 8-67).

Common fractures of the wrist include the Colles' fracture, a fracture of the distal radius with dorsal angulation of the distal fragment and an associated fracture of the ulnar styloid (Fig. 8-68). The mechanism of injury is typically falling on an outstretched hand with the palm facing down. A Smith fracture is essentially a reverse Colles' fracture, with the distal radial fragment angulated toward the palmar surface (Fig. 8-69).

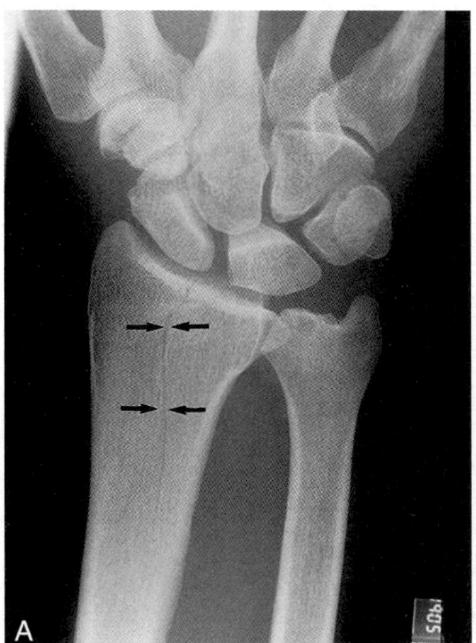

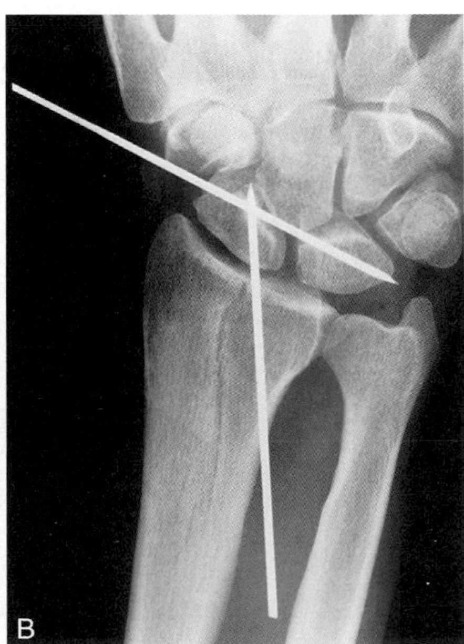

FIGURE 8-65 ■ Increasing fracture visibility with time. *A,* Initial PA view of the wrist shows a longitudinal fracture with intra-articular extension *(arrows)*. *B,* A film obtained 1 week later with fixation pins in place shows that the fracture line is much more evident owing to interval decalcification, which is a normal process. This may make fractures much more visible a week or so after the injury than on the initial films.

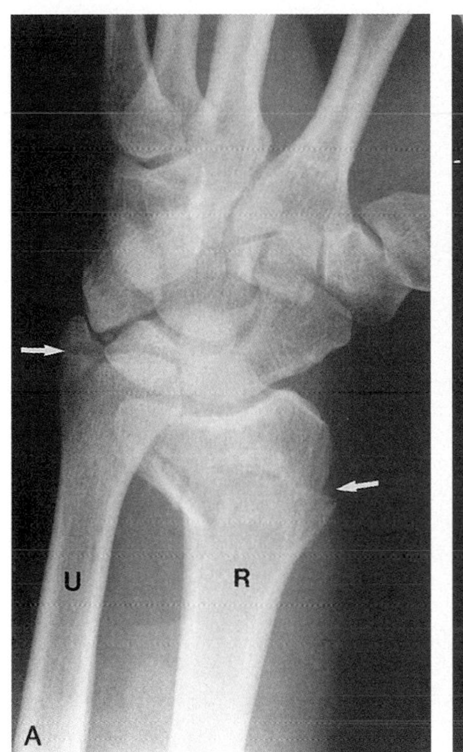

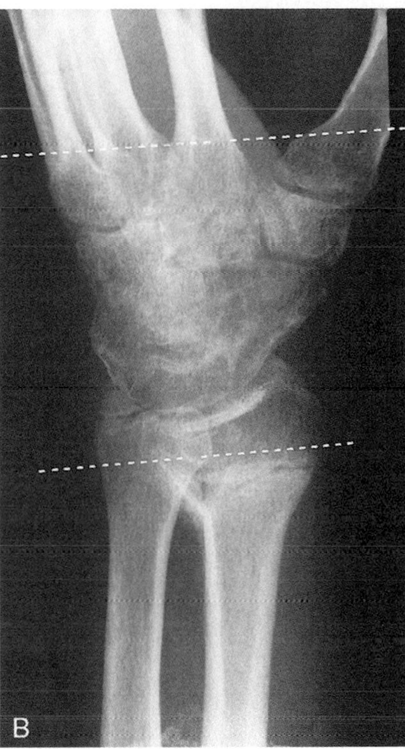

FIGURE 8-66 ■ **Interval disuse osteopenia.** *A,* An initial film demonstrates fractures of the distal radius and ulnar styloid *(arrows)*. The carpal bones are well mineralized and clearly delineated. *B,* A repeated film 3 weeks later shows marked resorption of calcium in a periarticular distribution *(between the dotted lines)*. This is due to disuse and increased blood flow.

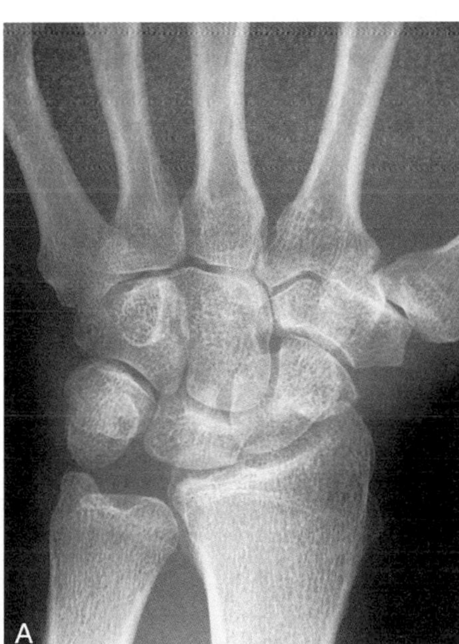

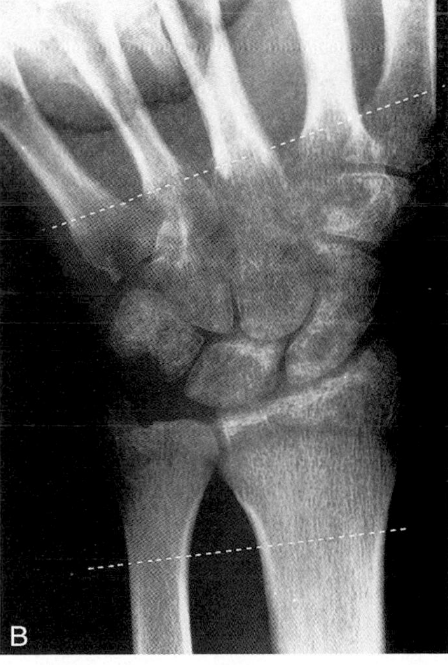

FIGURE 8-67 ■ **Reflex sympathetic dystrophy (RSD).** *A,* A film in this patient who had relatively minor forearm trauma does not demonstrate any abnormality. *B,* The patient continued to complain of pain over the next 2 months, and another film of the wrist shows periarticular and carpal decalcification due to increased blood flow. The exact cause of RSD is debatable.

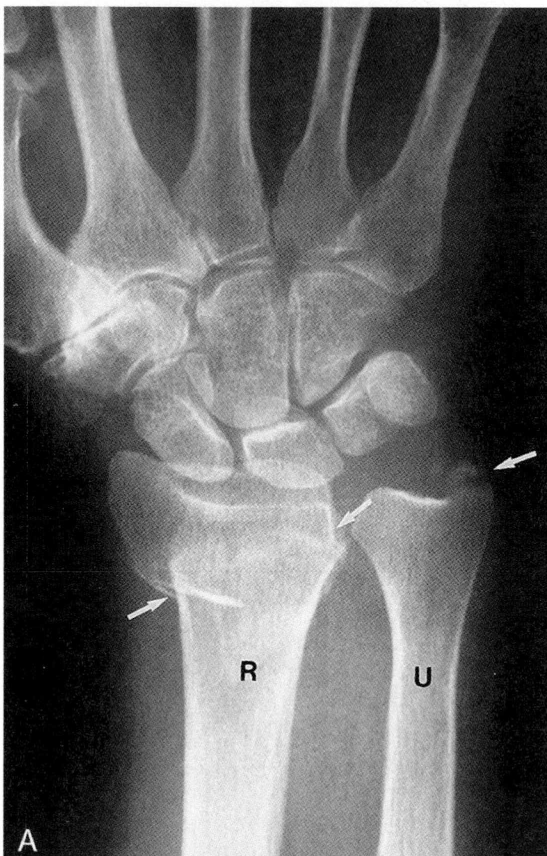

FIGURE 8-68 ■ **Colles' fracture.** *A,* An impacted distal radial fracture and a fracture of the ulnar styloid are identified on the posteroanterior view in this patient who fell on the outstretched hand. *B,* The lateral view of the wrist shows dorsal displacement and angulation as well as some impaction of the distal radius. If the fracture of the distal radius extended into the joint, it would be termed a Barton's fracture.

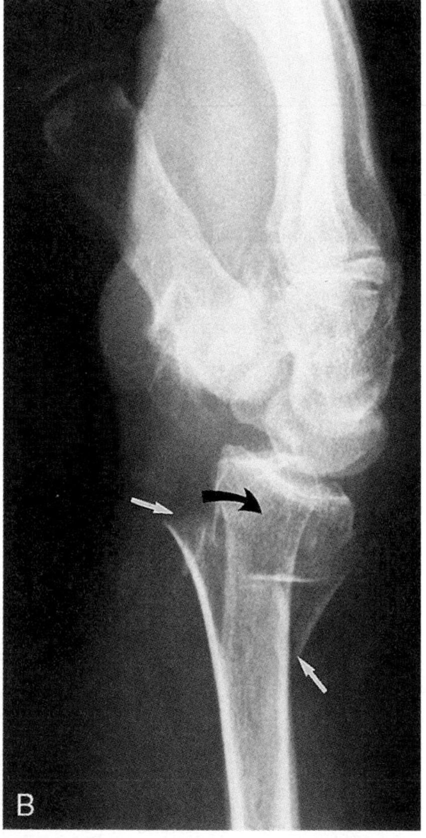

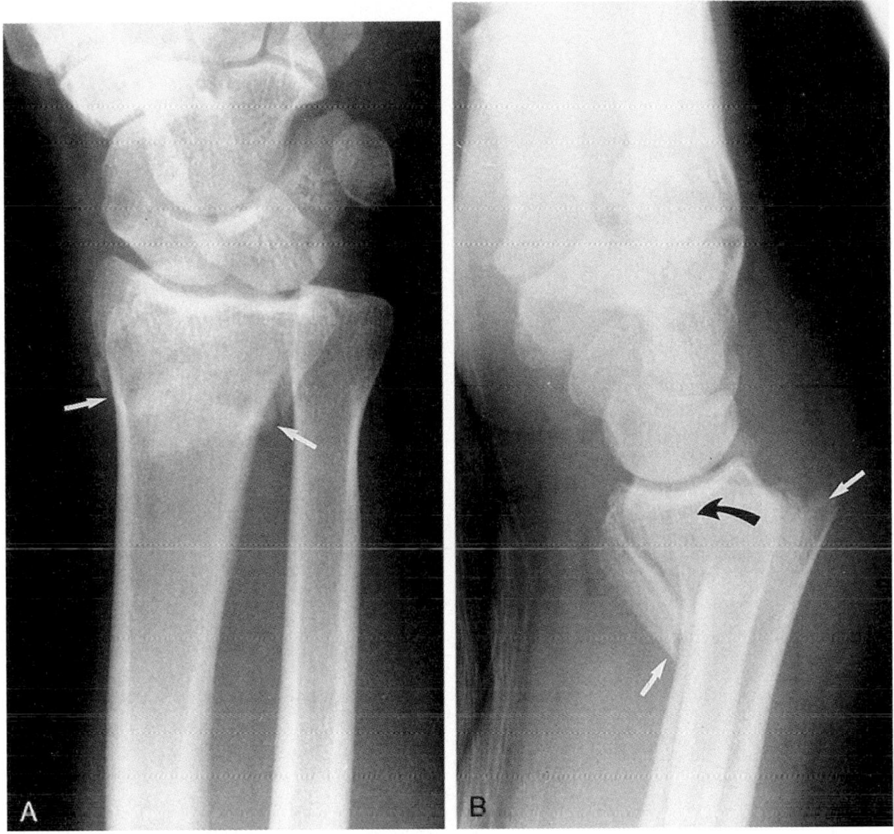

FIGURE 8-69 ■ Smith's fracture. *A,* An anteroposterior view of the wrist shows an impacted fracture of the distal radius. *B,* The lateral view shows volar displacement of the distal fragment. If the fracture had extended into the articular surface, it would have been called a reverse Barton's fracture.

The most common fracture of the carpal bones is a fracture of the midportion of the carpal navicular. The navicular has an unusual blood supply. The arteries supply the more distal aspect of the bone and then circle back to the more proximal portion. A fracture through the midportion of the navicular can disrupt the blood supply to the proximal portion and cause aseptic necrosis. When this occurs, the proximal portion of the navicular becomes dense or white relative to the rest of the carpal bones (Fig. 8-70).

An injury that can result from impaction of the distal radius and the carpal bones is disruption of the ligaments between the navicular and the lunate. Sometimes this can be a subtle finding, but remember that the space between the distal radius and the carpal bones should be about the same as the distance between the lunate and the navicular. If you have a question as to whether this space is widened, an AP image of the other wrist can be used for comparison (Fig. 8-71). Tenderness over the dorsal aspect of the wrist should raise the possibility of a triquetral fracture. This fracture is usually seen only on the lateral view and may be just a small avulsion fragment (Fig. 8-72).

Major falls can cause either lunate or perilunate dislocations of the carpal bones. The key to initial recognition of these dislocations on the AP view is that you no longer see a distinct proximal crescentic row of carpal bones and then a distal row. The lateral view usually makes the

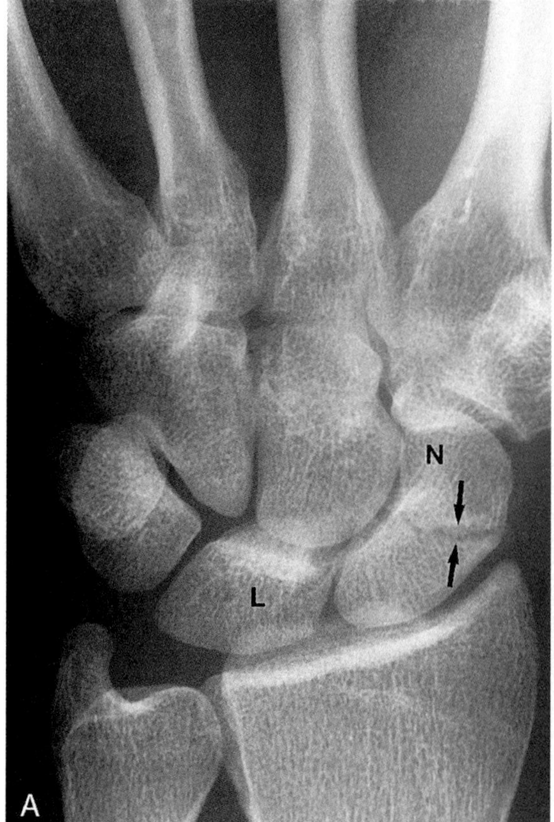

FIGURE 8-70 ■ Scaphoid or navicular fracture. *A,* A posteroanterior view of the wrist in a patient who fell on his outstretched hand shows a lucent line extending through the midportion of the navicular. *B,* A later complication in this patient is aseptic necrosis of the proximal fragment *(large arrow).* Note that this fragment has maintained normal mineralization because the blood supply has been interrupted. In contrast, the remainder of the carpal bones demonstrate loss of calcium due to hyperemia and disuse after the fracture.

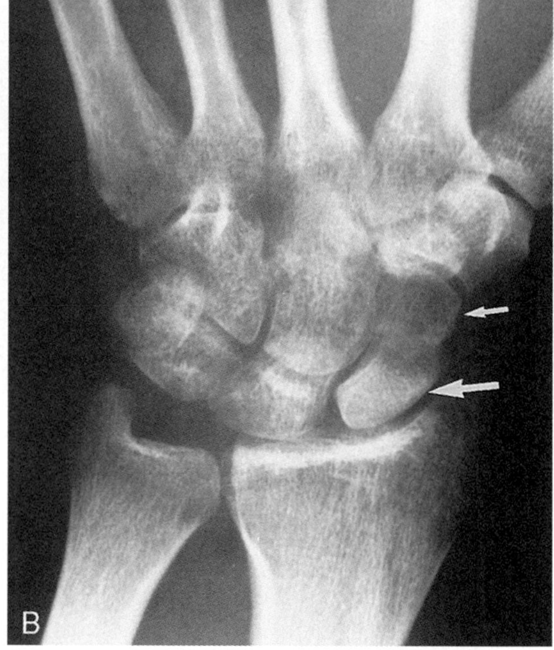

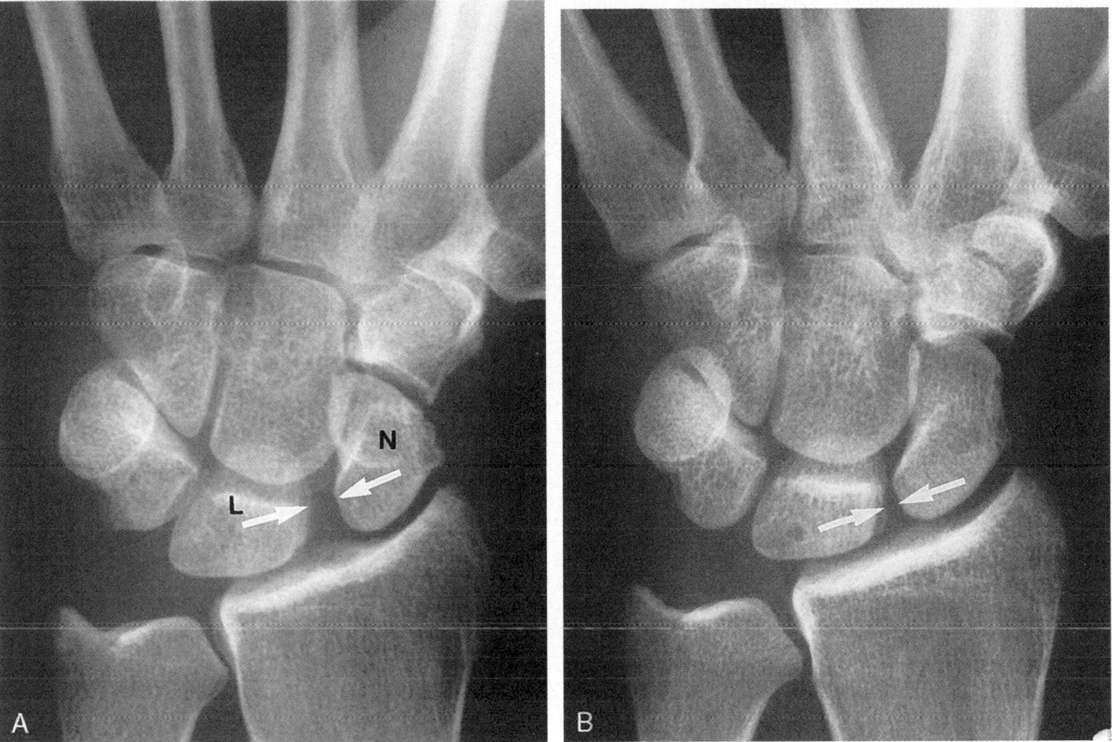

FIGURE 8-71 ■ Scapholunate disassociation. *A,* A posteroanterior view of the wrist demonstrates a widened space between the navicular and the lunate *(arrows)* due to ligamentous disruption from an impaction injury. *B,* A normal wrist shows that the typical distance between the navicular and lunate *(arrows)* should be about the same as that between the navicular and the radius.

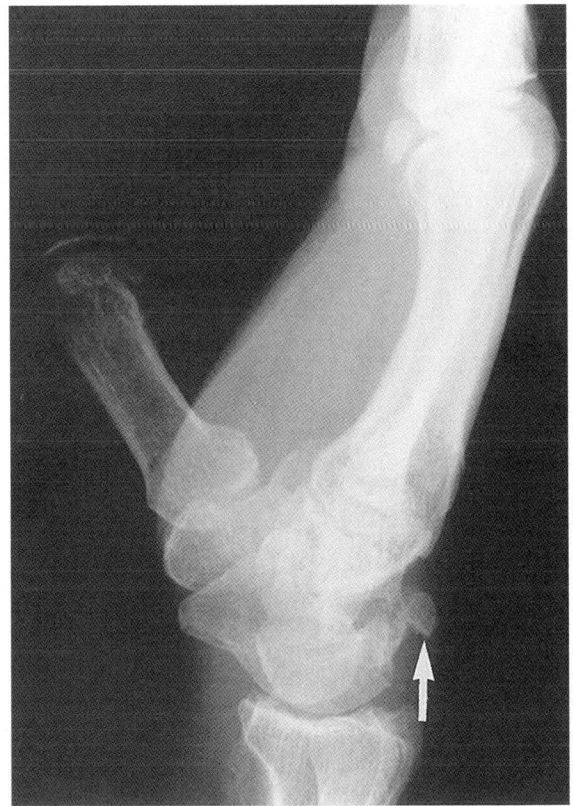

FIGURE 8-72 ■ Triquetral fracture. An avulsion fracture of the dorsum of the wrist that is typically seen only on the lateral view. You should look very carefully in this location, because this fracture is easily missed.

type of dislocation reasonably clear. In perilunate dislocation, the lunate is in normal position at the end of the radius, but the remainder of the carpals are dislocated posteriorly and are usually overriding with some shortening of the wrist (Fig. 8-73). In a lunate dislocation, the rest of the carpals remain in a line along the axis of the radius; however, the lunate is usually rotated and dislocated toward the palmar surface (Fig. 8-74). Trauma of the lunate also can result in aseptic necrosis. This is typically referred to as Kienbock's malacia. This may occur as a result of repeated minor traumas or one episode of trauma. The entity is recognized by irregularity and increased density of the lunate relative to the other carpal bones (Fig. 8-75).

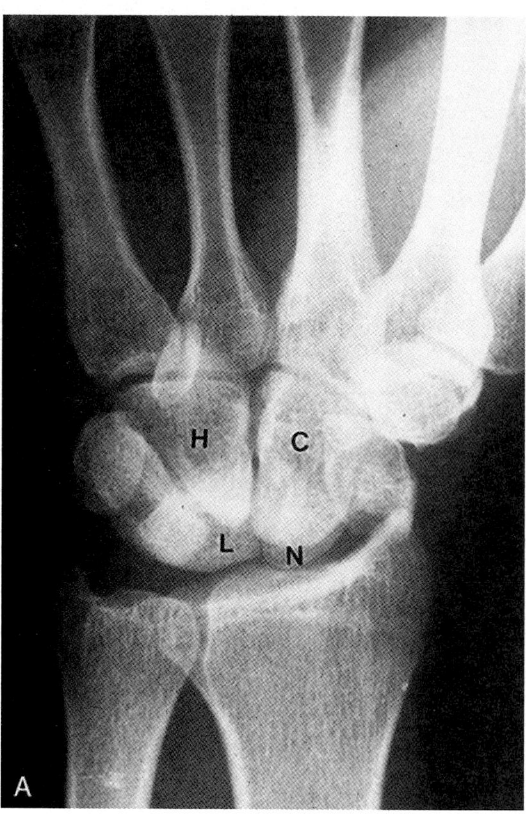

C = grand os
H = os crochu
L = semi lunaire
N = scaphoide.

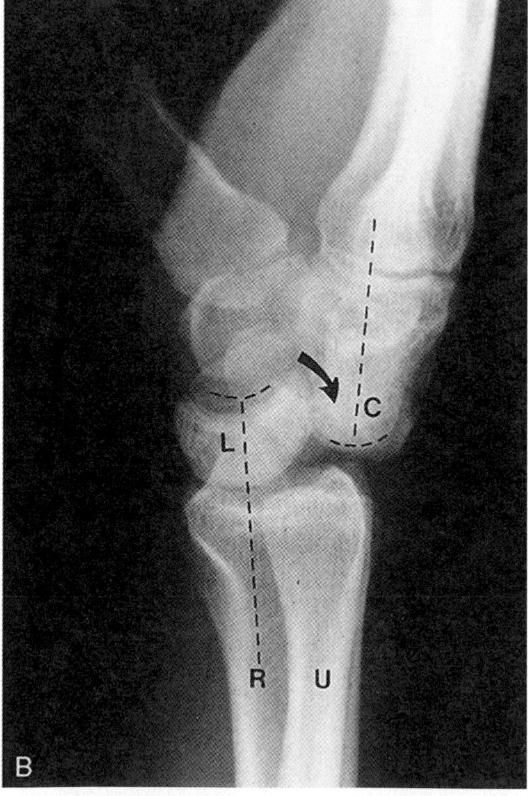

FIGURE 8-73 ■ Perilunate dislocation. *A,* A posteroanterior view of the wrist does not show the normal two crescentic rows of carpal bones but rather shows significant overlap of the hamate (H) and the lunate (L) as well as the capitate (C) with the navicular (N). *B,* A lateral view shows that the lunate remains in alignment with the end of the radius, but the remainder of the carpal bones have been dislocated dorsally.

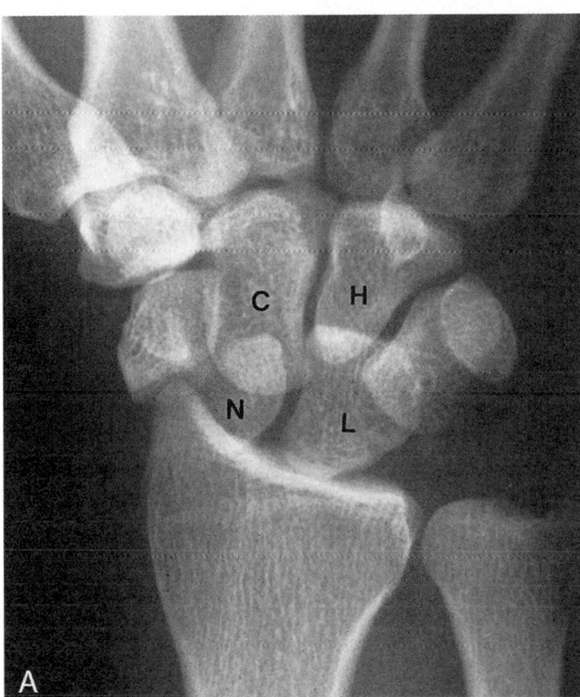

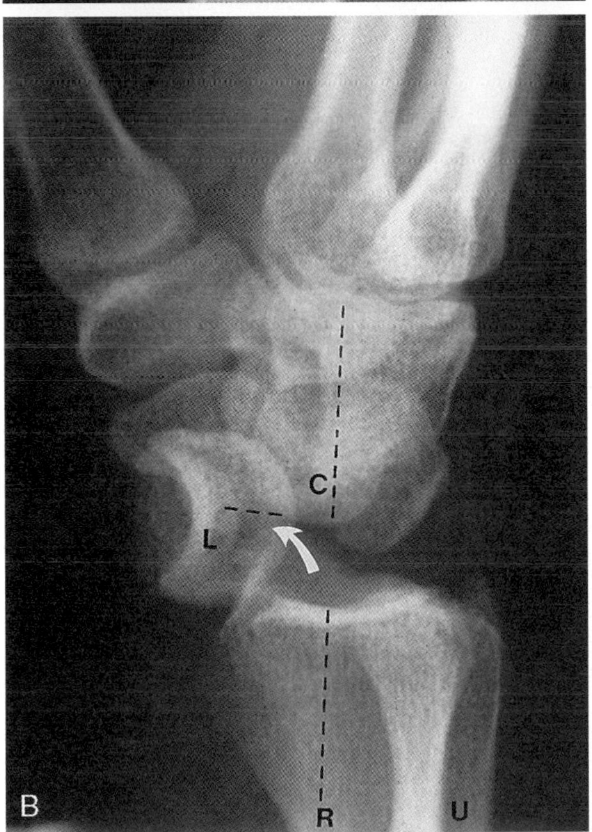

FIGURE 8-74 ■ Lunate dislocation. *A,* On the posteroanterior view of the wrist, significant overlap is seen of the capitate and navicular as well as the hamate and the lunate. Furthermore, clear overlap appears between the navicular and the radial styloid. All these findings suggest dislocation. *B,* On the lateral view, the carpal bones remain in alignment with the distal radius, but the lunate has rotated and dislocated in the palmar direction *(arrow).*

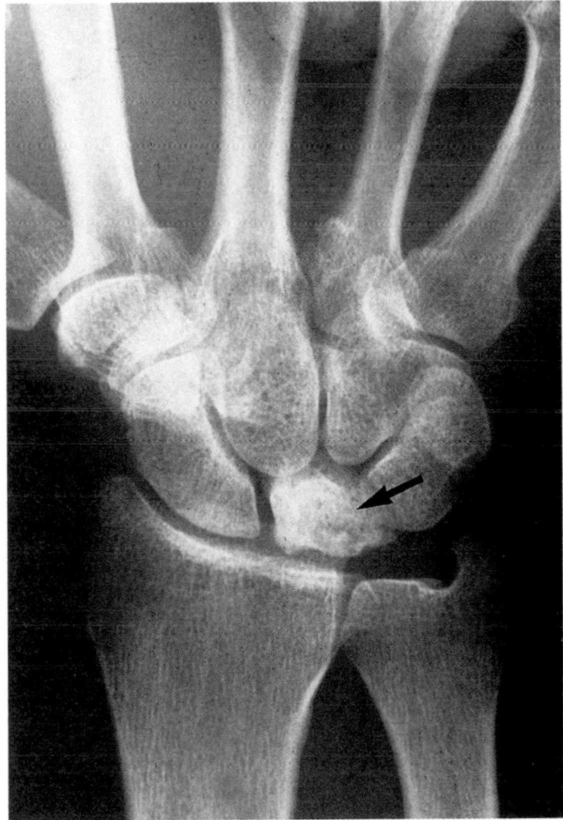

FIGURE 8-75 ■ Aseptic necrosis of the lunate. A posteroanterior view of the wrist shows irregularity and increased density or sclerosis of the lunate *(arrow),* also referred to as Kienbock's malacia.

HAND

Normal Anatomy and Imaging

Images of the hand and fingers taken for trauma should include AP, lateral (see Fig. 8-64), and oblique views. If the clinical issue is related to arthritis, an AP view of both hands is all that is needed. A relatively common finding in the hand involves shortening of a metacarpal, typically the fourth (Fig. 8-76). This is usually a normal variant, but the differential diagnosis includes Turner's syndrome, pseudohypoparathyroidism, and a few other much less common entities.

Trauma

Plain x-rays of the hands may be taken for evaluation of foreign bodies. The most common are glass, pencil lead, metallic slivers, and pieces of wood. Glass is usually somewhat radiopaque and can be recognized by its very sharp corners or a geometric shape (Fig. 8-77). Metallic fragments are, of course, easy to spot, because they are so dense. Wood and pencil lead are typically not visible on an x-ray. Pencil lead is not visible is because it is actually graphite and not lead.

Two relatively frequent fracture sites are found in the metacarpals. The most common of these is a fracture of the distal fifth metacarpal (the so-called "boxer's fracture"). The head of the fifth metacarpal is angled toward the palmar surface and may be somewhat impacted (Fig. 8-78).

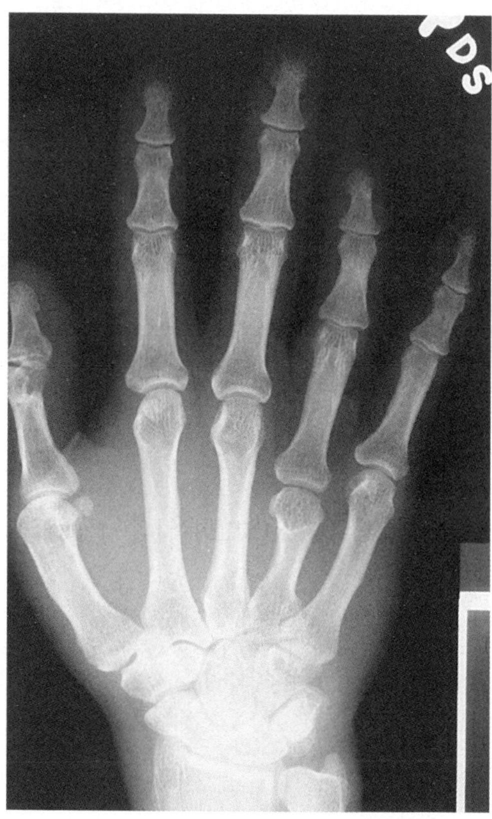

FIGURE 8-76 ■ Short fourth metacarpal. Although this can be a normal variant, it also has been associated with Turner's syndrome, sickle cell disease, infections, and some metabolic bone diseases, such as pseudohypoparathyroidism.

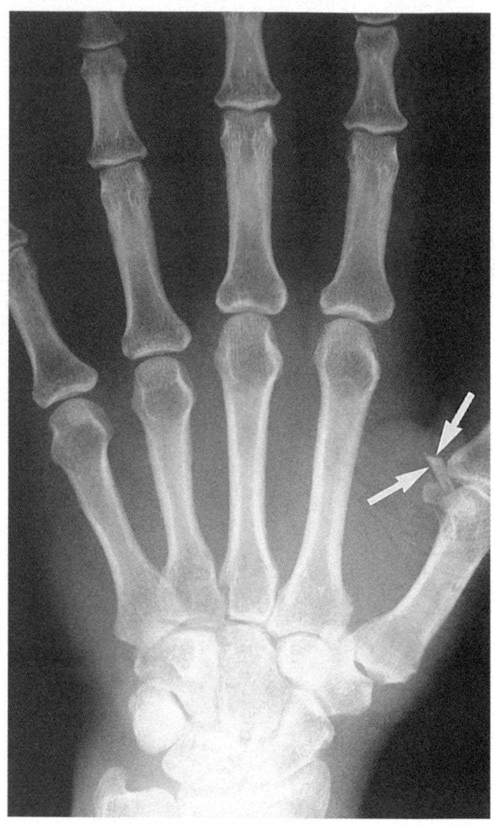

FIGURE 8-77 ■ Glass within the soft tissue of the hand. Most glass has enough density that it is radiopaque and can be recognized by the sharp corners *(arrows)* and the patient history. Remember that objects made of either wood or graphite usually are not visible on a radiograph.

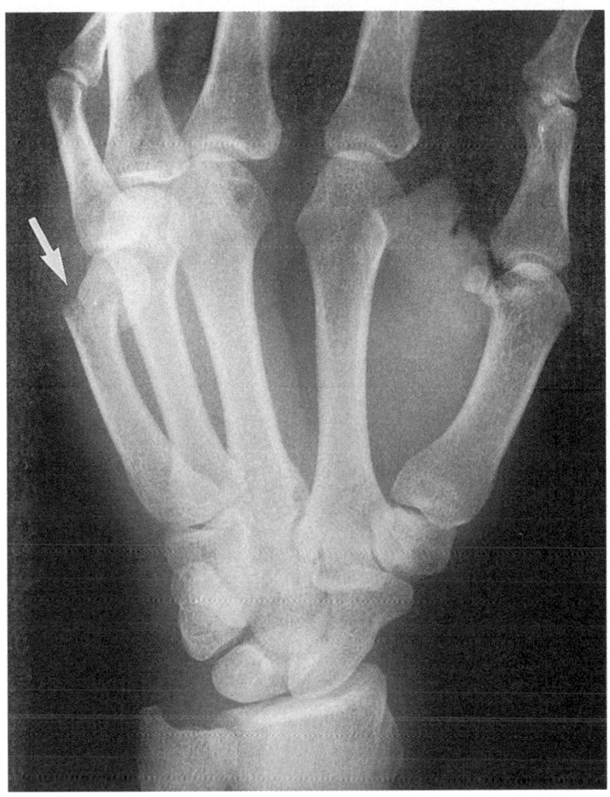

FIGURE 8-78 ■ Boxer's fracture. This hand film was obtained on a teenager who had hand pain after punching a wall. The fracture usually occurs at the neck of the fifth metacarpal, with volar angulation of the distal fragment. Contrary to its name, it is not often seen in professional boxers.

The second common location for hand fractures is the base of the thumb. Bennett's and Rolando's fractures are triangular fractures of the base of the first metacarpal, with extension into the articular surface. Oblique fractures of the first metacarpal base may not extend into the joint (Fig. 8-79). Another rather classic fracture of the thumb is an avulsion fracture of the base of the proximal phalanx. Although this is called a "gamekeeper's thumb," a common mechanism of injury is getting a ski pole caught in the snow with the thumb being pulled backward.

Fingers not only can be fractured but also can be dislocated. Often, on AP projection, dislocation cannot be appreciated except as slight joint-space narrowing and soft tissue swelling; however, on the lateral view, the dislocation is usually obvious (Fig. 8-80). All dislocations are clinically obvious, but if an unusual associated deformity or angulation is seen, it may be useful to get a prereduction image to see whether an associated fracture is present.

In children, fractures about articular surfaces can occur in a variety of ways. They may involve only the epiphyseal plates or various combinations of the epiphyseal plate and the metaphysis. The Salter-Harris classification, shown schematically in Figure 8-81, is used for describing childhood fractures about most joints. A Salter-Harris type II fracture of the fifth digit is shown in Figure 8-82. Another relatively

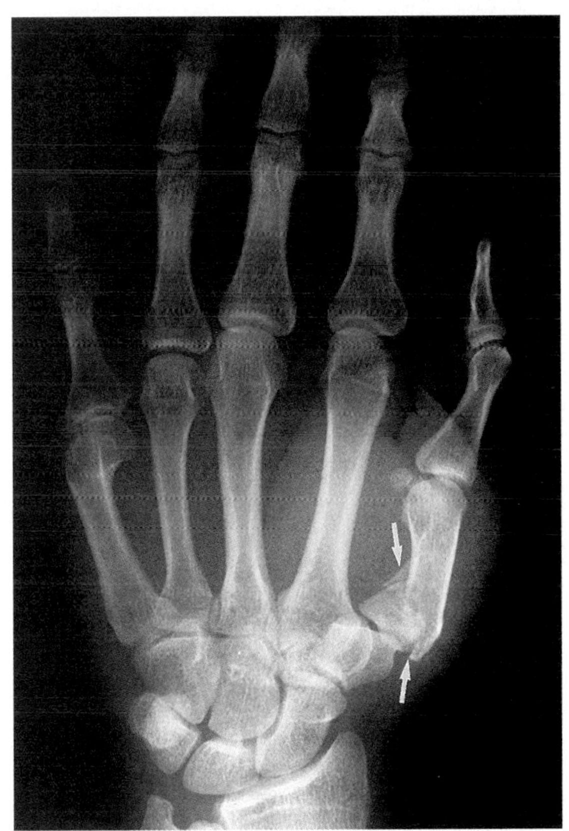

FIGURE 8-79 ■ Extra-articular fracture of the first metacarpal base. An oblique fracture is seen at the metacarpal base *(arrows)* but without extension into the joint space. If extension into the joint space with a single linear fracture had occurred, this would be termed a Bennett's fracture; if it were a comminuted fracture extending into the joint space, it would be termed a Rolando's fracture.

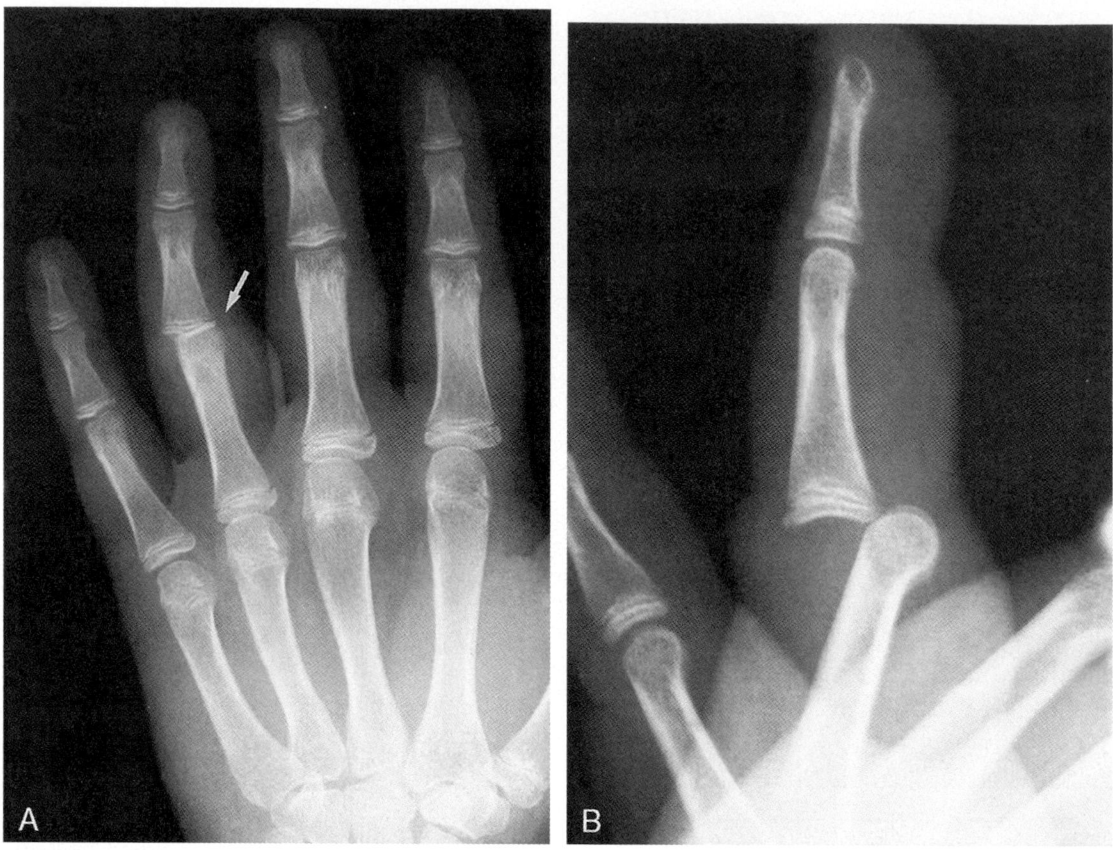

FIGURE 8-80 ■ Complete dislocation of a proximal interphalangeal joint. *A,* A posteroanterior view of the hand shows some soft tissue swelling in what looks like only narrowing of a joint space. *B,* A lateral view clearly shows the dislocation, although this, of course, would be clinically obvious. This case should serve as a lesson in why two views are needed before you come to a conclusion about the position of various structures on a radiograph.

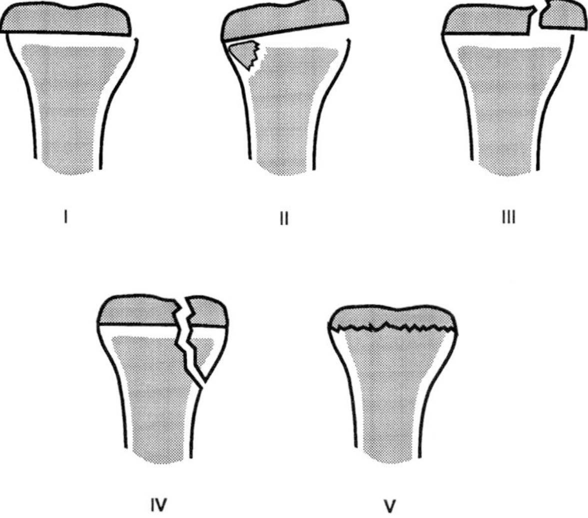

FIGURE 8-81 ■ Salter-Harris classification of epiphyseal fractures in children. A type I fracture is straight across the epiphyseal plate and may have some lateral displacement of the epiphysis. This occurs 5% of the time. A type II fracture involves a portion of the epiphyseal plate and a corner fracture through the metaphysis. This occurs 75% of the time. A type III fracture involving part of the epiphysis occurs only about 10% of the time. A type IV fracture involving part of the epiphysis and part of the metaphysis occurs about 10% of the time. A type V fracture is direct impaction and has the most serious consequences for further growth.

common fracture of the fingers involves the base of the middle phalanx on the palmar surface. This small avulsion fracture is referred to as a volar plate fracture (Fig. 8-83). It is easily missed unless you look carefully at the lateral view. Of course, fractures of the terminal tuft of the distal phalanges occur very frequently from people slamming their fingers in doors and other objects. These are quite obvious on the x-ray.

Infection

Infections are quite frequent in the hands as well as the feet. Often the clinical problem is differentiating between cellulitis, osteomyelitis, and septic arthritis. When the x-ray shows destruction of a single joint space with involvement of the bone on both sides of the joint, septic arthritis should be considered (Fig. 8-84). Osteomyelitis usually is radiographically identified by soft

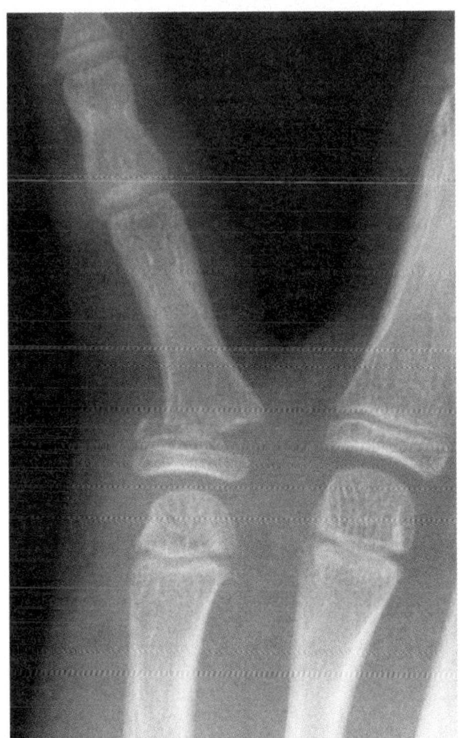

FIGURE 8-82 ■ A Salter-Harris type II fracture of the fifth proximal phalanx.

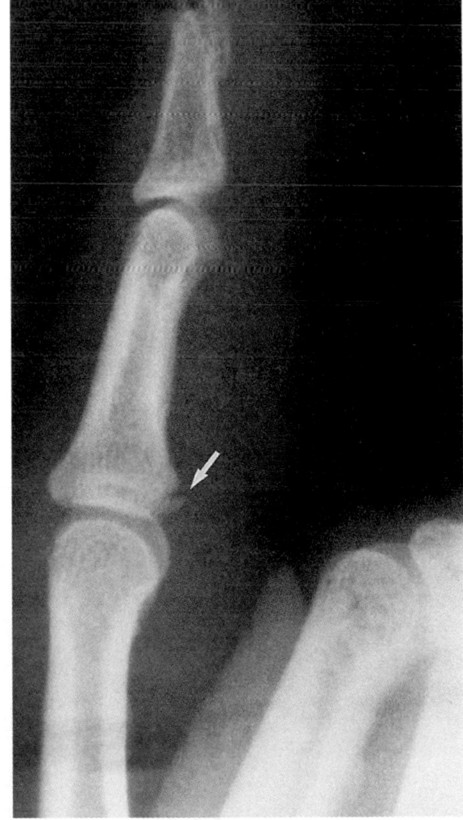

FIGURE 8-83 ■ **Volar plate fracture.** This fracture is seen only on the lateral view and is a small avulsion fracture, most commonly occurring at the base of the middle phalanx.

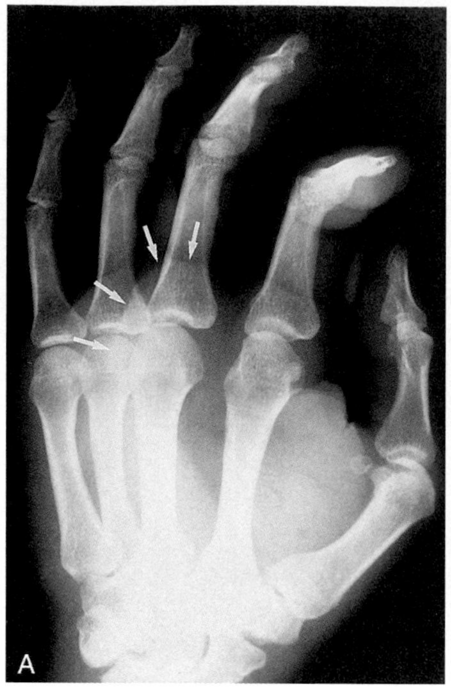

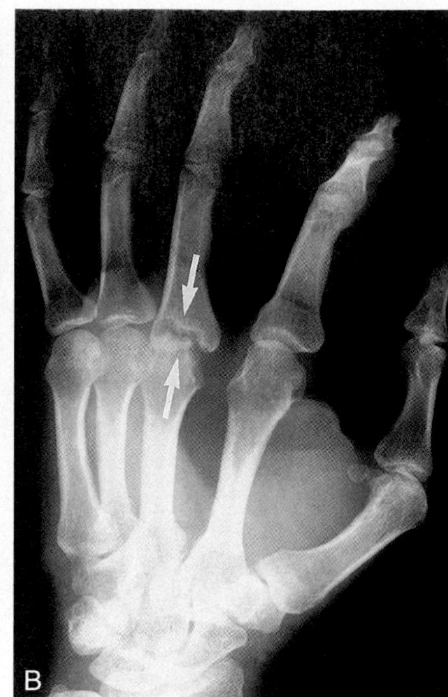

FIGURE 8-84 ■ Septic arthritis. *A,* A film obtained 1 day after a human bite over the third metacarpophalangeal joint shows only some soft tissue swelling *(arrows). B,* A repeated x-ray 4 weeks later shows destruction of both the distal metacarpal and the proximal phalanx because of an infection within the joint space.

tissue swelling, lucent or destructive areas within the bone itself, or focal periosteal reaction. An illustration of osteomyelitis of the foot appears later (Fig. 8-163). With cellulites, only soft tissue swelling occurs without bone or joint changes. An infection of a distal phalanx in a gardener should raise the possibility of sporotrichosis.

Arthritis

Evaluation of the hands for arthritis can provide some general ideas about the type of arthritis, although commonly a number of patients whose laboratory findings of rheumatoid arthritis conflict with the x-ray appearance that resembles degenerative arthritis. The reverse also is true. Thus the radiographic diagnosis should not be leaned on too heavily.

Rheumatoid arthritis (RA) occurs most frequently in female patients, and they initially are seen with morning stiffness, swelling of one or more joints, and subcutaneous nodules. General radiographic findings of RA include narrowing of the carpal joints, subchondral cysts, and erosion of the bones at the lateral edges of the joints. Patients with clinically obvious RA can often have normal-looking images of the hand and then undergo rapid progression. In addition to the findings already described, ulnar deviation at the metacarpophalangeal joints is relatively characteristic (Fig. 8-85), but it can occasionally occur with systemic lupus erythematosus (SLE). Any arthritis but RA can be seen with normal mineralization of bones. Diffuse osteoporosis is mostly seen with RA, but periarticular demineralization also is quite common.

In advanced RA, the patient's hands may develop the so-called "boutonniere deformity," which is hyperextension of the distal interphalangeal (DIP) joint and flexion in the peripheral interphalangeal (PIP) joint. Another deformity is almost the reverse of this. The "swan-neck" deformity also can result from hyperextension of the PIP joint and flexion of the DIP joint. If the metacarpophalangeal joints have been completely destroyed, it is possible to replace these with silicone prostheses.

Findings of RA in other bones include penciling or erosion of the distal clavicle and narrowing and erosions of the shoulder, hip,

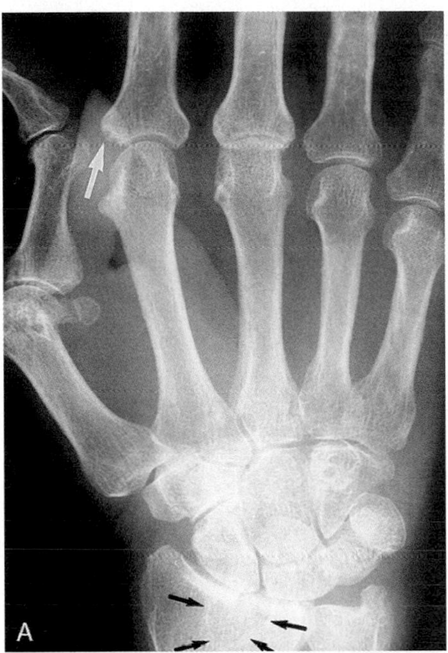

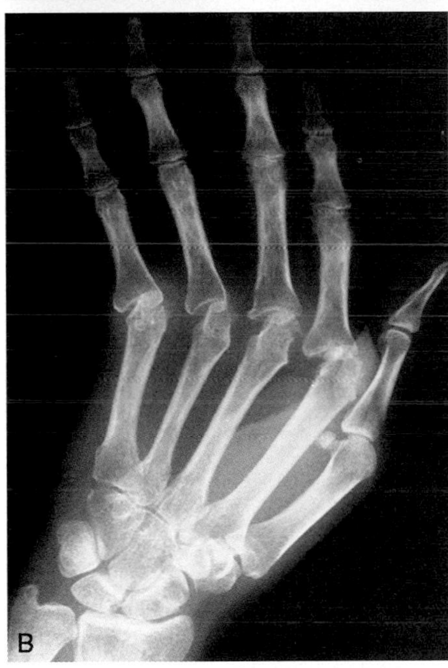

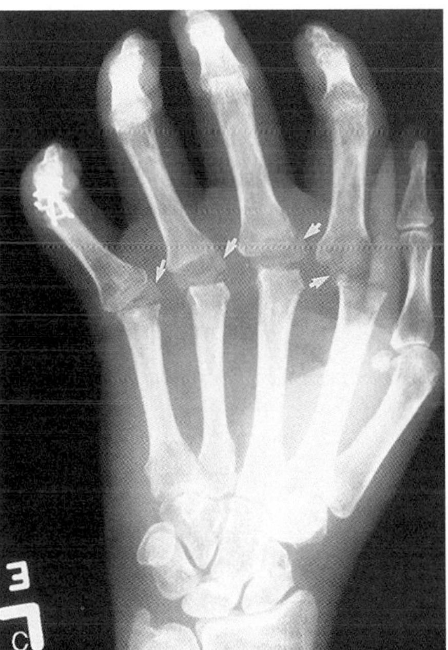

FIGURE 8-85 ■ Rheumatoid arthritis of the wrist and hands. *A,* Relatively classic findings include narrowing of the carpal joint with subchondral cyst formation *(dark arrows)* and periarticular erosions *(large white arrow).* This most commonly occurs in the second and third metacarpophalangeal joints; usually sparing of the distal interphalangeal joints is found. *B,* Late changes of rheumatoid arthritis include subluxation and ulnar deviation at the metacarpophalangeal joint. *C,* This patient's disease progressed rapidly and required silicone joint replacements *(arrows)* of the second to fifth metacarpophalangeal joints.

and knee joints, as well as atlantoaxial subluxation. Finally, a widened space between the carpal lunate and navicular bone can be seen (the Terry Thomas sign). Remember that these patients also can have interstitial lung changes, pulmonary nodules, and various forms of carditis.

When an arthritis involves DIP joints with relative sparing of the proximal ones, erosive osteoarthritis and psoriatic arthritis become the more likely diagnoses (Fig. 8-86). Pseudogout can cause calcification within cartilage (chondrocalcinosis). This is not a finding specific to pseudogout, because it also occurs in

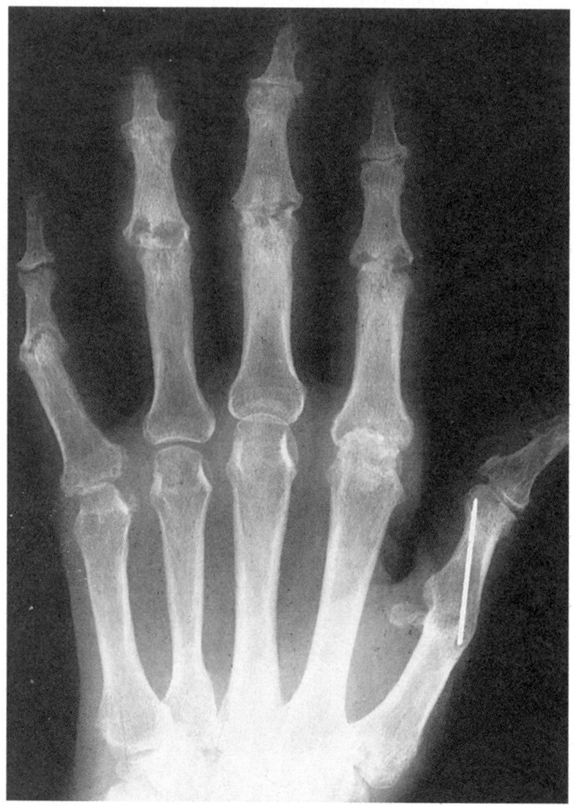

FIGURE 8-86 ■ **Psoriatic arthritis.** Involvement of the distal and proximal interphalangeal joints is most common. Asymmetrical changes also are common. Erosions can be aggressive and usually involve the intra-articular joint spaces.

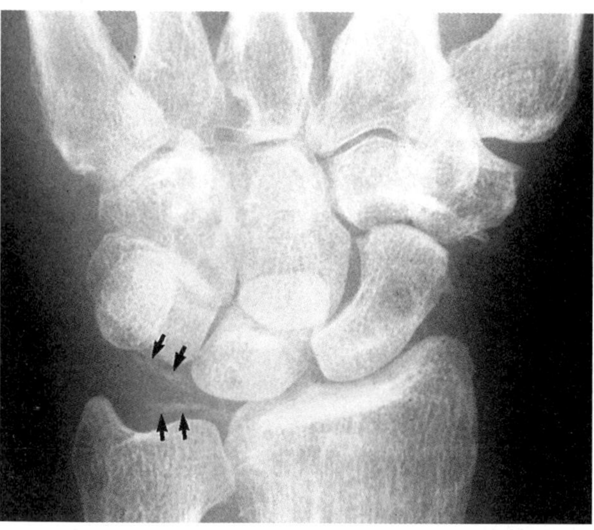

FIGURE 8-87 ■ **Calcium pyrophosphate deposition disease.** Acute synovitis, sometimes called pseudogout, may be found. Here, calcification is seen in the cartilage of the wrist.

hypercalcemic states. In the wrist and hand, the calcification is most often seen in the ulnar carpal region (Fig. 8-87). The other common site is the knee joint.

Tumors

Tumors of the hand and wrist are quite rare. The most common tumor is a benign enchondroma. This typically occurs in either the metacarpals or the proximal phalanges. It causes a lucent area in the central portion of the shaft with some expansion and inner table thinning of the cortex. Pathologic fractures through these areas may occur as a result of the bone thinning (Fig. 8-88).

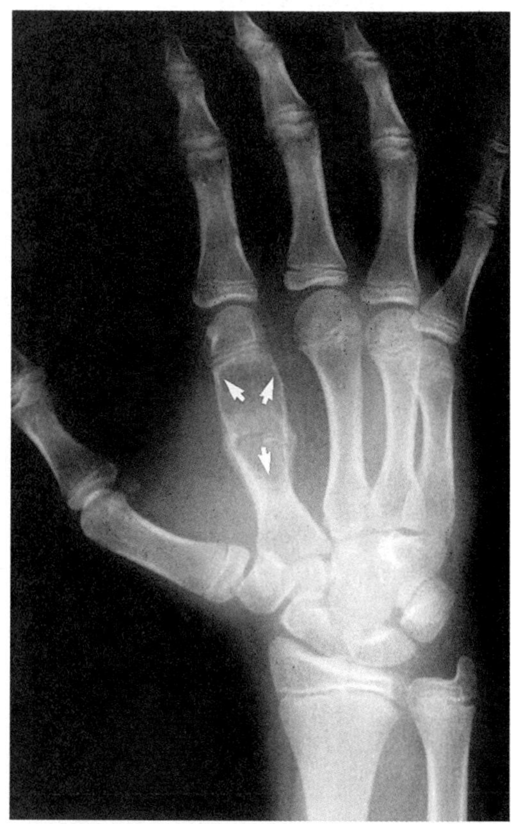

FIGURE 8-88 ■ **Enchondroma.** A lucent lesion in a metacarpal or phalanx is most likely to be an enchondroma. It may be somewhat expansile *(arrows),* and fracture may be noted through the area of weakened bone. A healing fracture with some periosteal reaction is seen in the midportion of this lesion.

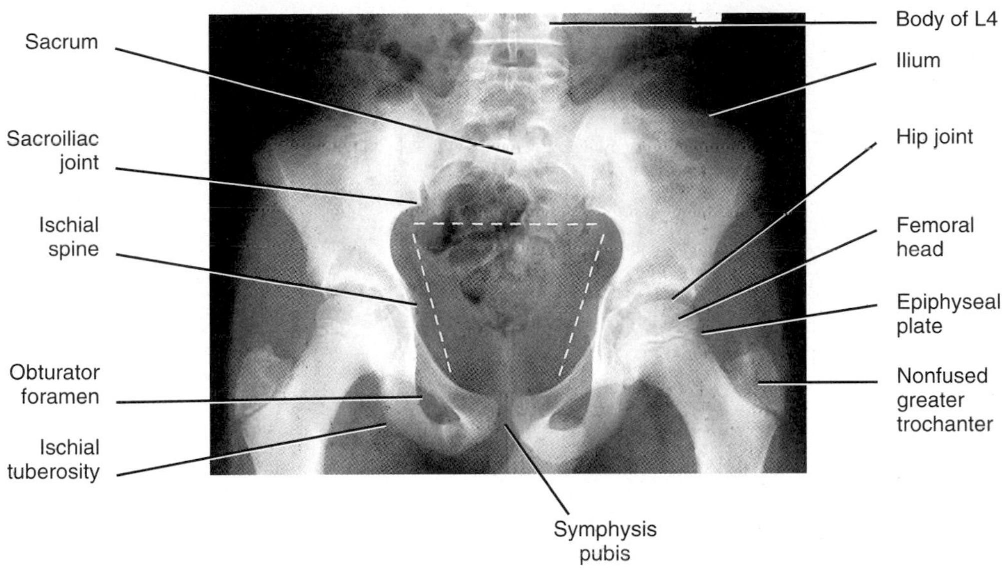

FIGURE 8-89 ■ Normal anatomy of the teenage male pelvis. Note the generally triangular (android) shape of the pelvic inlet.

PELVIS

Normal Anatomy and Imaging

When you order a plain x-ray of the pelvis, only an AP view normally is obtained. On the AP view, clear demonstration exists of the iliac wings, ischium, pubis, and both hips as well as the lower lumbar spine. You should be able to look at the image and determine not only whether the person is male or female but also the general age of the patient. The inlet of the male pelvis is generally somewhat triangular (Fig. 8-89), whereas the female pelvis has a much more ovoid shape (Fig. 8-90). Occasionally the genitalia are included on the film.

The general age of the patient is ascertained by the presence or absence of degenerative changes in the lower lumbar spine and hip joints. In children, incomplete fusion of the acetabulum is present; in slightly older children, you will be able to see clearly the apophysis of the greater trochanter and the epiphyseal plate of the hip. In the middle to late teens, an apophysis appears on the iliac crest as well as on the inferior ischium (Fig. 8-91). Although these apophyses can sometimes be mistaken for avulsion fractures, the symmetry from one side of the pelvis to another and their location are usually enough to identify them clearly. Several normal variants or results of very common conditions are found. These are symmetric sclerotic areas (white) about the pubis or the sacroiliac (SI) joint. These are essentially normal findings and occur much more commonly in women, probably as the result of pelvic widening during childbirth (Fig. 8-92).

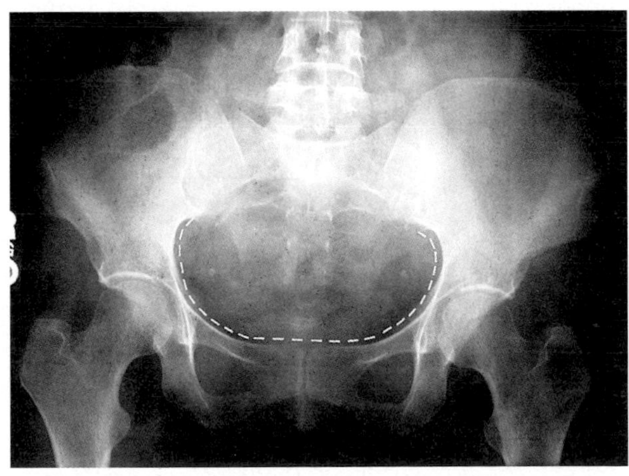

FIGURE 8-90 ■ Normal anatomy of the adult female pelvis. Note the general ovoid (gynecoid) shape of the pelvic inlet.

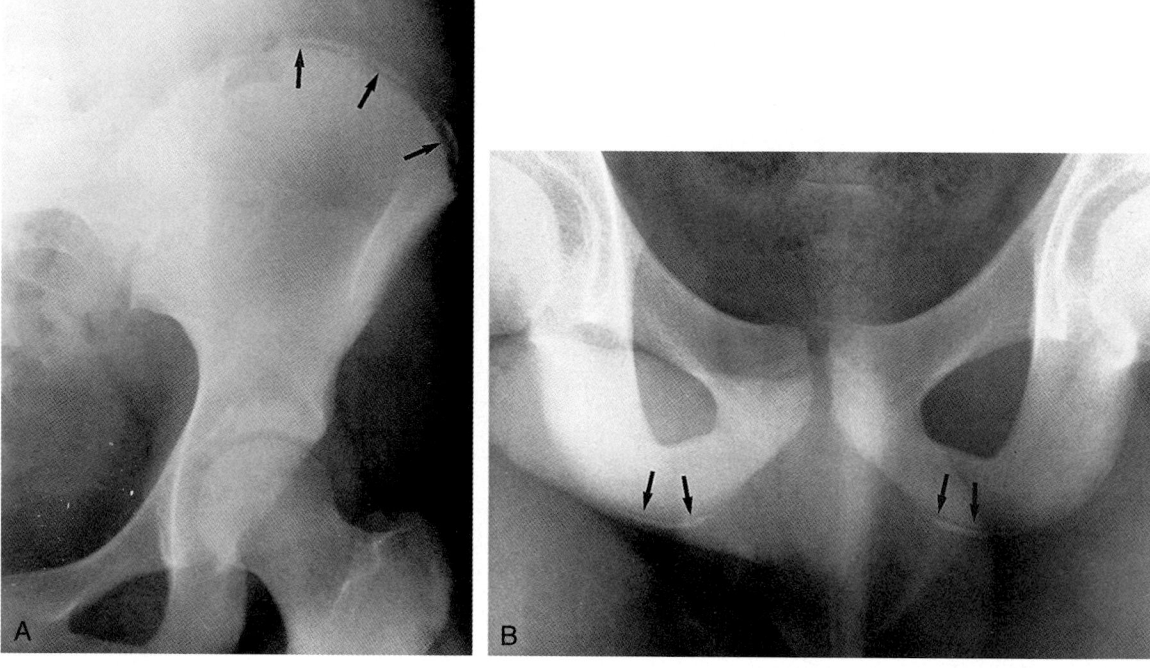

FIGURE 8-91 ■ Normal apophyses. During the mid- and late teen years, an apophysis can be seen over the iliac crest *(A)* and along the inferior aspect of the ischium *(B)*. These should not be mistaken for avulsion fractures.

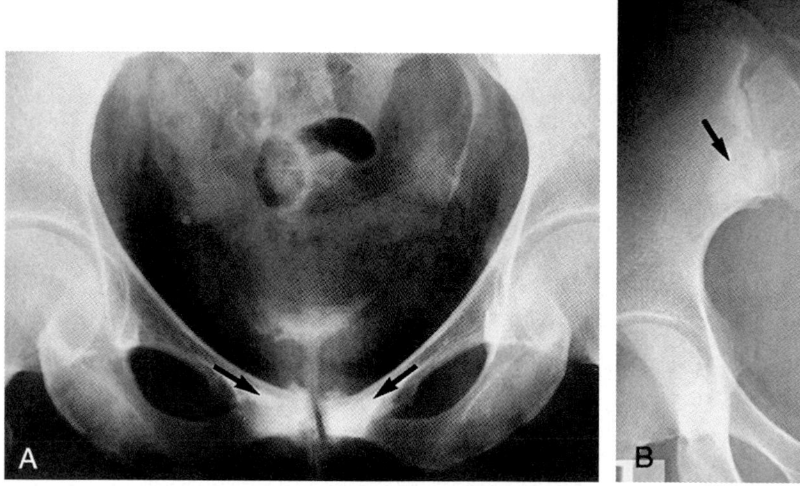

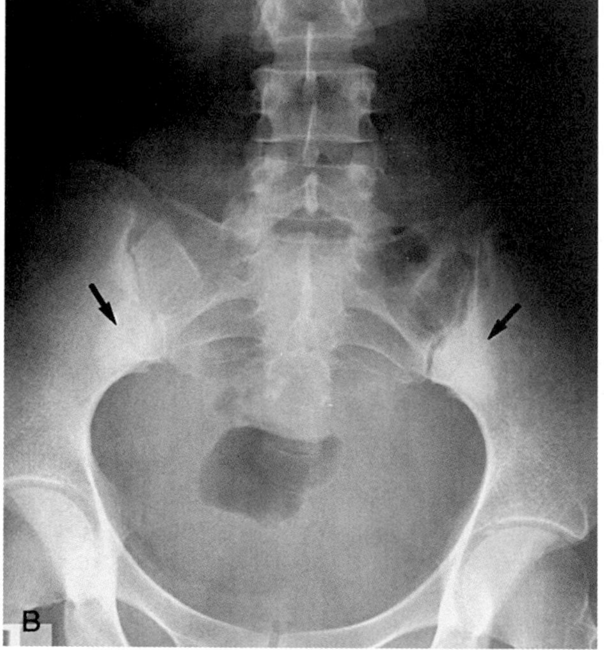

FIGURE 8-92 ■ Benign sclerotic pelvic lesions. *A,* Osteitis condensans pubis with sclerosis along both sides of the pubis *(arrows)*. This condition commonly occurs in women and is believed to be the result of childbirth trauma. This film is from a postvoid view of an intravenous pyelogram, accounting for the contrast in the bladder and left ureter. *B,* Osteitis condensans ilii is seen in a different patient as sclerosis lateral to both sacroiliac joints *(arrows)*.

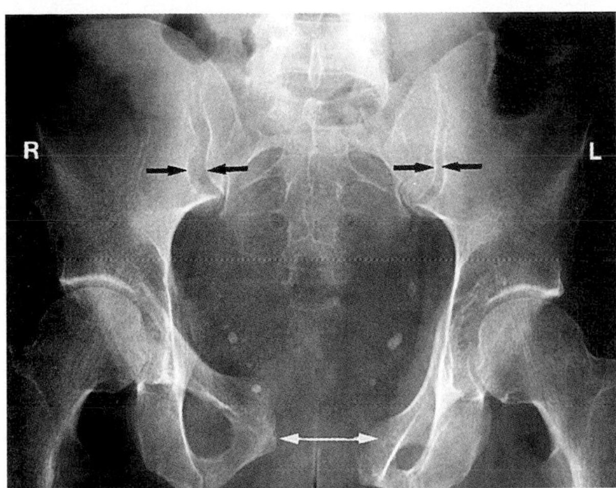

FIGURE 8-93 ■ **Pelvic fracture.** Marked diastasis of the pubis *(white arrow)* and widening of both sacroiliac joints is present, but the right is greater than the left *(black arrows)*. Whenever the pelvic ring is interrupted (as in this case), the fracture is unstable.

Trauma

A number of traumatic lesions can occur in the pelvis. A relatively common, and probably inappropriate, examination to order is a view of the coccyx. Demonstration of a coccyx fracture does not change treatment. When a pelvic fracture is suspected, an AP x-ray is the initial view to order. You should examine the symphysis pubis. A widening of the symphysis of more than 1 cm is definitely abnormal. If the symphysis is widened, also look for widening of one of the SI joints (Fig. 8-93) or the sacrum itself (Fig. 8-94). The reason is that the pelvis is essentially a bony ring, and it is difficult to widen it or break it in one place without causing a traumatic injury elsewhere. Many pelvic fractures are accompanied by internal pelvic hematomas. When a fracture in the pubic region is identified, you should

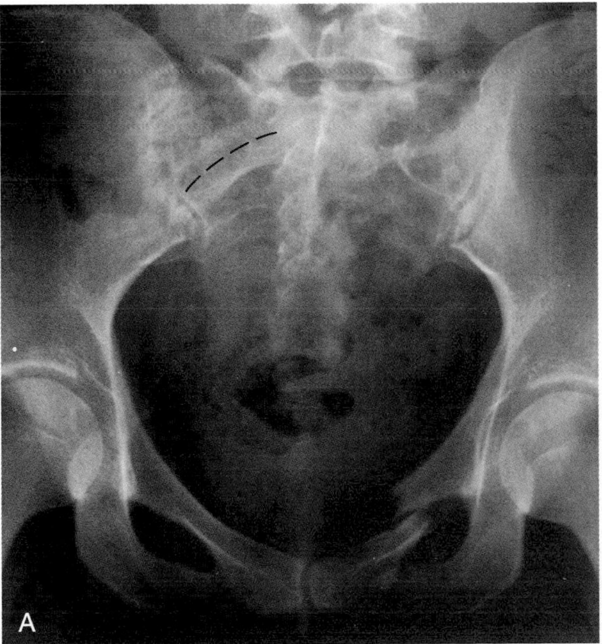

FIGURE 8-94 ■ **Pelvic and sacral fracture.** An anteroposterior image of the pelvis *(A)* clearly shows a left lower pelvic fracture. Not initially obvious is a sacral fracture. Note that the sacral arcuate lines are intact on the right *(dashed line)*, but they are discontinuous on the left. The fracture is confirmed on a computed tomography scan *(B)* of the pelvis *(arrows)*.

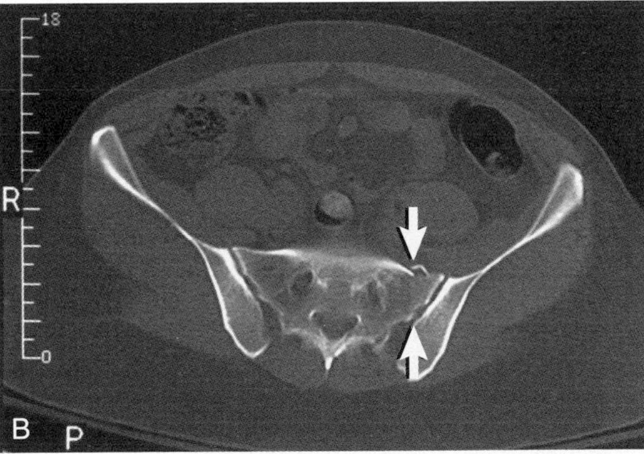

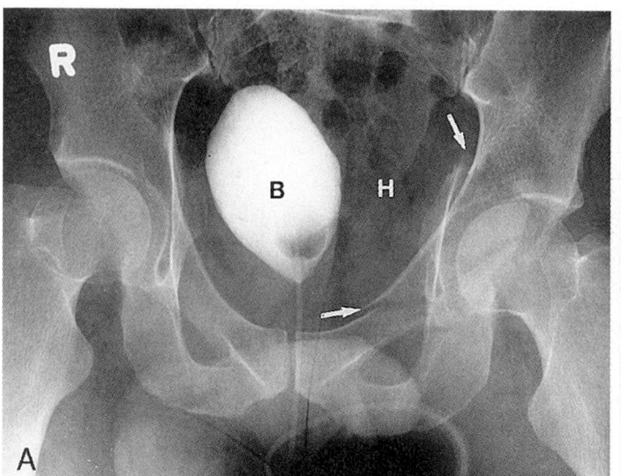

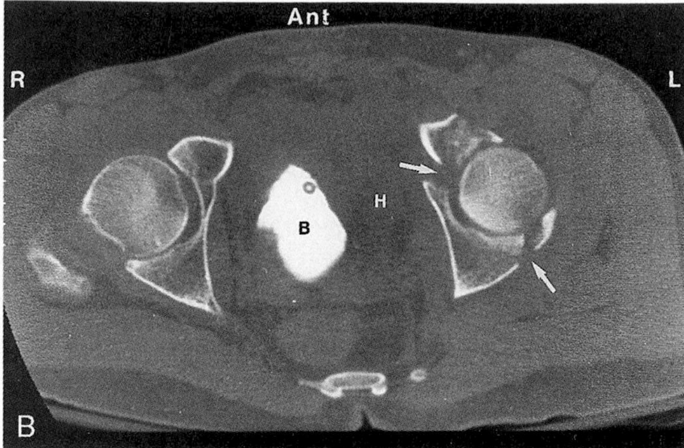

FIGURE 8-95 ■ **Fracture of the acetabulum.** An anteroposterior view of the pelvis *(A)* clearly shows the corners of the fracture *(arrows)* as well as a hematoma displacing the bladder to the right. To see the exact nature of the acetabular injury, often a computed tomography scan *(B)* is required; in this case, it shows a complex fracture involving both the anterior and the posterior portions of the acetabulum.

exclude urethral and bladder injury. A cystogram is often performed to rule out bladder rupture. Sometimes the resultant hematoma is large enough to displace the bladder superiorly and laterally (Fig. 8-95).

Benign Lesions

Paget's disease is a common benign lesion of the pelvis, usually with involvement of only the right or left half of the pelvis. The iliopectineal

FIGURE 8-96 ■ **Paget's disease.** *A,* On an anteroposterior view of the pelvis, enlargement of the left iliac crest with cortical thickening *(arrowheads)* and sclerosis and thickening of the left iliopectineal line *(arrows)* can be seen. These findings typically affect only one side of the pelvis. A posterior view from a nuclear medicine bone scan *(B)* shows markedly increased activity in the left hemipelvis as a result of the increased blood flow that occurs in this disease.

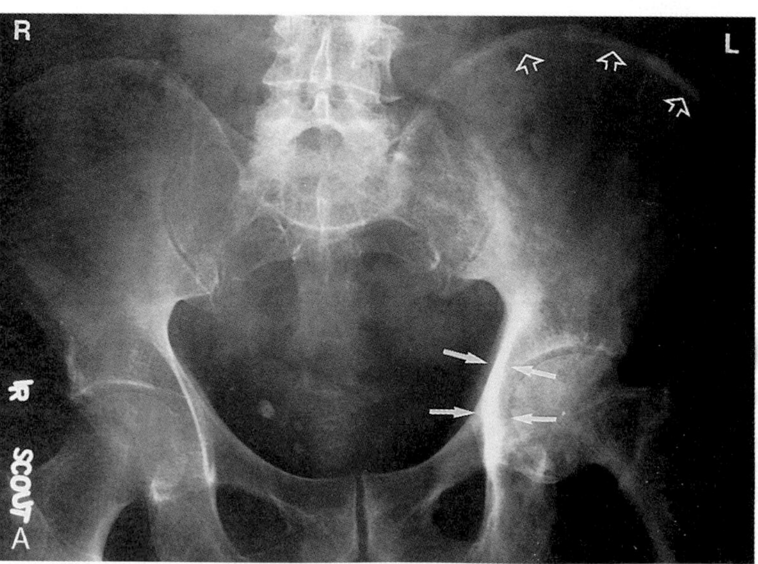

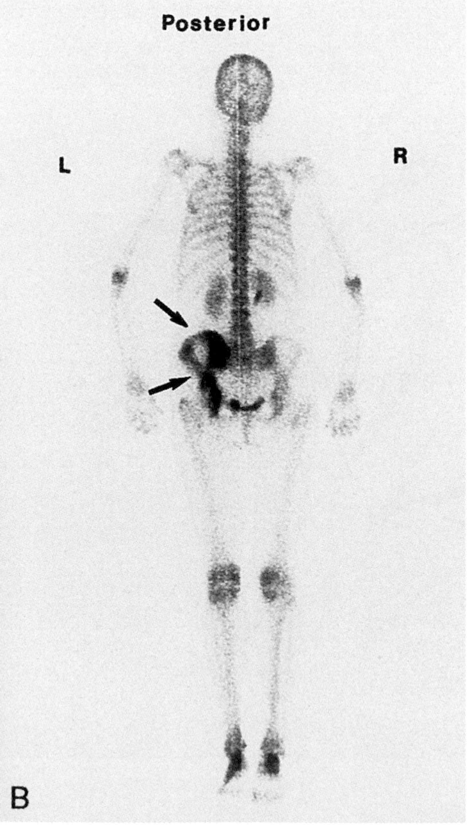

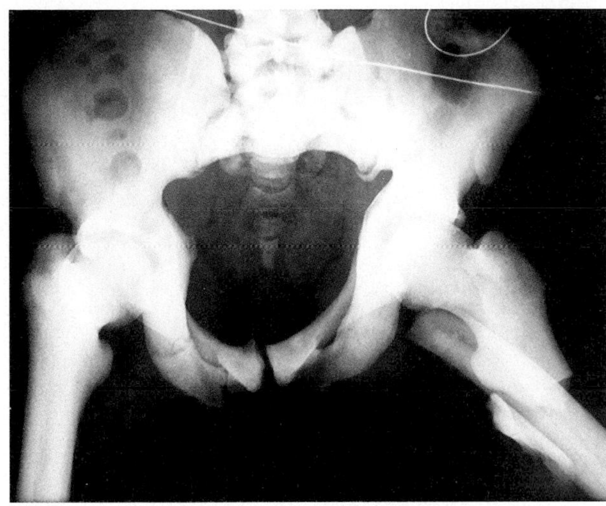

FIGURE 8-97 ■ Osteopetrosis. In this disease, also called "marble bone" disease, an abnormality in osteoclast function occurs. As a result, the bones become very dense or white, but they are almost chalklike and fracture easily. The patient broke his femur by just falling out of bed. Differential diagnoses of uniformly increased bony density would include fluorosis and myelofibrosis.

line becomes thickened; coarsening of the trabecular pattern is seen; and the bone expands as the cortex becomes thickened (Fig. 8-96). If a nuclear medicine bone scan is done, markedly increased blood flow to the bone will result in increased radioactivity in the affected areas. A generalized coarse trabecular pattern and patchy sclerosis of the whole pelvis and other bones can be due to renal failure. A diffuse increase in bone density can occur as a result of myelofibrosis, fluoride poisoning, osteopetrosis ("marble bone" disease) (Fig. 8-97), or diffuse sclerotic metastases.

Malignant Lesions

Gas within the bowel commonly projects over the pelvic bones. These gas bubbles can sometimes be difficult to tell from a lytic bone lesion. If a question remains, oblique views will show the gas rotating anteriorly. True focal lesions of the flat bones of the pelvis are often malignant. The differential diagnosis depends to a large extent on the age of the patient. In a young patient, you may suspect Ewing's sarcoma (Fig. 8-98). Chondrosarcomas tend to arise in the pelvis of adults. On an x-ray, these tumors often have cauliflower or popcorn calcifications extending from the bone (Fig. 8-99). In older patients, favorite choices for multiple lytic or destructive lesions are metastases from lung, breast, or renal cell carcinoma and multiple myeloma (plasmacytoma). Dense or sclerotic lesions of the pelvis include metastases from prostate carcinoma (Fig. 8-100) and occasionally breast cancer.

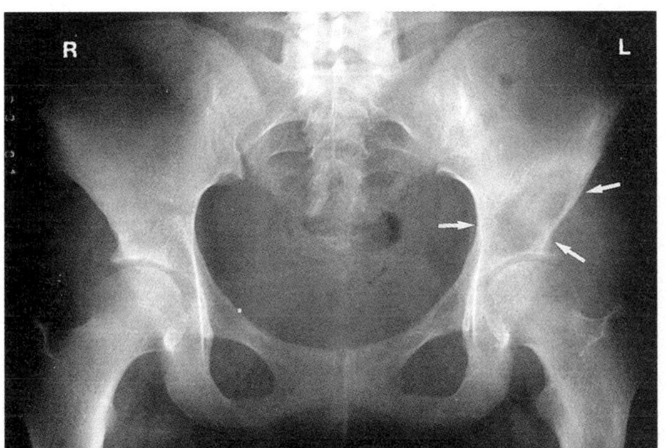

FIGURE 8-98 ■ Ewing's tumor. An anteroposterior view of the pelvis in this 17-year-old girl shows a destructive lesion above the left acetabulum with some surrounding sclerosis *(arrows)*. In a young individual, Ewing's tumor should be considered when a tumor is noted in any flat bone, such as pelvis, ribs, scapula, or skull.

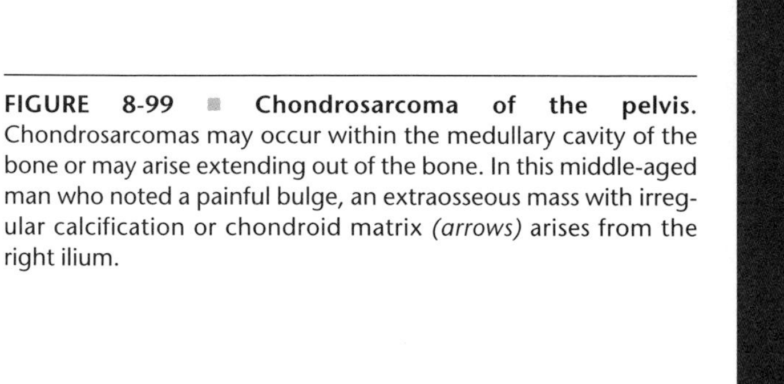

FIGURE 8-99 ■ Chondrosarcoma of the pelvis. Chondrosarcomas may occur within the medullary cavity of the bone or may arise extending out of the bone. In this middle-aged man who noted a painful bulge, an extraosseous mass with irregular calcification or chondroid matrix *(arrows)* arises from the right ilium.

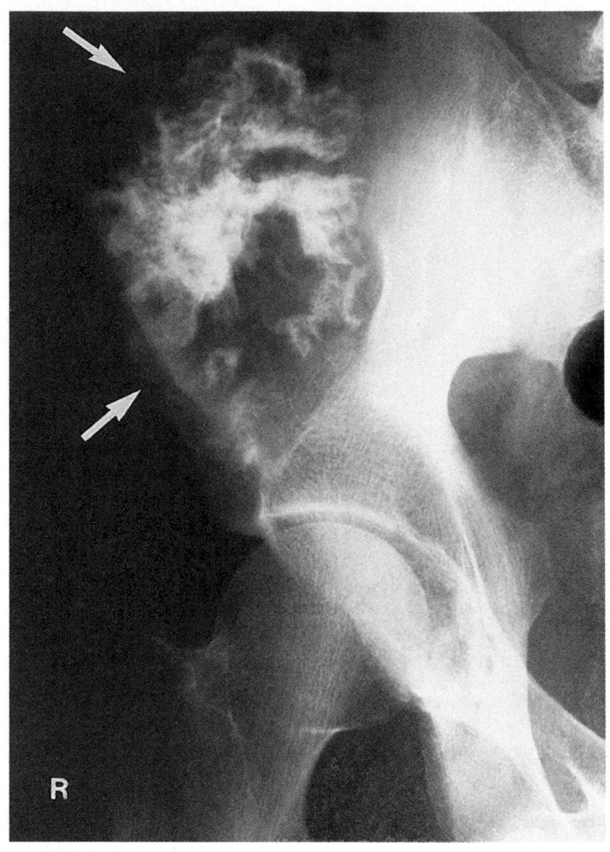

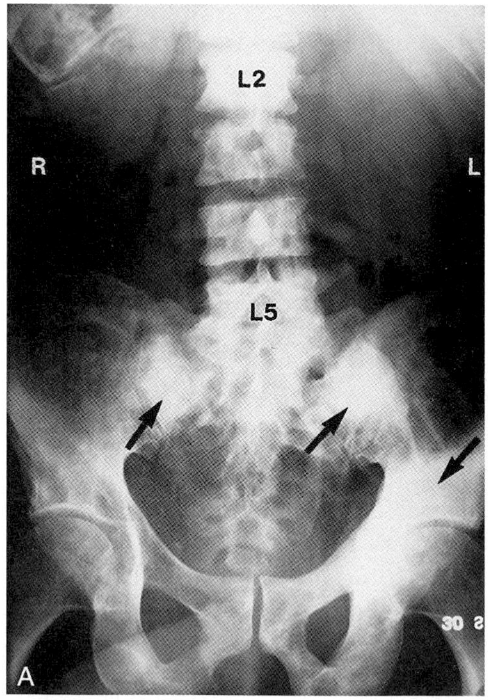

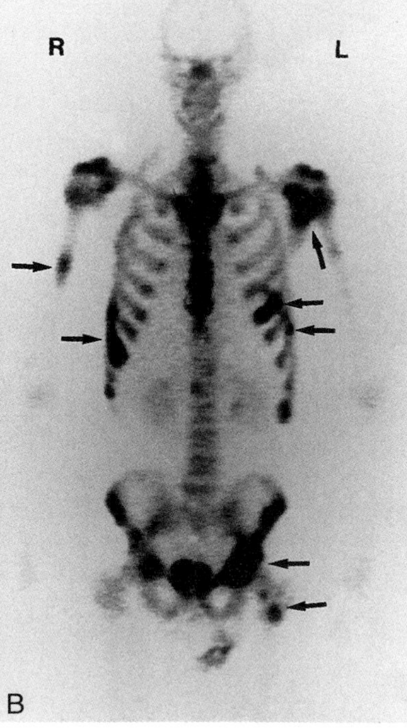

FIGURE 8-100 ■ Metastatic prostate cancer. *A,* An anteroposterior view of the pelvis and lumbar spine demonstrates multiple areas of increased density *(arrows)* in a patchy distribution. Vertebrae L2 and L5 also are abnormally white or increased in density. *B,* A nuclear medicine whole-body bone scan most commonly shows the metastatic deposits as areas of increased activity *(arrows).*

HIP

Images of the hip are done in the AP and "frog-leg" (abducted) projections. Lateral views usually are difficult to obtain and even more difficult to interpret. You should examine the relation of the femoral head to the acetabulum, look for cortical discontinuities to suggest fractures, and examine the trabecular pattern to look for potential osseous lesions. In young teenagers, notice the apophysis of both the greater and the lesser trochanter. Children younger than 10 or 12 years will not have fusion of the midportion of the acetabulum (Fig. 8-101).

Hip Pain

Acute hip pain can be due to inflammatory arthritis, septic arthritis, trauma, and tumors. These entities were discussed earlier. Chronic hip pain can result from a number of conditions. The most common is degenerative arthritis. Complaints are typically of groin or thigh pain or loss of mobility. Physical examination initially shows a loss of internal rotation, and as the disease advances, external rotation is lost. The initial workup should include plain x-rays, even though symptoms may be present before radiographic changes occur. Conversely, about 90% of persons older than 40 years have degenerative changes of the hip, but only about 30% of them have symptoms. Degenerative changes include joint-space narrowing, subchondral cyst formation, and bone spurs. Advanced imaging techniques are usually not needed. Follow-up imaging examinations are indicated if hip rotation has decreased by 20% or more or if function has changed dramatically. Pain in the upper outer thigh and tenderness in the midtrochanteric region should suggest trochanteric bursitis.

Aseptic necrosis of the hip is most commonly manifested by flattening, irregularity, and sclerosis of the superior aspect of the femoral head. It can have a number of causes, and a mnemonic is ASEPTIC. This refers to anemia (sickle cell), steroids, ethanol, pancreatitis, trauma, idiopathic, and Caisson's disease (Fig. 8-102). The most sensitive imaging study for early aseptic necrosis is MRI. If this is not available, a nuclear medicine bone scan can be used. Late changes of aseptic necrosis with femoral head deformity can easily be seen on plain x-rays.

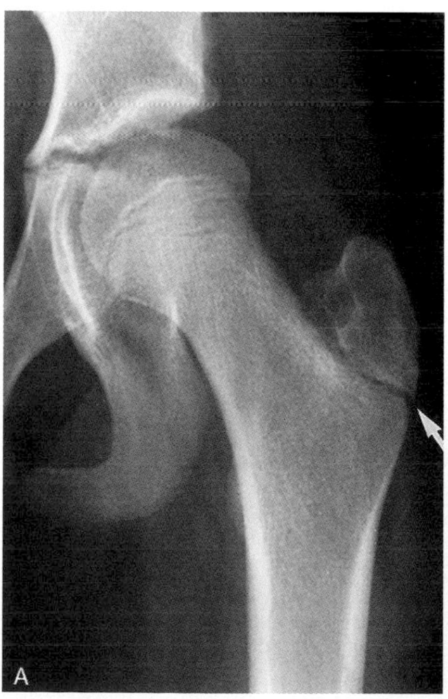

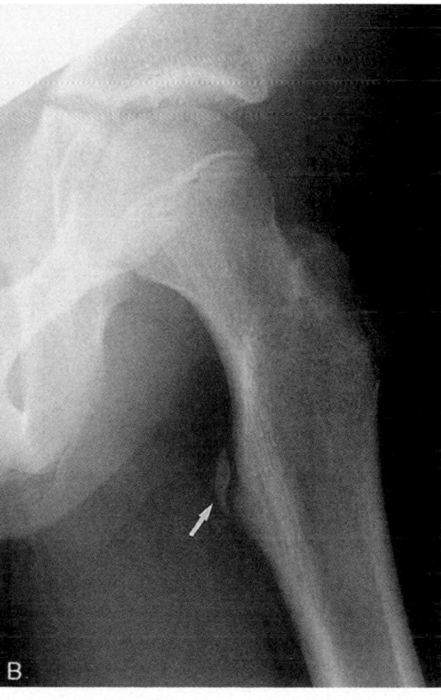

FIGURE 8-101 ■ **Normal apophyseal structures in a 10-year-old child.** *A,* An anteroposterior view of the hip clearly shows the apophysis of the greater trochanter. *B,* An oblique view shows another apophysis of the lesser trochanter. Also notice that at this age, the acetabulum is not completely fused.

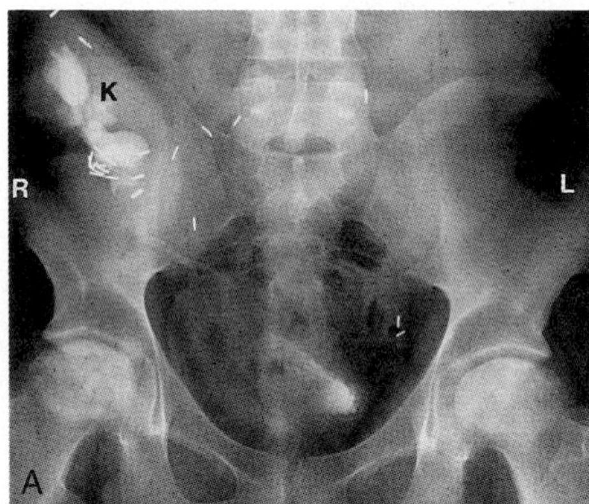

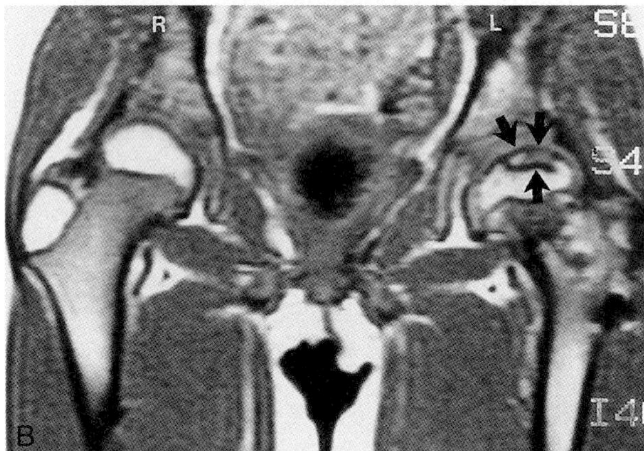

FIGURE 8-102 ■ Aseptic necrosis of the hips. *A,* Aseptic necrosis can occur from a number of causes, including trauma and steroid use. In this patient, an anteroposterior view of the pelvis shows a transplanted kidney (K) in the right iliac fossa. Use of steroids has caused this patient to have bilateral aseptic necrosis. The femoral heads are somewhat flattened, irregular, and increased in density. *B,* Aseptic necrosis in a different patient is demonstrated on a magnetic resonance imaging scan as an area of decreased signal in the left femoral head. This is the most sensitive method for detection of early aseptic necrosis.

A common problem associated with a prosthetic hip is pain due to loosening, infection, or dislocation. Dislocations are easily visualized on a plain x-ray examination. Pain may occur with loosening of the prosthesis or infection. If the prosthesis is loose and wiggling, the distal tip moves more than the rest of the shaft. A plain x-ray examination may show thinning of the bone cortex near the tip of the prosthesis. With loosening, a nuclear medicine bone scan shows increased activity near the distal tip of the prosthesis. A nuclear medicine abscess (labeled *white blood cells*) scan can be ordered to exclude infection.

Trauma

Table 8-6 shows the high-yield areas to examine for lower extremity trauma. Dislocations of the hip are usually the result of motor vehicle accidents. By far the most common dislocation is posteriorly, and on the AP image, the head of the

TABLE 8-6 ■ **Examination of an X-ray of the Lower Extremity Done for Trauma**

Hip
AP and frog-leg view
Widening of joint space
Posterior dislocation (femoral head up and out)
Anterior dislocation (femoral head in and down)
Fractures, femoral neck or intertrochanteric
Pelvic or acetabular fracture
Knee
AP view
Tibial plateau fracture
Tibial spine fracture
Patellar fracture
Lateral view
Joint effusion above patella
Fat fluid level in effusion
Patellar fracture
Ankle
AP view
Medial and lateral malleolus for soft tissue swelling and fracture
Ankle mortise for asymmetrical widening
Lateral view
Posterior malleolar fracture
Distal fibular fracture
Bulging of fat planes about joint (effusion)
Talar neck for fracture
Calcaneus for fracture
Base of 5th metatarsal fracture
Foot
AP view
Base of 5th metatarsal fracture
Fracture of distal portions of 2nd–5th metatarsals
Widening of the space between the base of the 1st and 2nd metatarsal base
Lateral view
Dislocations of the toes

Note: All images that are done for trauma involving a joint should have an oblique view as well. Many fractures are seen only on the oblique view.

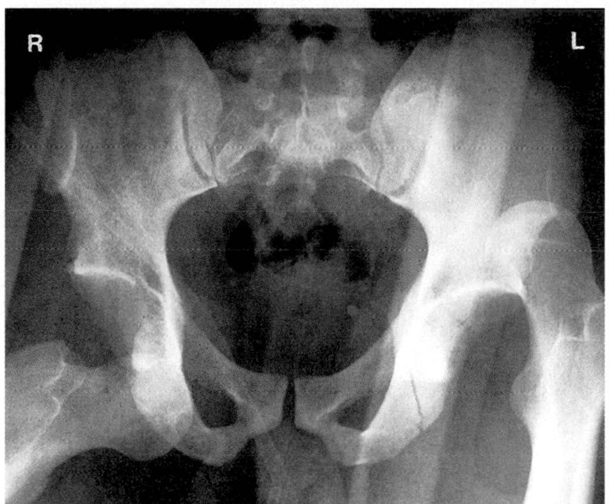

FIGURE 8-103 ■ Hip dislocation. This patient. who was in a motor vehicle accident, has both an anterior and a posterior dislocation of the hips. Posterior dislocation occurs 90% of the time and is seen here on the left, with the femoral head displaced superior and lateral to the acetabulum. On the right, an anterior dislocation appears, with the femoral head displaced inferiorly and medially.

femur appears to be superiorly and laterally displaced. When the hip is anteriorly dislocated, the femoral head appears inferior and medial to the acetabulum (Fig. 8-103). With any dislocation, associated fracture fragments from the rim of the acetabulum may be found. As the hip is relocated, these small fragments may be caught in the joint space. Sometimes they are difficult to see on a plain x-ray, but if the fragment is in the joint, the distance from the head of the femur to the acetabulum will be widened. CT scanning can be of value in such cases (Fig. 8-104).

Fractures of the hip are most common in the region of the femoral neck and in the intertrochanteric region (Fig. 8-105). Stress fractures of the femoral neck may appear only as an ill-defined sclerotic (white) band extending across the femoral neck. In older persons, a hip fracture may be difficult to see because so little calcium exists in the bone.

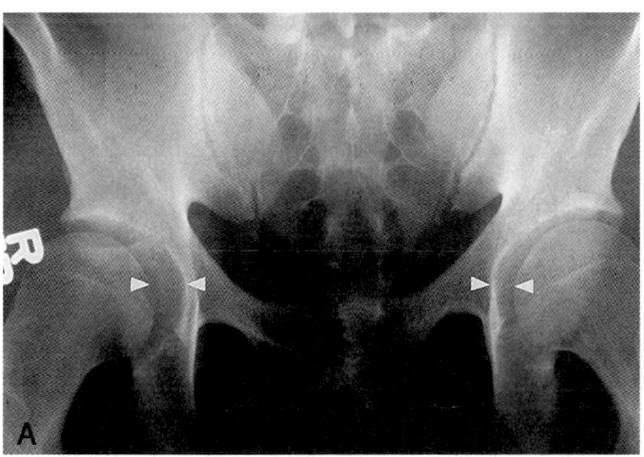

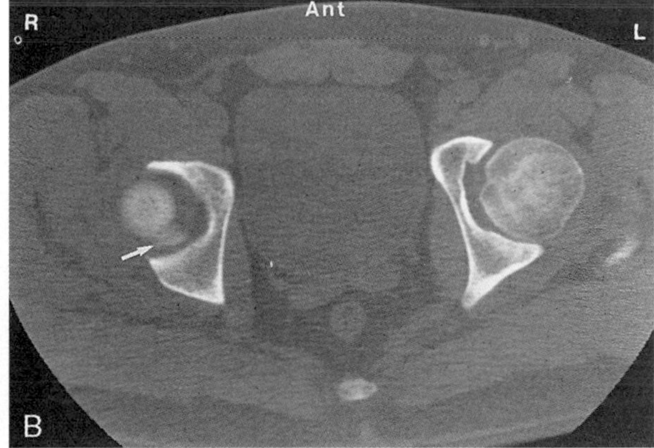

FIGURE 8-104 ■ Fracture fragment after hip dislocation. *A,* In this patient with a posterior right hip dislocation, pain and limitation of motion occurred after relocation. Asymmetrical widening is noted on the right between the femoral head and the acetabulum. No fracture fragment could be seen; however, with a transverse computed tomography scan *(B),* a bony fracture fragment could be seen in the joint space *(arrow).*

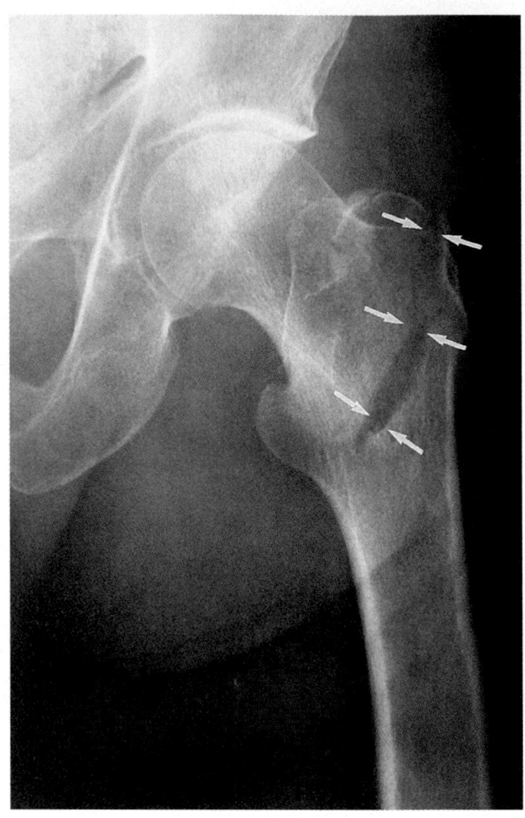

FIGURE 8-105 ■ Intertrochanteric fracture of the hip. With extracapsular hip fractures, an intertrochanteric fracture *(arrows)* occurs 70% of the time, whereas a subtrochanteric fracture occurs 30% of the time. Intracapsular fractures most commonly affect the femoral neck.

A number of orthopedic devices are used to fix hip fractures. These include plate and screws or multiple pins through the femoral neck. Prosthetic replacement of the femoral head and neck (Fig. 8-106) is often necessary for degenerative changes. The prosthetic devices may or may not use cement in the femoral shaft. Depending on the degree of degenerative change in the acetabulum, orthopedic surgeons also may use an acetabular component or an articulating (bipolar) section in the prosthetic femoral neck.

FEMUR

Normal Anatomy

The normal osseous anatomy of the femur is quite obvious and is not discussed here. The normal image projections are AP and lateral. Fractures of the femur also are very obvious. As expected, they may be transverse, spiral, or comminuted, with various degrees of angulation and overriding of the fragments.

Benign Lesions

It is important to be able to assess bone lesions and the likelihood of their being benign or malignant. Signs that a bone lesion may be benign are as follows: (1) it is small; (2) it does not have associated reaction of the periosteum; (3) it has a narrow zone of transition between the normal bone and the lesion; and (4) it has a thin, well-defined sclerotic (white) margin.

The bones of the leg are favored places for a benign fibrous cortical defect. These are usually located near but not at the ends of the bones and are usually well marginated. As the name suggests, they are present predominantly in the cortex of the bone rather than having their epicenter in the marrow space (Fig. 8-107). Another lesion, called a *nonossifying fibroma*, has the same characteristics, but it is bigger. Whether

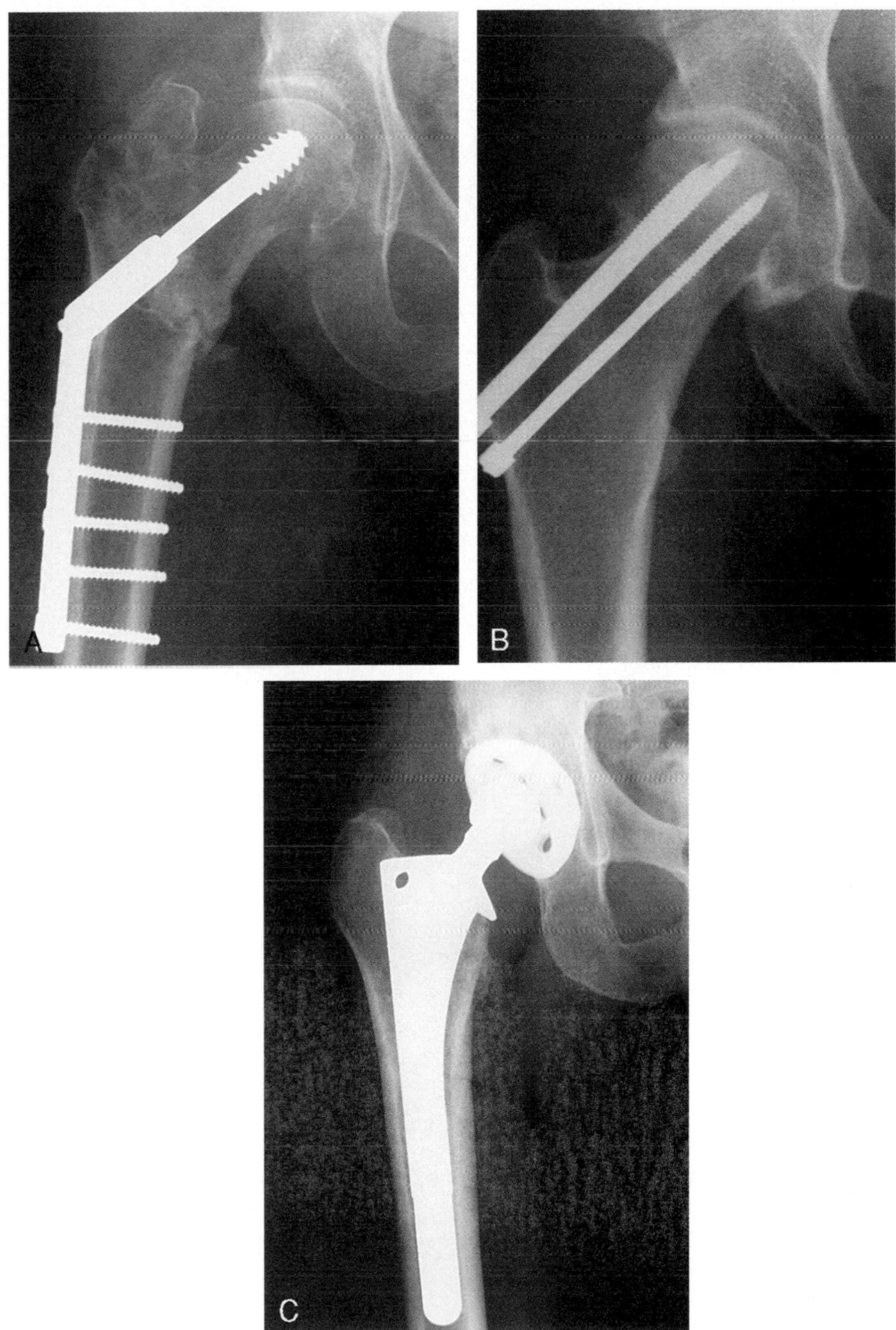

FIGURE 8-106 ■ Orthopedic fixation devices after hip fracture. *A,* A sliding hip screw is often useful for an intertrochanteric fracture. This can be recognized by the side plate, barrel, and lag screw. *B,* Knowles hip pins have been used in a different patient to repair an intracapsular femoral neck fracture. *C,* After failed healing of a femoral neck fracture, a noncemented articulating (bipolar) femoral hip prosthesis was placed.

these lesions are truly different or simply a spectrum of the same lesion is unknown.

Fibrous dysplasia usually is a lytic lesion that looks like a hole in the bone. Fibrous dysplasia may present as a single lesion (monostotic) (Fig. 8-108), or it may be in multiple areas throughout the skeleton (polyostotic). It is centered in the marrow cavity and can be single or lobular. Lytic fibrous dysplasia thins the cortex on the inner margins. Most fibrous dysplasia lesions are found in children or young adults. In addition to the lucent, sort of cystic, variety, a form is found in which the bone is diffusely involved and softened. When this happens in the femur, deformity occurs with lateral bowing. This is referred to as a "shepherd's crook" deformity.

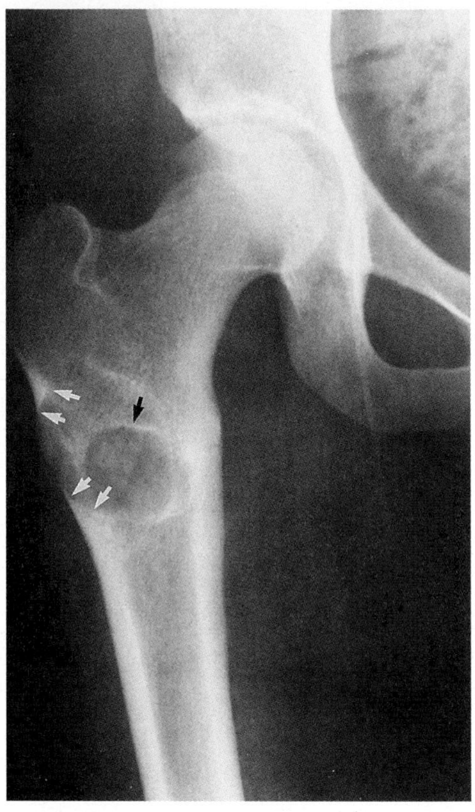

FIGURE 8-108 ■ Fibrous dysplasia. Bone lesions of fibrous dysplasia can be single (monostotic) or multifocal (polyostotic) and represent a benign developmental anomaly with fibrous tissue in the medullary space. Typically, there is a very narrow zone of transition between the lesion and normal bone *(black arrow)*, and the lesion may scallop or thin the normal cortex from the inner side *(white arrows)*. The bone also may be slightly expanded.

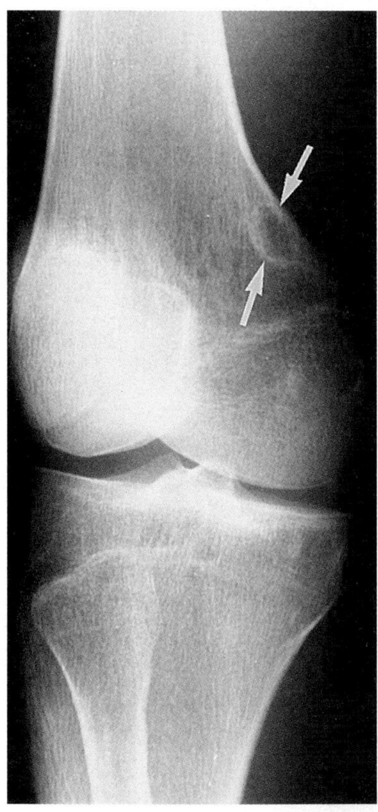

FIGURE 8-107 ■ Fibrous cortical defect. This is probably the same lesion as a nonossifying fibroma. These are most commonly seen in the lower extremity of teenagers, particularly the femur and tibia. Here the lesion is lucent and seen to have a sclerotic or dense margin. These lesions will fill in and become dense with time, and they are clinically insignificant.

Amorphous or scattered calcifications projecting within the marrow space are usually the result of benign lesions, such as enchondroma (Fig. 8-109) or bone infarcts (Fig. 8-110). Bone infarcts are relatively common in patients with sickle cell disease and also can be a result of decompression sickness from diving.

Malignant Lesions

A lytic (destructive) lesion of bone that does not have a sclerotic margin in an adult should be regarded as a malignancy until proven other-

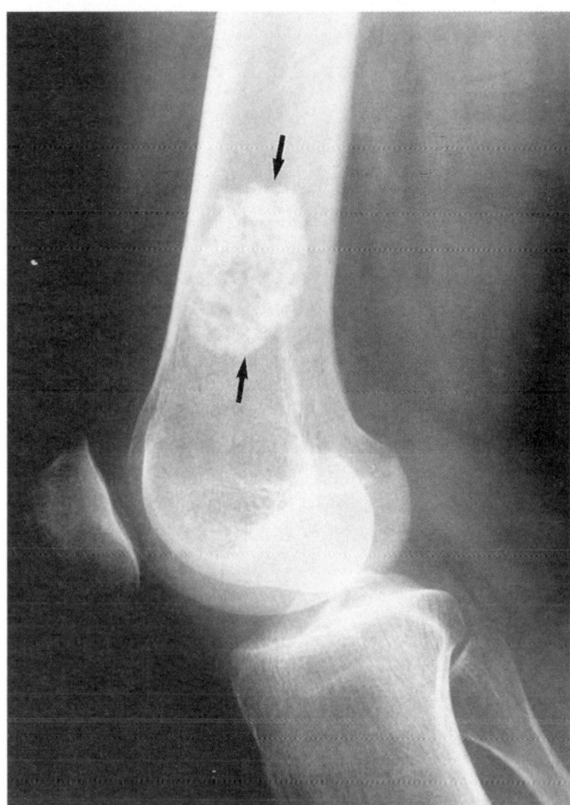

FIGURE 8-109 ■ Enchondroma. This lateral view of the knee shows a dense lesion that is somewhat amorphous and projects within the medullary space of the bone. A well-defined lesion such as this is most likely an enchondroma, although a low-grade intramedullary chondrosarcoma also must be considered.

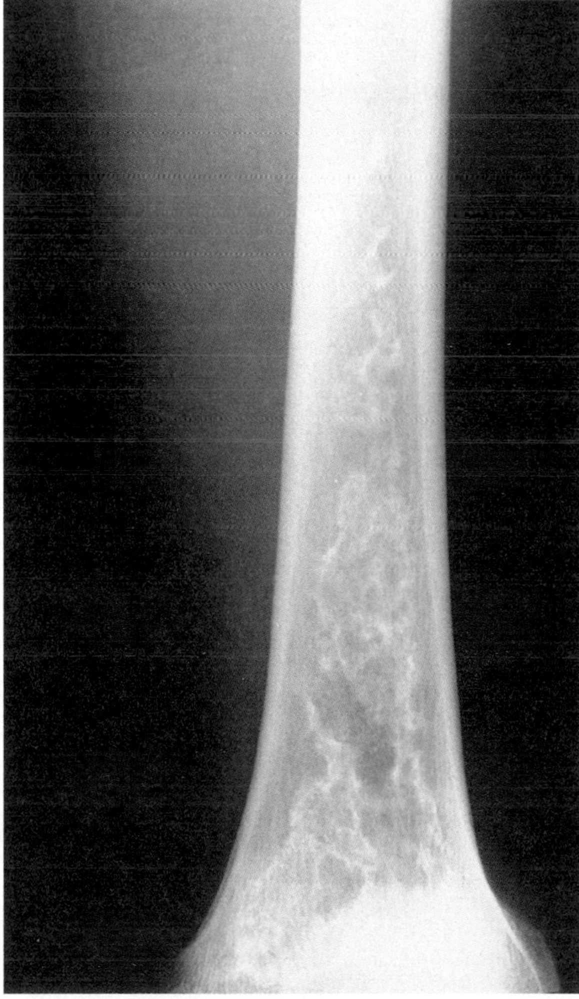

FIGURE 8-110 ■ Bone infarcts. Diffuse and amorphous calcification within the medullary space is seen here in the distal femur. Bone infarcts such as this can occur in patients with sickle cell disease or as a result of decompression sickness after underwater diving accidents.

wise. Breast cancer, lung cancer, and a host of other neoplasms commonly produce lytic lesions of bone. A number of primary bone lesions can produce this appearance, including plasmacytoma and eosinophilic granuloma.

Chondrosarcomas tend to occur in the femur, pelvis, and ribs. In the femur, they are most common in the metaphysis. They can be very variable in appearance from purely destructive, destructive with a chondroid (irregular calcification) matrix, to exostotic, or projecting from the cortex of a bone. The mean age for occurrence is 40 to 45 years.

Even if a patient has known metastatic disease elsewhere, it is important to identify metastatic sites in the pelvis and lower extremities. This is because these sites are weight bearing and are susceptible to pathologic fractures that can disable the patient (Fig. 8-111). Early detection can allow placement of a medullary rod or radiation therapy, which will allow a terminal patient to ambulate rather than being bedridden for the remaining months of life.

Periosteal Reaction

Periosteal reaction can be due to either benign or malignant lesions. Obviously, local periosteal reaction will be seen about a healing fracture. However, this is normally quite obvious and does not cause any confusion in interpretation. Generalized periosteal reaction can occur along the long bones of the extremities in patients with lung cancer. This condition is known as hypertrophic pulmonary osteoarthropathy (HPO). The reason for the periosteal reaction is unclear.

Infections also can cause periosteal reaction. Osteomyelitis that has been present for several weeks can cause minimal periosteal reaction, and chronic osteomyelitis that has been present for months and years can cause a florid calcified periosteal reaction (Fig. 8-112).

In young patients (age 5 to 20 years), periosteal reaction in the midportion (diaphysis) of a long bone should raise the suspicion of a Ewing's tumor; if located around the joint such

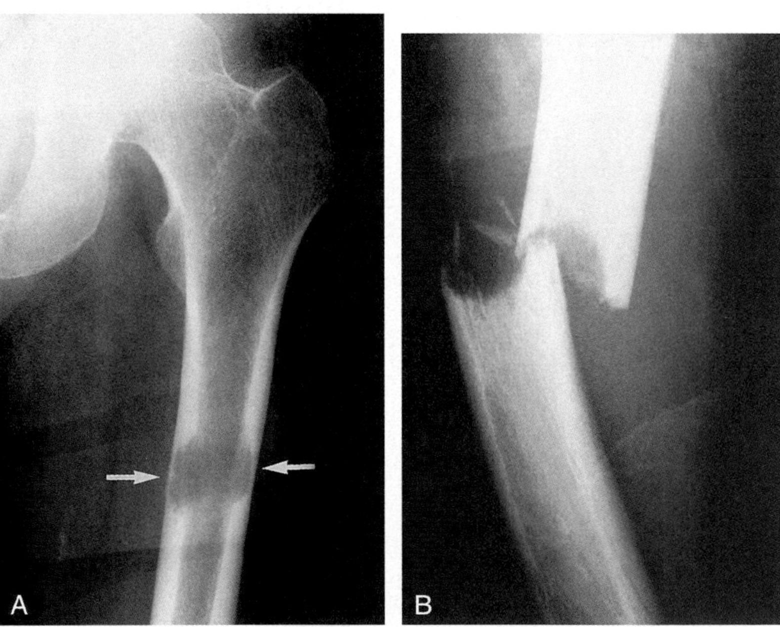

FIGURE 8-111 ■ Lytic bone metastases. *A,* A view of the femur in this patient with known lung carcinoma shows a destructive lesion expanding from the marrow space and thinning the cortex *(arrows).* This lesion has no clear margin or white rim to distinguish it from normal bone. Lesions such as this in weight-bearing bones are important to find so that therapy can be undertaken to prevent pathologic fracture. *B,* A view of the femur in the same patient, who returned 2 weeks later with a pathologic fracture.

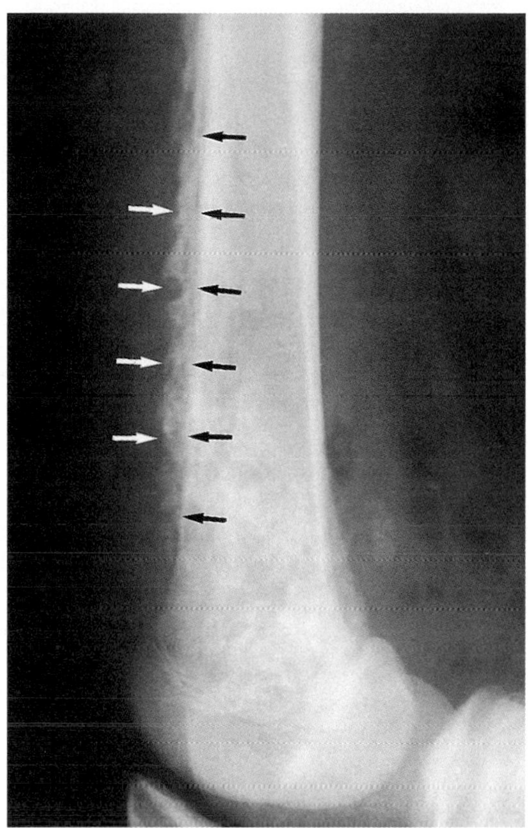

FIGURE 8-112 ■ Chronic osteomyelitis. A lateral view of the knee shows florid periosteal reaction *(arrows)*. The periosteal reaction that is dense and extends over a long area suggests chronic osteomyelitis. The bone of the distal femur has a mottled appearance as a result of the infection. Note also that the distal femoral epiphysis is not fused; given the periosteal reaction, the location in the distal femur, and the patient's age, also consider an osteogenic sarcoma.

as the knee, it should raise the suspicion of an osteogenic sarcoma (Fig. 8-113). Sunburst (radiating)-type periosteal reaction is particularly worrisome for malignancy.

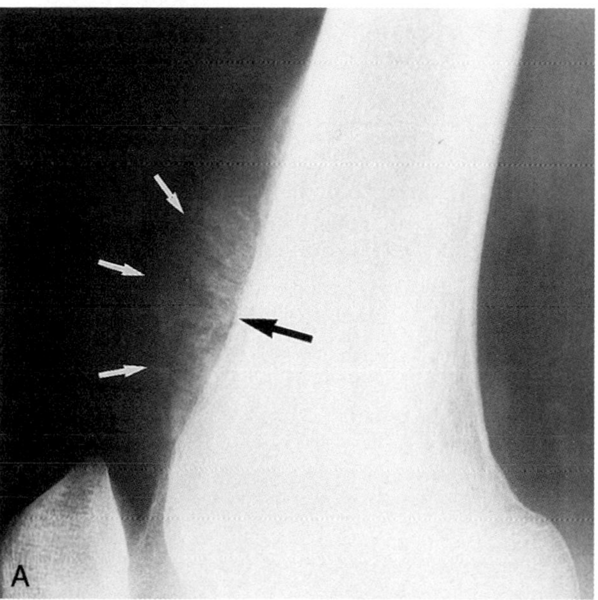

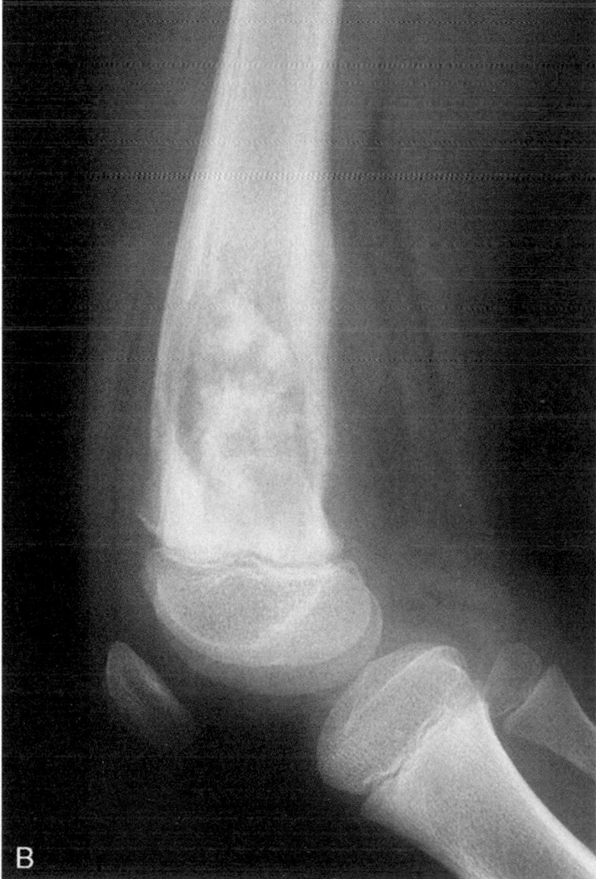

FIGURE 8-113 ■ Osteogenic sarcoma of the knee. A lateral view of the knee *(A)* in a 19-year-old man shows a sunburst-type periosteal reaction *(arrows)*. Knowing that the distal femur is the most common site of osteogenic sarcoma, that periosteal reaction is a feature, and that this patient is a teenager should make osteogenic sarcoma very high on your differential diagnostic list. Another common presentation *(B)* is a predominantly destructive central lesion seen here in the distal femur of an 8-year-old girl.

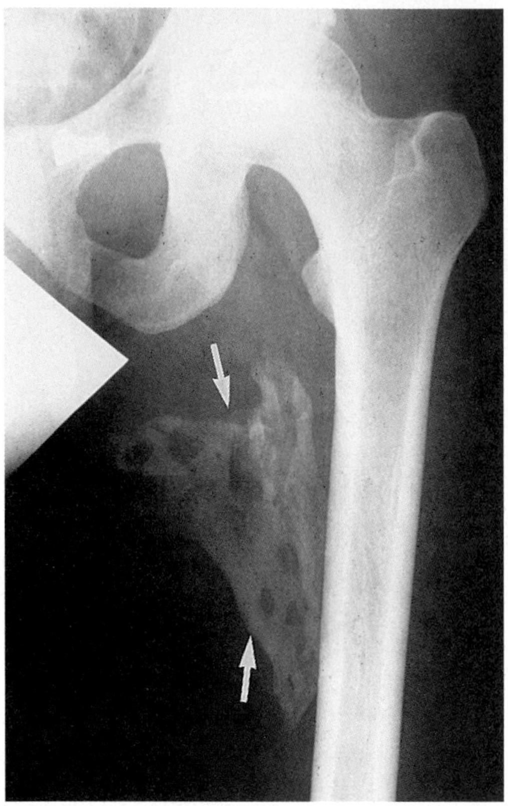

FIGURE 8-114 ■ **Myositis ossificans.** The soft tissues of the thigh are a common location for blunt traumatic injury. In this case, dystrophic calcification has developed within the soft tissue *(arrows),* significantly limiting the range of motion of this young soccer player.

Myositis Ossificans

Calcification can occur in soft tissues. The muscles of the thigh are particularly prone to trauma, and bleeding within the soft tissue can subsequently calcify. This condition is referred to as myositis ossificans (Fig. 8-114) and may require surgery after the calcification has matured.

KNEE

Normal Anatomy

The normal imaging projections that are obtained of the knee are AP and lateral views (Fig. 8-115). The lateral view is taken with the knee partially flexed. The AP view is important for assessing whether joint-space narrowing is present. This view also will show whether calcification of the cartilage has occurred in the joint space. Sometimes the tibial plateaus are at slightly different angulations so that the x-ray beam does not go horizontally through both medial and lateral compartments.

The lateral view is used to evaluate the patella and to determine whether a joint effusion is present. Both views are used to assess degenerative changes, fractures, and the general matrix of the bone of the distal femur, proximal tibia, and proximal fibula. Both views also are needed to see whether a bony fragment lies within the joint space. This is necessary because in order to be sure that the fragment or loose body is within the joint space, it must be triangulated by using both projections.

Two special views of the knee are commonly requested. The first of these is the "sunrise" view, a tangential view of the anterior portion of the flexed knee, looking from the top down. The advantage of this view is that the relation of the patella to the anterior femur is clearly shown. Another view is the "tunnel" view. In this, the knee is flexed more than on the routine lateral view, and the x-ray beam is directed horizontally across the tibial plateau through the "tunnel" created by the femoral condyles. This affords a very good look at the anterior and posterior tibial spines as well as the femoral condyles.

In children, the epiphyseal plate of the distal femoral epiphysis and the proximal tibial epiphysis is well seen until at least age 10 years. Complete fusion typically occurs in girls at about the age of 15 years, and in boys, several years later (Fig. 8-116). In teenagers, it is important to note on the lateral view that the anterior portion of the proximal tibial epiphysis folds down to form the attachment for the inferior aspect of the patellar tendon. It almost looks like a horn projecting downward from the anterior portion of the proximal tibia, and this is normal. A fairly common normal variant is the fabella. This is a small sesamoid bone in the tendons posterior to the knee joint, easily

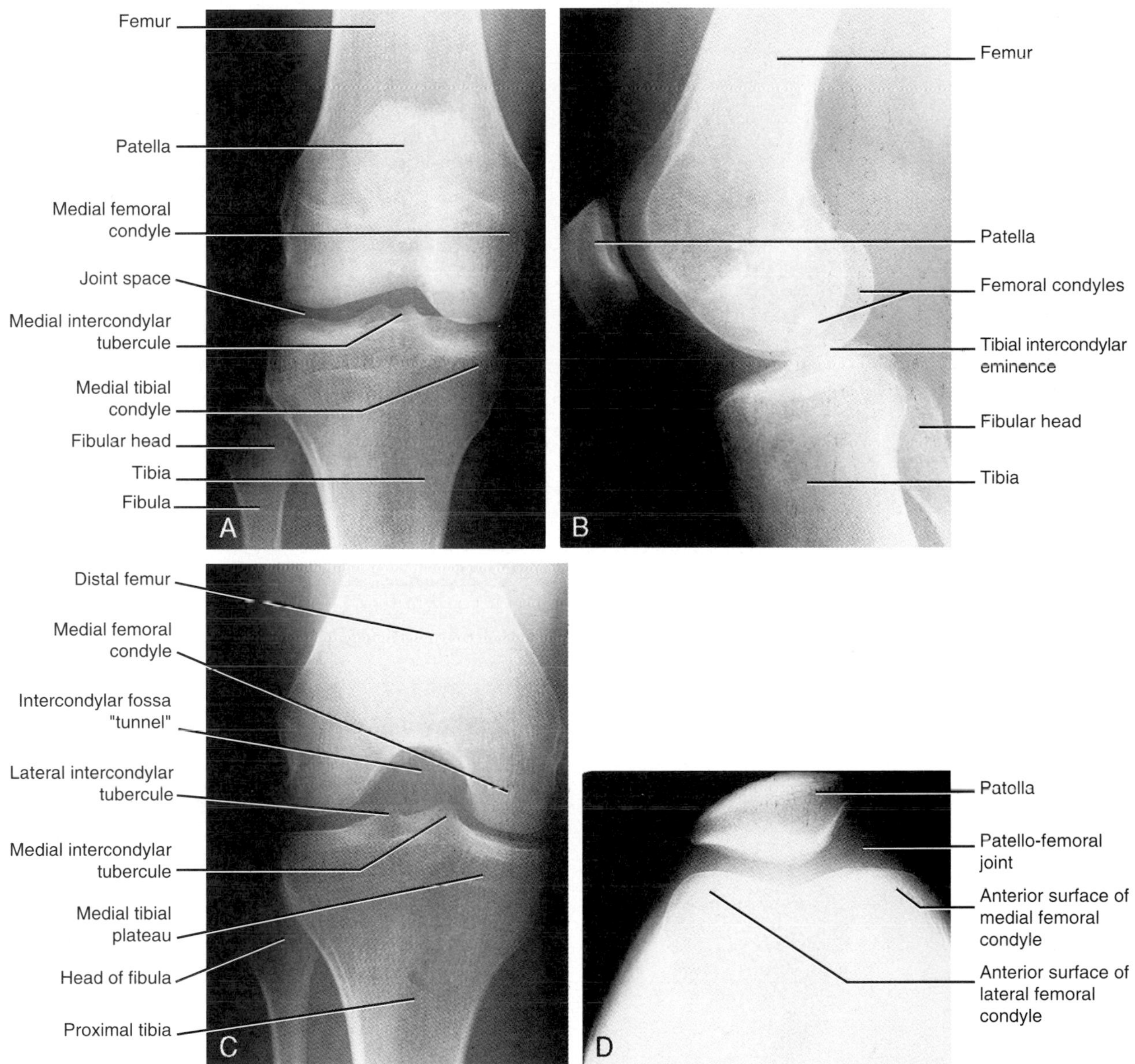

FIGURE 8-115 ■ Normal anatomy of the knee in the anteroposterior projection *(A),* lateral projection *(B),* tunnel view *(C),* and sunrise view *(D).*

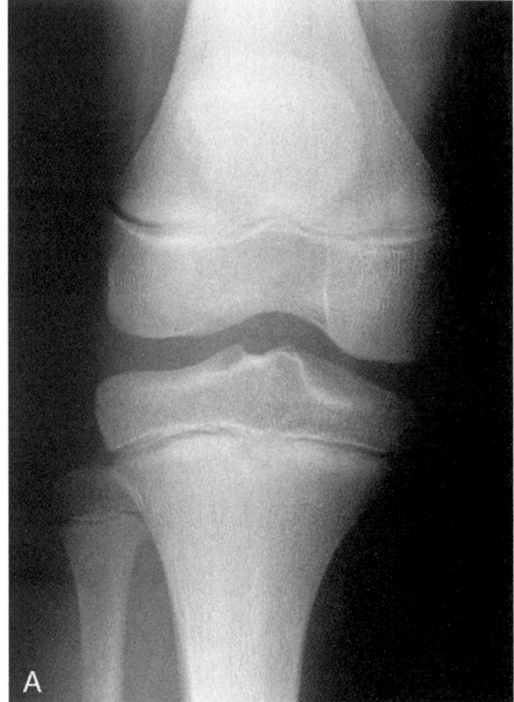

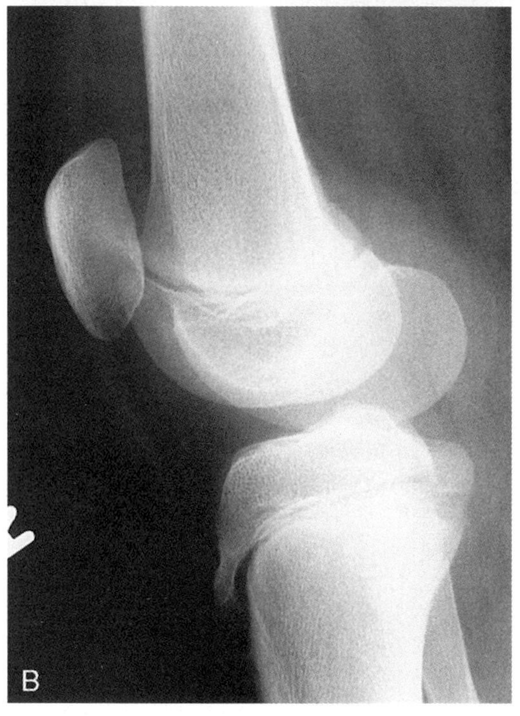

FIGURE 8-116 ■ Normal knee in an 11-year-old child. *A,* An anteroposterior view clearly demonstrates the epiphyses of the distal femur, proximal tibia, and fibula. *B,* A lateral view shows the normal downward projection of the proximal tibial epiphysis along the anterior portion of the tibia to form the tibial tubercle.

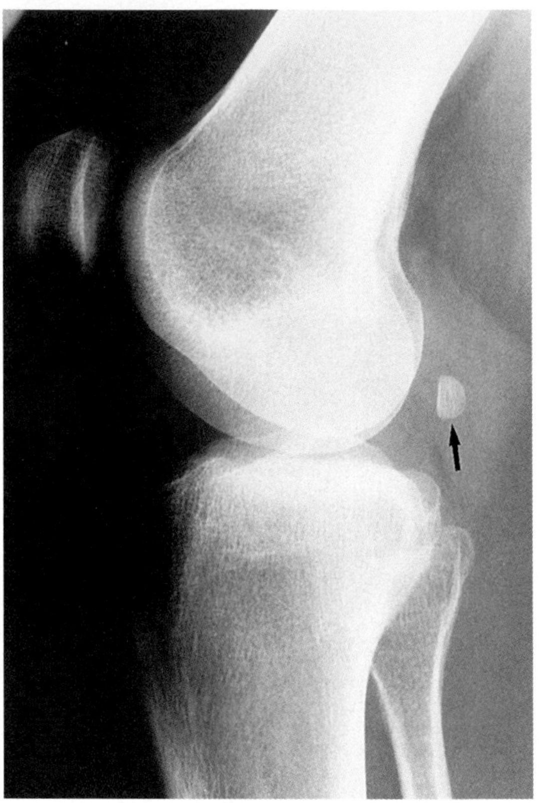

FIGURE 8-117 ■ Fabella. On the lateral view of the knee, a small oval bone can be seen posterior to the knee joint *(arrow).* This essentially is a sesamoid bone and is a normal variant of no clinical significance.

seen on the lateral view (Fig. 8-117). With MRI, the soft tissues, including the tendons, ligaments, and cartilage of the knee, can be exquisitely visualized (Fig. 8-118). Structures of particular interest on these images are those that are commonly involved in trauma, such as the cruciate ligaments and the medial and lateral menisci.

Knee Pain and Degenerative Changes

The diagnosis of chronic meniscal tear is based on a history of pain, knee catching, locking, giving way, snapping, or clicking. On physical examination, tenderness may be found along the joint line and reproduction of the clicking sound by manipulation (McMurray's sign).

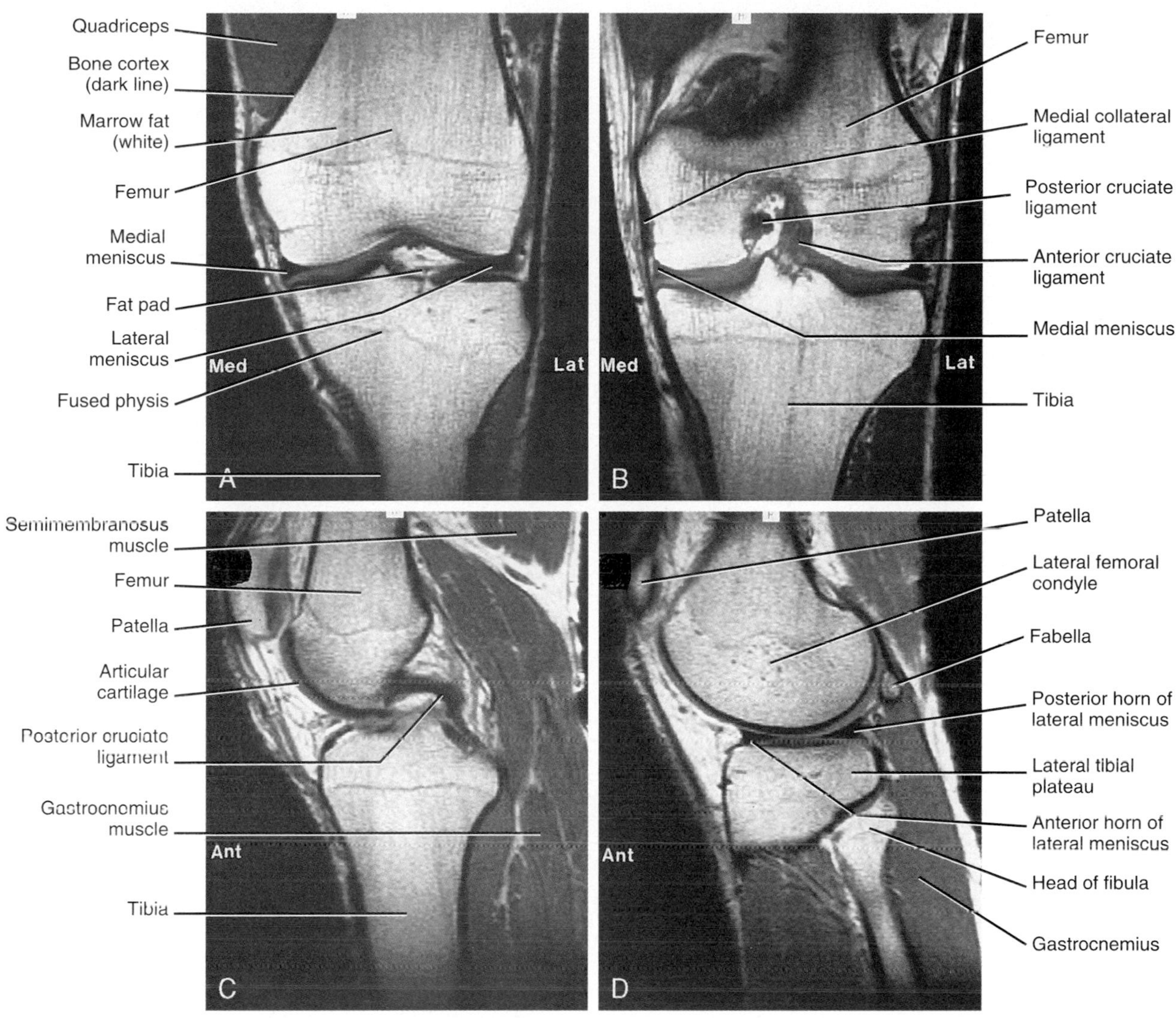

FIGURE 8-118 ■ **Normal anatomy of the knee on a magnetic resonance scan.** Images are presented in the coronal view near the front of the knee *(A)* and in the midportion of the knee *(B)*. Additional sagittal or lateral magnetic resonance views are identified through the middle of the knee *(C)* and in the lateral compartment *(D)*.

Radiography is indicated to exclude significant osseous injury. With acute meniscal injury, often loss of motion, joint effusion, and acute muscle spasm are found. Again, an x-ray is indicated to exclude a fracture. A difference of opinion exists as to whether to then proceed with arthroscopy or to do an MRI scan. Both approaches are used.

Chronic knee pain may be due to degenerative change. On physical examination, usually limited motion or pain with motion is seen and, unlike RA, no systemic symptoms are noted. Redness or swelling over the joint appear, as well as deformity. Laboratory tests are not needed. Plain radiographs are indicated for initial workup to determine the extent of disease, even though radiographic findings often do not correlate with symptoms. Degenerative changes of the knee are manifested by joint-space narrowing and sclerosis of the bony articular margins. It is quite common to have only the medial or

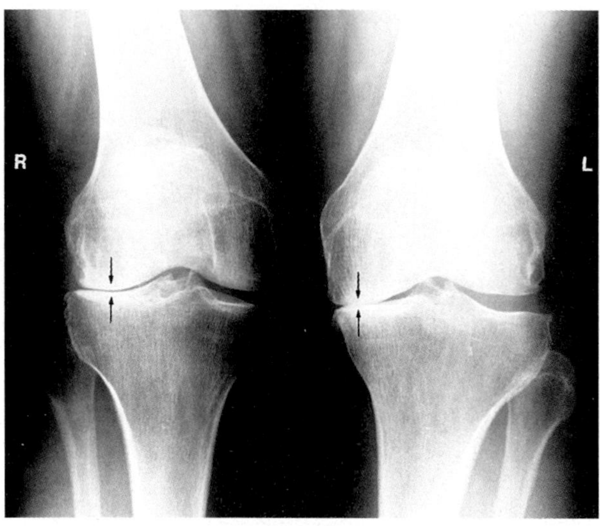

FIGURE 8-119 ■ Degenerative osteoarthritis. In this standing view of both knees, significant narrowing and sclerosis of the medial compartment of the left knee and of the lateral compartment of the right knee are noted.

lateral compartment involved while the other compartment appears quite normal (Fig. 8-119). Other signs of degenerative change are small overhanging spurs at the edges of the joints. No other imaging is indicated unless symptoms significantly progress or surgery is planned, and then plain x-rays are again ordered.

Occasionally, degenerative changes of the joint can involve disruption of pieces of cartilage that come loose and are a nidus calcification. These calcifications are often within the joint space and can be single or multiple. If they are single, they are called a "loose body." If they are multiple and extensive, the condition is termed synovial chondromatosis (Fig. 8-120). Internal derangement of the knee is usually suspected on the basis of clinical findings (clicking, locking, giving way, limitation of motion, or pain with passive range of motion). An MRI is indicated if plain x-rays are nonspecific and only if some form of therapy is anticipated.

Trauma

A knee joint effusion is easiest to identify superior to the patella and anterior to the distal femur. You should look for this on the lateral view (Fig. 8-121). The effusion is basically water or blood, which has the same density as muscle, and it is visualized only because anterior displacement of the normal fat line is present. It is not appropriate to order a knee x-ray to exclude or identify an effusion, because this is much better done by clinical examination. Knee effusions are usually identified as an incidental finding in patients who have had trauma and for whom the examination was ordered because a fracture was suspected.

The two most common soft tissue injuries of the knee involve the cruciate ligaments and the menisci. As mentioned earlier, the imaging study of choice for these is MRI, with which the cruciate ligaments can be well seen, and tears or par-

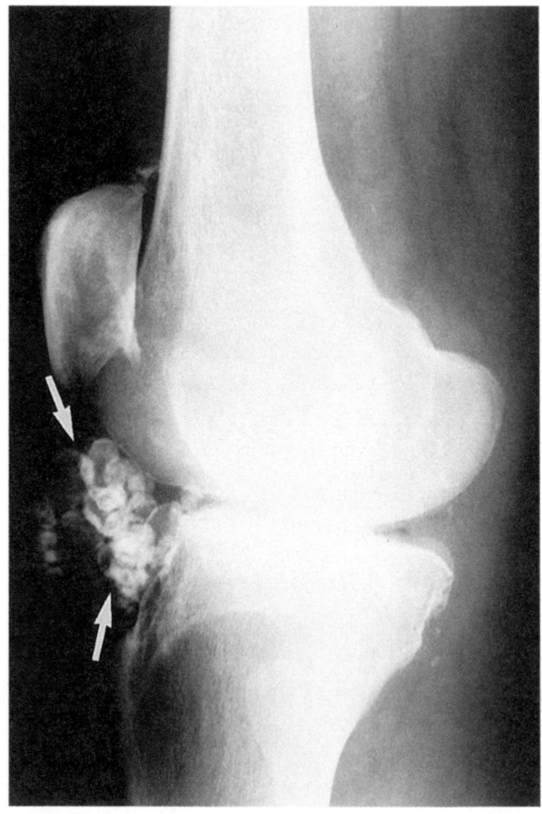

FIGURE 8-120 ■ Synovial osteochondromatosis. These are small calcified loose bodies within the joint space *(arrows)*. This is sometimes referred to as "housemaid's knee" or "nun's knee."

tial tears of these ligaments can be easily identified (Fig. 8-122). Repair of cruciate ligaments often involves transplantation of a tendon and insertion of a bone plug. The x-rays that are obtained in follow-up of these patients demonstrate several screws in the femoral intracondylar notch and proximal tibia.

Normal cartilage looks quite black on MRI, and it typically is triangular. When tears are present within the cartilage, an area of increased signal (white) can be seen (Fig. 8-123). Not all areas of increased signal represent a tear, and a number of subtle criteria are used by radiologists to differentiate between degenerative change and a tear.

Patellar fractures are usually caused by a direct blow to the patella during a fall. The fractures are seen as dark lines across the bone, with sharp corners and edges (Fig. 8-124). A normal variant that is often confused with a patellar fracture is the bipartite patella. It is an abnormality in growth and results in a rounded or oval bony fragment in the upper and outer portion of the patella (Fig. 8-125). It usually is not a problem to differentiate from a fracture because of its location (upper outer portion) and its rounded and well-marginated edges.

Tibial plateau fractures are best visualized on the anterior view. They are reasonably common, and you should look for a vertical lucent line located slightly lateral to the center of the tibial spines. Sometimes, if the fracture is oblique to the x-ray beam, it can be difficult to see, but you may notice depression of one of the

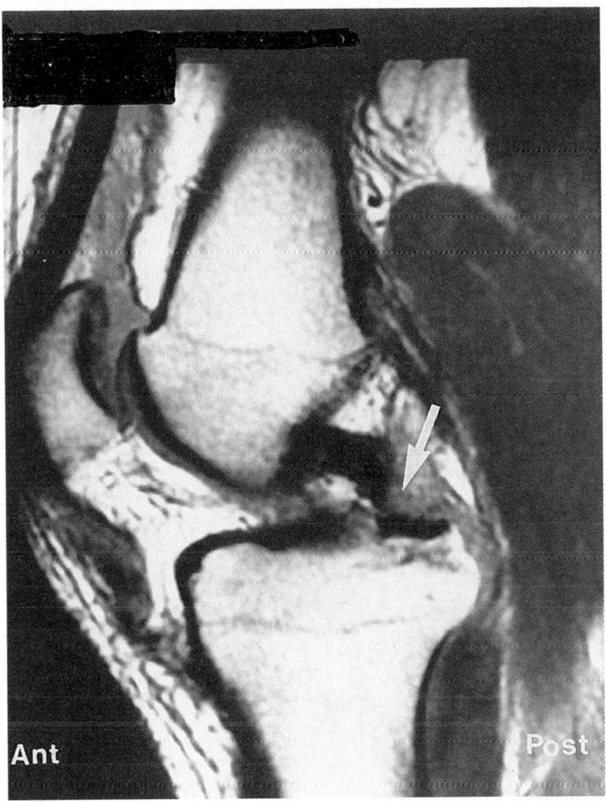

FIGURE 8-122 ■ **Posterior cruciate ligament tear.** A lateral or sagittal view of the knee on magnetic resonance imaging scan demonstrates disruption *(arrow)* of the normal dark posterior cruciate ligament.

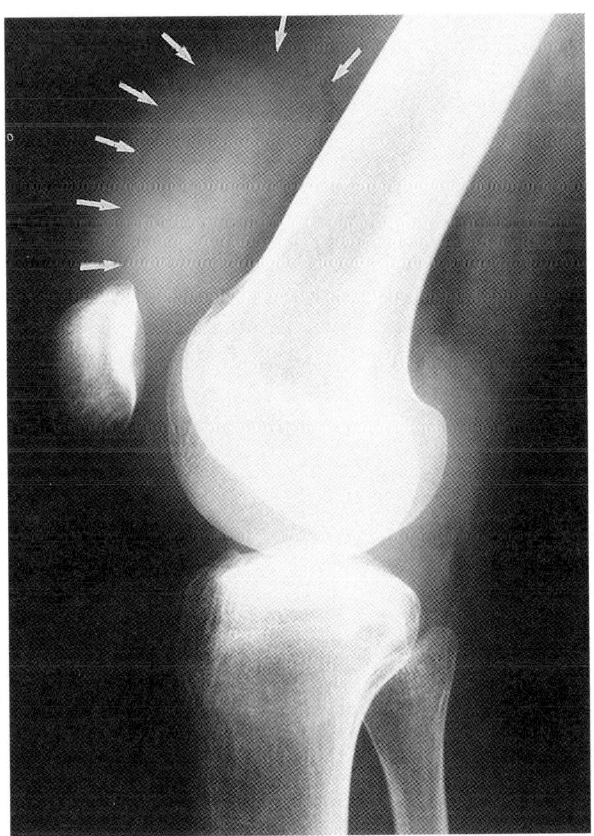

FIGURE 8-121 ■ **Large knee effusion.** Knee effusions are best detected on the lateral view by looking above the patella and seeing anterior displacement of the dark fat line by soft tissue or water density *(arrows)*. Knee effusions are even more easily and accurately detected by clinical examination.

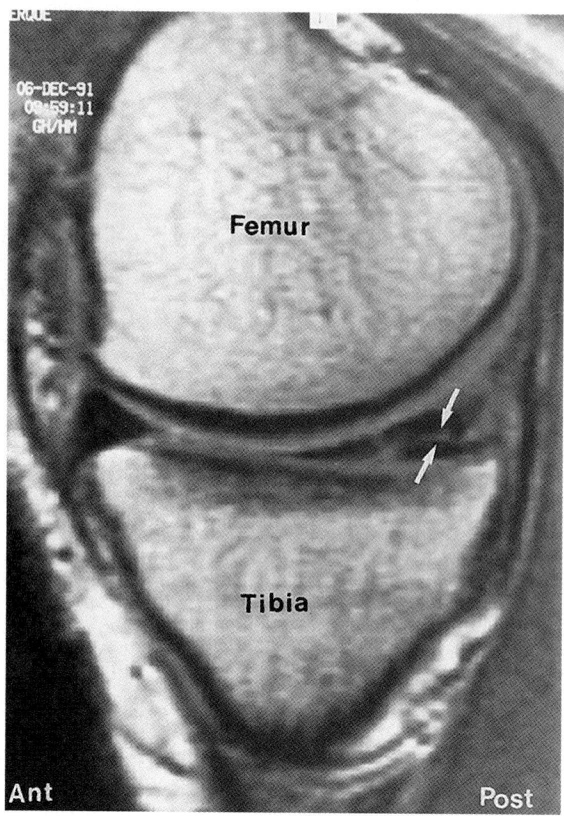

FIGURE 8-123 ■ **Tear in the posterior horn of the lateral meniscus.** A sagittal view of the lateral knee on a magnetic resonance imaging scan shows increased signal *(arrows)* extending to the edges of the normally black or dark meniscus.

tibial plateaus, and you may see a step-off as you trace the tibial cortex along the joint surface. With tibial plateau fractures, a collection of fluid is often seen above the patella. Remember that because lateral knee images for trauma are done with the patient lying down, you can often see a horizontal "fat/fluid" level above the patella (Fig. 8-126). This probably does not represent fat from the marrow space coming from the site of the fracture, but rather represents layering of the various components of blood into cells and serum in a hemorrhagic effusion. Because tibial plateau fractures can sometimes be difficult to see, if you see a fat/fluid level on the lateral knee image, you should look very hard to find a tibial plateau fracture.

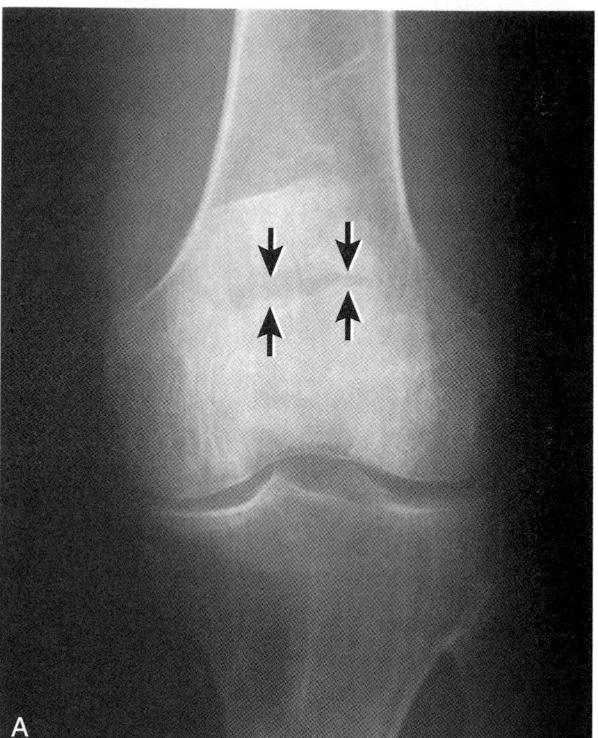

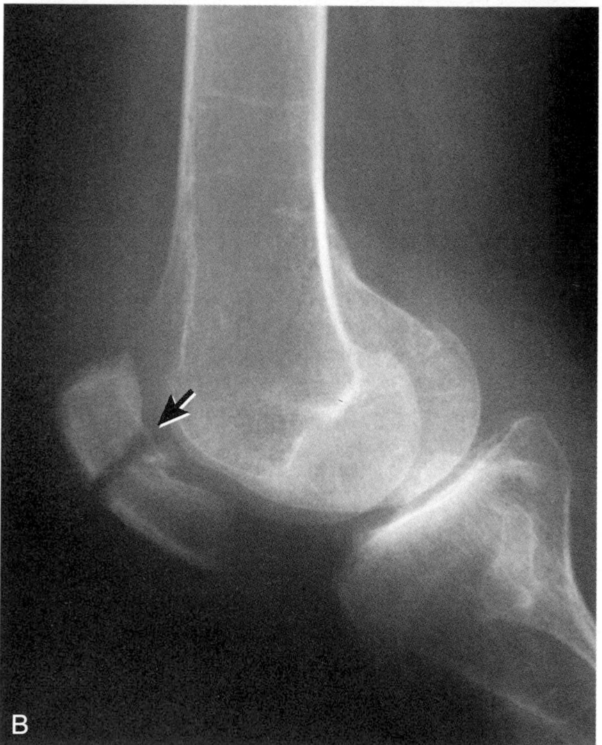

FIGURE 8-124 ■ **Patellar fracture.** An anteroposterior view and *(A)* and lateral view *(B)* of the knee shows lucent or dark lines *(arrows)* with sharp corners along the mid portion of the patella.

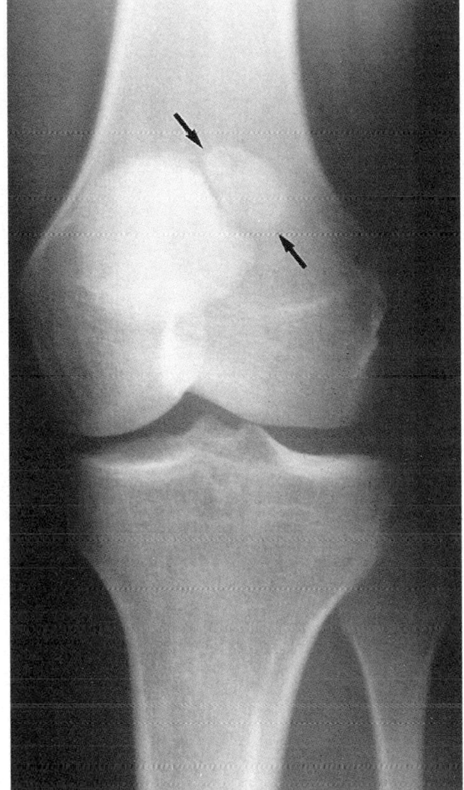

FIGURE 8-125 ■ Bipartite patella. On this anteroposterior view of the knee, a fragment can be seen in the upper outer portion of the patella *(arrows).* Note that this is rounded and that the location in the upper outer portion of the patella indicates that this is a normal variant of no clinical significance; it should not be mistaken for a patellar fracture.

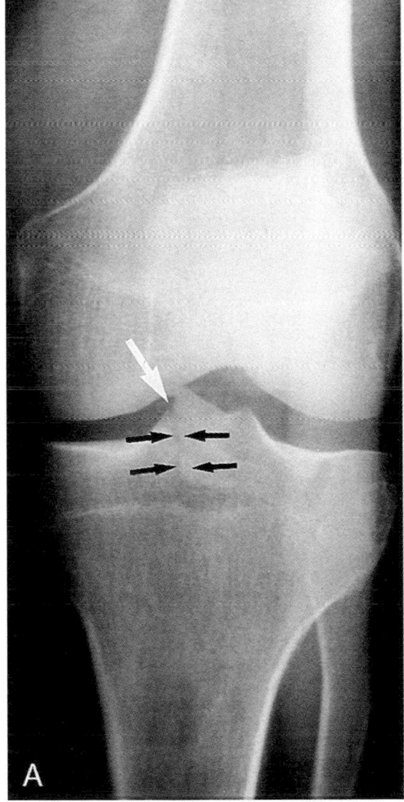

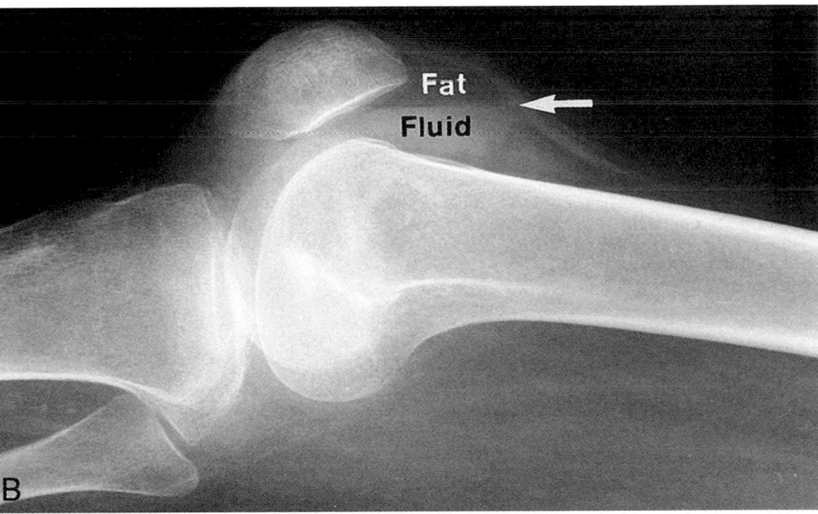

FIGURE 8-126 ■ Tibial plateau fracture. An anteroposterior view *(A)* shows a vertical lucent line extending into the upper portion of the tibia. A cortical step-off *(white arrow)* also is seen just medial to the intercondylar tubercle. The true extent of these fractures may be difficult to appreciate on plain films. A lateral cross-table view of the knee *(B)* shows a typical fat/fluid level in the suprapatellar region. This actually is not fat but settling blood in a hemarthrosis.

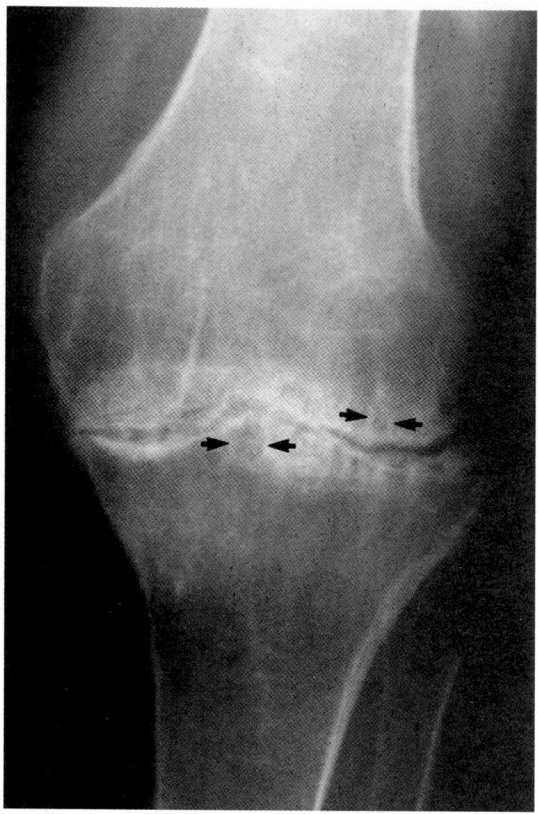

FIGURE 8-127 ■ Rheumatoid arthritis of the knee. Diffuse joint space narrowing with subchondral cyst formation is present *(arrows)*. A distinguishing feature between this and degenerative arthritis is that in rheumatoid arthritis, degenerative osteophytes or spurs are not usually seen.

Arthritis

A number of arthritides can affect the major joints. RA is a major player and can cause synovial destruction with joint-space narrowing. One of the tip-offs to RA is the presence of subchondral cysts just under the bony cortex on both sides of the joint space (Fig. 8-127).

Sometimes calcification can be seen within the articular cartilage of the knee. This finding is called chondrocalcinosis (Fig. 8-128); it is usually easy to distinguish from loose bodies within the joint space, because it is calcification in a horizontal linear fashion. Chondrocalcinosis may be due to degenerative change, hypercalcemic states, and pseudogout, as well as some other less common entities.

When degenerative changes of the knee are extensive enough, a prosthetic knee replacement may be required (Fig. 8-129). A number of prostheses are available, but, in general, they have a femoral condylar component as well as a proximal tibial and patellar component. Sometimes the patellar component is not installed. On the AP view, these prostheses may look as if they are not touching each other when they are in contact. This is because of a plastic surface that is not visible on the x-ray. Abnormalities to look for with a prosthesis involve infection and loosening. Both are seen as a lucent line or rarefaction of bone around the screws or the base of the implant.

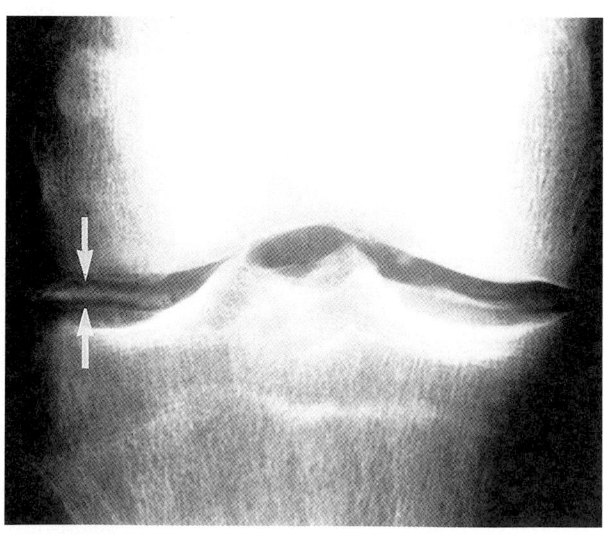

FIGURE 8-128 ■ Chondrocalcinosis. Calcification of the cartilage in this knee is seen particularly well in the lateral compartment *(arrows)*. This is due to calcium pyrophosphate deposition disease (CPPD). Calcification is not seen in all patients with CPPD, and not all patients with chondrocalcinosis have CPPD.

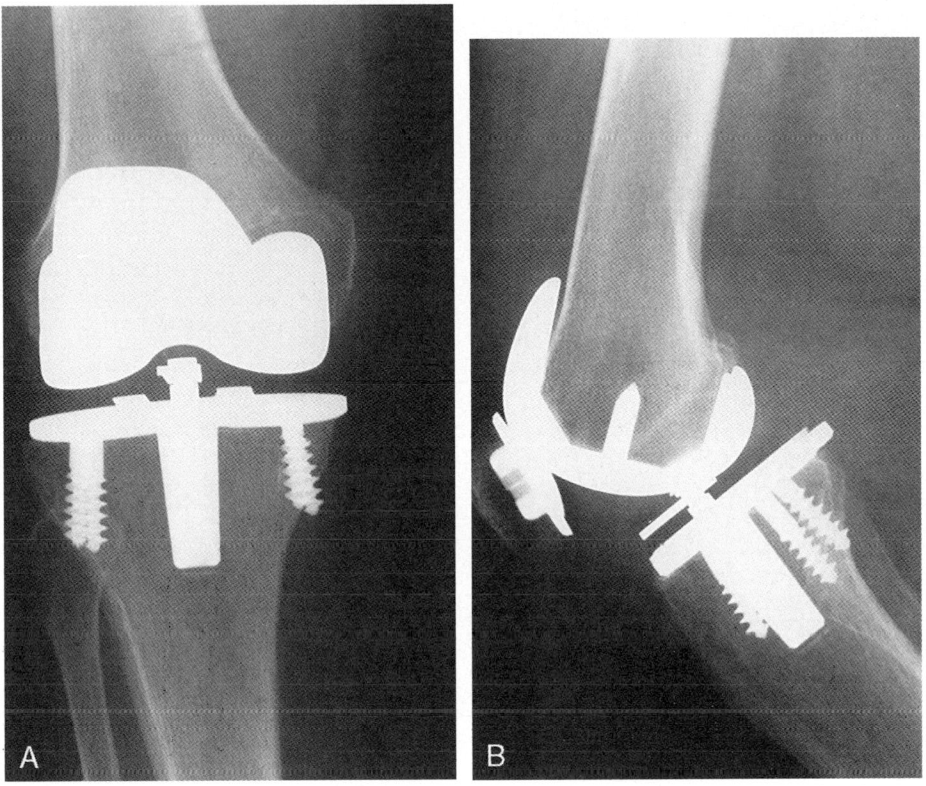

FIGURE 8-129 ■ Total knee replacement. An anteroposterior view of the knee *(A)* demonstrates the distal femoral and proximal tibial portions of a semiconstrained prosthesis. The two pieces do not appear to sit directly on each other, because a plastic or Teflon spacer in between is not seen on the x-ray. The lateral view *(B)* demonstrates that this is a tricompartment replacement with a prosthetic posterior patellar portion as well.

Tumors

A benign tumor, called a giant cell tumor, commonly occurs around the knee, particularly in the proximal tibia. It is a lytic lesion that is often quite large and characteristically occurs between the ages of 20 and 35 years. The tumor appears to arise from the old epiphyseal plate and to extend in both directions. It is not seen before epiphyseal closure, and when it is present, it typically crosses the fused epiphyseal plate (Fig. 8-130). Usually it is not confused with a malignant lesion, because it typically occurs during the late teens or in young adults. This is beyond the age for most osteogenic sarcomas and before the age for most metastatic lesions. In addition, its single focus and location peripherally in an extremity would be very unusual features of a metastatic lesion.

Osteogenic sarcoma is discussed later in the pediatric section of this chapter. A few unusual forms of osteogenic sarcoma do occur at older ages. Periosteal osteosarcomas, which constitute about 4% of all osteosarcomas, are broadly based, typically in the posterior aspect of the femoral shaft. They occur in persons aged about 40 years. Periosteal osteosarcomas are about half as common, have a saucer-shaped depression of the cortex, and occur at 10 to 20 years of age. Remember that osteosarcomas in older adults can be produced by malignant degeneration of Paget's disease and may occur at any age as a consequence of radiation therapy.

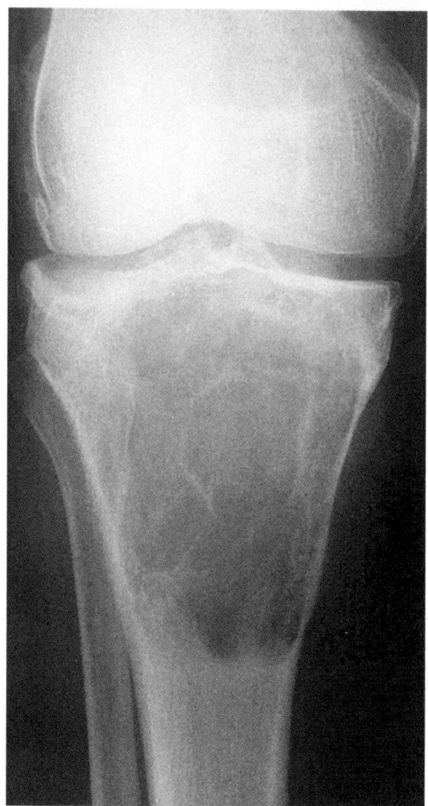

FIGURE 8-130 ■ **Giant cell tumor.** An anteroposterior view of the knee in this 25-year-old man demonstrates a destructive lesion that is centered at the fused epiphyseal plate and has extended into the metaphysis and the epiphysis. These lesions most commonly occur in the tibia or femur. The lesion is often expansile and can be locally aggressive. About one third of these patients will have a pathologic fracture.

TIBIA AND FIBULA

Normal Anatomy

Typical imaging views include AP and lateral projections. You should be sure that the image includes the entire length from the tibial plateau to the ankle joint. The anatomy is fairly obvious.

Trauma

A few points about tibial fractures should be discussed. Spiral fractures usually involve the distal tibia and often occur as the result of boot-top ski injuries. When a spiral tibial fracture is present, you should look very carefully to see if overriding of the fragments is present (Fig. 8-131). Many times, only an ankle x-ray has been ordered, and the tibial fracture is clearly identified. Notice that it is not possible to shorten the tibia without associated trauma of the fibula, because the two bones are essentially hooked together at both ends. If you see only a tibial fracture, you should order a complete view of the tibia and fibula, and often you will find an associated fracture of the proximal portion of the fibula. Typical orthopedic hardware used in the fixation of frac-

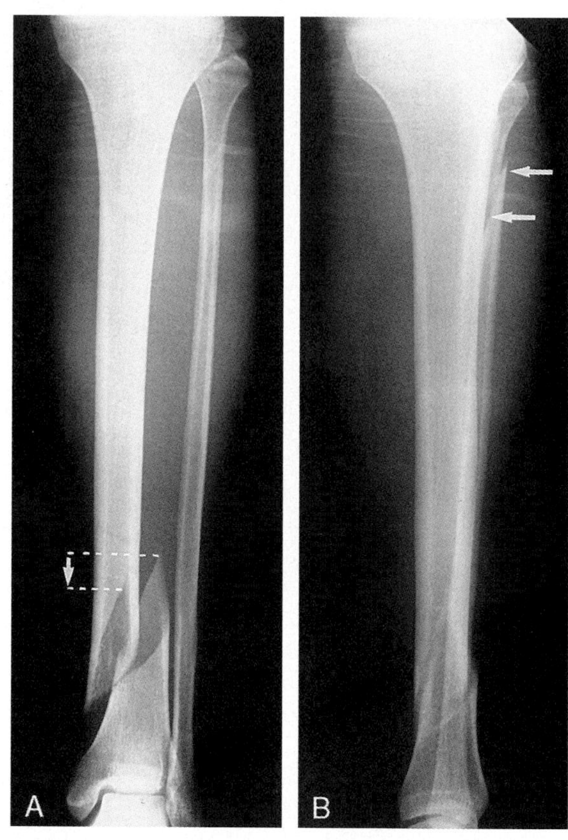

FIGURE 8-131 ■ **Spiral fracture of the distal tibia.** An anteroposterior view of the tibia *(A)* in a skier shows a spiral fracture, but note that there has been override of the fragments, causing shortening *(arrow).* This cannot possibly happen if the fibula is entirely intact. A lateral view *(B)* shows an accompanying fracture of the proximal fibula with override as well. This fibular fracture would have been missed if only ankle views had been ordered and the significance of the override had not been appreciated.

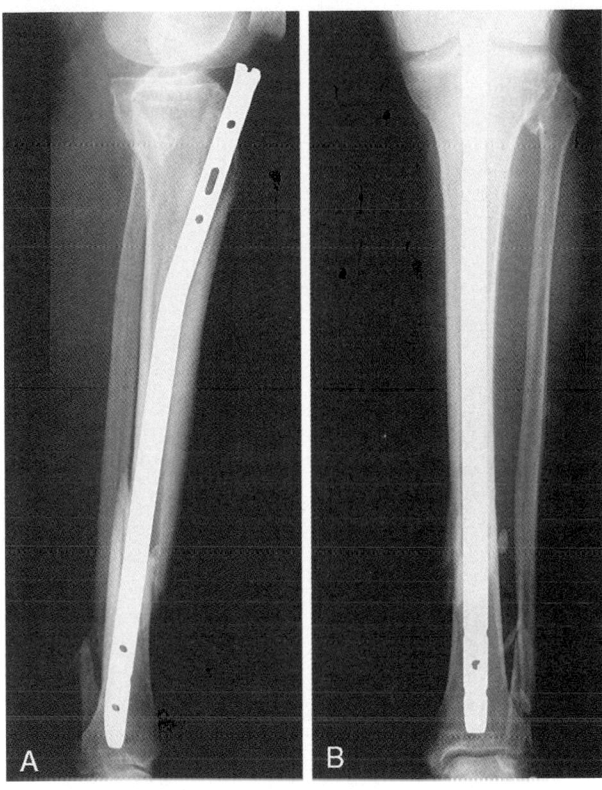

FIGURE 8-132 ■ Intramedullary fixation of a tibial fracture. *A,* A lateral view and *(B)* an anteroposterior view of the tibia demonstrate an intramedullary rod that has been placed down through the anterior and proximal portion of the tibia. The holes at the top and bottom of the rod provide a place for cross-linking screws. A rod (as opposed to a plate and screws) is necessary because this is a weight-bearing bone with a lot of stress on it.

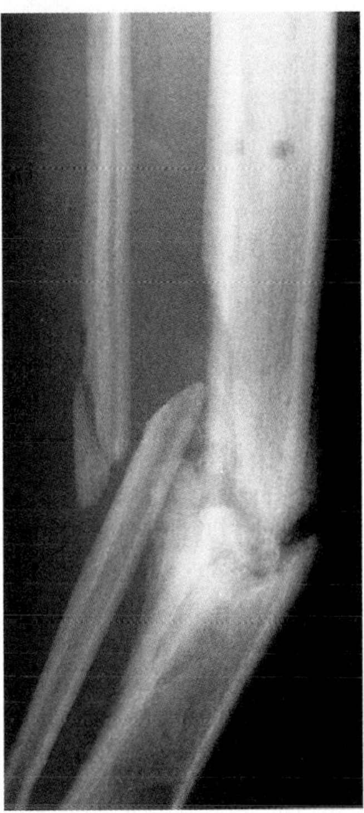

FIGURE 8-133 ■ Nonunion of a tibial fracture. This anteroposterior view of the distal tibia and fibula obtained 3 months after the fracture occurred shows no significant periosteal reaction bridging the fractures. A dark lucent line remains across the original fracture site as a result of fibrous tissue having grown in and preventing healing.

tures of the middle or distal tibia includes intramedullary rods (Fig. 8-132). These rods also can be used for fractures in the midportion of the femur. Occasionally fractures of long bones do not heal because fibrous tissue grows between the ends of the bone. This is called a nonunion. It can be identified by the presence of a lucent line on the image that is persistent and extends across the fracture site several months after the fracture occurred (Fig. 8-133).

Tumors

Some benign bone tumors occur in long bones, particularly in the lower extremity. The first of these is simply an outgrowth of bone and is called an osteochondroma. The cortex of the bone typically sticks out on a stalk and has a bulbous or mushroom-shaped cap. The cap is covered with cartilage. This growth almost invariably arises near a joint, with the stalk always pointing away from the joint (Fig. 8-134). These lesions are usually asymptomatic unless they stick out far enough to be traumatized easily. If there is enlargement of such a lesion or associated pain without previous trauma, malignant transformation should be suspected. In a form of hereditary multiple exostoses, the number of exostoses may vary from a few to hundreds, but they are usually bilaterally symmetrical.

An osteoid osteoma usually occurs along the cortex of a bone. It has a central area of lucency with a little sclerotic (white) nidus within it (Fig. 8-135). About 75% of cases occur in persons

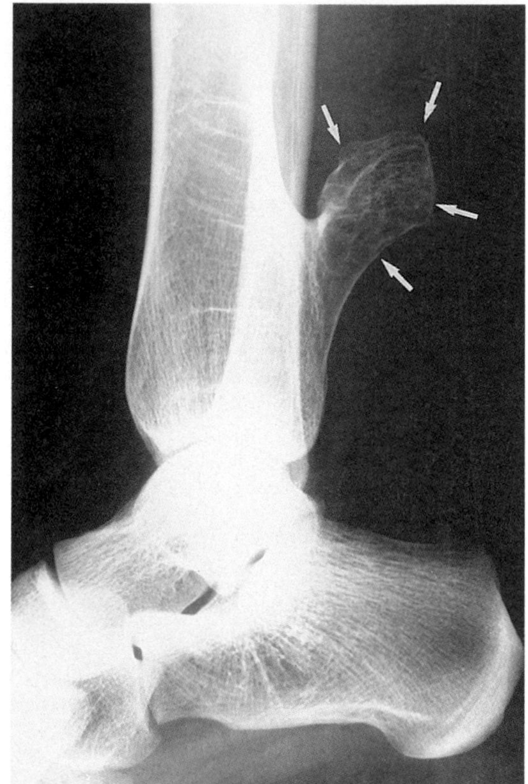

FIGURE 8-134 ■ Osteochondroma. On this lateral view of the ankle, a benign osteochondroma is seen projecting posteriorly on a stalk. The end *(arrows)* is often covered with a cartilaginous cap. These lesions always occur near a joint but point away from it.

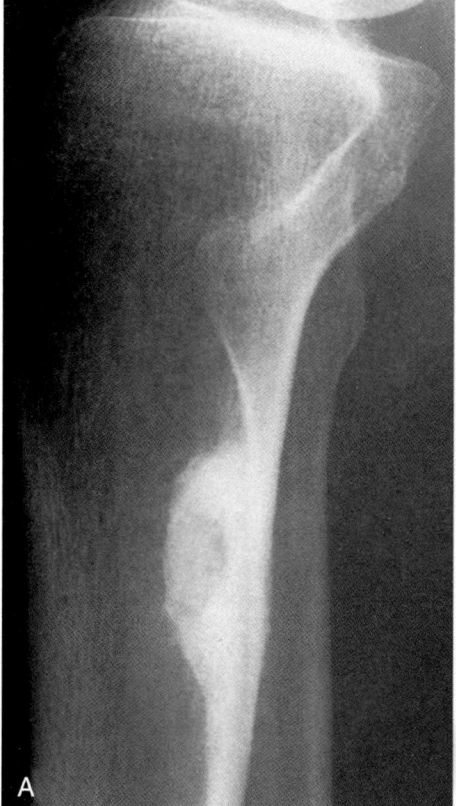

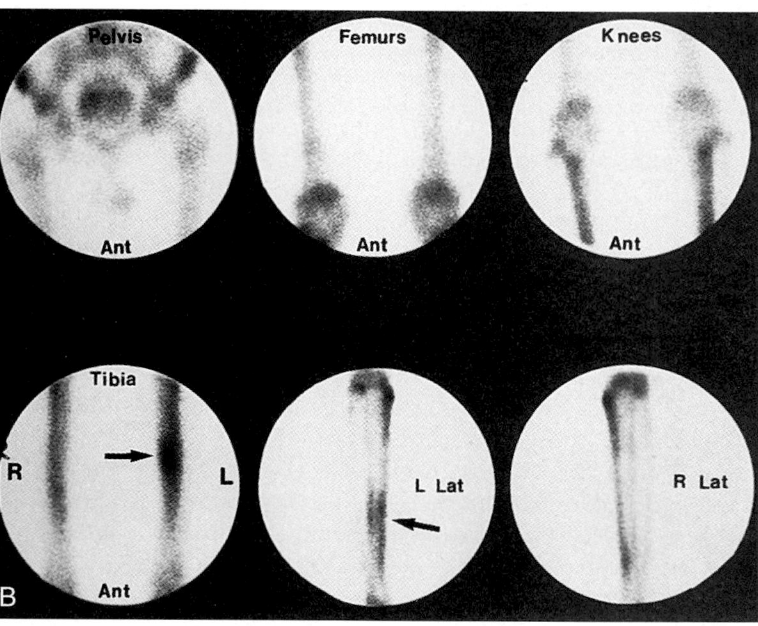

FIGURE 8-135 ■ Osteoid osteoma. A lateral view *(A)* of the proximal tibia shows a very dense lesion in the posterior cortex. A darker central area contains a white nidus. This lesion in a 20-year-old man caused pain in this area, relieved by aspirin. Fifty-five percent of these lesions occur in the femur and tibia. *B,* A nuclear medicine bone scan in a different patient with an osteoid osteoma in the left lower tibia shows increased activity *(arrows)* at the site of the lesion.

between the ages of 11 and 26 years. This lesion incites a large amount of reaction, causing dense surrounding bone and sometimes local periosteal reaction. It is typically painful, and the pain is relieved by aspirin. On a nuclear medicine bone scan, these lesions are intensely hot. If all you see is an area of dense sclerosis near the cortex of a bone and you are unable to visualize a nidus or central lucent area, sometimes a CT scan can demonstrate the nidus.

With the exception of metastatic disease, most bone tumors are quite obvious and quite rare. Because the differential diagnosis depends on the age, location, imaging characteristics,

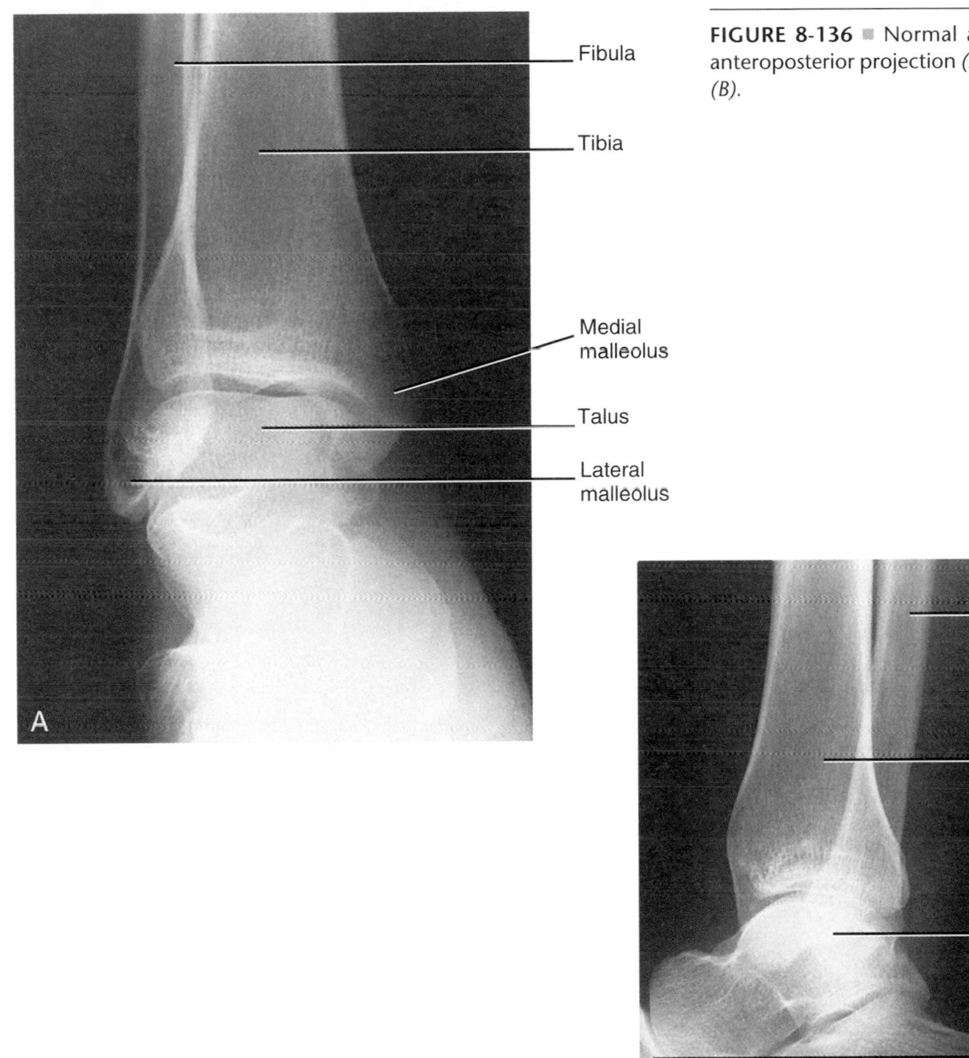

FIGURE 8-136 ■ Normal anatomy of the ankle in the anteroposterior projection *(A)* and in the lateral projection *(B)*.

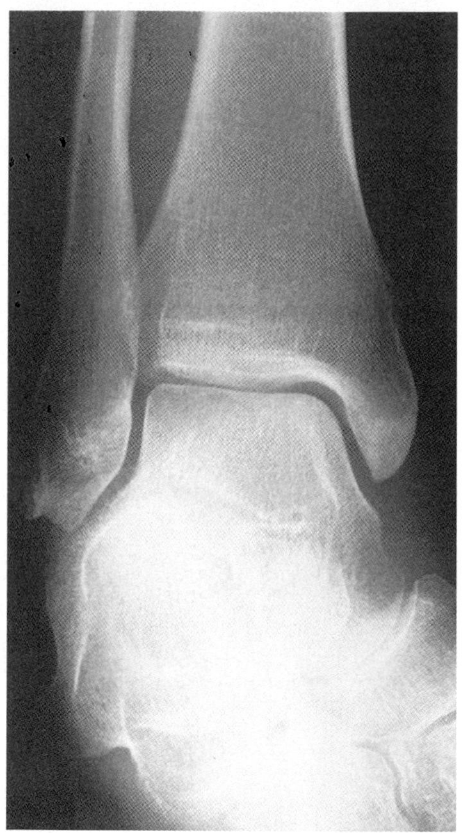

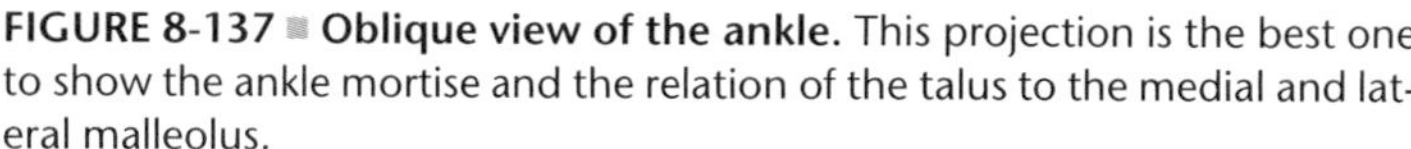

FIGURE 8-137 ■ Oblique view of the ankle. This projection is the best one to show the ankle mortise and the relation of the talus to the medial and lateral malleolus.

and clinical history, always seek consultation with a radiologist before assuming that the lesion you are looking at is benign.

ANKLE

Normal Anatomy

Normal imaging projections of the ankle are AP, lateral, and oblique. Although oblique views of most bones and joints are not normally obtained, this is important in the traumatized ankle because a number of oblique fractures that occur in the ankle are not easily seen on the AP or lateral view. The oblique view also allows a better look at the ankle mortise (Figs. 8-136 and 8-137).

An interesting phenomenon occurs often on ankle x-rays but also can occur on any image on which the dense cortex of bones overlaps. Where the cortices of two bones cross, occasionally a dark or lucent line will appear along the anterior edge of one cortex, and this dark line looks as though it is actually extending through the cortex of the other bone. This is an artifact called the "Mach effect." The point is that if you see a lucent line through the cortex of a bone, you should make sure that another overlapping bone at this exact point is not causing a pseudofracture artifact (Fig. 8-138*A*). Sometimes a lucent line can be seen extending through the cortex of a bone as a result of a blood vessel passing through a nutrient canal (Fig. 8-138*B*), and this should not be mistaken for a fracture.

The ankle of a child demonstrates an epiphysis in the distal tibia and fibula. In children between the ages of 7 and 12 years, you also will see a calcaneal apophysis on the lateral view. This is seen as a crescentic density over the posterior aspect of the heel, and it should not be mistaken for a fracture (Fig. 8-139).

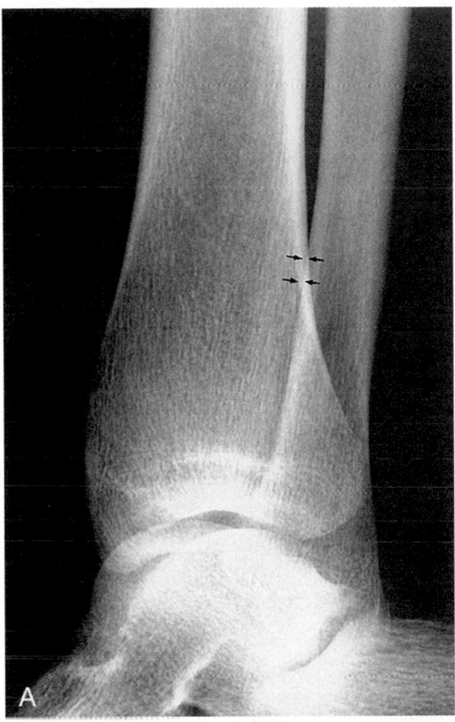

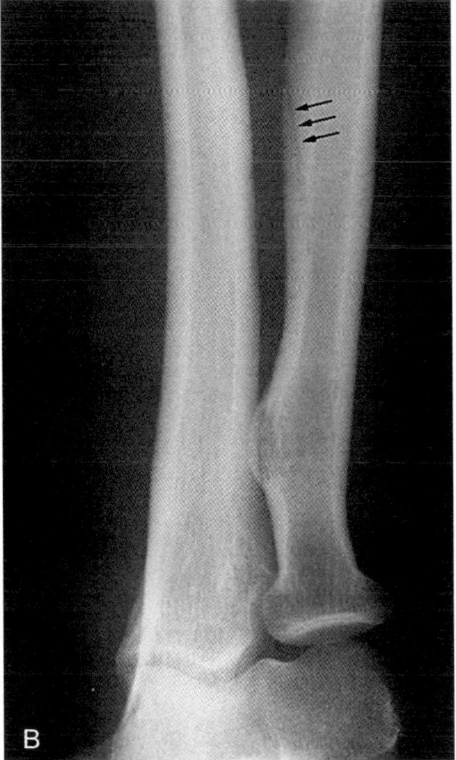

FIGURE 8-138 ■ **Pseudofractures.** *A,* A Mach effect is an optical illusion that can be seen anywhere two bones cross each other. On this lateral view of the ankle where the cortex of the fibula and tibia project crossing each other, the dark line *(arrows)* is an artifact and can be mistaken for a fracture of the posterior tibial cortex. *B,* A nutrient canal is seen in the radius as a dark oblique line *(arrows)* extending through one side of the bony cortex.

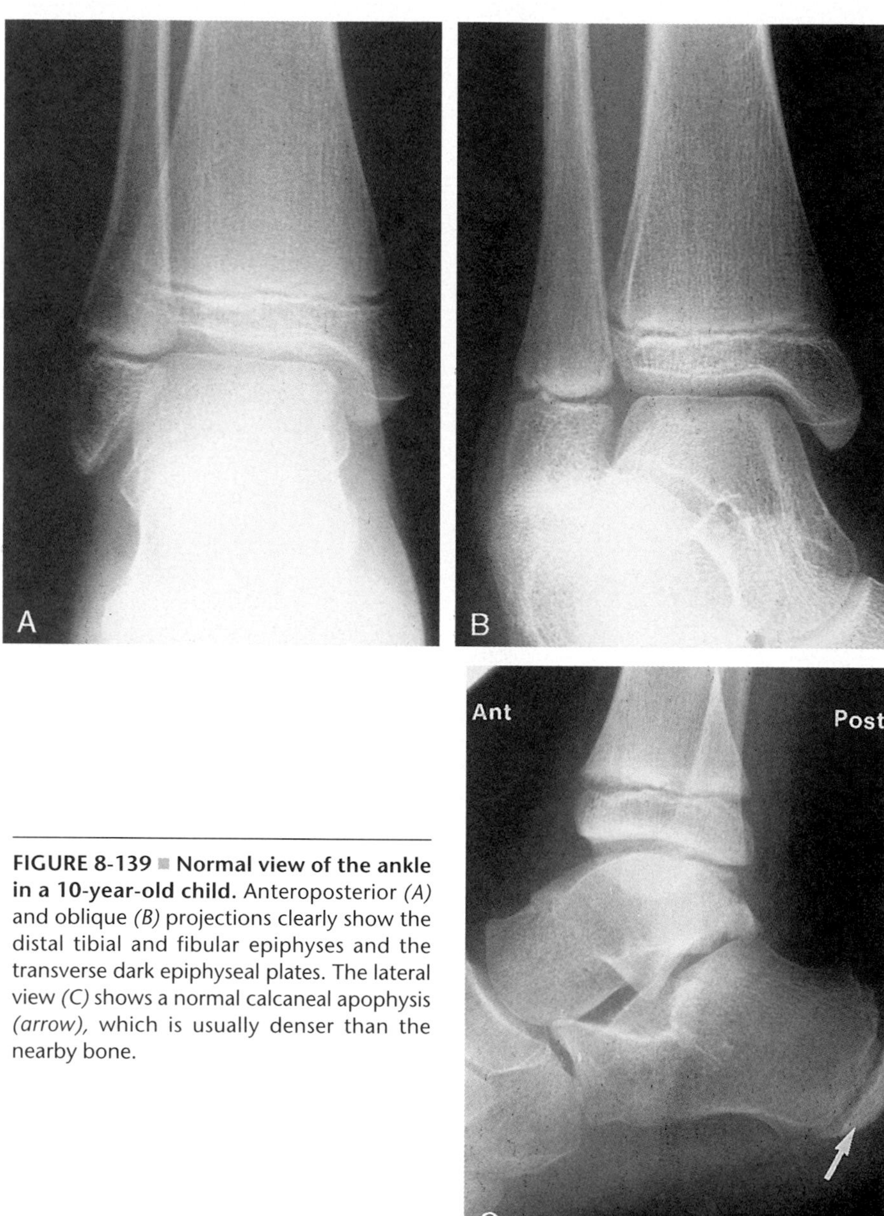

FIGURE 8-139 ■ Normal view of the ankle in a 10-year-old child. Anteroposterior *(A)* and oblique *(B)* projections clearly show the distal tibial and fibular epiphyses and the transverse dark epiphyseal plates. The lateral view *(C)* shows a normal calcaneal apophysis *(arrow),* which is usually denser than the nearby bone.

Trauma

The vast majority of ankle x-rays are obtained to evaluate the effects of trauma. On the lateral view of the ankle, look for an anterior thin, dark fat line right in front of the joint space. If it is displaced or bowed forward, an effusion, hemorrhage, or infection is present in the ankle joint (Fig. 8-140).

The most common fractures of the ankle involve either the medial or the lateral malleolus. Less commonly, fractures are found of the

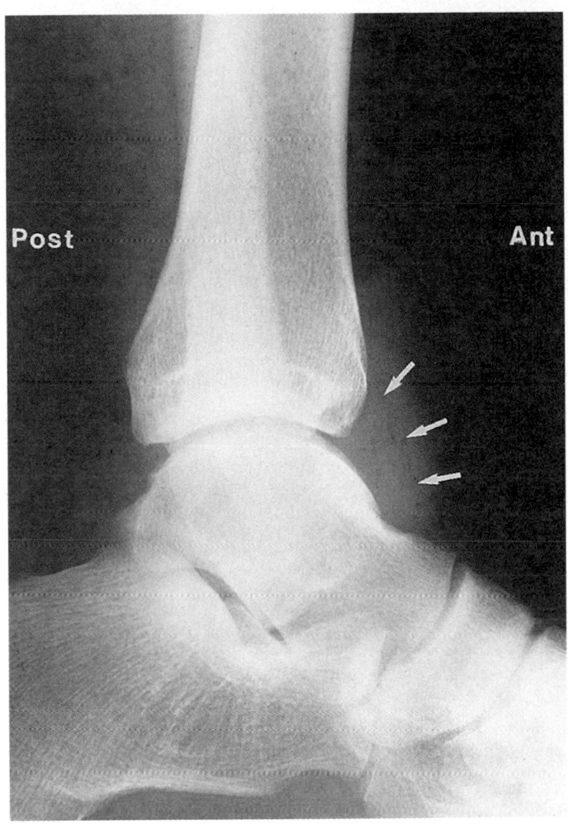

FIGURE 8-140 ■ Ankle effusion. An ankle effusion is best seen on the lateral view. The dark fat stripe *(arrows)* is displaced and bowed anteriorly by fluid within the joint.

medial and lateral malleolus (bimalleolar fracture; Fig. 8-141*A*). With very severe trauma, fractures are noted not only of both medial and lateral malleoli but also of the posterior aspect of the tibia (trimalleolar fracture). Whenever the posterior malleolus is fractured, almost always an associated medial or lateral malleolar fracture is seen. The extreme force and disruption necessary to cause a trimalleolar fracture disrupts ligaments as well, often causing subluxation of the distal tibia relative to the talus (Fig. 8-141*B*).

The Weber classification is usually used to describe fractures of the fibula. It allows evaluation of the severity of injury to the tibiofibular ligament. This ligament is located just slightly above the ankle joint. A fracture of the fibula below the ligament is a Weber A fracture. When the fracture is at the ligament level, it is a Weber B, and above the ligament, it is a Weber C fracture. The most common fracture is a Weber B, caused by supination and external rotation.

Malleolar fractures can be treated in a number of ways, including screws and pins (particularly in the medial malleolus) and sometimes plates and screws. Occasionally, in the case of a compound fracture, antibiotic beads will be placed in the wound. These can be visualized on the plain x-ray (Fig. 8-142). As with other joints, when orthopedic hardware is present and follow-up images are performed, you should look for destructive areas along the shafts of the screws as well as sclerosis that is not associated with the fracture itself. These are findings that suggest infection and osteomyelitis (Fig. 8-143).

Just because the bony structures of the ankle look normal on the plain x-ray does not mean that no soft tissue pathology is present. Significant ligamentous disruption may not be appreciated. If clinical suspicion persists about ligamentous disruption and laxity of the ankle, stress views can be performed. These are images taken while the ankle is being twisted, and they can show widening of the ankle joint (Fig. 8-144). MRI is rarely indicated for most ankle trauma.

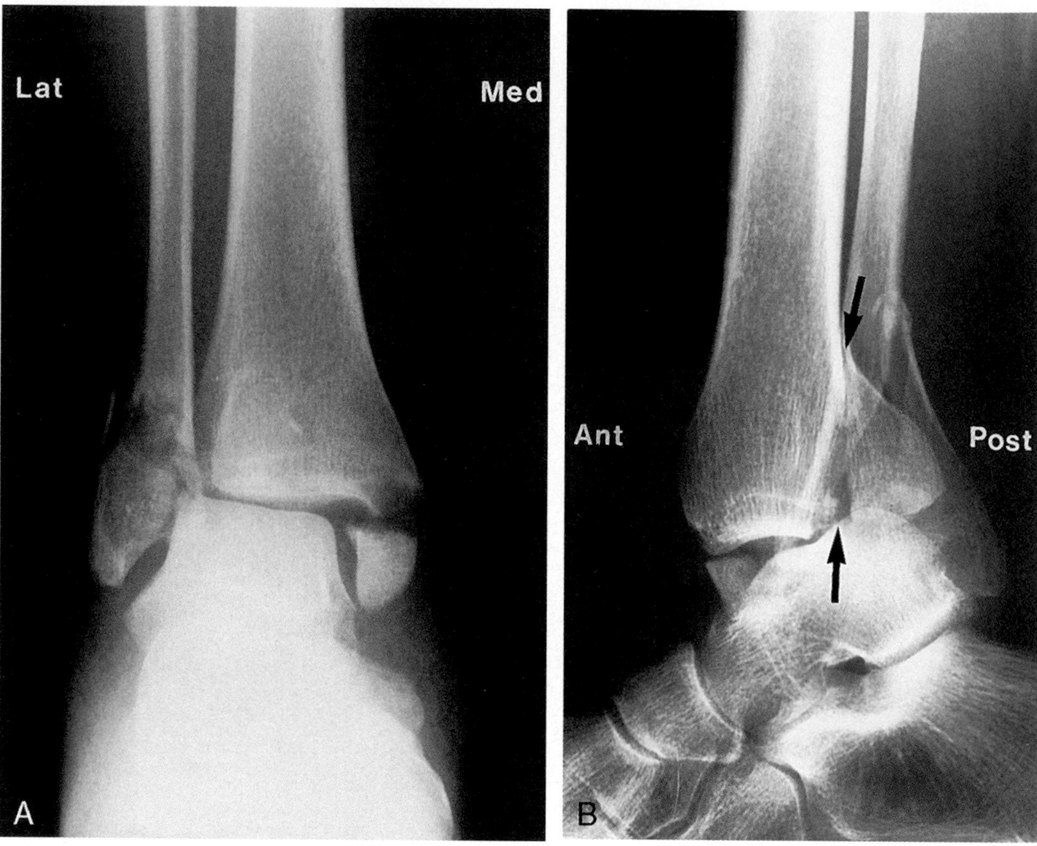

FIGURE 8-141 ■ Ankle fractures. *A,* In this bimalleolar fracture, the horizontal fracture medially and an oblique fracture laterally mean that this was an eversion injury. An inversion injury usually results in a horizontal fibular fracture and oblique fracture of the medial malleolus. *B,* Trimalleolar fracture in a different patient. The lateral view is necessary to show a fracture of the posterior malleolus *(arrows).* Also note that the anterior subluxation of the distal tibial on the talus.

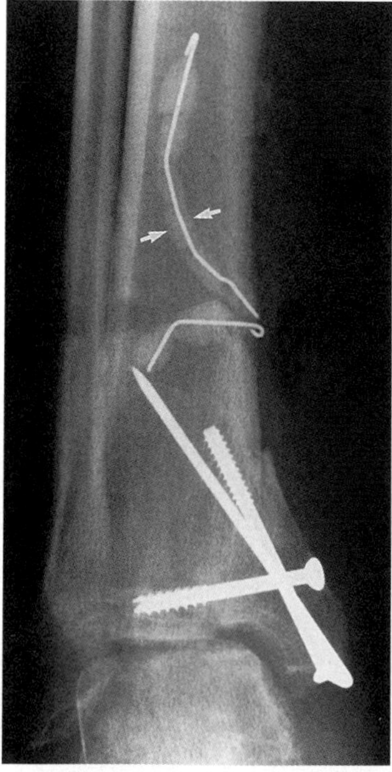

FIGURE 8-142 ■ Antibiotic beads. This anteroposterior view of the ankle demonstrates fixation screws and pin through the medial malleolus. The wire with beads *(arrows)* represents local antibiotic therapy, which may be used for open fractures.

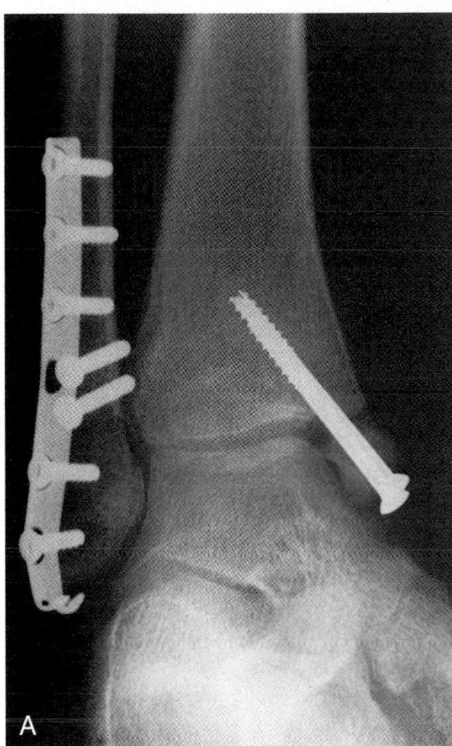

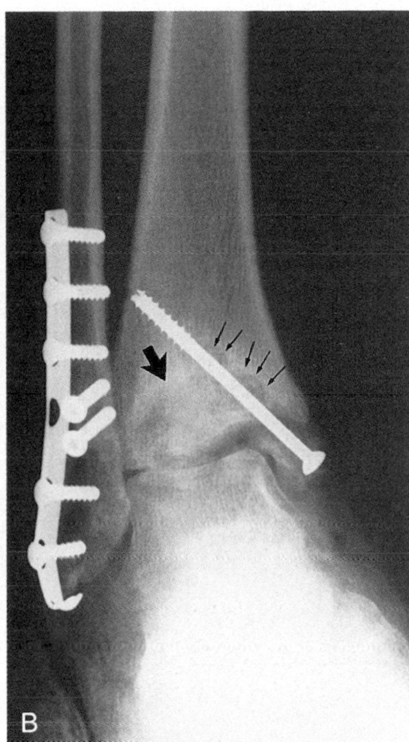

FIGURE 8-143 ■ Developing osteomyelitis. *A,* An oblique view of the ankle immediately after repair of a bimalleolar fracture shows two screws through the medial malleolus and a plate and screws in the lateral malleolus. *B,* A repeated examination 6 weeks later, when a low-grade fever and pain had developed, demonstrates destruction of bone around the edge of the screw *(small arrows)* and a larger destructive lesion *(large arrow)* of the distal tibial extending to the joint surface.

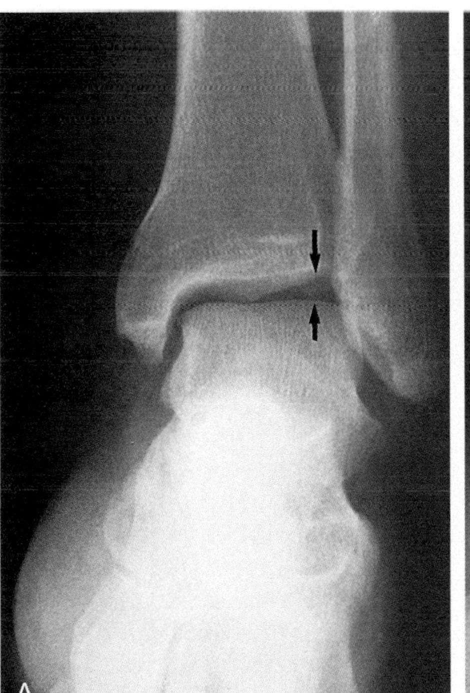

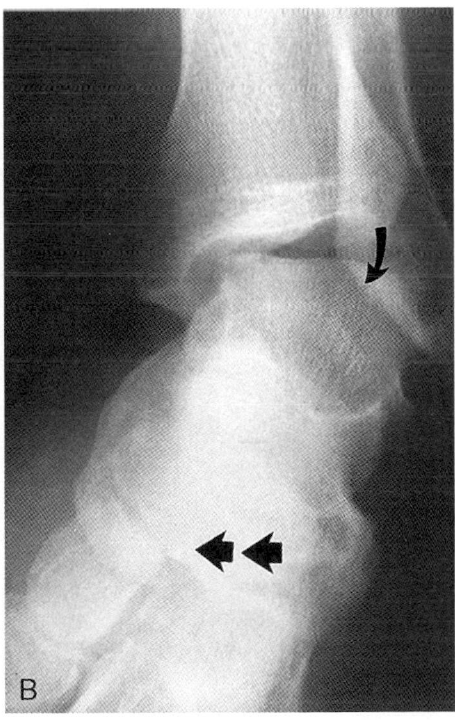

FIGURE 8-144 ■ Ankle instability. *A,* An anteroposterior view of the ankle demonstrates slight widening of the lateral aspect of the ankle mortise *(arrows)*. *B,* A stress view was obtained by inverting the foot (in the direction of the *large arrows*). This makes the ligamentous injury much more obvious by opening the ankle mortise even farther *(curved arrow)*.

Benign Nontraumatic Abnormalities

Three fairly common dense bone abnormalities are seen typically in the distal tibia. These lesions do occur in other bones, but the ankle is imaged so frequently that questions about them come up more often relative to the ankle. The first of these are horizontal dense lines in the metaphysis of the tibia (Fig. 8-145). These are called "growth arrest" lines, and they represent a time when some interference occurred with the normal longitudinal growth process of the bone, perhaps periods of sickness during the individual's life. Occasionally, dense lines such as these reflect heavy metal ingestion (lead poisoning or ingestion of bismuth or phosphorus). Growth arrest lines are of no clinical significance whatever at the time they are seen, because they are a representation of a historic event.

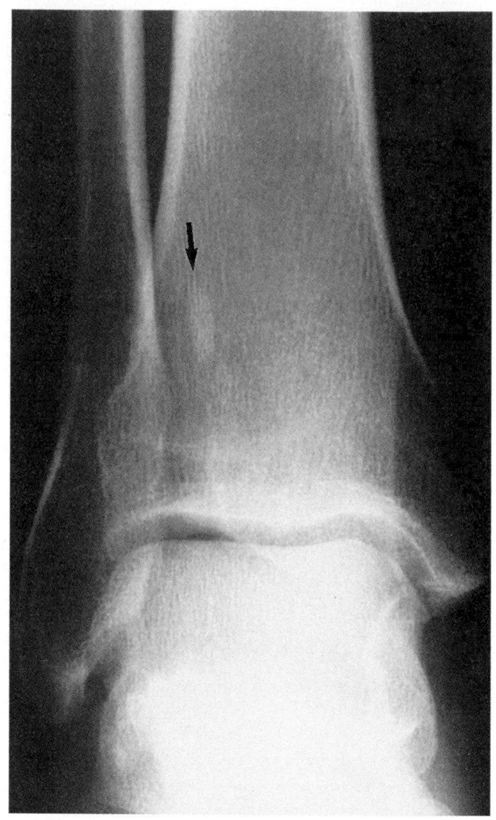

FIGURE 8-146 ■ Bone island. This small oval dense area *(arrow)* of bone is essentially a normal variant. It is often incidentally seen around the ankle because the ankles are x-rayed so frequently for trauma. These benign lesions almost always are <1 cm in the longest axis, and the long axis of the elliptical lesion is parallel with the long axis of the bone.

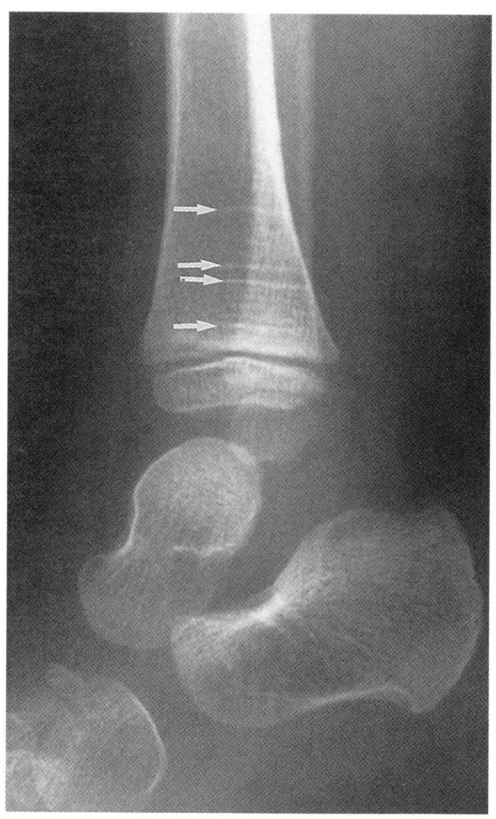

FIGURE 8-145 ■ Growth-arrest lines. These transverse dense lines in the metaphysis of a long bone are due to bouts of illness this child had in the past. Similar horizontal lines can be due to episodic heavy metal ingestion, such as lead poisoning.

Small oval sclerotic or dense lesions can occur in most bones. These are called bone islands, and their origin is uncertain. They are completely benign lesions and should be regarded as a normal variant. They rarely measure more than 5 or 6 mm in width and 1 cm in length. The long axis of the oval is always in the long axis of the bone or aligned with the trabecular pattern (Fig. 8-146). Benign fibrous cortical defects and nonossifying fibromas have been discussed in relation to the femur (see Fig. 8-107). If the lesions are large, they may fracture, but many heal spontaneously during young adult life, leaving behind an area of dense bone (Fig. 8-147).

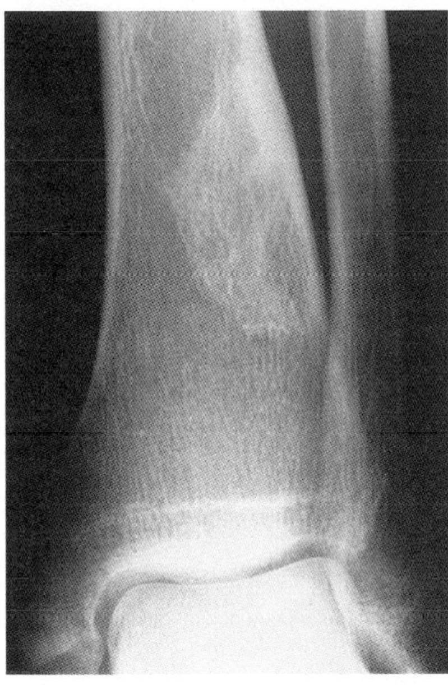

FIGURE 8-147 ■ **Healed nonossifying fibroma.** These lesions are usually discovered incidentally in young adults. Ninety percent are found near the metaphysis of the tibia or fibula. The dense nature and lack of periosteal reaction indicate that this is a benign lesion, and no further workup is called for.

FOOT

As with the ankle, typical imaging projections of the foot after trauma include AP, lateral, and oblique. For purposes of an arthritis workup, AP and lateral views are sufficient (Fig. 8-148). A special view of the foot called the calcaneal view is taken when a fracture of the calcaneus is suspected. The foot is flexed, and the x-ray beam is angled down through the posterior aspect of the heel. This provides a good view of at least the posterior half of the calcaneus (Fig. 8-149).

You should be aware of a few congenital and developmental abnormalities of the foot, such as fusion or a bony bridge across the proximal bones, for example, between the talus and the calcaneus or between the calcaneus and the navicular. Many times these can be seen on plain films, although occasionally CT scanning is needed to identify the abnormality.

A wide variety of small accessory bones are seen about the ankle and tarsal bones (Fig. 8-150). These are variable but usually can easily

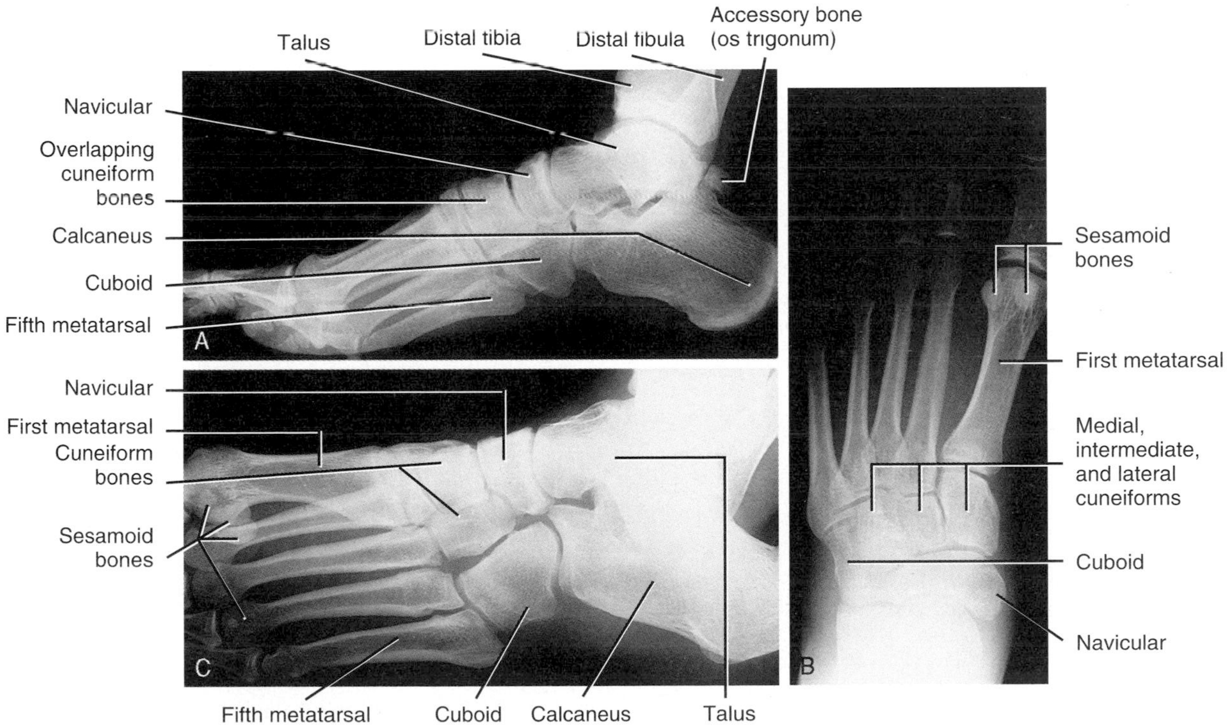

FIGURE 8-148 ■ Normal anatomy of the foot in the lateral projection *(A)*, anteroposterior projection *(B)*, and oblique projection *(C)*.

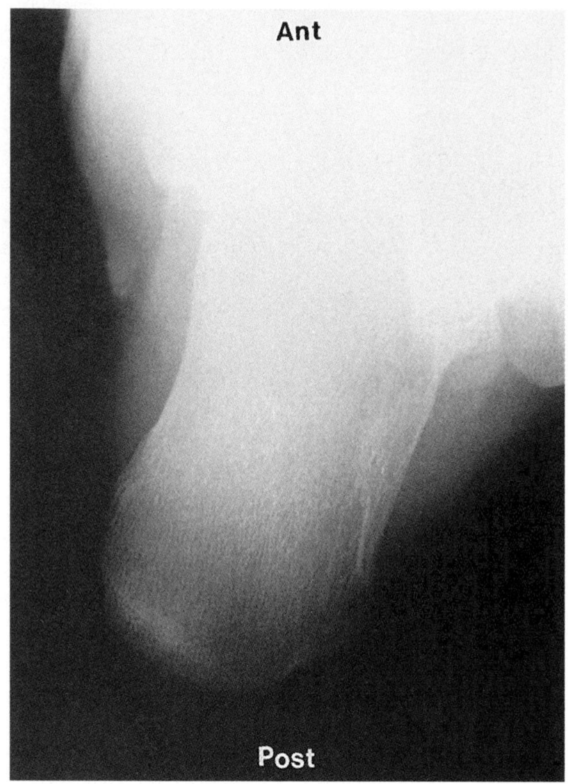

FIGURE 8-149 ■ **Calcaneal view.** This view is taken to look for subtle fractures of the posterior aspect of the calcaneus by placing the foot on a film and shooting down along the backside of the ankle.

be distinguished from fractures, because accessory bones are well corticated and typically round or oval. Another common developmental abnormality is a cystic-looking area that occurs in the anterior and midportion of the calcaneus. Although this sometimes is called a calcaneal cyst, MRI has shown that a large number of them are intraosseous lipomas. Why they tend to occur in this location is unknown (Fig. 8-151). Generally they are not clinically significant, but if they are large, the weakened bone may result in a pathologic fracture.

Trauma

A number of foot x-rays are ordered to look for foreign bodies that the patient stepped on. If the suspected object is metallic, it can normally be visualized (Fig. 8-152). As was discussed in the section on the hand, most glass also can be seen. If the object is not visible externally, a radiologist may operate a fluoroscope while another physician is locating the object. Digging around in the sole of the foot often causes residual painful scars, and the more easily an object can be located, the less scarring should occur. Remember that wooden objects or graphite from pencils will not be visualized by x-ray examination.

Fractures of the foot can involve any bone. Fractures of the talus are rare but almost always involve the neck of the talus (Fig. 8-153). This is the so-called "aviator's fracture," because it occurred when early pilots crashed and

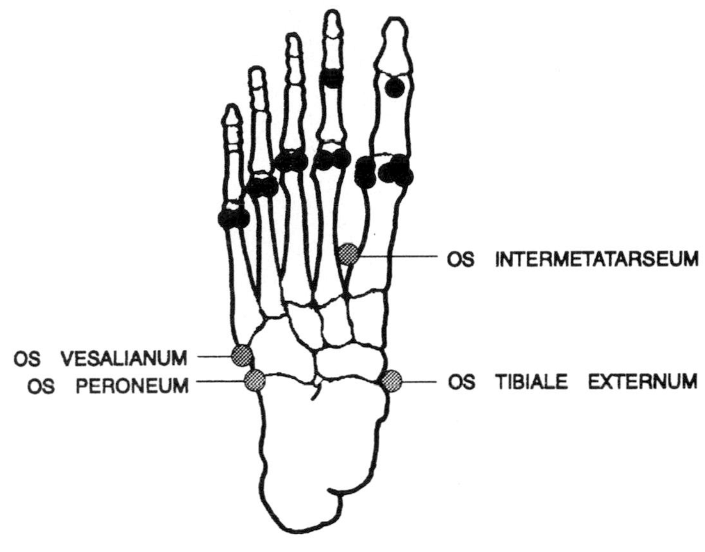

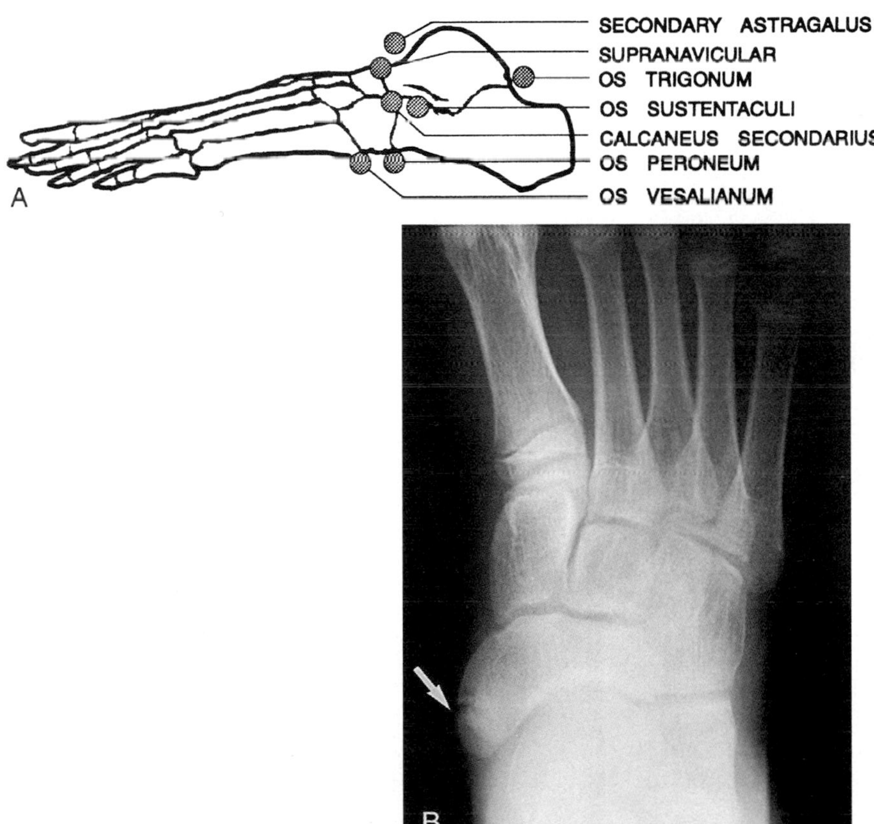

FIGURE 8-150 ■ Accessory bones of the foot. *A,* Schematic representation of normal accessory and sesamoid bones. *B,* An image of the foot of a child shows an accessory os naviculare *(arrow).*

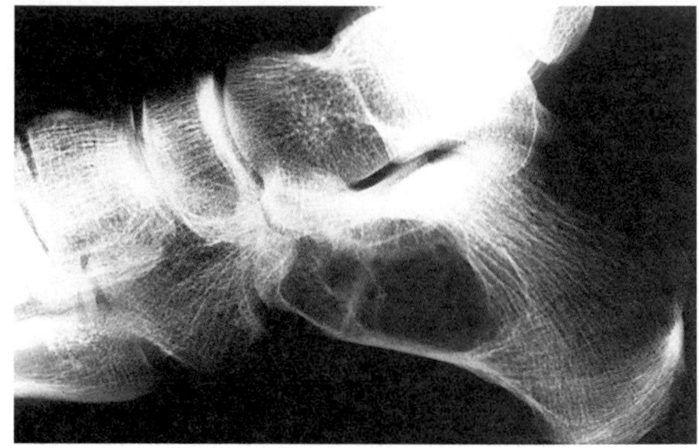

FIGURE 8-151 ■ Calcaneal cyst. This lateral view of the foot shows a large well-defined lucent area in the anterior portion of the calcaneus. Although this has been referred to as a calcaneal cyst, often it has been shown to contain fat and to be an intraosseous lipoma. These lesions almost never occur at any other location.

slammed their feet into the front of the cockpit. Obviously, today the fracture is much more often due to motor vehicle accidents. Calcaneal fractures often can be difficult to appreciate on the lateral view and are almost impossible to see on an AP view. For this reason, the calcaneal view that we discussed earlier should also be ordered (Fig. 8-154). Sometimes patients with persistent foot pain have normal plain x-rays. A nuclear medicine bone scan can sometimes localize a bone in which an occult fracture is present (Fig. 8-155).

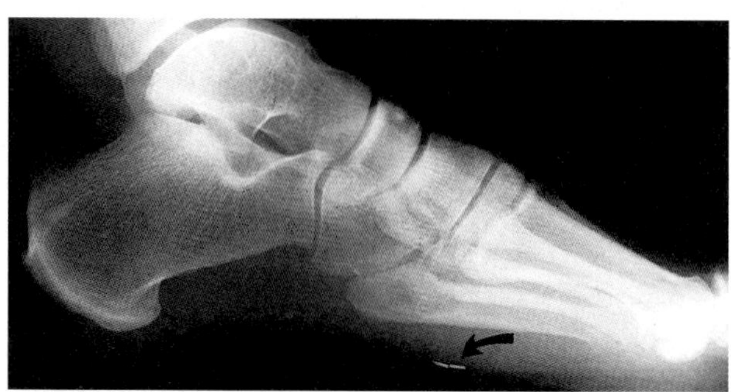

FIGURE 8-152 ■ Sewing needle in the foot. The lateral view of the foot shows two metallic needle fragments *(arrow)* in the sole of the foot.

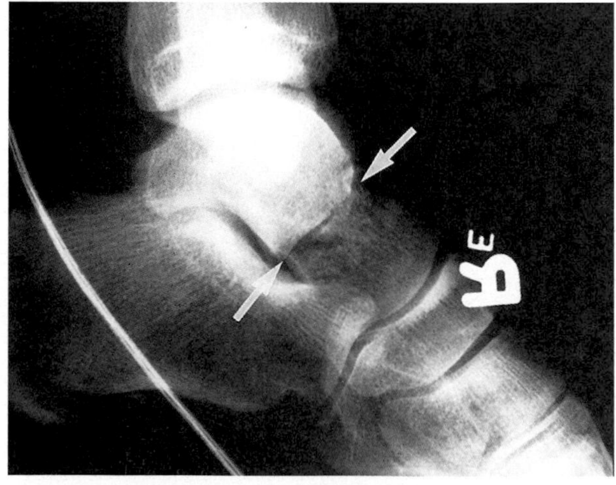

FIGURE 8-153 ■ Talar neck fracture. A lucent line can be seen extending through the talus *(arrows)*. This is the second most common fracture of the proximal foot, and historically it is referred to as an aviator's fracture.

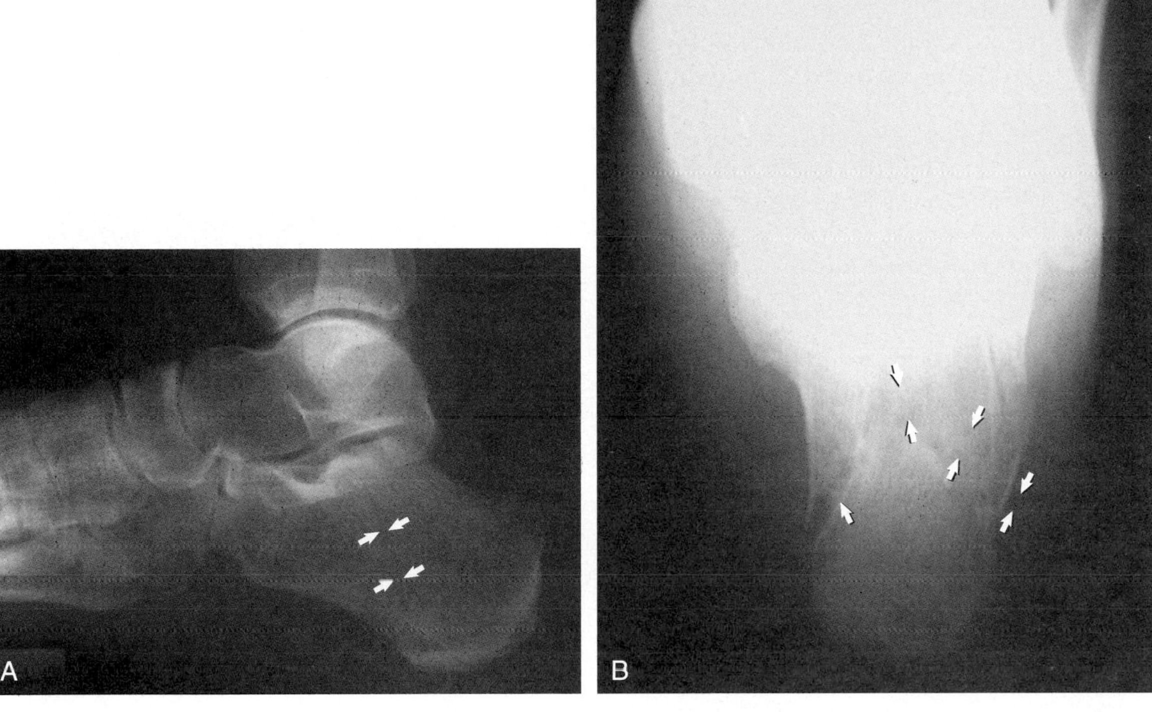

FIGURE 8-154 ■ Calcaneal fracture. The lateral view of the calcaneus *(A)* shows a subtle lucent (*dark*) line through the calcaneus. This extends into the subtalar joint about 75% of the time. This fracture also has been called a lover's fracture (probably from tales of disappointed lovers jumping off buildings or bridges). A calcaneal view *(B)* in the same patient makes the fracture much more obvious *(arrows),* particularly at the lateral margins.

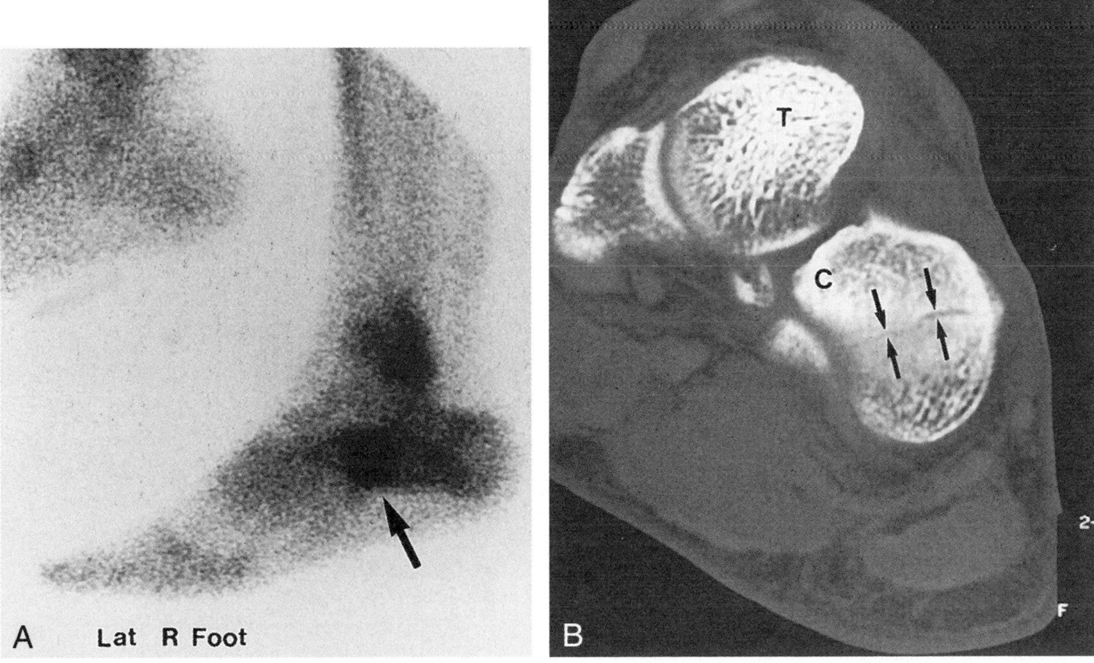

FIGURE 8-155 ■ Occult calcaneal fracture. *A,* In this patient who had a normal x-ray of the foot and continued to have pain, a nuclear medicine bone scan was performed. A lateral image of the foot shows an area of markedly increased activity *(arrow)* along the anterior portion of the calcaneus. *B,* A computed tomography scan was then performed with thin sections over the area of interest, and the calcaneal fracture was identified *(arrows).*

A very common fracture of the foot involves the base of the fifth metatarsal. Frequently an apophysis on the lateral aspect of the fifth metatarsal base is found, and this is often confused with a fracture. The way to tell the two apart is by noting that the long axis of the apophysis is parallel to the long axis of the metatarsal. Fractures, conversely, typically are transverse or perpendicular to the long axis of the bone (Fig. 8-156).

Most fractures of the metatarsals are fairly easy to recognize. Two unique fractures can occur in this region. The first is the so-called Lisfranc fracture, actually a fracture and lateral dislocation of the second, third, fourth, and fifth metatarsals relative to the tarsal bones. This usually happens as a result of falling out of a saddle while horseback riding and getting a foot caught in the stirrup (Fig. 8-157).

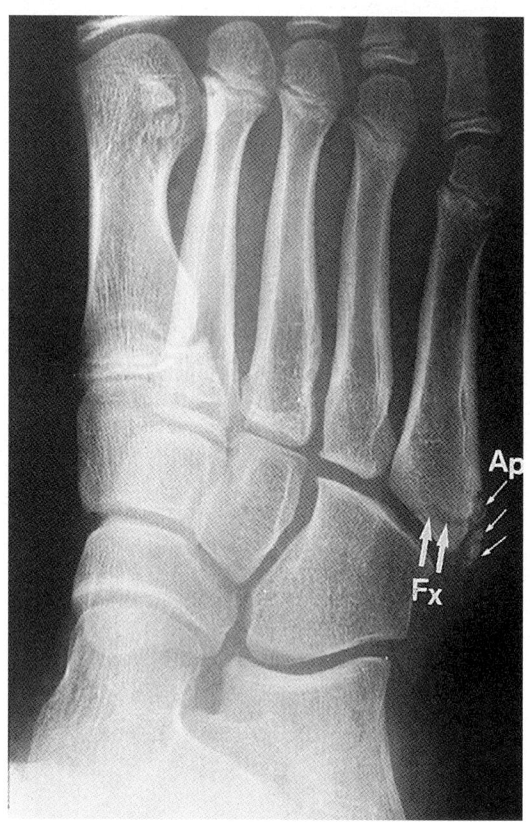

FIGURE 8-156 ■ Fracture of the fifth metatarsal base. This fracture usually occurs from inversion of the foot and is transverse across the base of the metatarsal. This should not be confused with a normal fifth metatarsal apophysis, also present in this patient. The fracture is always transverse and is referred to as a Jones fracture. The apophysis is always parallel with the long axis of the metatarsal.

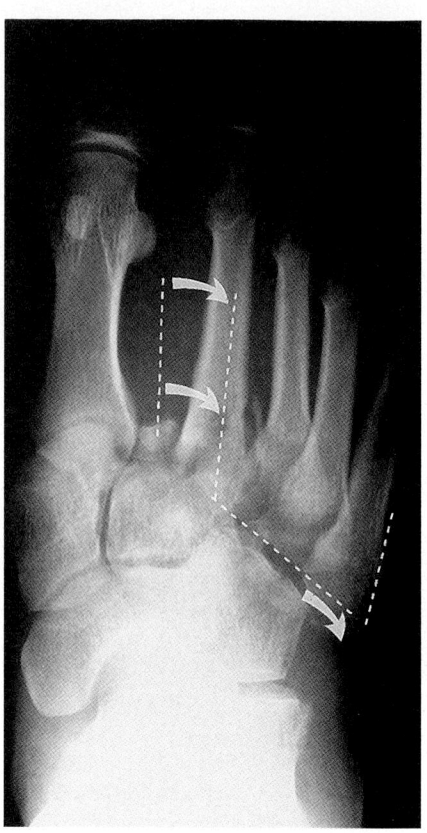

FIGURE 8-157 ■ Lisfranc fracture/dislocation. In this fracture/dislocation, the second through fifth metatarsals are fractured and/or subluxed laterally *(arrows).*

Another classic fracture of the metatarsals is the so-called "march" fracture. This is a stress fracture that typically occurs in army recruits who have to march long distances and are not used to it, but it also is seen in athletes and dancers. The distal third of the second, third, or fourth metatarsal is the usual location. If you look very carefully in this region, sometimes you can see slightly increased sclerosis or periosteal reaction (Fig. 8-158). If the x-ray is normal, a stress fracture may still be present, and in this circumstance, it is usually easily visualized as an area of intensely increased activity on a nuclear medicine bone scan.

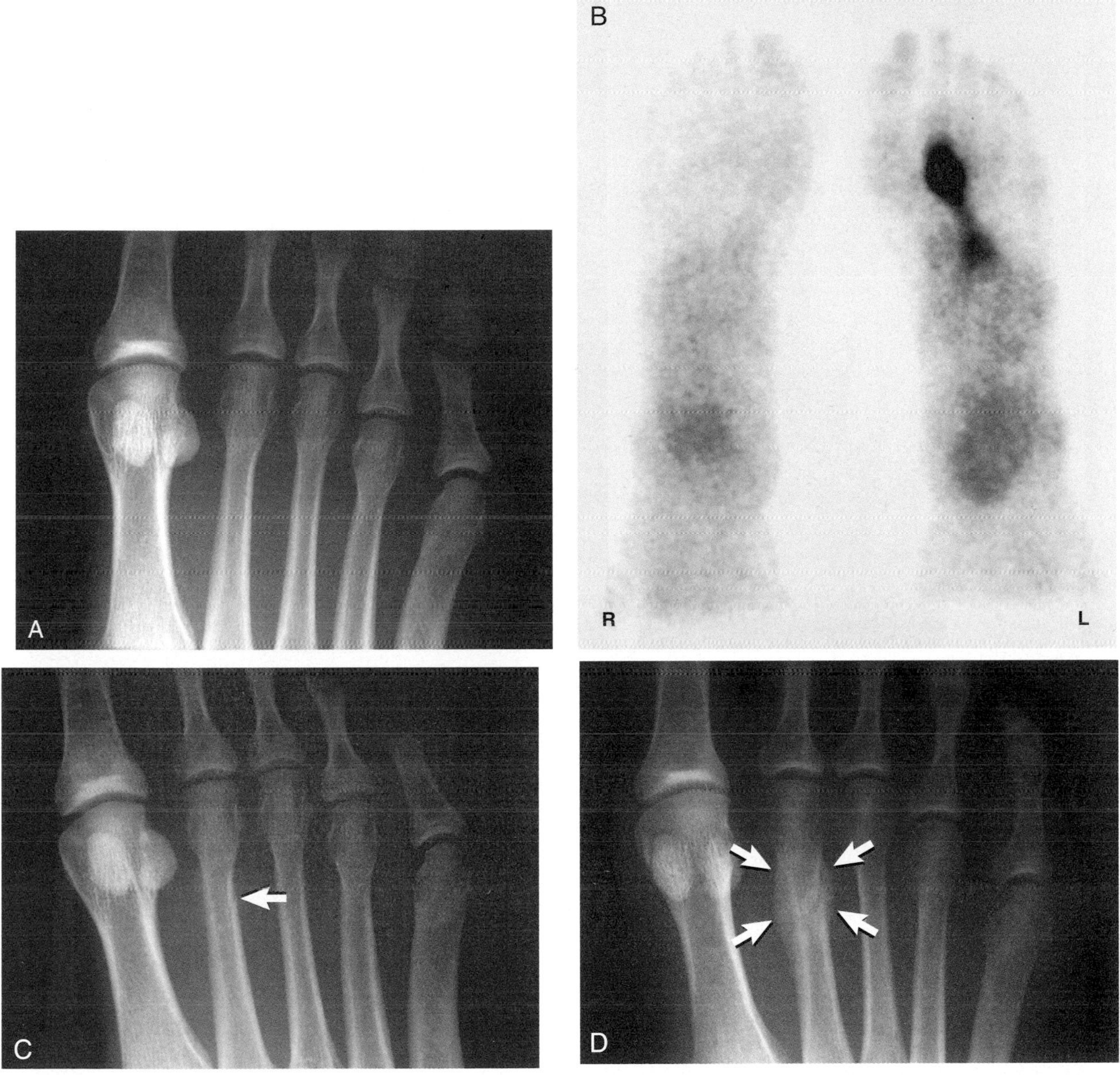

FIGURE 8-158 ■ Stress fracture. *(A)* A college student who had walked 400 km in Spain during the summer and had foot pain had a negative initial x-ray. A nuclear medicine bone scan *(B)* at the same time was intensely positive. Another x-ray 10 days later *(C)* showed a subtle cortical fracture *(arrow)*. A follow-up examination 3 weeks later *(D)* clearly shows developing callus *(arrows)*. This also is referred to as a "march" fracture. They can be very difficult to appreciate even when you know where to look.

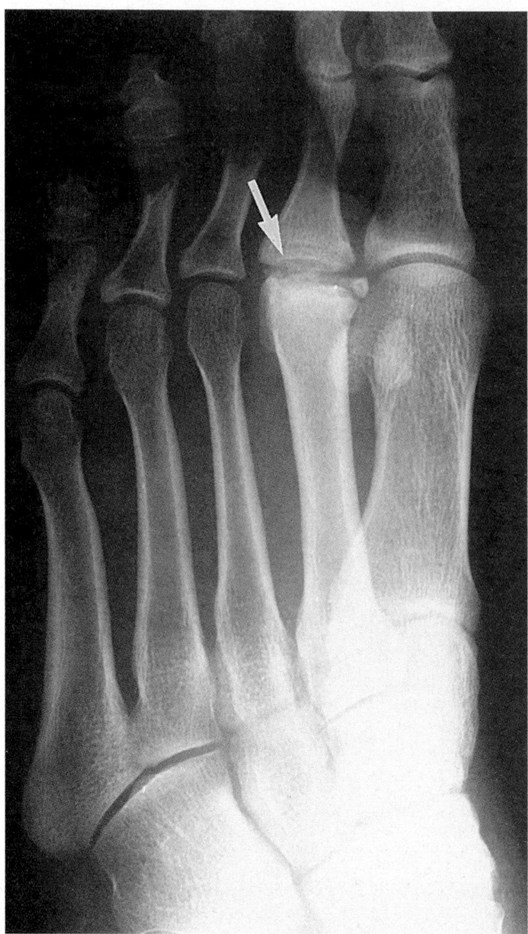

FIGURE 8-159 ■ Aseptic necrosis of the second metatarsal head. This usually occurs in teenagers and is referred to as a Freiberg osteonecrosis. Subsequent degenerative arthritis in this region is common.

A form of aseptic necrosis most commonly involves the head of the second metatarsal. This is manifested as flattening of the articular surface with associated sclerosis (Fig. 8-159) and is called a Kohler-Freiberg infarction. The lesion is seen less frequently in the head of the third or first metatarsal. This injury is believed to be a type of stress fracture, and it is often found during late adolescence. Degenerative joint disease is a late complication of this condition.

Degenerative and Arthritic Conditions

Views of the feet obtained for arthritis evaluation are often unrevealing or nonspecific, and if any imaging is ordered for arthritis evaluation, the highest yield usually is obtained with an AP view of the hands. As pointed out earlier, the radiographic findings, although somewhat characteristic, are not as specific as laboratory findings. The major metabolic abnormality that occurs in the foot is gout (Fig. 8-160), typically manifested as swelling over the first metatarsophalangeal joint. On plain x-ray, these are erosions in the periarticular region with overhanging edges. These are late findings, and again the diagnosis is best made by laboratory analysis.

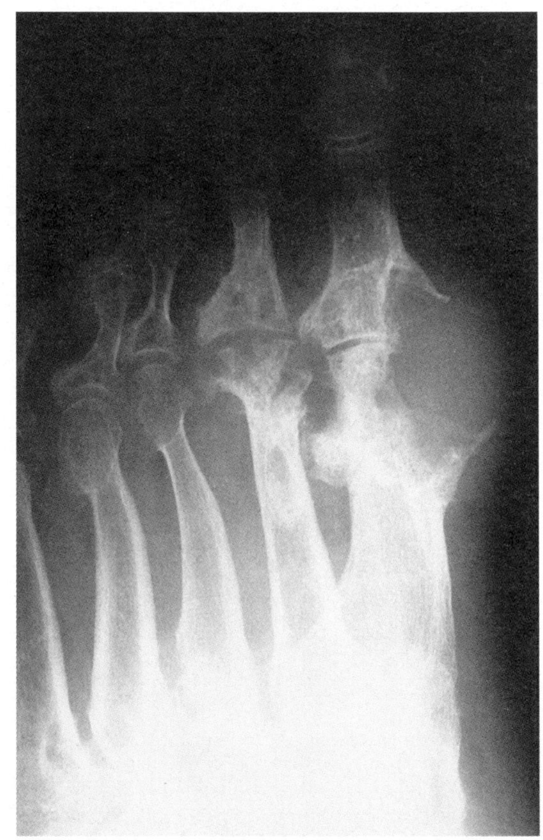

FIGURE 8-160 ■ Gout. The first metatarsal phalangeal joint is the most commonly affected. This large tophus has caused erosion at the margins of the joints; in general, however, the joint space itself is reasonably well preserved.

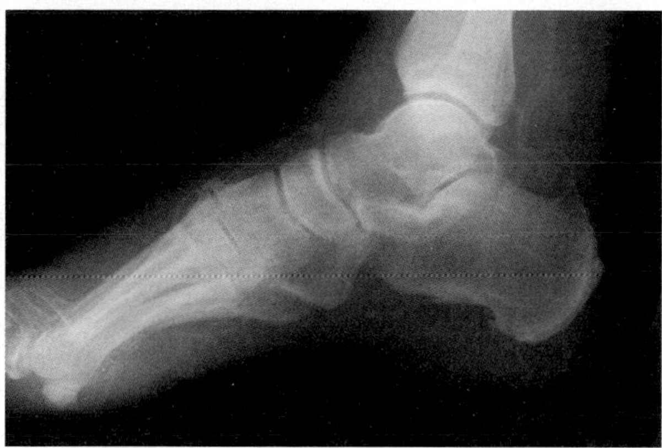

FIGURE 8-161 ■ Vascular calcifications. A lateral image of the foot shows extensive vascular calcifications. When this is seen, the patient almost always has diabetes.

Diabetes and Complications

In patients with diabetes, peripheral neuropathy as well as vascular insufficiency may develop (Figs. 8-161 and 8-162). The latter is particularly acute in the toes, and often concomitant infection is found. X-rays of the feet can demonstrate changes of osteomyelitis to help distinguish it from cellulitis. The characteristic signs of osteomyelitis include soft tissue swelling, focal loss of trabecular pattern, periosteal reaction, and frank bone destruction (Fig. 8-163). The differentiation of osteomyelitis from cellulitis is important because the therapy for osteomyelitis involves weeks of intravenous therapy. If the bone changes that have been described are found, you can conclude that osteomyelitis is present. Osteomyelitis, however, can be present with a normal x-ray, and if clinical suspicion is high, evaluation with a three-phase nuclear medicine bone scan is often useful. Other plain x-ray changes that are characteristic of diabetic involvement of the foot include marked vascular calcification and occasionally air within the soft tissue due to infection and gangrene.

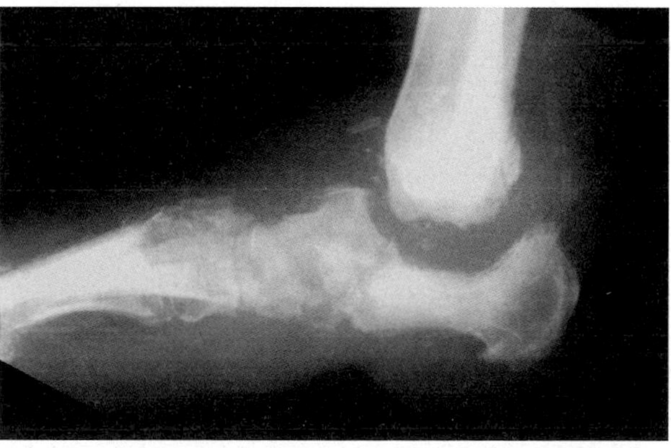

FIGURE 8-162 ■ Neuropathic ankle and foot secondary to diabetes. On a lateral view of the foot and ankle, extensive destruction of the ankle joint and tarsal bones is seen. Note that in spite of the destruction, the bones are not demineralized, indicating use, and by inference, the absence of pain.

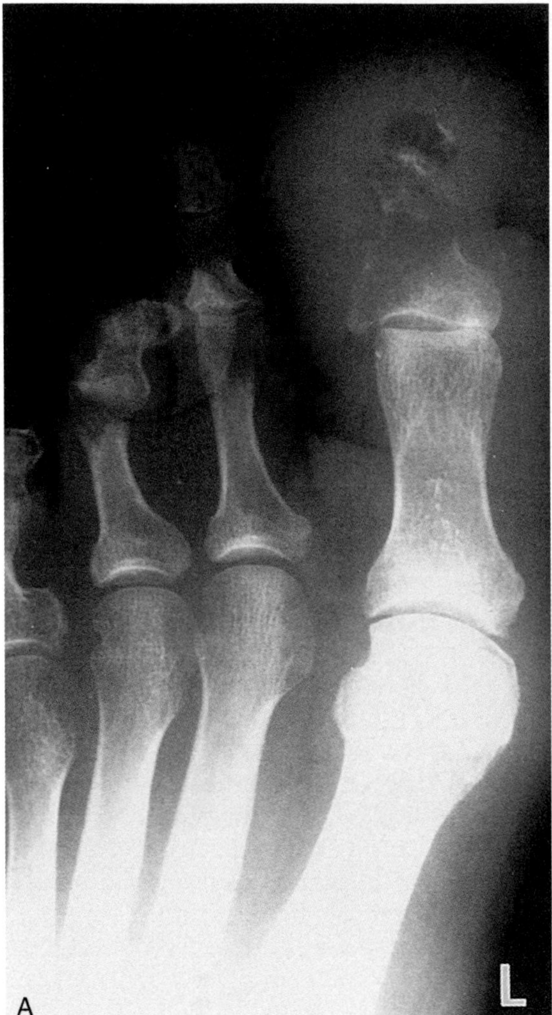

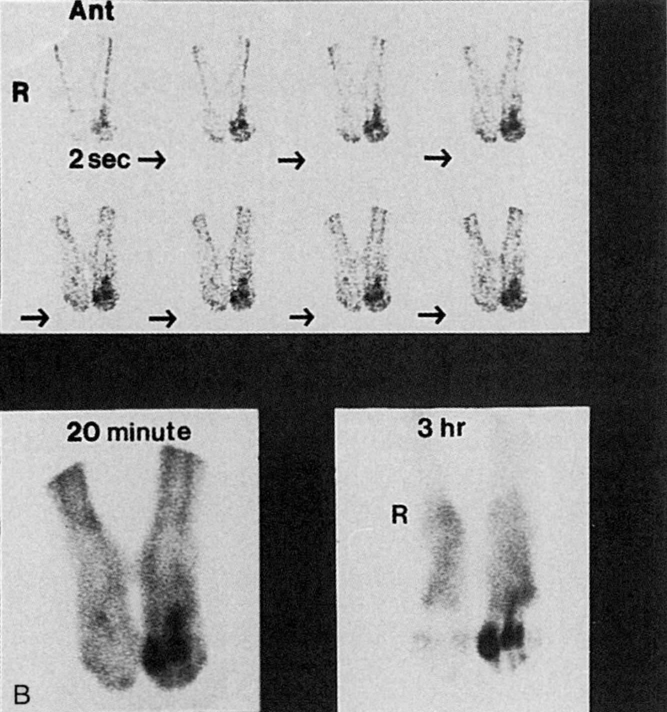

FIGURE 8-163 ■ **Osteomyelitis of the foot.** *A,* In this diabetic patient, significant soft tissue swelling and destruction of the bony structure of the distal phalanx of the great toe are noted. *B,* Even when x-rays are normal, osteomyelitis may be present. A nuclear medicine bone scan is more sensitive and will show increased blood flow in the first seconds after radionuclide injection, increased blood pooling at 20 min, and more focal and intense radioactivity on the 3-hour images.

PEDIATRIC MUSCULOSKELETAL IMAGING

Skull

Anatomy. Typical views of the skull in a child are the same as in adults: AP and lateral. The differences in normal anatomy consist of dark or lucent lines that represent the cranial sutures (Fig. 8-164) and a small face in comparison with the cranium. Cranial sutures usually remain partially open until at least midlife, and it is particularly important that they remain open in the early years of life to allow growth of the brain. The sutures of the skull can close prematurely (craniosynostosis). The sagittal suture is most commonly involved, and the coronal suture less so. Premature closure of the sagittal suture results in growth of the skull in the areas where the coronal and lambdoid sutures remain open, and the skull becomes much longer than normal (scaphocephaly) (Fig. 8-165). If the coronal suture closes prematurely, growth continues to occur along the sagittal suture, and the skull becomes much wider than normal. A skull film is often not necessary, because the shape of the skull and a ridge of bone over the closed suture are clinically apparent. On a skull film, the prematurely closed suture may be dense (white) at the edges or may just be difficult to see.

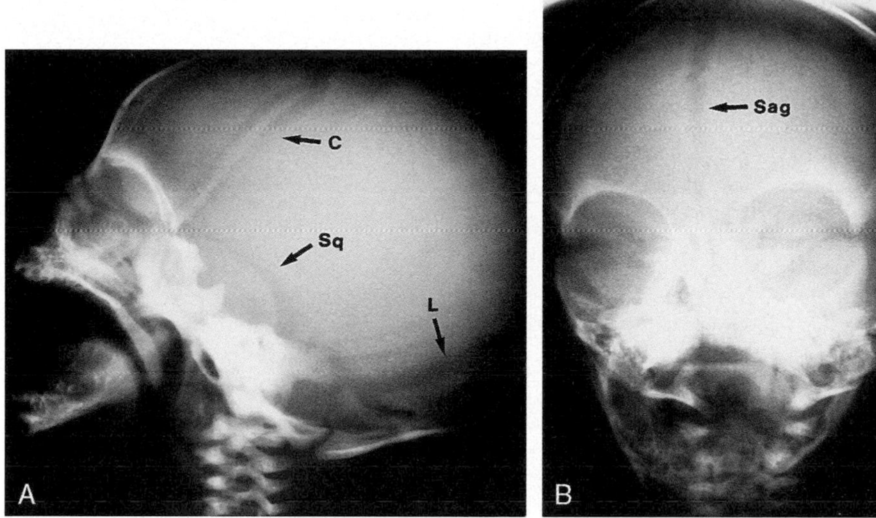

FIGURE 8-164 ■ **Normal newborn skull.** *A,* The lateral view clearly shows the lambdoidal (L), squamous (Sq), and coronal (C) sutures. *B,* An anteroposterior view clearly shows the sagittal suture.

Trauma. Fractures are seen as very sharply defined lucent lines that do not correspond to sutures. The margins of the sutures are somewhat wiggly, especially as they near closure. Sometimes it can be difficult to differentiate between a fracture and a vascular groove. Most vascular grooves are seen on the lateral view of the skull and radiate superiorly and posteriorly from a position just above the ear. In addition, if you look carefully, the vascular groove is a lucent line that is bounded by a sclerotic (white) margin before you reach the normal bone of the skull. A skull fracture will be a lucent line (dark) and then normal skull.

Occasionally a fracture line will widen progressively during the first weeks or months after injury. The widening is due to formation of an underlying leptomeningeal cyst, which causes pressure and subsequent atrophy of the bone at the edges of the fracture line. The dura is torn at

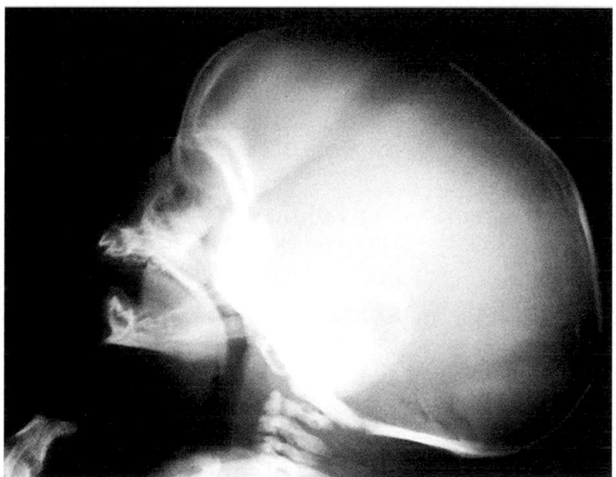

FIGURE 8-165 ■ **Premature closure of the sagittal suture.** Closure of the sagittal suture has allowed growth of the skull only in the anteroposterior direction; here the coronal and lambdoidal sutures can be seen to be widened.

the time of injury, allowing this process to occur. Sometimes this lesion is referred to as a growing skull fracture of childhood, and it usually will not heal without surgery (Fig. 8-166).

Another common traumatic lesion of childhood is a cephalohematoma. These are caused by traumatic hemorrhage into the neonatal scalp during labor, although they also can occur after cephalic injury during infancy or childhood. With healing, usually a new shell of subperiosteal bone is seen over the hematoma, which then thickens and calcifies. Clinically, cephalohematomas can disappear in weeks to months, although the x-ray finding(s) may persist long afterward (Fig. 8-167).

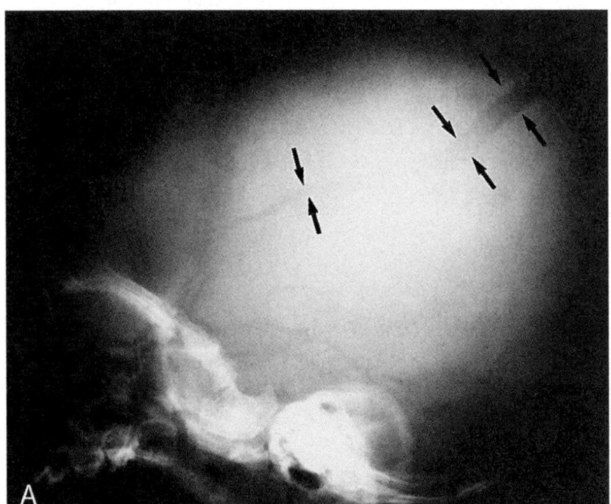

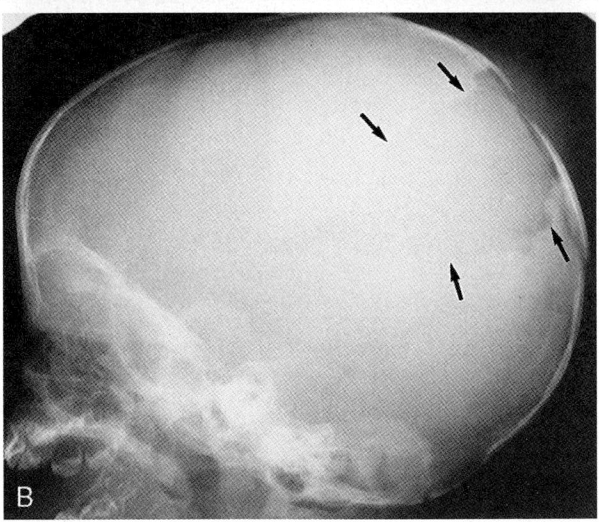

FIGURE 8-166 ■ **Growing skull fracture of childhood.** *A,* A parietal skull fracture is easily seen on this lateral view of the skull *(arrows)*. *B,* A repeated skull film 2 months later shows that the fracture line has become very wide *(arrows)* due to a leptomeningeal cyst and continued pressure erosion of the bone.

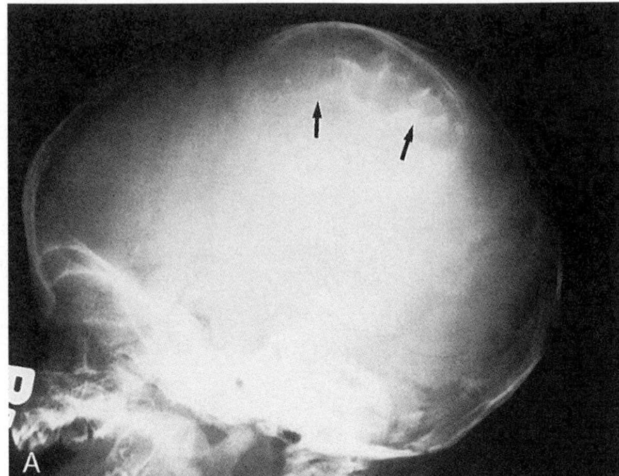

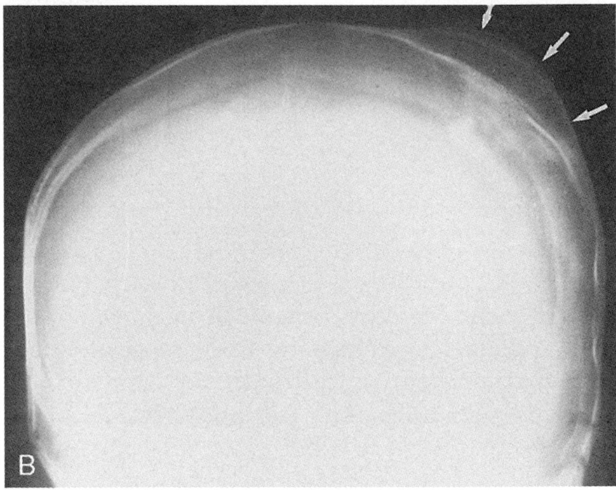

FIGURE 8-167 ■ **Cephalohematoma.** *A,* A lateral view of the skull shows a lucent multilocular and expansile lesion *(arrows)*. *B,* An anteroposterior tangential view of the skull shows that this lesion is primarily bulging out from the normal skull cortex because of calcification of the hematoma.

Neoplastic lesions of the skull can occur during childhood. Almost all appear as multiple lucent holes (Fig. 8-168). Typical malignant lesions in very young children are due to histiocytosis X, although with slightly older children, metastatic lesions occur from neuroblastoma.

Many clinicians order sinus views to look for sinusitis. This is often the result of parental concern rather than medical need. You should

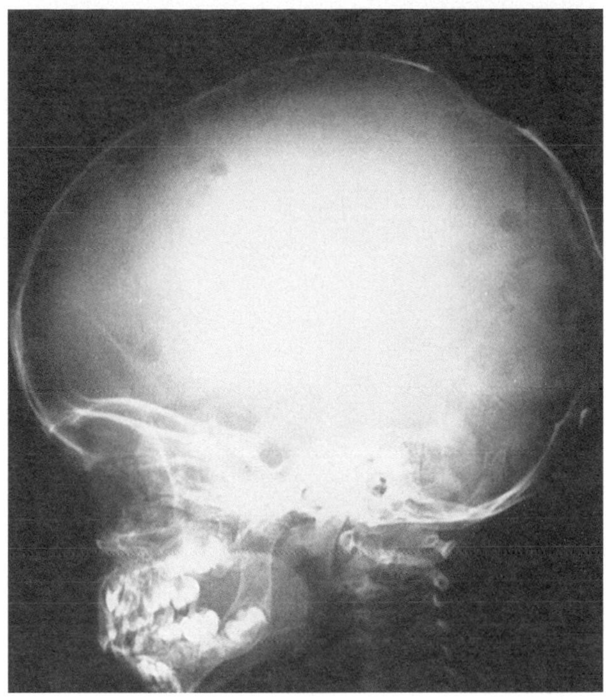

FIGURE 8-168 ■ Histiocytosis X of the skull. Multiple lucent holes of varying sizes are seen in this lateral projection of the skull. A large scalloped lesion has destroyed the cortex over the posterior aspect of the skull and has beveled edges, characteristic of this disease.

remember that the sinuses are not developed at birth and are progressively pneumatized over the first 10 years of life. The first sinuses to appear are the maxillary sinuses; the frontal sinuses come much later. For both children and adults, it is inappropriate to order sinus views for what clinically appears to be routine sinusitis (Fig. 8-169).

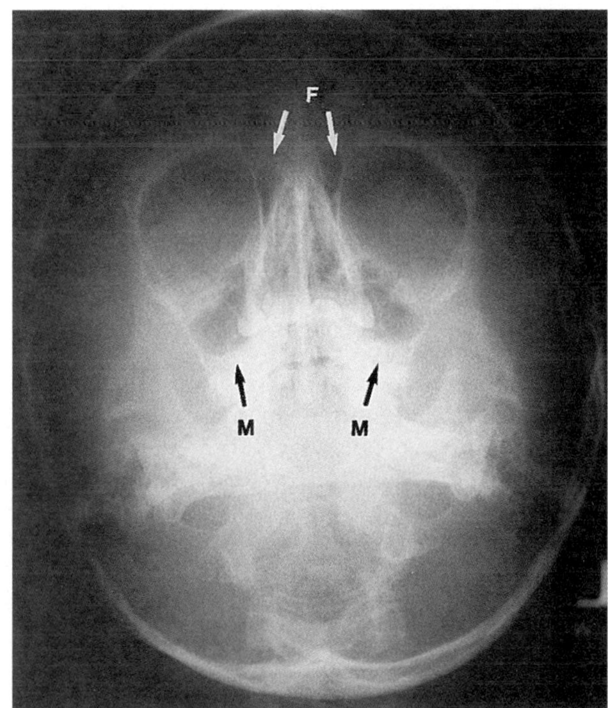

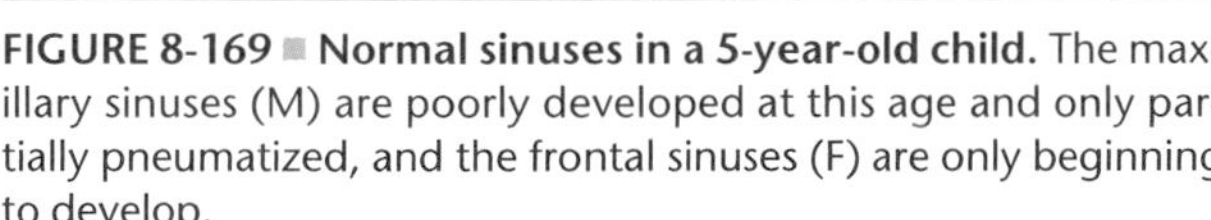

FIGURE 8-169 ■ Normal sinuses in a 5-year-old child. The maxillary sinuses (M) are poorly developed at this age and only partially pneumatized, and the frontal sinuses (F) are only beginning to develop.

Spine

Two items cause confusion in interpretation of cervical spine views in children. The first is that the odontoid process and the body of C2 form as separate ossification centers, and fusion occurs in the first year or so of life (Fig. 8-170*A*). Occasionally nonfusion can persist into adulthood. The differentiation from an odontoid fracture can be made by the absence of sharp, angulated corners and the absence of soft tissue swelling. Another surprising but common finding in children is a pseudosubluxation at C2 and C3. This is simply a normal variant and occurs when the child has his or her neck slightly flexed (Fig. 8-170*B*). If this occurs in children older than approximately 5 years, you should suspect a traumatic cause rather than a normal variant.

A number of congenital spinal abnormalities occur, including hemivertebra and butterfly vertebra, which often result in scoliosis. Severe abnormalities are usually diagnosed soon after birth, but more minor abnormalities may not be found until a scoliosis workup is performed in adolescence or adulthood.

A rather unusual spinal abnormality of childhood is called diskitis. This usually occurs in the lumbar spine and appears radiographically as a decreased disk space (Fig. 8-171). On a nuclear medicine bone scan, increased activity of the vertebral body is noted both above and below the affected level. The origin of this entity is uncertain, but it may represent a low-grade infection.

Upper Extremity

Humerus. Lesions in the proximal humerus that are lytic, somewhat expansive, and quite well demarcated are usually unicameral bone cysts (see Fig. 8-55). Care should be taken, however, in the diagnosis, because the third most common site of osteogenic sarcoma is the proximal humerus.

Elbow. The pediatric elbow can cause difficulties in interpretation owing to the development of various ossification centers. The epiphysis of the radial head initially appears at ages approxi-

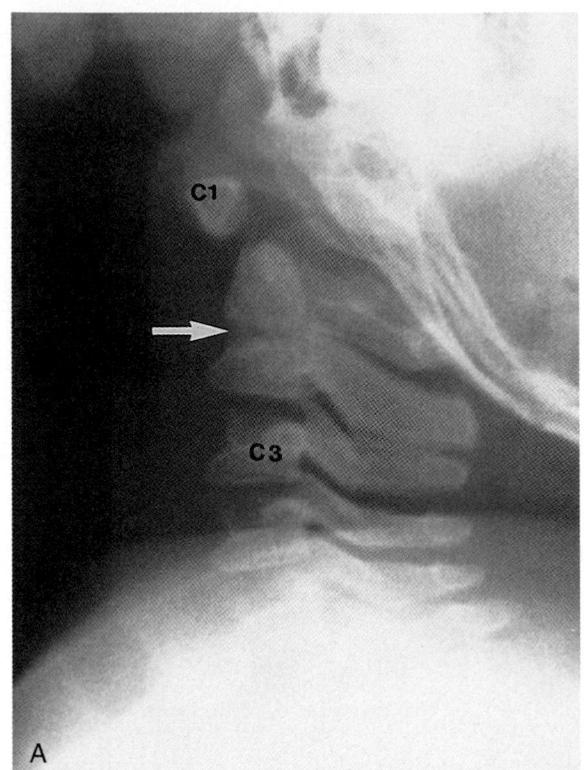

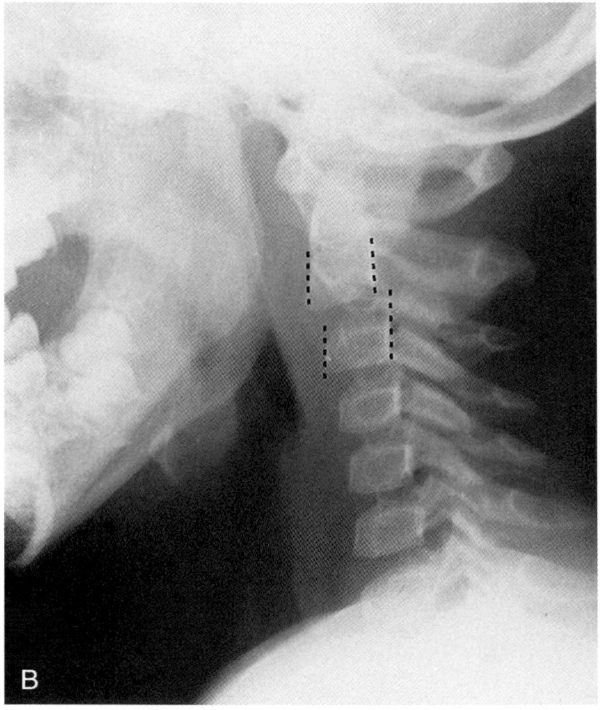

FIGURE 8-170 ■ Normal variations of the cervical spine in children. *A,* A lateral view in a newborn child shows a cleft where the odontoid is not yet completely fused to the body of C2. This is normal. *B,* Pseudosubluxation of C2 on C3 is a very common normal variant in children; it occurs only at this level, particularly when the neck is straight or slightly flexed.

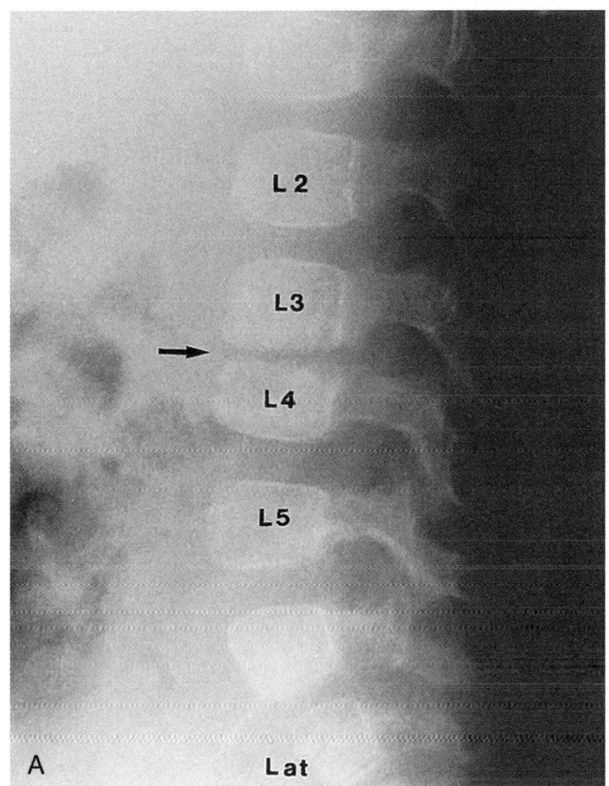

FIGURE 8-171 ■ Diskitis. *A,* A lateral view of the lumbar spine in this child with back pain shows a decreased disk space at L3-L4 *(arrow).* Sometimes the disk space is not appreciably narrowed, and the diagnosis can sometimes be made with a nuclear medicine bone scan *(B).* Here, on an anterior view of the lumbar spine, increased radioactivity is seen at L3 and L4, compatible with the diagnosis of diskitis.

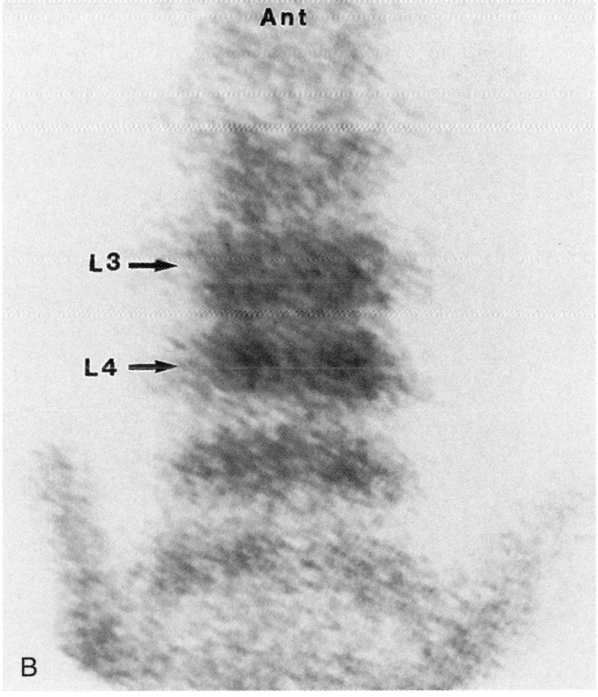

mately 3 to 5 years, and the olecranon appears between 8 and 11 years. The capitulum of the distal humerus appears at younger than 1 year, the medial epicondyle at 3 to 6 years, the trochlea at 7 to 9 years, and the lateral epicondyle at 12 to 14 years. The development may even be asymmetrical between right and left, depending on which arm is dominant (Fig. 8-172). The asymmetrical appearance of the lateral condylar ossification center can often be mistaken for a fracture, and clinical correlation is essential. Note should be made that avulsion fractures of the lateral condyle are quite rare, whereas avulsion fractures of the medial condyle are much more common. When this occurs, it is sometimes called "Little Leaguer's elbow" (Fig. 8-173).

In examining the elbow for fracture, remember that visualization of the anterior fat pad lying up against the anterior aspect of the distal humerus is a normal finding. A posterior fat pad should never be seen, and the anterior fat pad should not be displaced or bowed forward (Fig. 8-174*A*). In addition, the apophysis of the olecranon should not be mistaken for a fracture.

A relatively common fracture in children is a supracondylar fracture that extends across the distal aspect of the humerus. When this occurs, there is almost always bowing forward of the anterior fat pad and visualization of the posterior fat pad. You should evaluate the anterior humeral line. This line should extend down into the middle third of the capitellum (Fig. 8-174*B*).

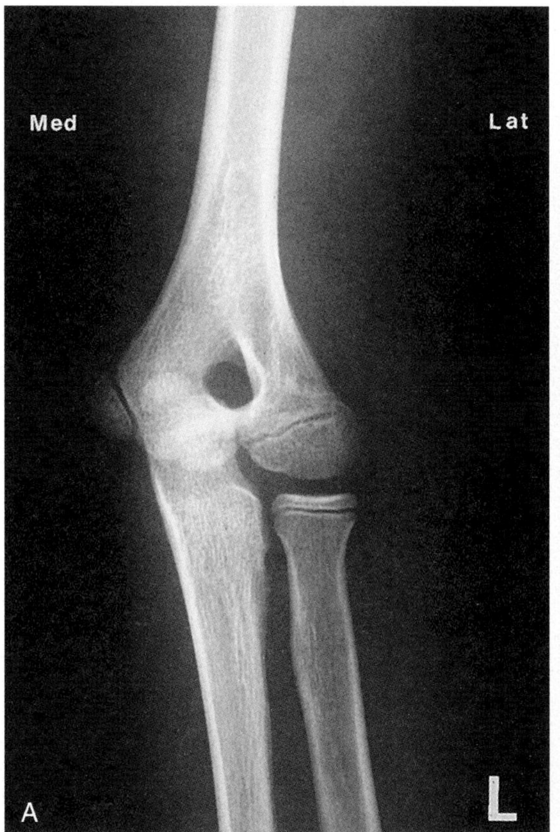

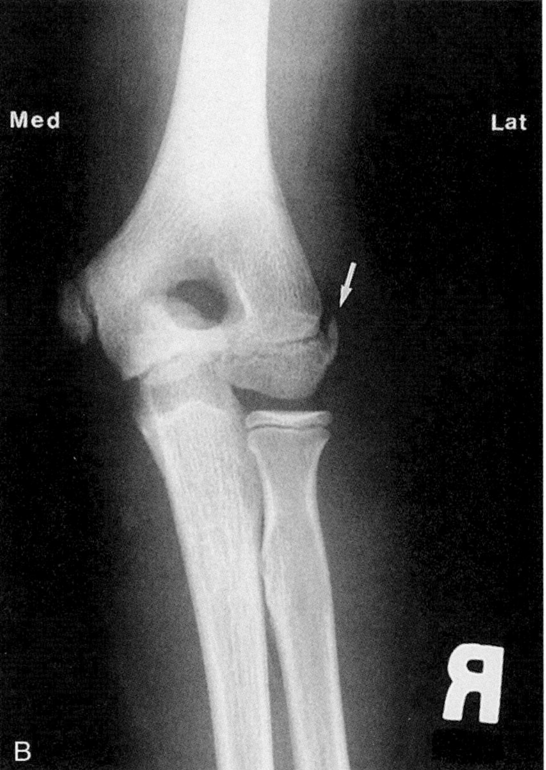

FIGURE 8-172 ■ Normal variation and development of the elbow in children. *A,* On an anteroposterior view of the left elbow, the medial epicondyle is visualized, but the lateral is not. *B,* On the right side, the lateral epicondyle is seen. This asymmetrical development from one side to the other can occur normally. Because lateral epicondyle fractures are rare, you should suspect that this is an apophysis.

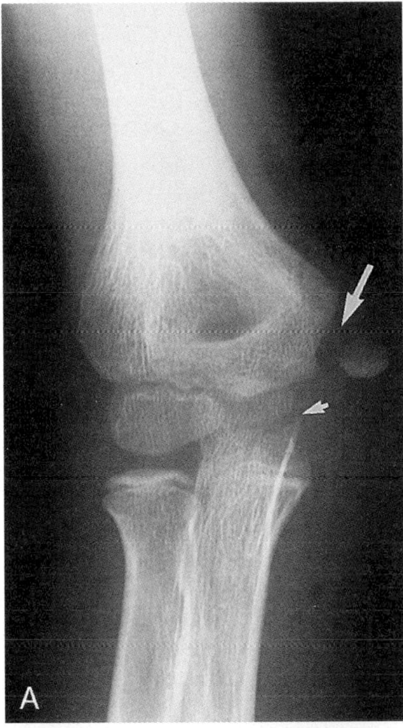

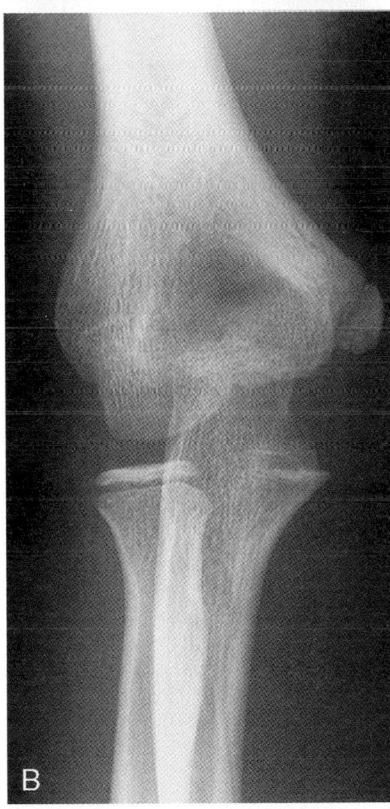

FIGURE 8-173 ■ **"Little Leaguer's elbow."** *A,* An anteroposterior view of the elbow shows an abnormally wide space between the medial epicondyle and the distal humerus *(large arrow).* An olecranon fracture also is seen *(small arrow). B,* The opposite elbow is shown for comparison with the normal position of the medial epicondyle.

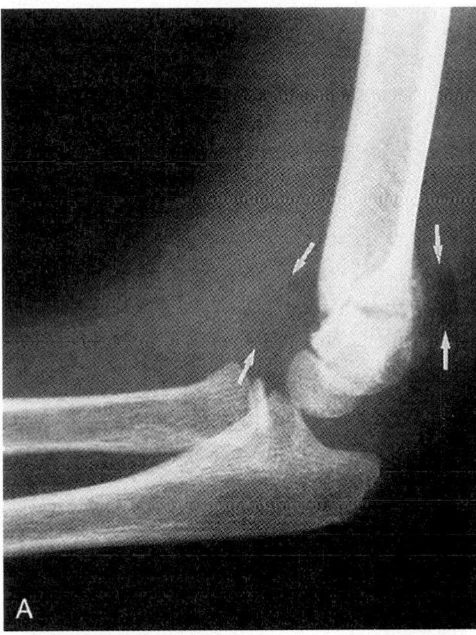

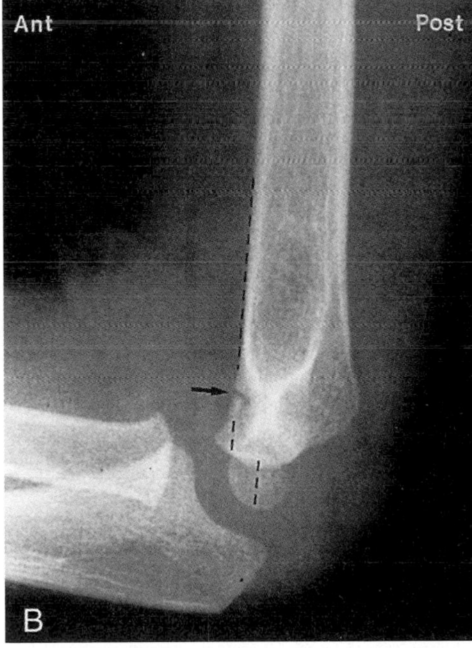

FIGURE 8-174 ■ **Supracondylar fractures.** This is the most common elbow fracture in children. *A,* A lateral view of the elbow shows marked anterior displacement of the anterior fat and visualization of the posterior fat pad *(arrows),* a sign that a fracture is almost certainly present. *B,* In a younger child, a fracture is seen because of the posterior displacement of the capitellum from the anterior humeral line. An incomplete cortical fracture also is seen *(arrow).*

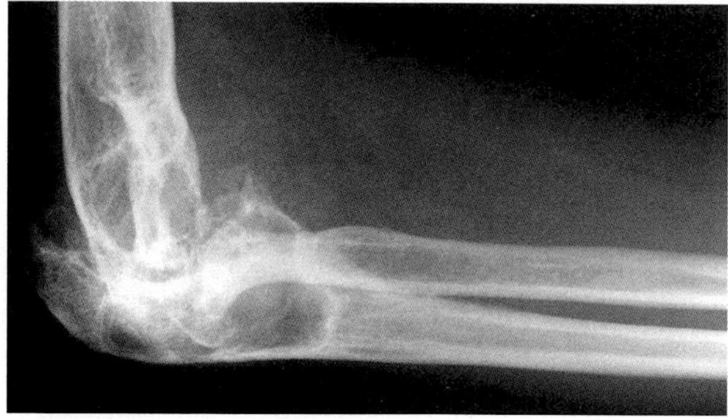

FIGURE 8-175 ■ Hemophilia. A lateral view of the elbow shows marked destruction of the joint space. Chronic bleeding within the joint has destroyed the cartilage. Similar findings may be seen with juvenile rheumatoid arthritis.

Destructive lesions involving a joint space usually are produced by inflammatory lesions. They may be the result of infection in the joint space (septic arthritis) or of other chronic inflammatory processes, such as inflammation due to intermittent bleeding within the joint in patients with hemophilia (Fig. 8-175). Significant joint involvement also occurs in children who have juvenile rheumatoid arthritis.

Forearm, Wrist, and Hand. Fractures of the forearm and wrist are very common in children; a number of the types that occur in adults have already been discussed. Whenever multiple fractures are found, especially those that appear to be in different stages of healing, child abuse should be suspected. The fact that the fractures are of different ages can be ascertained by periosteal reaction or callus around some, but not around other, fracture sites. If child abuse is suspected, additional views of the skull, ribs, pelvis, and both upper and lower extremities should be obtained (Fig. 8-176).

Young children have bones that are relatively plastic, and two unique childhood fractures occur as a result of this plasticity. The first is a "buckle" or "torus" fracture. Sometimes, on

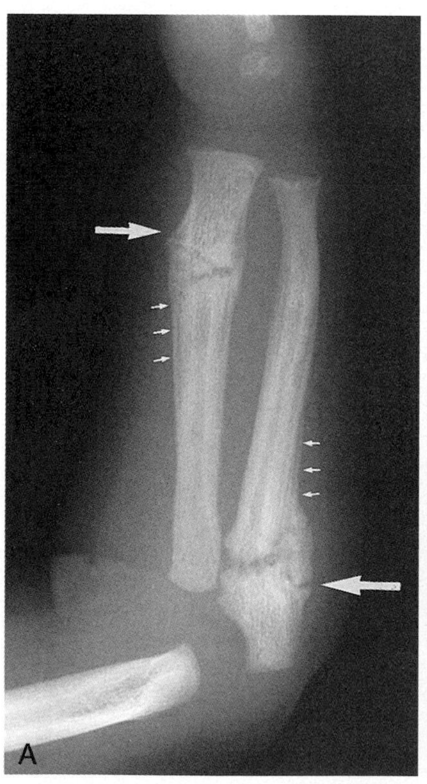

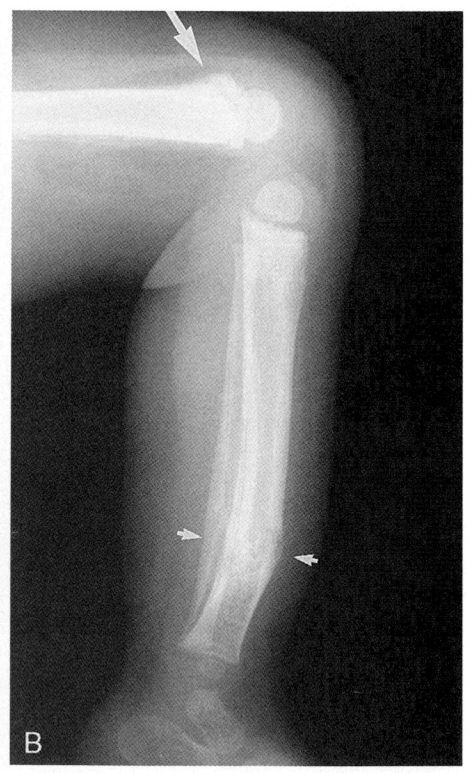

FIGURE 8-176 ■ Child abuse. *A,* A view of the forearm in this child shows extensive periosteal reaction *(small arrows)* and transverse fracture lines *(large arrows).* Fractures of long bones in children, particularly with different stages of healing, are very suggestive of a battered child. *B,* A lateral view of the lower extremity in the same child also reveals fractures of the distal fibula and tibia *(small arrows)* as well as a metaphyseal corner fracture *(large arrow)* of the distal femur. This latter fracture also is typical of child abuse.

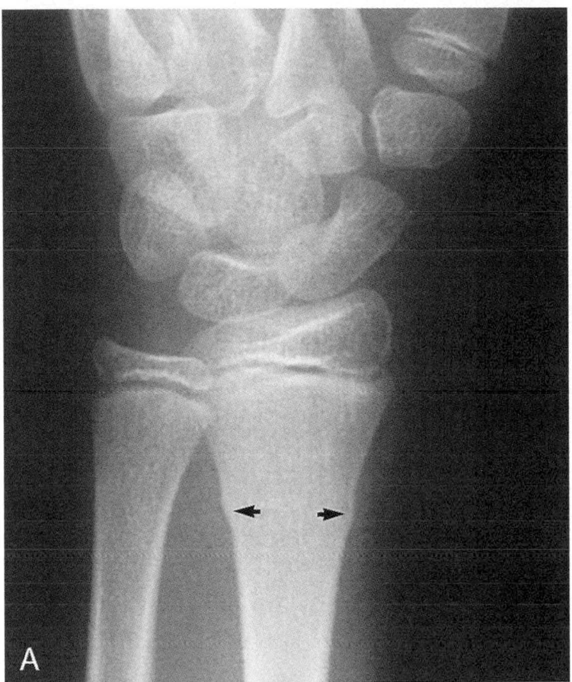

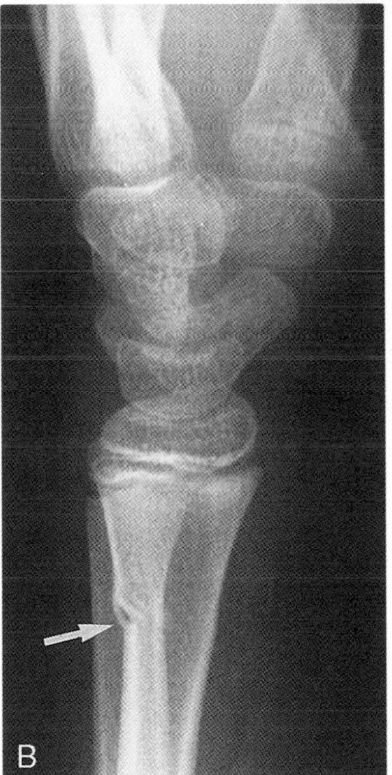

FIGURE 8-177 ■ **Torus or buckle fracture.** *A,* An anteroposterior view of the wrist shows slight bulging of the cortex in the metaphyseal region *(arrows). B,* A lateral view of the wrist shows buckling of the dorsal cortex.

a single view, all you will identify is a slight outward bulge of the cortex, whereas on other views, you may actually see a buckling of the cortex (Fig. 8-177). The other fracture is the so-called greenstick fracture. In this, the bone is bent but typically fractured only on one side of the cortex, similar to the breaking of a green twig (Fig. 8-178).

At the end of any long bone, a number of the Salter-Harris–type fractures described earlier can be seen (see Fig. 8-81). One of the most difficult fractures to see is a nondisplaced, or very minimally displaced, Salter-Harris type I fracture through the epiphyseal plate. Often the x-ray at the time of injury will be normal; however, a repeated examination 1 to 2 weeks later will reveal increasing sclerosis (white lines) across the epiphyseal plate, indicating a healing fracture (Fig. 8-179). Fortunately, nondisplaced Salter-Harris type I fractures are not important clinically.

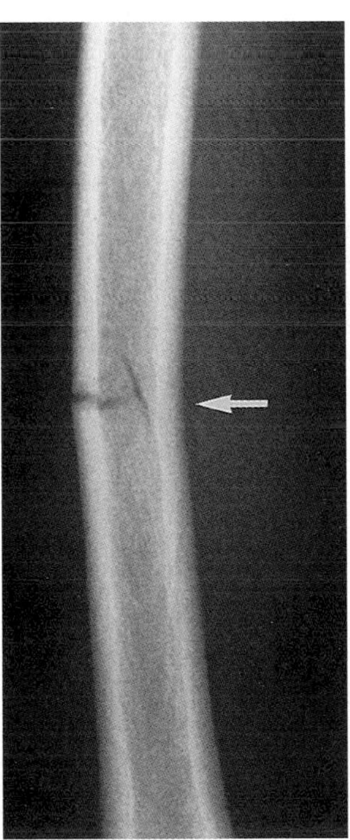

FIGURE 8-178 ■ **Greenstick fracture.** In the humerus of this elementary school child, a direct blow from the direction of the *arrow* has caused an incomplete transverse fracture.

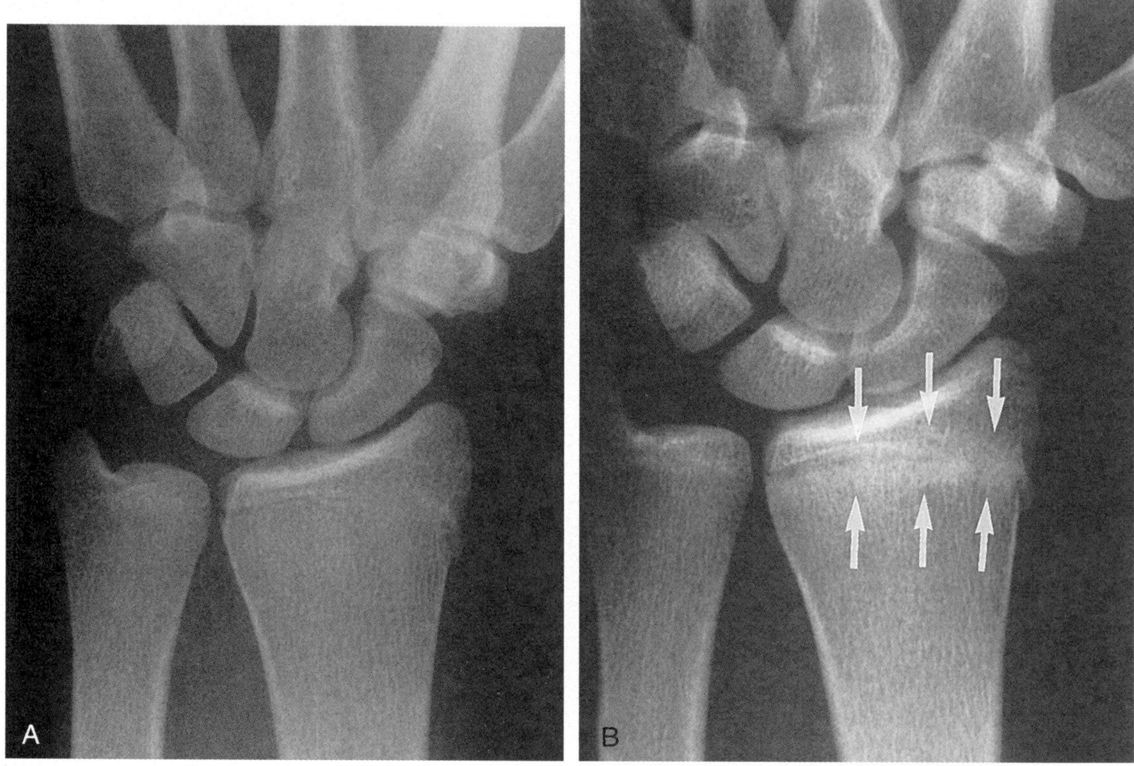

FIGURE 8-179 ■ Occult Salter-Harris fracture of the distal radius. *A,* An anteroposterior view of the wrist at the time of the injury does not show any cortical disruption or displacement. *B,* A repeated examination 10 days later shows sclerosis across the epiphyseal plate, indicating healing of an occult Salter-Harris type I fracture.

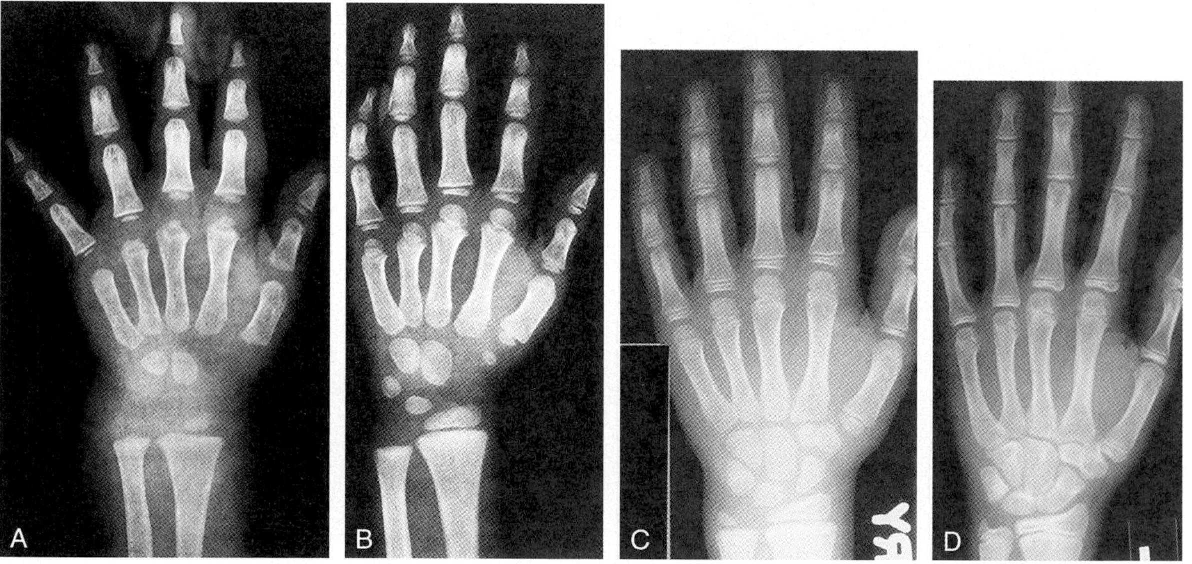

FIGURE 8-180 ■ Normal development anatomy of the hand during childhood. A 2-year-old boy *(A),* 5-year-old boy *(B),* 7-year-old boy *(C),* and 15-year-old boy *(D).* In general, the approximate age can be guessed, because the number of carpal bones usually is close to the child's age in years up to about 7 years.

Normal growth of the bones in the hand includes appearance and development of the carpal bones and of epiphyses at the end of the radius and ulna, the distal second through fourth metacarpals, the proximal first metacarpal, and the proximal aspects of the phalanges. At birth, essentially no ossification centers of the carpal bones or epiphyses are seen in the hand. As a general rule, one carpal bone appears each year from age 1 year to about age 7 years (Fig. 8-180). Variation may occur in the appearance of the epiphyses and ossification centers between the two hands, and the growth pattern is usually somewhat more advanced in girls than in boys of the same age.

In a child younger than 10 years, it is very rare to have fractures of the carpal bones. Typical hand fractures in children involve either Salter fractures of the fingers or fractures of the terminal phalanges (because children usually get their fingers caught in doors and other objects).

Osteomyelitis in very young children often involves both the distal metaphysis and the epiphysis of a bone because the epiphysis receives its blood supply from the shaft of the bone. In older children, the epiphysis has its own separate blood supply, and osteomyelitis usually involves the metaphysis just proximal to the epiphyseal plate. With hematogenous spread of bacteria, multiple bones can be involved. The x-ray findings of osteomyelitis include soft tissue swelling, bone destruction, and periosteal reaction. As with adults, if a clinical question remains about the presence of osteomyelitis or even septic arthritis, a radionuclide bone scan is often helpful (Fig. 8-181).

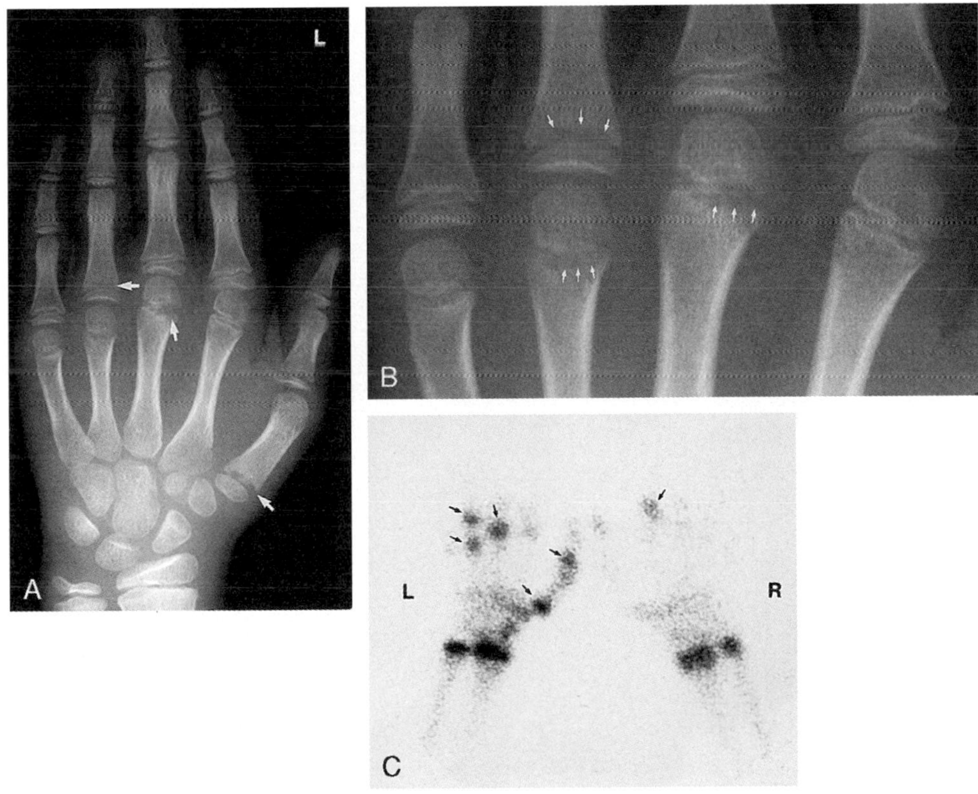

FIGURE 8-181 ■ **Multifocal osteomyelitis.** *A,* An anteroposterior view of the hand demonstrates metaphyseal destruction of at least three sites. This hematogenously spread osteomyelitis usually will not cross the epiphyseal plate if the child is more than several years old. *B,* Detailed view of the hand showing the areas of metaphyseal destruction *(arrows)*. *C,* A nuclear medicine bone scan of both hands in this child shows additional areas of abnormality *(arrows)* that were clinically unsuspected.

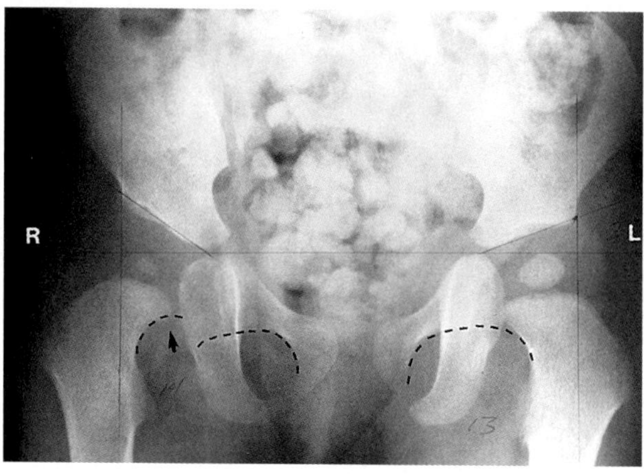

FIGURE 8-182 ■ **Congenital dislocation of the hip.** An anteroposterior view demonstrates dislocation of the right hip. The *dotted line*, which should be continuous, is called Shenton's line. The right acetabulum also is at a steeper angle on the right than on the left. Diagnosis of congenital dislocation of the hip should be made on the basis of clinical examination.

Pelvis and Hips. Dislocation of the hip in children is usually congenital and occurs more often in girls than in boys. The radiographic diagnosis may be made in a number of ways. Radiographic diagnosis of a congenital hip dislocation is unreliable in the neonate because the ossification center for the femoral head is not developed. Perhaps the simplest imaging method is evaluation of Shenton's line, which is formed by the medial aspect of the obturator foramen and the medial aspect of the femoral neck. Together, these should form a nice smooth, curved arc (Fig. 8-182). A frog-leg view with the legs abducted is useless, because in this position, the hip is reduced. X-ray diagnosis of congenital hip dislocation should be done rarely, if ever, because the clinical finding of an audible click when the hips are abducted should be sufficient to make the diagnosis. If any doubt remains, ultrasound examination should be obtained.

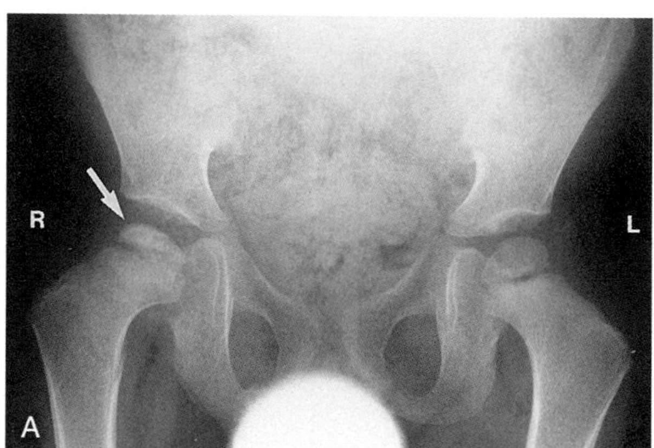

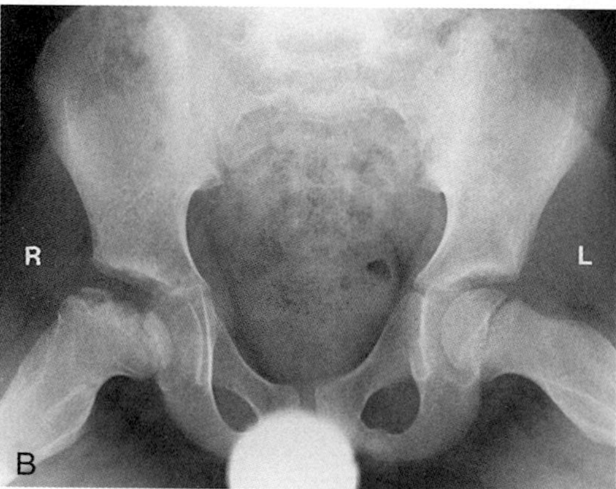

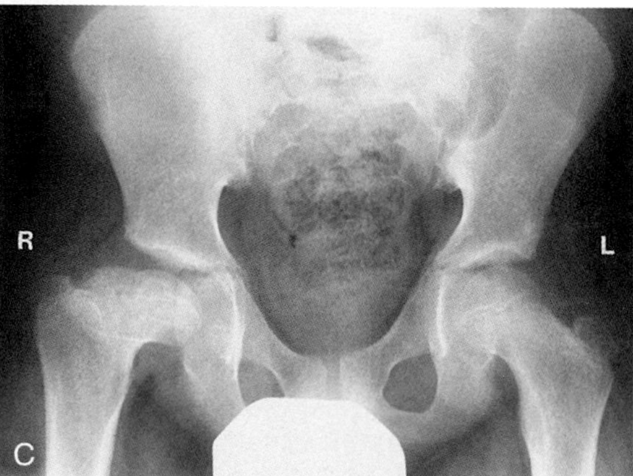

FIGURE 8-183 ■ **Legg-Perthes disease.** *A,* An anteroposterior view of the pelvis demonstrates fragmentation and sclerosis of the right femoral epiphysis in this 6-year-old boy. *B,* A follow-up film obtained 8 years later shows continuing deformity due to the osteonecrosis. Significant degenerative arthritis *(C)* developed by age 12 years.

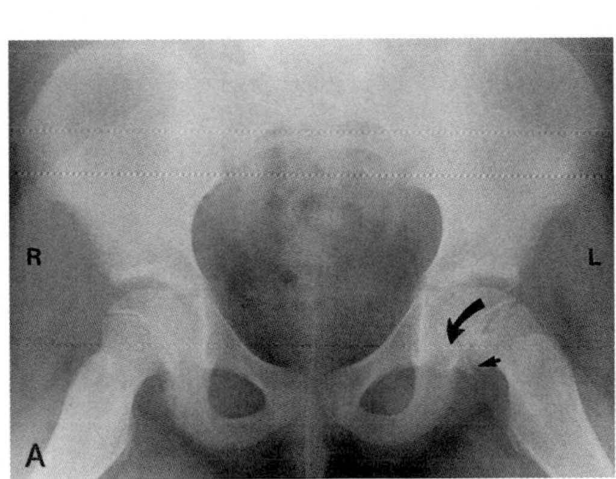

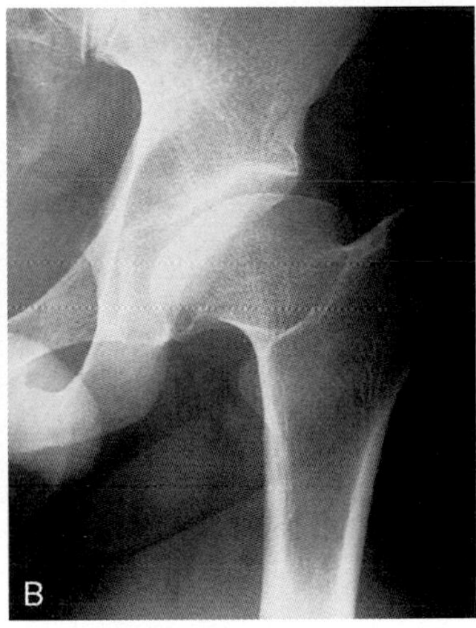

FIGURE 8-184 ■ Slipped capital femoral epiphysis. *A,* An anteroposterior view of the pelvis in this overweight teenage boy shows slipping of the left femoral epiphysis relative to the femoral neck *(arrows).* This essentially is a Salter-Harris type I fracture. *B,* Follow-up film of the left hip 10 years later shows significant deformity, which will result in degenerative arthritis.

Occasionally aseptic necrosis of the epiphysis of the femoral head (Legg-Perthes disease) can develop in children. Boys are more commonly affected than girls. Clinical signs are a limp and pain, with limitation in motion of the hip. The imaging findings are irregularity, sclerosis (increased density), and fragmentation of the epiphysis. Often a resulting deformity is followed by a disabling osteoarthritis decades later (Fig. 8-183).

Another pediatric hip abnormality is slipping of the epiphysis of the femoral head. The cause of this is unknown, and it usually does not happen in children younger than 9 years. The diagnosis is made from the images by noting a thickened epiphyseal plate and medial displacement of the femoral head relative to the femoral neck (Fig. 8-184). The lateral or abducted frog-leg view of the hip offers the best view of these findings. When the epiphysis fuses, no more slippage occurs, but the deformity that has occurred will be permanent, and later degenerative disease will be a complication.

Lower Extremities

Although systemic bone diseases are quite rare in children, two entities are important to be aware of. The first is osteogenesis imperfecta. This is a hereditary disease, with abnormal collagen fibers and a disorder of the osteoblasts. Fragile bones or teeth, thin skin, and sometimes blue sclera are noted. Two forms of the disease are found, one noted immediately at birth and one appearing later. The disease is characterized on imaging by multiple healing fractures and bowing deformities of the bone (Fig. 8-185).

Arthritic changes in children are very rare, with the exception of juvenile rheumatoid arthritis and hemophilia. Both these diseases can cause fluid collections within the joint and destruction of the cartilage, followed by degenerative change. Hyperemia also may result in overgrowth of the epiphyseal region of the bone. The joint effusions, irregularity of the articular surface, and subsequent degenerative changes are easily visualized on x-rays (Fig. 8-186).

Ewing's tumor typically occurs in the shaft of the long bones or in flat bones, such as the pelvis, scapula, and ribs. In contrast, osteogenic sarcomas occur most commonly in the distal femur, less commonly in the proximal tibia and proximal humerus, and rarely elsewhere. An osteogenic sarcoma may initially appear as a destructive lesion in the central

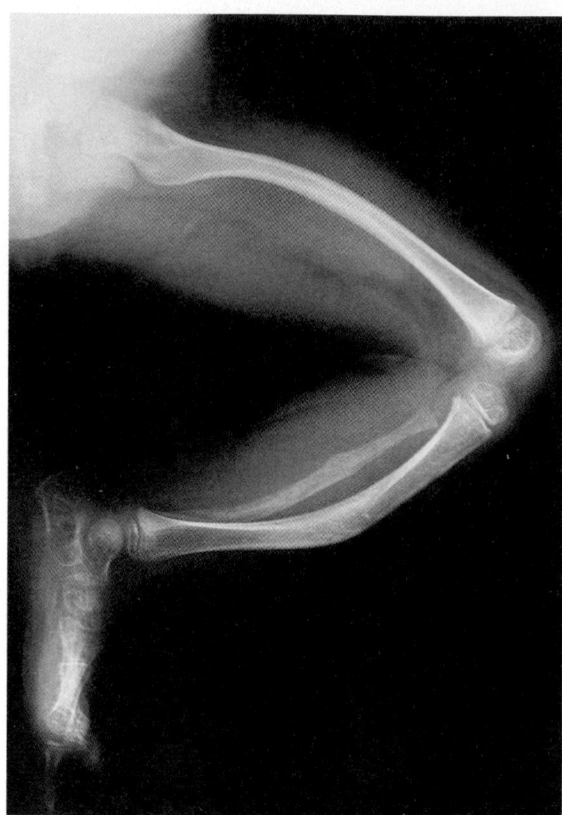

FIGURE 8-185 ■ Osteogenesis imperfecta. This lateral view of the lower extremities shows marked bowing of the bones due to softening and multiple fractures that occur as a result of this congenital bone dysplasia.

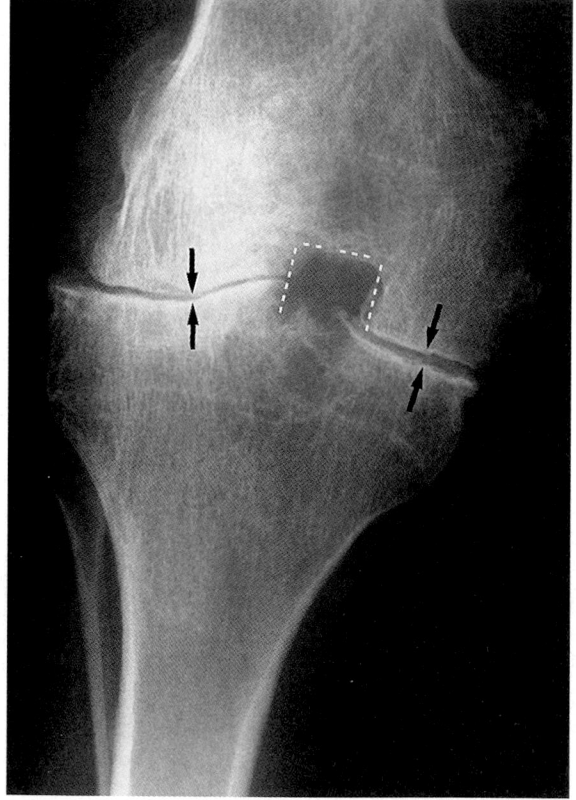

FIGURE 8-186 ■ Hemophilia. An anteroposterior view of the knee shows marked joint-space narrowing with destruction due to repeated bleeding into the joint space; a very square intercondylar notch is present. Similar findings are seen in juvenile rheumatoid arthritis.

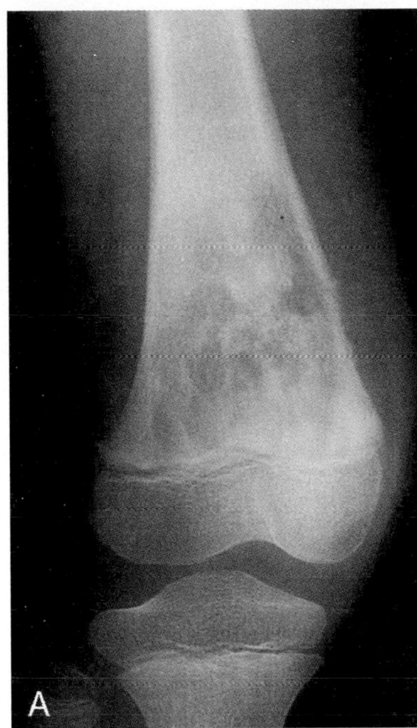

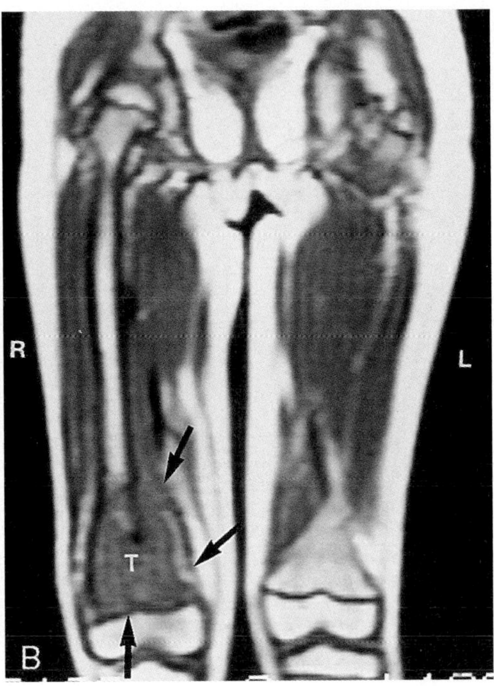

FIGURE 8-187 ▪ Central osteosarcoma. *A,* A destructive lesion is seen in the metaphysis on this anteroposterior view of the knee in a young teenager with pain. *B,* A magnetic resonance scan of both legs shows the soft tissue extent of the tumor *(arrows).*

portion of the bone or with periosteal reaction and soft tissue swelling (Fig. 8-187). Often an MR scan is useful to show the soft tissue extent of the tumor.

A number of characteristic traumatic tibial lesions occur in children. As mentioned earlier, the proximal tibial epiphysis normally has an anterior projection that slopes down over the front of the tibia. On plain x-rays, this is best seen on the lateral view (see Fig. 8-116). This appearance can look a little bit irregular, however, if a small fragment is pulled off, and if the patient has pain, this is consistent with the diagnosis of Osgood-Schlatter injury. This is relatively frequent in children age 10 to 15 years, particularly in boys who participate in active sports. It probably represents a partial avulsion of the anterior tubercle by the inferior patellar tendon, and it heals with rest (Fig. 8-188).

In children between the ages of 3 and 5 years, a spiral or oblique fracture of the mid- or distal tibia may occur. It is usually referred to as a toddler's fracture. Sometimes a history of twisting the leg or jumping off a chair is found, but often these injuries are found in children who simply refuse to bear weight on the extremity. If this particular entity is suspected, AP, lateral, and oblique views of the tibia should be obtained (Fig. 8-189).

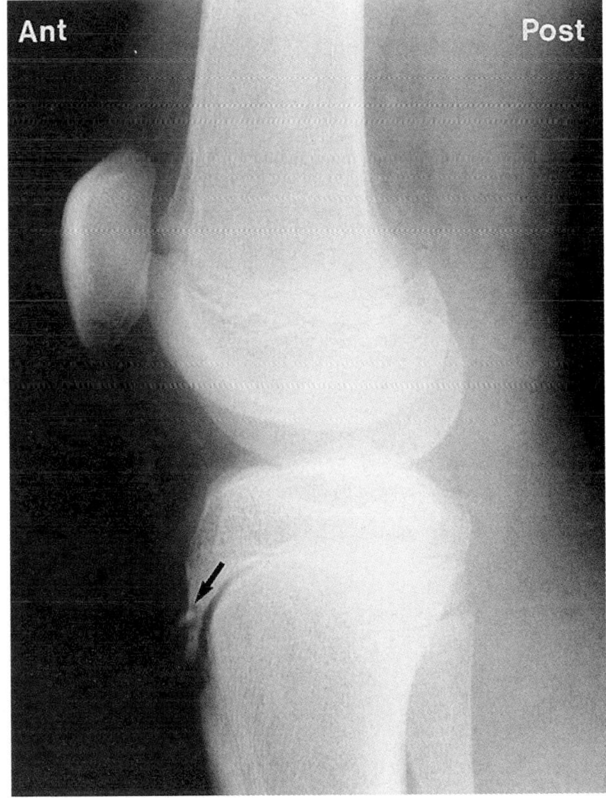

FIGURE 8-188 ▪ Osgood-Schlatter disease. A lateral view of the knee demonstrates a tiny avulsion fracture of the anterior tibial tuberosity in this young male athlete. This disease is quite common and usually is self-limited.

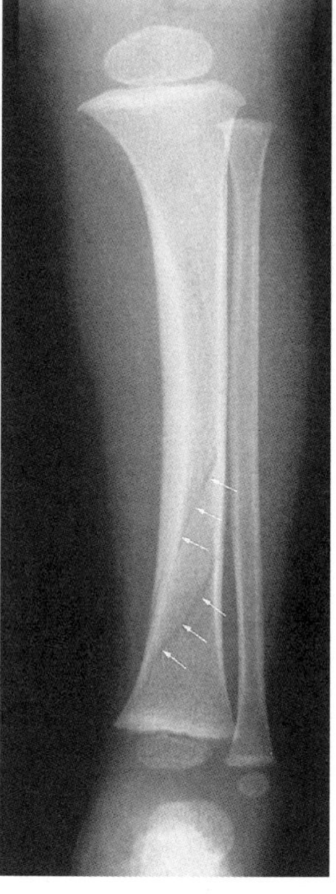

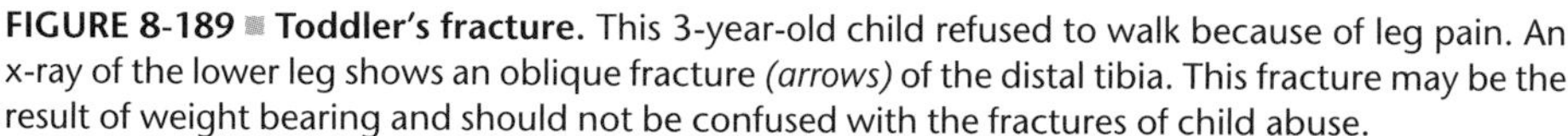

FIGURE 8-189 ■ Toddler's fracture. This 3-year-old child refused to walk because of leg pain. An x-ray of the lower leg shows an oblique fracture *(arrows)* of the distal tibia. This fracture may be the result of weight bearing and should not be confused with the fractures of child abuse.

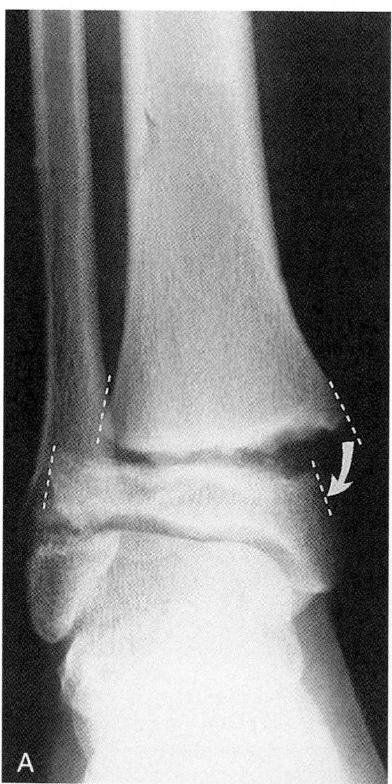

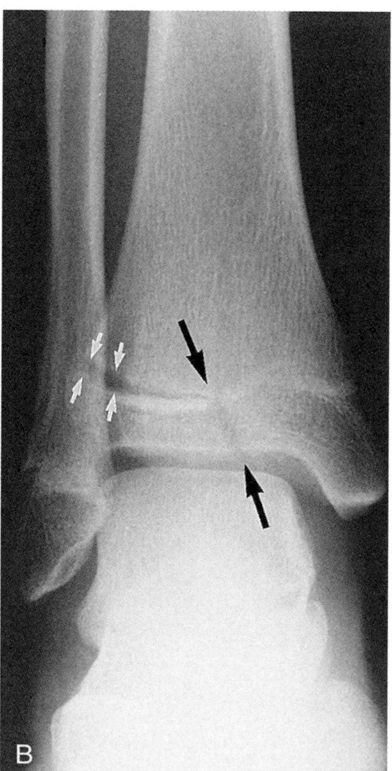

FIGURE 8-190 ■ Salter-Harris fractures of the ankle. *A,* A Salter type I fracture is seen with marked lateral displacement of the epiphysis relative to the tibial metaphysis. *B,* A Salter type III fracture of the lateral tibial epiphysis. This also is called a Tillaux fracture and probably occurs because the growth plate fuses from medial to lateral, making the medial side stronger.

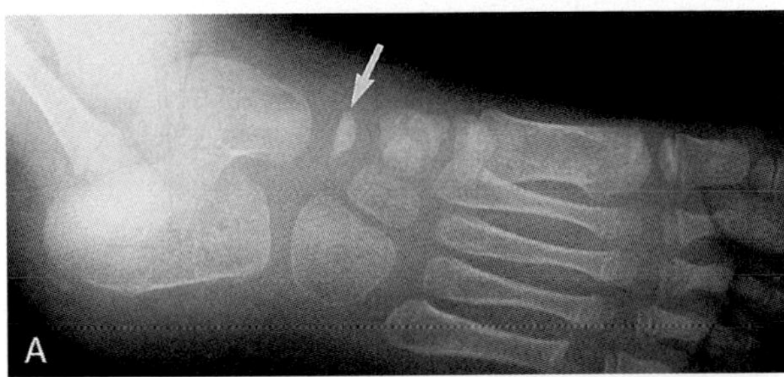

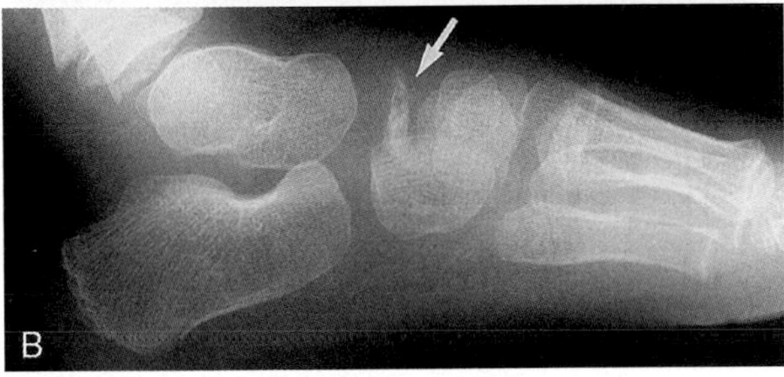

FIGURE 8-191 ■ **Aseptic necrosis of the tarsal navicular.** This usually occurs between the ages of 4 and 8 years and most commonly is recognized incidentally. Increased density *(A)* or irregularity *(B)* of the tarsal navicular may be found. This also is called Kohler's osteonecrosis. The abnormality is almost always self-limited and requires no therapy.

Salter Harris–type fractures are common in the ankle. As mentioned in the discussion of the wrist, the Salter-Harris type I fractures may not be displaced and may be seen only as increased density about the epiphyseal plate 1 or 2 weeks after the injury. If significant displacement and disruption of the epiphyseal plate is found, the diagnosis is usually not a problem. Sometimes even a Salter-Harris type III fracture can be subtle (Fig. 8-190). The fractures with the worst prognosis are the impacted Salter-Harris type V (see Fig. 8-81).

Occasionally, in a patient who has a history of foot trauma or pain, you may notice irregularity and increased density or sclerosis of the tarsal navicular (Fig. 8-191). This is referred to as Kohler's disease. Whether this condition is a result of trauma or aseptic necrosis is uncertain; it is often seen incidentally in a child with a twisted ankle. The patient occasionally may have pain over the navicular. This condition essentially always heals without any intervention. For some reason, the other tarsal bones are rarely, if ever, involved in this process. You should almost regard this finding as a normal variant.

Suggested Textbooks on the Topic

El-Khoury GY, Bennett L, Stanley M: Essentials in Musculoskeletal Imaging. Philadelphia, WB Saunders, 2003.

Kaplan P, Helms CA, Dussault RD, Anderson M, Major N: Musculoskeletal MRI. Philadelphia, WB Saunders, 2001.

Resnick D: Diagnosis of Bone and Joint Disorders, 4th ed. Philadelphia, WB Saunders, 2002.

Rogers LF: Radiology of Skeletal Trauma, 3rd ed. Philadelphia, WB Saunders, 2002.

9 Nonskeletal Pediatric Imaging

Pediatric musculoskeletal imaging of bone was covered in a special section at the end of Chapter 8. Congenital cardiac lesions were covered in Chapter 5. This chapter discusses imaging techniques, and Table 9-1 shows the appropriate imaging test for common pediatric problems.

HEAD

Imaging Techniques

Imaging of the fetal and infant brain can be done by using ultrasound as long as the fontanels remain open. Structures that can normally be visualized include the lateral ventricles, choroid plexus, thalamus, temporal lobes, and posterior fossa (Fig. 9-1). The two most common indications for ultrasound of baby heads are (1) evaluation of ventricular enlargement (hydrocephalus) and (2) hemorrhage either within the parenchyma of the brain or within the ventricles (Fig. 9-2). The major advantages of ultrasound in this application are that the imaging can be done in the neonatal intensive care unit and that ionizing radiation is not used. This is important, because these studies are repeated multiple times for continuing evaluation. If the fontanels are closed, computed tomography (CT) is usually used for evaluation of suspected hydrocephalus or hemorrhage.

Brain tumors in children are evaluated by CT or magnetic resonance imaging (MRI). With MRI, sedation is necessary, and pediatric monitoring of respiration and other functions in a very high magnetic field is difficult. CT scanning is easier to perform. About half of brain tumors in children are astrocytomas; medulloblastomas (20%), ependymomas (10%), and craniopharyngiomas (5% percent) are less common.

Childhood Seizures

Seizures may be provoked by infection, trauma, toxins, metabolic abnormality, tumor, hypoxia, cerebrovascular disease, cerebral malformation, or congenital abnormality. They also may occur without obvious cause. Febrile seizures usually occur between the ages of 6 months and 4 years, and most are generalized tonic/clonic seizures. Imaging is recommended for children with new-onset seizures who have experienced head trauma or partial seizures and for those who have an abnormal neurologic examination or an abnormal electroencephalogram. Imaging is not necessary for uncomplicated febrile seizures or in a patient with an obvious provoking cause. MRI is the usual imaging modality of choice, although noncontrasted CT is used initially if intracranial hemorrhage or recent trauma is suspected. For those children with a history of seizures, imaging usually is done only if the seizures are poorly controlled or are associated with a new neurologic deficit, or to follow up known abnormalities such as a tumor.

TABLE 9-1 ■ **Imaging of Pediatric Problems**

Suspected Problems	Imaging Test of Choice
Neonatal hydrocephalus or intracranial hemorrhage	Cranial ultrasound
Uncomplicated febrile seizure	No imaging needed
Seizure (neurologic deficit, partially unresponsive to therapy, new without obvious provoking factor)	MRI
Seizure (post-trauma)	Noncontrast CT
Croup or epiglottitis	Lateral soft tissue view of neck
Suspected inhaled foreign body	Inspiration/expiration or decubitus chest
Difficulty breathing	Chest x-ray
Esophageal atresia or tracheoesophageal fistula	Lateral radiograph with soft feeding tube in place
Asthma (uncomplicated)	No imaging needed
Asthma (poor response to therapy, complicated)	Chest x-ray
Suspected pneumonia	Chest x-ray
Congenital heart disease or congestive heart failure	Chest x-ray, echocardiogram
Gastroesophageal reflux	Barium swallow or nuclear medicine reflux study
Pyloric stenosis	Ultrasound
Duodenal atresia, stenosis, or midgut volvulus	Plain x-ray (use air as contrast)
Meconium ileus	Plain x-ray and Gastrografin enema
Appendicitis	Plain x-ray followed by ultrasound or CT
Intussusception	Plain x-ray followed by reduction using air or Gastrografin enema
Necrotizing enterocolitis	Plain x-ray of the abdomen and possible left lateral decubitus views (to look for free air)
Hirschsprung's disease	Barium or Gastrografin enema
Biliary atresia or neonatal hepatitis	Nuclear medicine hepatobiliary scan
Abdominal mass	Plain x-ray of abdomen and ultrasound or CT
Meckel's diverticulum	Nuclear medicine Meckel's scan
Rectal bleeding	See text
Child abuse	X-ray bone survey and possibly nuclear medicine bone scan
Osteomyelitis, cellulitis, or septic arthritis	Plain x-ray, MRI or three-phase nuclear medicine bone scan

CT, computed tomography; MRI, magnetic resonance imaging.

NECK

Croup and Epiglottitis

Lateral soft tissue views of the neck are often done for evaluation of the pediatric airway. This is important in cases of suspected croup or epiglottitis. As you evaluate these lateral images, you should look to see that the child's neck has been extended. In a young child, when the neck is flexed, the trachea can buckle forward, causing the appearance of a retropharyngeal mass. To avoid this artifact, simply extend the neck and lift the chin (Fig. 9-3).

Acute epiglottitis usually occurs in older children (between ages 2 years and 7 years) and most commonly is due to *Haemophilus influenzae*. This can be a life-threatening disease, and the clinical findings are severe sore throat, high fever, a muffled voice, and stridor. The patients often can breathe more easily sitting up, and they drool because they cannot swallow. This is a true pediatric emergency. Because intubation can be necessary on very short notice, a physician should accompany the child to the x-ray department. The lateral soft tissue view of the neck shows a thickened epiglottis, often appearing bulbous (in the shape of a thumb) (Fig. 9-4). Remember that the normal epiglottis is a delicate, thin, curved structure. Other findings include ballooning of the hypopharynx and subglottic edema in about one fourth of cases.

Croup typically occurs in young children (between ages 6 months and 3 years), and it usually has a respiratory syncytial viral (RSV) origin. The children often have a brassy cough (like the barking of a seal) and inspiratory stridor.

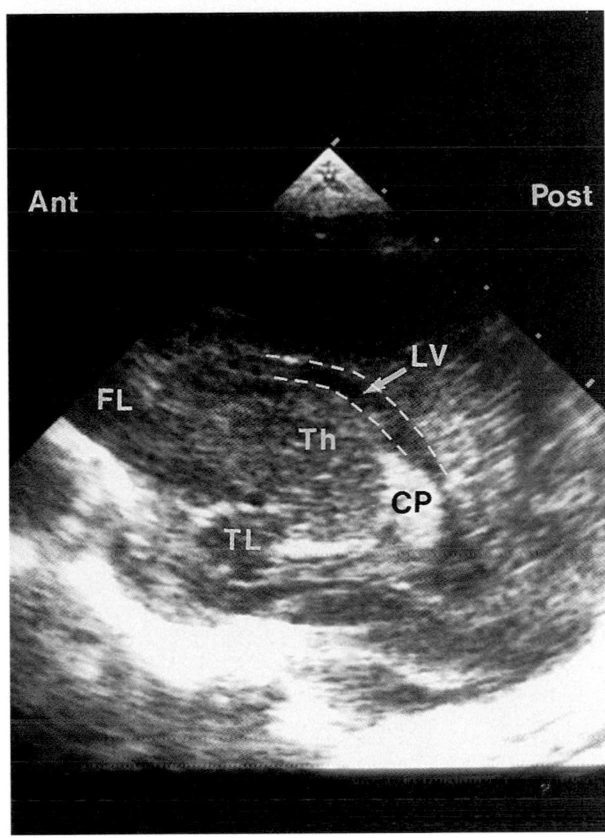

FIGURE 9-1 ■ Ultrasound of normal neonatal head. A sagittal view obtained through an open fontanel clearly shows the frontal lobe, lateral ventricle (LV), thalamus (Th), temporal lobe (TL), and choroid plexus (CP).

Occasionally the airway may have enough edema that placement of an artificial airway is necessary. The findings on the lateral view are marked ballooning of the pharynx and hypopharynx. On the anteroposterior (AP) view, the upper portion of the trachea is shaped like a steeple (Fig. 9-5). The "steeple sign," caused by subglottic edema, is not pathopneumonic, because it also can occur in some children who have epiglottitis.

CHEST

Normal Anatomy and Imaging

One of the major differences between the normal chest of an adult or child and a neonate is

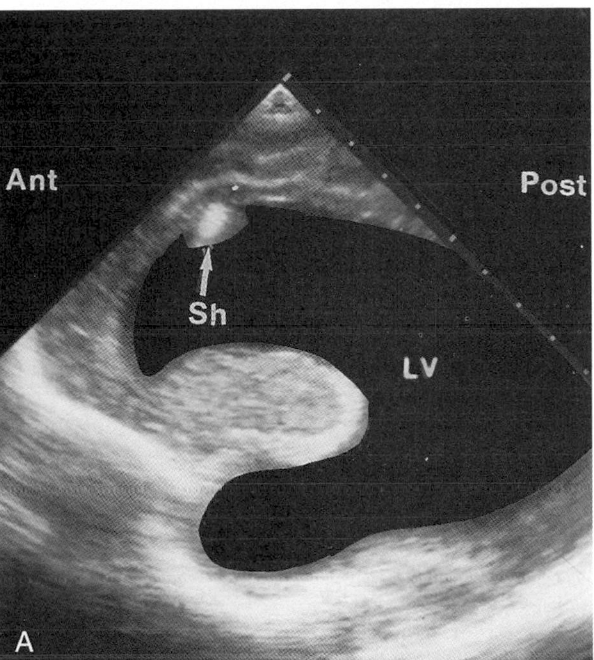

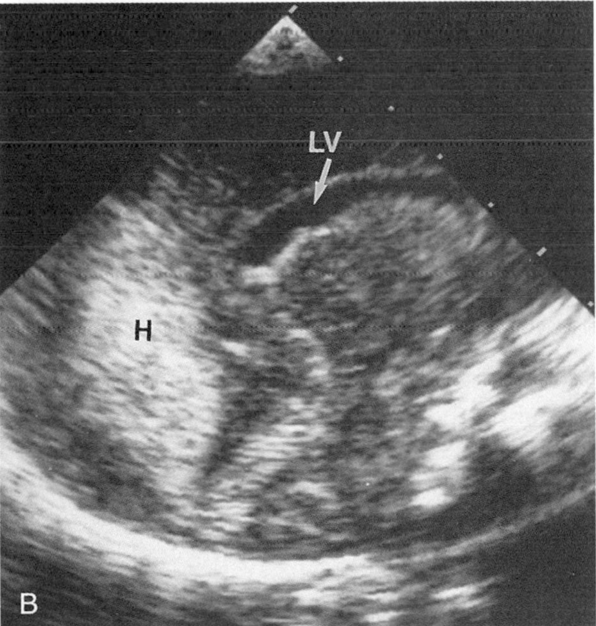

FIGURE 9-2 ■ Ultrasound of abnormal neonatal head. *A,* Sagittal view of the brain in a neonate with hydrocephalus. A dilated lateral ventricle (LV) is seen as well as the shunt (Sh) catheter. *B,* Intraparenchymal hemorrhage. A sagittal view of the brain in a different infant shows a normal-sized lateral ventricle but an area of increased echoes representing hemorrhage (H) within the substance of the brain.

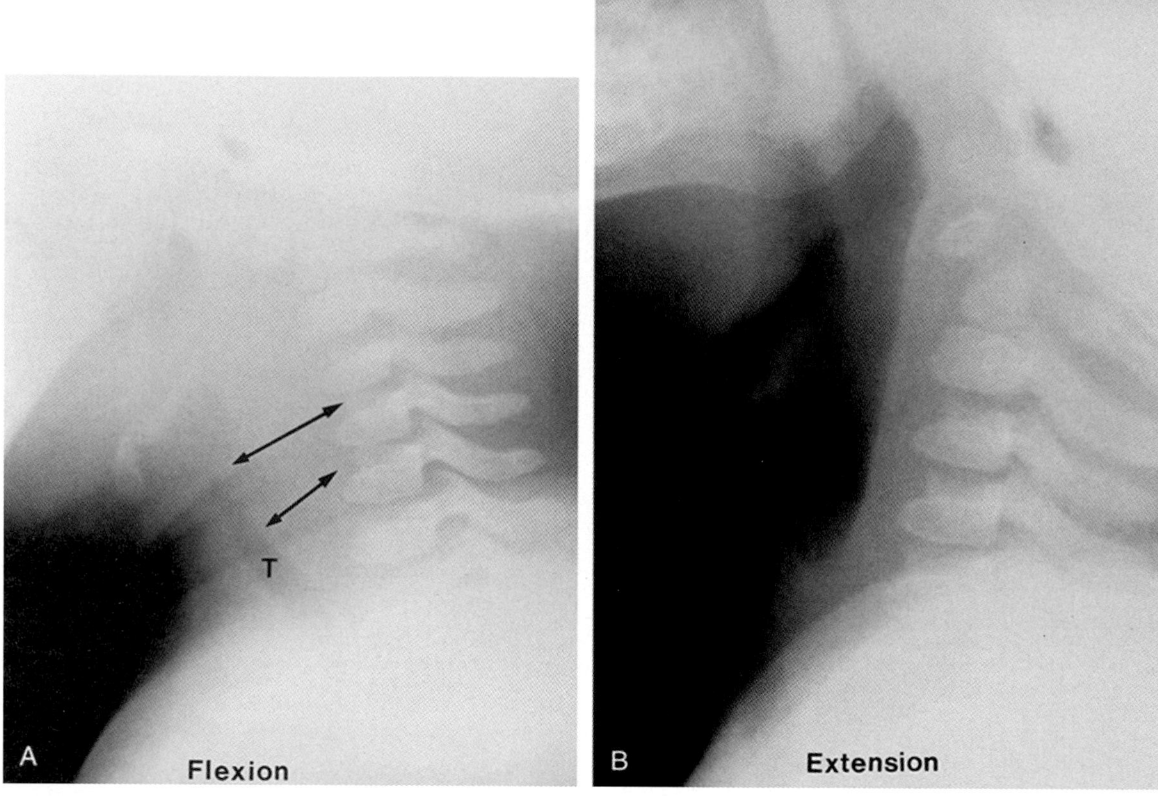

FIGURE 9-3 ■ **Pseudoretropharyngeal abscess.** *A,* Lateral soft tissue view of the neck in a child with the neck slightly flexed shows the trachea (T) bowed forward, which suggests that a retropharyngeal soft tissue mass is present *(arrows)*. *B,* A lateral view taken a few minutes later of the same child with the neck extended shows a normal prevertebral soft tissue pattern.

the presence of the thymus. It is routinely identified on chest x-rays from birth to approximately age 2 years. The thymus is usually seen as a widening of the soft tissues of the upper mediastinum, although occasionally it may appear to project out into the lung (the "sail sign") (Fig. 9-6). Some people mistakenly think that the "sail sign" is an indication that a pneumothorax is present. This is not true.

Imaging of the chest in infants and children can be difficult because of their uncooperative nature, especially when they are sick. In neonates, portable x-rays are usually obtained in the intensive care unit in a supine anteroposterior (AP) projection. Somewhat older children can be placed in a holder or restrained with Velcro straps while an image is obtained. In most of these instances, the image is taken randomly with respect to inspiration and expiration. Amazingly enough, hypoinflation of the chest is usually not a problem in interpretation of pediatric chest x-rays.

Most children with pneumonias, bronchiolitis, or reactive airway disease have hyperinflation. In most normal young children, the most superior portion of the hemidiaphragm is at the level of the posterior eighth rib. If the diaphragms are lower than this, hyperinflation should be considered, and pathology may well be present. Rotation of the patient can cause problems in interpretation. As the patient is rotated to the left, the right cardiac border projects over the spine, and the right lower lobe pulmonary vessels are indistinct and can mimic an infiltrate (Fig. 9-7).

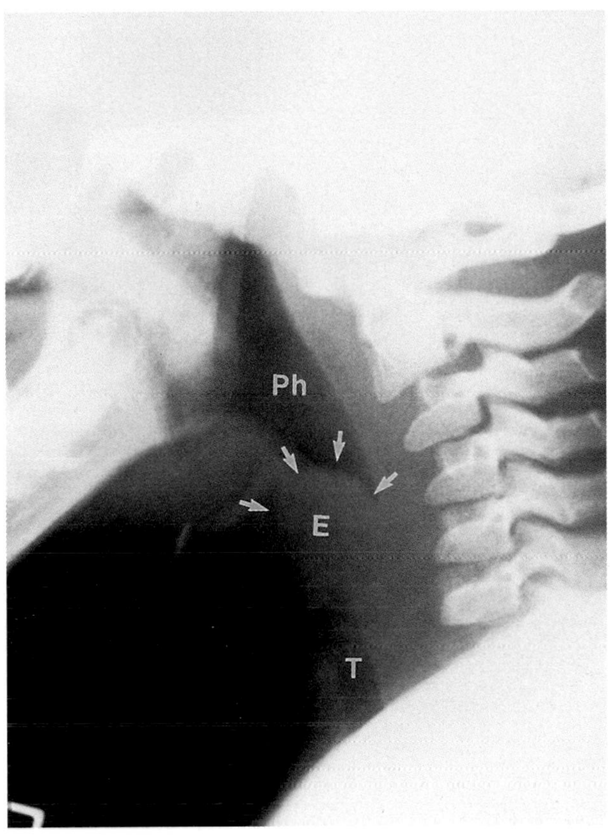

FIGURE 9-4 ■ **Epiglottitis.** A lateral soft tissue view of the neck shows a ballooned pharynx (Ph) with a swollen epiglottis (E) in the shape of a large thumbprint *(arrows)*.

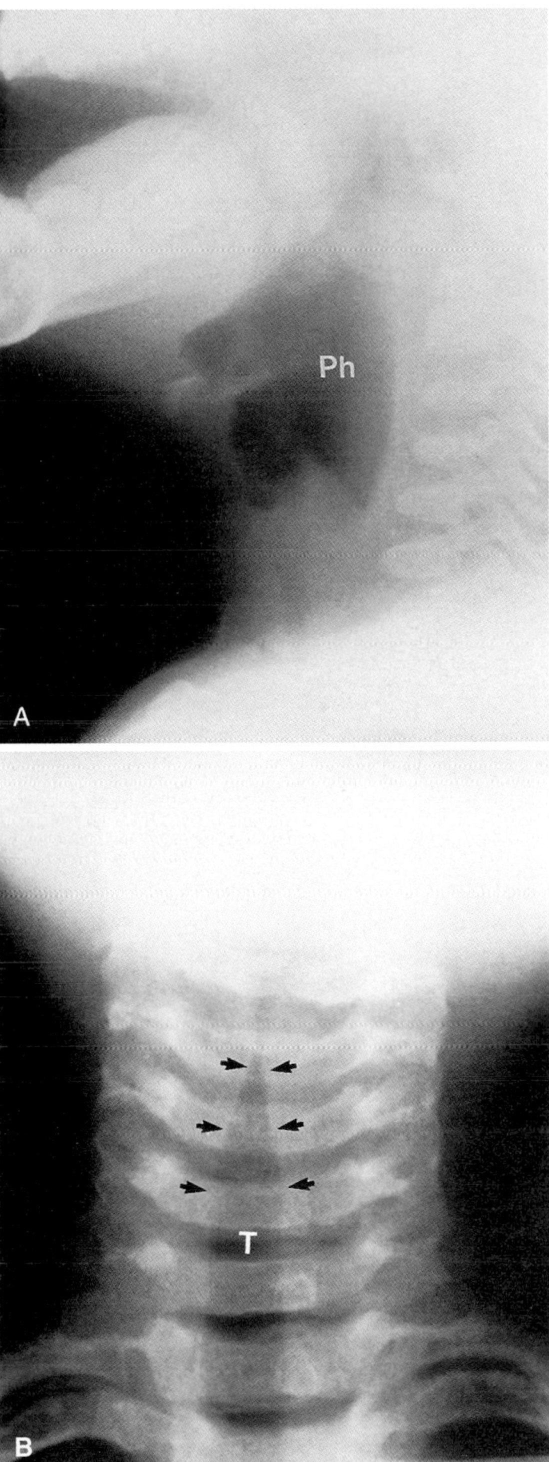

FIGURE 9-5 ■ **Croup.** In a child with a "barking" cough, a lateral soft tissue view of the neck *(A)* demonstrates a markedly ballooned pharynx (Ph). *(B)* An anteroposterior (AP) view of the neck shows a steeple-shaped trachea (T) *(arrows)* caused by subglottic edema.

A favorite x-ray examination is the "babygram." This is an AP view of both the chest and the abdomen. In very small babies, the x-ray exposure can be adequate to visualize pulmonary vasculature, bowel gas, and skeletal structures. Conversely, if you are interested only in the chest, a chest x-ray is what you should order to avoid unnecessary radiation exposure.

Foreign Bodies

Foreign bodies can be either aspirated or ingested. Most foreign bodies consist of vegetable material (such as peanuts) or plastic. Remember that vegetable and plastic items are usually not visible on a plain x-ray. When a foreign body is aspirated into a bronchus, two possibilities exist. The first is that the object will

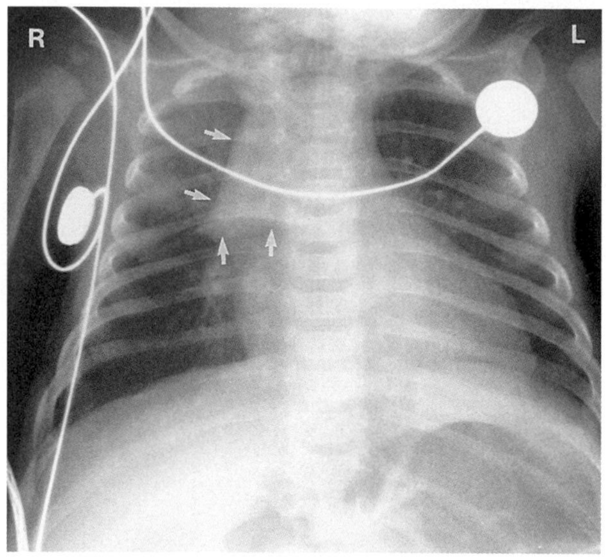

FIGURE 9-6 ■ Normal thymic shadow. A posteroanterior (PA) view of the chest shows a very prominent thymic shadow *(arrows)*. Sometimes referred to as the sail sign, this is a normal finding.

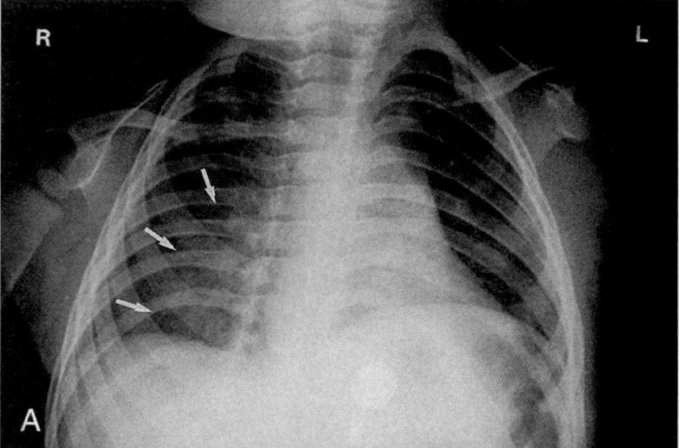

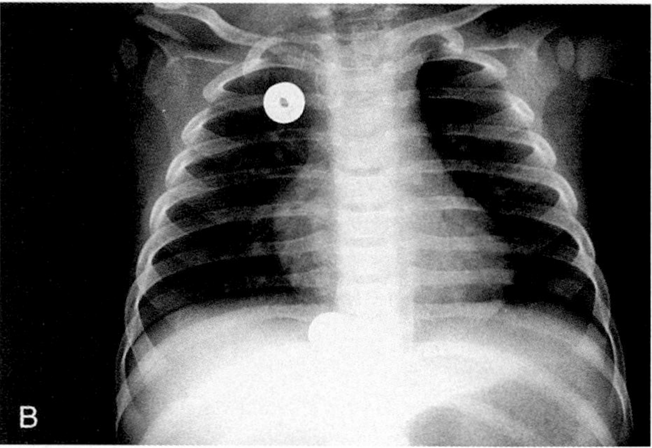

FIGURE 9-7 ■ Pseudoinfiltrate due to poor positioning. A, An anteroposterior (AP) view of the chest was obtained but is slightly rotated. This throws the heart shadow to the left and makes the right pulmonary vascularity appear prominent, creating the impression of a right middle or lower lobe infiltrate *(arrows)*. B, A repeated view obtained on the same infant within 10 min shows that the chest is perfectly normal.

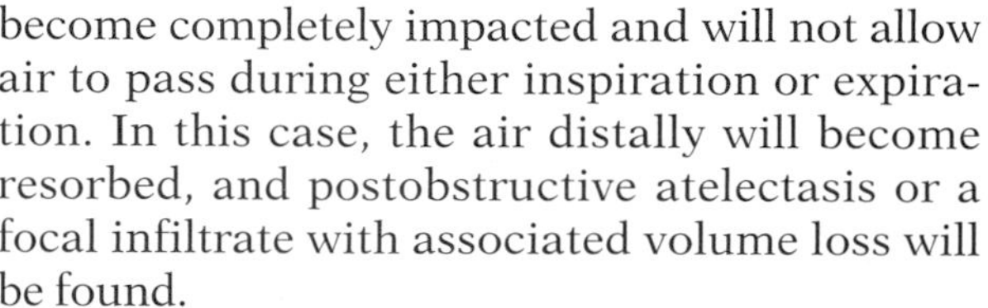

become completely impacted and will not allow air to pass during either inspiration or expiration. In this case, the air distally will become resorbed, and postobstructive atelectasis or a focal infiltrate with associated volume loss will be found.

The second possibility is that the object is only incompletely obstructing the bronchus. This occurs because, during inspiration, the bronchus becomes larger in diameter, and air can pass around the object. During expiration, the bronchus becomes narrower due to pressure in the lung, and the air distal to the object cannot escape. The object acts as a ball-valve. Thus if you are suspicious of the presence of an inhaled foreign body, be sure to order an inspiration and an expiration image. On the inspiration film, you may see postobstructive atelectasis, or the chest x-ray may be normal. If the chest is normal, a ball-valve phenomenon may still exist, and on the expiration view, air will be trapped on the affected side, whereas the unaffected lung will decrease in volume. When this happens, a resultant shift of the mediastinum toward the normal unaffected side will be seen (Fig. 9-8).

Swallowed objects may be caught within the esophagus. In children, the objects that are large enough to remain in the esophagus are typically coins. These may be lodged at the level of the thoracic inlet, or they may sit in the esophagus just above the level of the aortic arch (Fig. 9-9). Another common foreign object that may lodge in either the hypopharynx or the esophagus is a fish bone or chicken bone. Chicken bones may be visualized on plain x-rays, but most fish

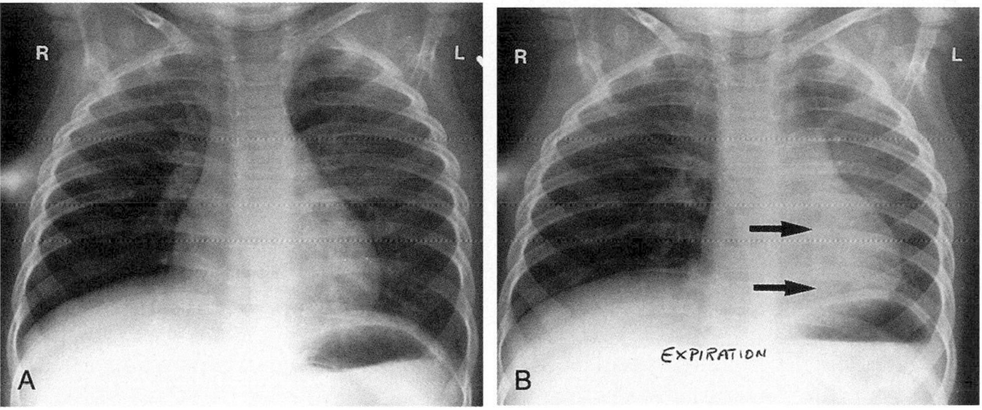

FIGURE 9-8 ■ **Foreign body in right main-stem bronchus.** *A,* An inspiration view of the chest looks essentially normal. *B,* An expiration view shows that the left lung has decreased in volume (as expected) but that a shift of the heart to the left has occurred. The right lung remains hyperinflated due to the inability of the air to escape the ball/valve phenomenon caused by the foreign body.

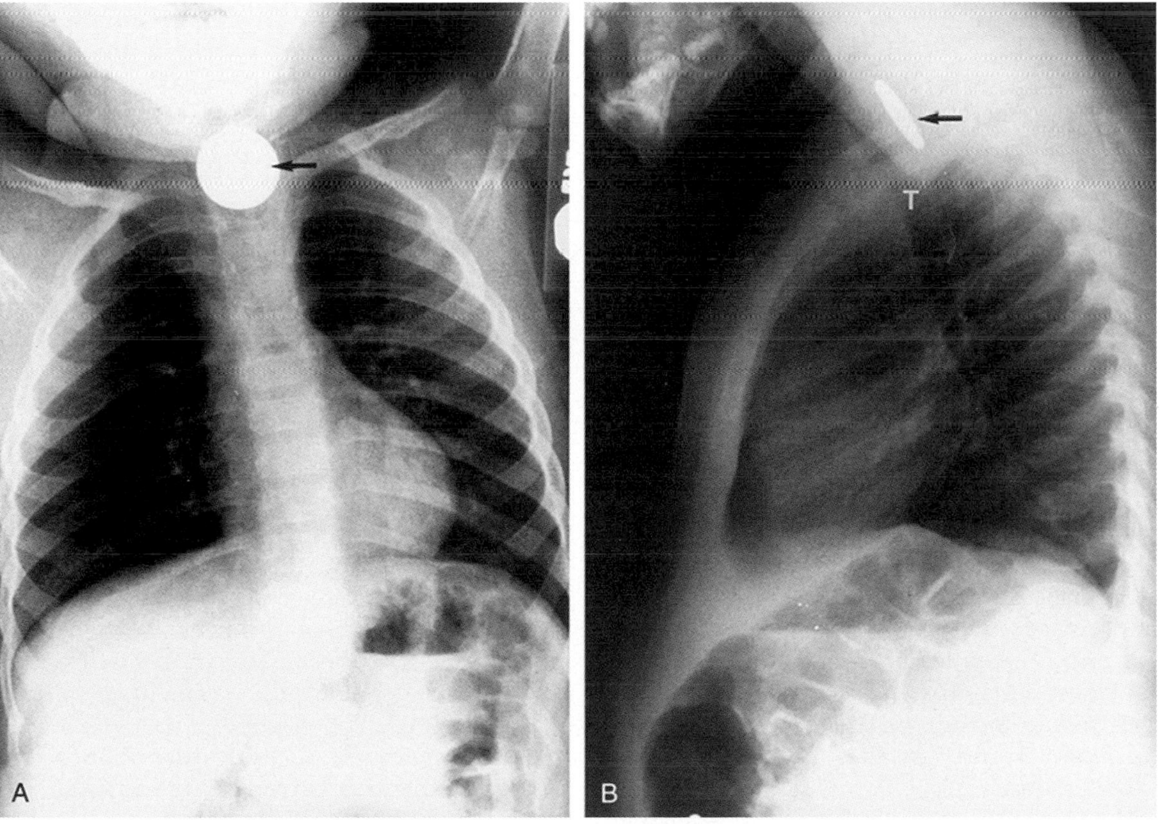

FIGURE 9-9 ■ **Coin in the esophagus.** *A,* A posteroanterior (PA) view of the chest demonstrates a quarter *(arrow)* that is lodged in the esophagus just at the thoracic inlet. *B,* The lateral view also shows the coin behind the trachea in the esophagus.

bones are composed of cartilage and are essentially invisible.

Tubes and Lines

A discussion of central venous catheters, jugular catheters, and pleural tubes has been included in Chapter 3. The tubes and catheters that are of specific interest in children are endotracheal tubes and umbilical artery and vein catheters. The tip of an endotracheal tube should be at least as far down as the level of the medial clavicles or at the level of the vertebral body of T1 or T2. The endotracheal tube also should have its tip located 1 or 2 cm proximal to the carina. If the carina cannot be easily visualized, you should remember that on an AP or a posteroanterior (PA) chest x-ray, a tube with its tip projecting over the vertebral body of T5 is probably too low. Endotracheal tubes that are too low usually will go down the right main-stem bronchus, because this is more vertical in orientation than the left main-stem bronchus. Initially, an endotracheal tube positioned in the right main-stem bronchus may demonstrate a relatively normal-appearing lung. With time, however, selective obstruction of the right upper lobe bronchus will cause right upper lobe atelectasis with progressive collapse (Fig. 9-10) or generalized left lung collapse.

Umbilical artery and vein catheters are easily differentiated on the lateral view of the abdomen and chest. The umbilical artery catheter (UAC) proceeds inferiorly from the umbilicus down into the pelvis and then turns and comes up the aorta (Fig. 9-11). Usually the tip of a UAC is positioned at approximately the level of the vertebral body of T8. If a UAC is advanced too far, it can proceed up into the great vessels of the head and neck or go anteriorly in the aortic arch. An umbilical vein catheter (UVC) also is best identified on the lateral view. It can be seen progressing immediately superiorly from the umbilicus and then posteriorly along the liver and into the inferior vena cava and right atrium.

If both a UAC and a UVC are present on an AP view, it is not often easy to tell them apart, especially because you will be seeing the portions of the catheters that are inside and outside the baby. What you should do is imagine where the umbilicus should be. A catheter that goes straight up and slightly to the right of the midline is a UVC, and one that goes down toward the pelvis and then toward the head is a UAC.

Another catheter that can sometimes be confusing is a ventriculoperitoneal shunt catheter. These shunts, which are placed for relief of hydrocephalus, extend from the lateral ventricle of the brain down along the soft tissues of the neck and anterior chest wall and then into the peritoneal cavity (Fig. 9-12). Less commonly, the distal shunt tip may be placed in the region of the right atrium.

Respiratory Disease in the Newborn

A number of entities can cause neonatal respiratory difficulty (Table 9-2). You should be able to recognize a congenital diaphragmatic hernia, because it is a cause of respiratory distress in the neonatal period, and it carries a mortality rate well in excess of 50%. Clinical manifestations are a scaphoid abdomen and bowel sounds in the chest. Cyanosis due to pulmonary hypoplasia and pulmonary hypertension also may be present. These hernias occur more commonly on the left and will displace the heart and tracheal structures to the right. An opacity within the chest often has visible bowel or at least air-filled spaces within it (Fig. 9-13).

At birth, meconium aspiration can occur. Meconium is the term used for the first stool evacuated after birth, and it is composed of mucus, epithelial cells, bile, and debris. In fetal distress, evacuation of meconium into the amniotic fluid may occur. Only about 10% of the time does this cause respiratory problems. At birth, as a result of this, coarse patchy infiltrates as well as hyperinflation of the lungs may be found, which clears in about 3 to 5 days. Pneumothorax or pneumomediastinum occurs in about 25% of cases.

Another cause of respiratory distress within 48 hours of birth is transient tachypnea of the newborn (TTN). Lung volumes may be larger than normal, and there may be linear or streaky opacities that usually clear within 2 days. TTN is

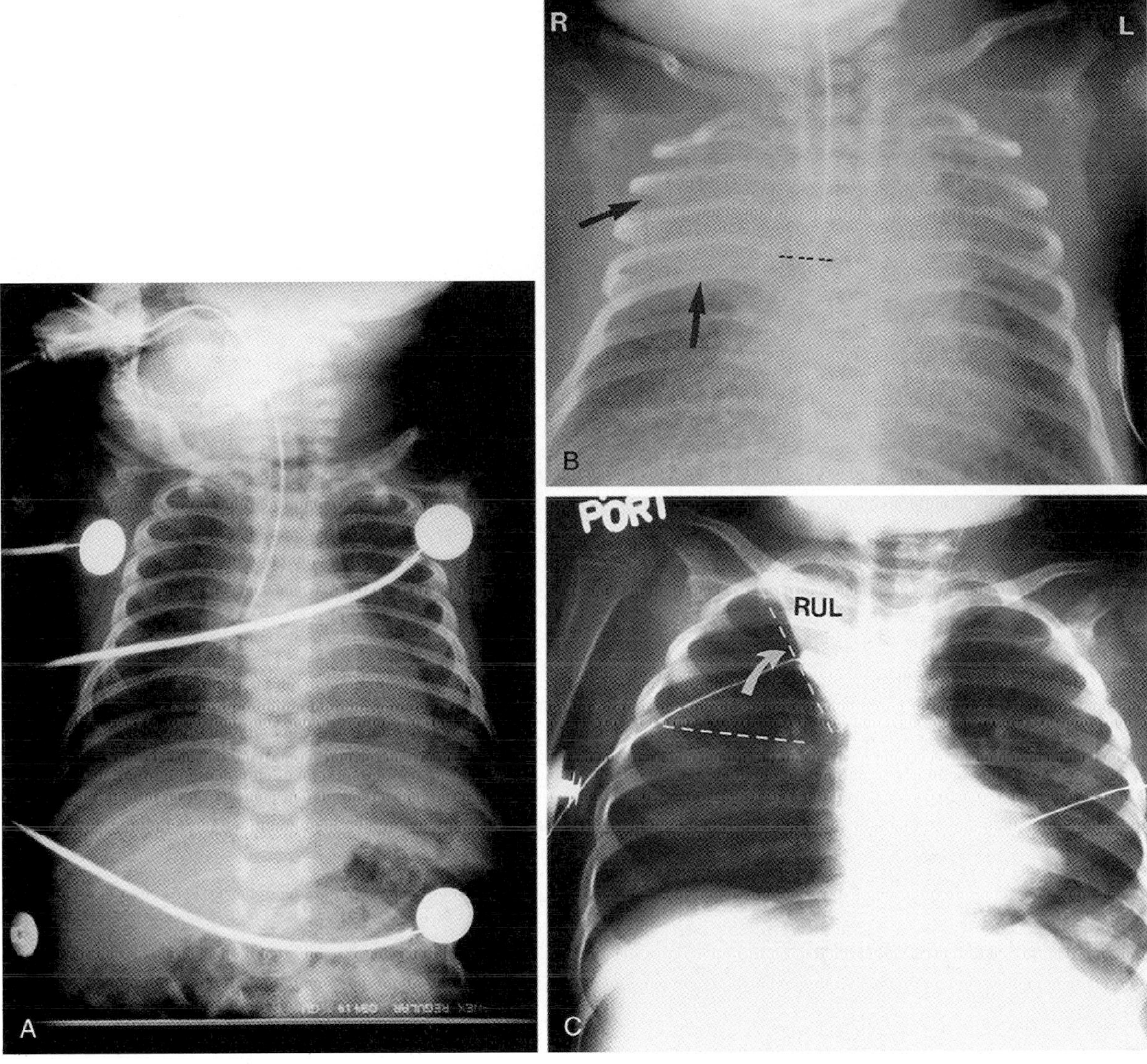

FIGURE 9-10 ■ Progressive right upper lobe atelectasis. *A,* A posteroanterior (PA) view of the chest demonstrates an endotracheal tube with the tip down in the right main-stem bronchus. This will often obstruct the right upper lobe bronchus. *B,* Early atelectasis of the right upper lobe occurs with resorption of air, causing consolidation *(arrows)* and slight upward bowing of the minor fissure. C, As collapse of the right upper lobe becomes complete, the minor fissure rotates upward and medially, and the completely collapsed right upper lobe (RUL) remains as a small density along the right paratracheal region.

really a clinical and not a radiographic diagnosis; it is due to delayed resorption of intrauterine pulmonary liquid.

Hyaline membrane disease (HMD) is caused by surfactant deficiency and results in low lung volumes (unless the infant is intubated) and granular or ground-glass opacities of both lungs. Any opacity in the lungs of a premature infant should be considered to be HMD until another cause is established. Air bronchograms are often present, and, rarely, a pleural effusion is found. Hyaline membrane disease typically becomes

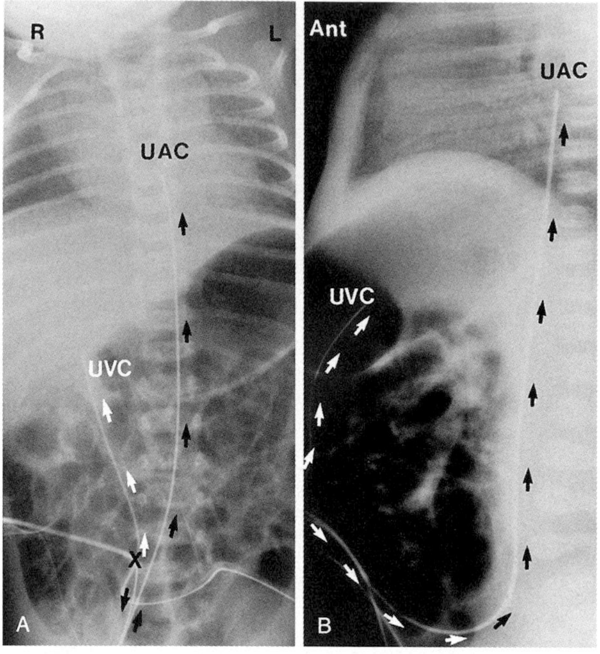

FIGURE 9-11 ■ Differentiation of umbilical artery from umbilical vein catheters. *A,* On the anteroposterior (AP) view babygram, if you imagine the position of the umbilicus (at the position of the X), the catheter, which initially goes inferiorly and then turns and goes superiorly just to the left of midline, is the umbilical artery catheter (UAC) *(black arrows).* A catheter that goes into the umbilical region and immediately progresses cephalad and slightly to the right of the midline *(white arrows)* is the umbilical vein catheter (UVC). *B,* A lateral view of the same infant demonstrates the inferior and then the posterior and superior course of the umbilical artery catheter, and the immediate superior course of the umbilical vein catheter progressing toward the inferior portion of the liver.

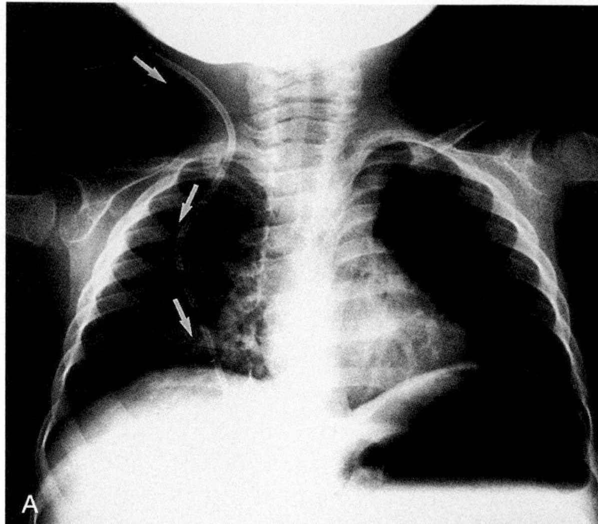

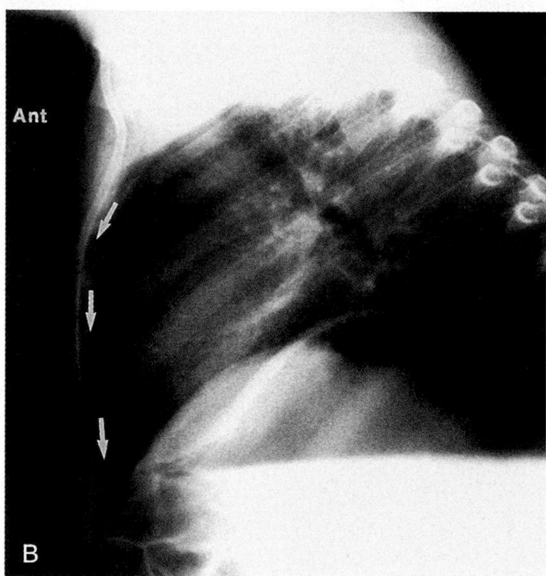

FIGURE 9-12 ■ Ventricular peritoneal shunt for hydrocephalus. *A,* An anteroposterior (AP) view of the chest shows a catheter coming down from the cervical region and progressing across the chest, but not in a pathway that would represent vascular or other mediastinal structures. *B,* The lateral view of the chest shows the catheter progressing along the anterior soft tissues down into the abdomen.

radiographically apparent at 4 to 6 hours after birth.

With HMD or pneumonia, infants may need positive-pressure ventilation. The complications of this respiratory therapy include pulmonary interstitial emphysema and bronchopulmonary dysplasia. Pulmonary interstitial emphysema (PIE) refers to accumulation of air outside of alveoli and in interstitial or perivascular spaces. The imaging features include tortuous linear lucencies that radiate outward from the hilum and may extend all the way to the periphery of the lung. If you look carefully, these do not resemble the pattern of a typical bronchial tree but are more tortuous (Fig. 9-14). You should be able to recognize PIE, because it may rapidly result in life-threatening complications, such as pneumothorax, pneumomediastinum, or pneumopericardium (Fig. 9-15).

Because the AP chest x-rays of newborns or neonates are usually obtained with the infant in

TABLE 9-2 ■ **X-ray Findings of Respiratory Distress in the Newborn**

Entity	Time	Lung Volume	Lung Findings
Diaphragmatic hernia	At birth	Compressed	Bowel in chest
Meconium aspiration	At birth	Increased	Coarse, patchy infiltrates
Transient tachypnea	0–2 days	Normal or increased	Homogeneous diffuse or linear infiltrates
Hyaline membrane disease	0–7 days	Decreased*	Granular infiltrates
Neonatal pneumonia	Variable	Variable	Granular or patchy infiltrates
Pneumothorax	Variable	Decreased	Lucent dark area at lung edge†

* Can be increased if the patient is on positive-pressure ventilation (PEEP).
† Pneumothorax is much more common in children who are on PEEP.
Look carefully for a basilar, medial, or anterior pneumothorax, because the films are usually done supine.

a supine position, a pneumothorax may be difficult to appreciate. This is because the air is usually located anteriorly (and not superiorly or laterally) in the pleural space. You may be able to see lucencies either at the base of the lung or along the medial aspect of the lung. Often a lateral projection taken with the child lying on the back is necessary to show you the (anterior) pneumothorax (Fig. 9-16).

Bronchopulmonary dysplasia (BPD) is thought to be the result of oxygen toxicity or barotrauma associated with respiratory therapy. BPD usually progresses as either HMD or neonatal pneumonia is resolving. BPD is usually seen progressing from approximately 1 week to 1 month of life. The lungs typically become hyperinflated, although they may have diffuse opacity

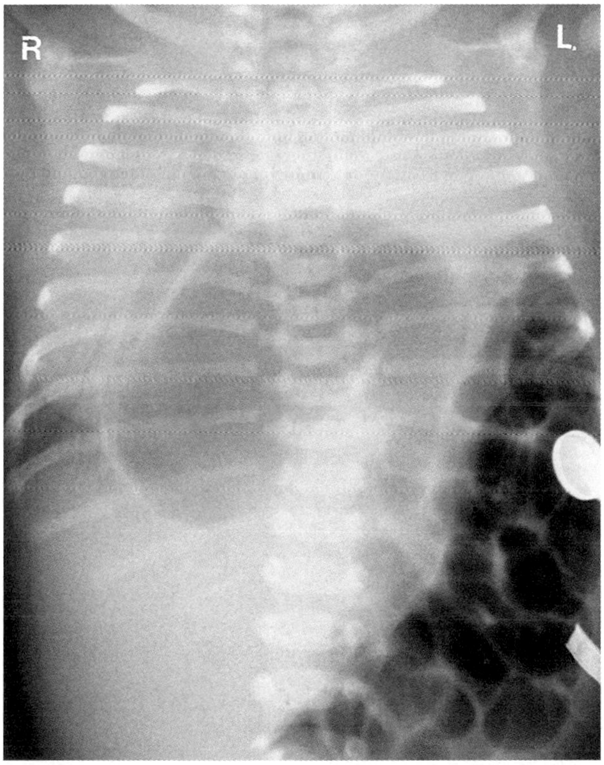

FIGURE 9-13 ■ **Diaphragmatic hernia.** This newborn had significant respiratory difficulty. An anteroposterior (AP) view of the chest and abdomen demonstrates opacification of the left hemithorax, with bowel loops pushing up into the opacified left hemithorax. This condition carries a high fatality rate and should be recognized immediately.

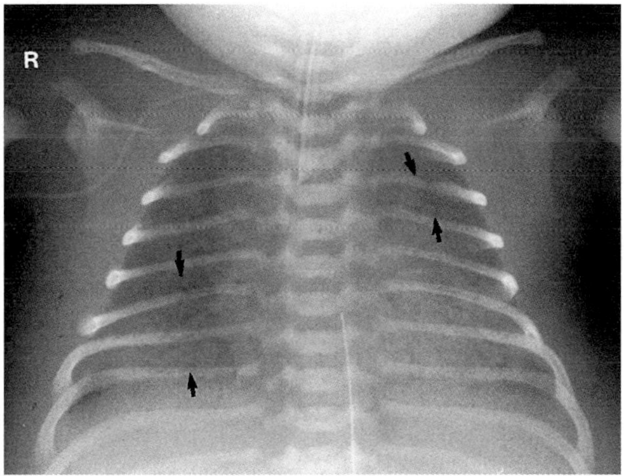

FIGURE 9-14 ■ **Pulmonary interstitial emphysema (PIE).** This anteroposterior (AP) view of the chest shows generalized opacification of both lungs in a child with hyaline membrane disease. The *arrows* indicate linear air collections that do not follow the normal branching bronchial pattern and represent air in the interstitium. These patients often quickly progress to having a pneumothorax.

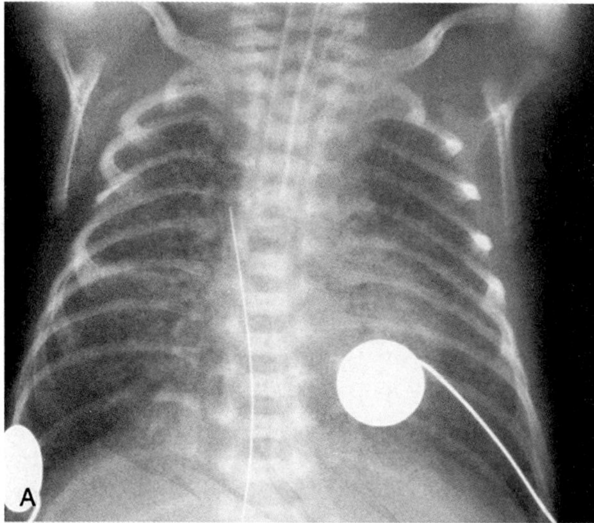

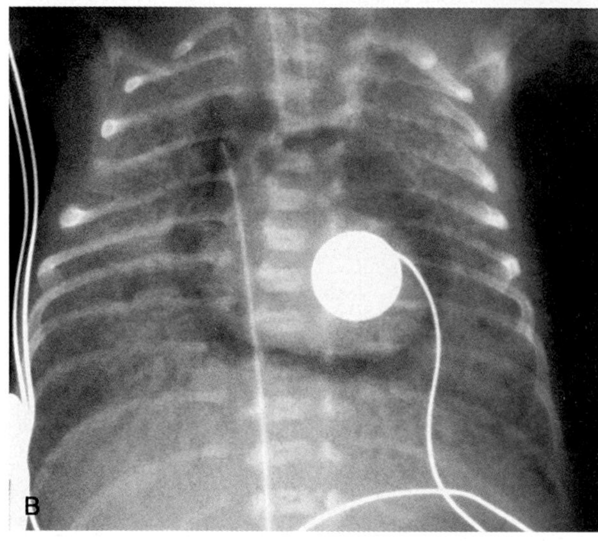

FIGURE 9-15 ■ Complications of hyaline membrane disease. *A,* Most patients with hyaline membrane disease have low lung volume and bilateral infiltrates. This patient is hyperinflated, with the diaphragms down to the level of the posterior tenth ribs because of the need for positive-pressure ventilation. *B,* A subsequent anteroposterior (AP) chest x-ray demonstrates development of a pneumopericardium, seen as a dark collection of air surrounding the heart.

with linear densities caused by fibrosis. Areas of rounded lucency may appear within the lung.

Bronchiolitis, Reactive Airway Disease, and Pneumonia

Neonatal pneumonia may result in a lung that is low in volume, normal, or hyperinflated. The lung opacities are typically granular, and the time course is variable. Neonatal pneumonias are due to transplacental infection (from toxoplasmosis, other [congenital syphilis and viruses], rubella, cytomegalovirus, herpes simplex virus [TORCH]) or from perineal flora acquired as a result of premature rupture of the membranes or while passing through the birth canal.

Very young children (from several weeks to 1 year of age) may have a viral pneumonia caused either by RSV or by *Haemophilus influenzae*. With these, the early stage is bronchiolitis. About 15% of children younger than 2 years will develop bronchiolitis and will initially have rhinorrhea, sneezing, cough, and low-grade fever followed by the rapid onset of tachypnea and wheezing. Most cases occur during winter and early spring. These patients will not have infiltrates on the chest x-ray, and hyperinflation is the only radiographic clue. Bronchiolitis most commonly is due to RSV. As these viral pneumonias progress, perihilar or peribronchial opacities also may develop. This can be seen as peribronchial cuffing or hilar adenopathy. Again, many of these patients show associated hyperinflation. The peribronchial cuffing can be seen by looking for an outline of a bronchus in the region of the hilum and noting that the bronchial wall is thicker than a line traced by a fine lead pencil.

As children get somewhat older (age 1 to 3 years), they develop bacterial pneumonias during this period. *Pneumococcus* is a common pathogen, whereas *Staphylococcus aureus* and *H. influenzae* are usually seen during infancy. Bacterial pneumonias typically cause alveolar infiltrates with lobar or segmental consolidations, often with effusion. Staphylococcal pneumonias may cause pneumothorax and also may cavitate. Most of the bacterial pneumonias have appearances similar to those already described for adults. The two exceptions are the cavitating staphylococcal pneumonias and, occasionally, what is termed a *round pneumonia*. A round pneumonia is usually a bacterial pneumonia in an early stage and later may develop into typical lobar consolidations (Fig. 9-17).

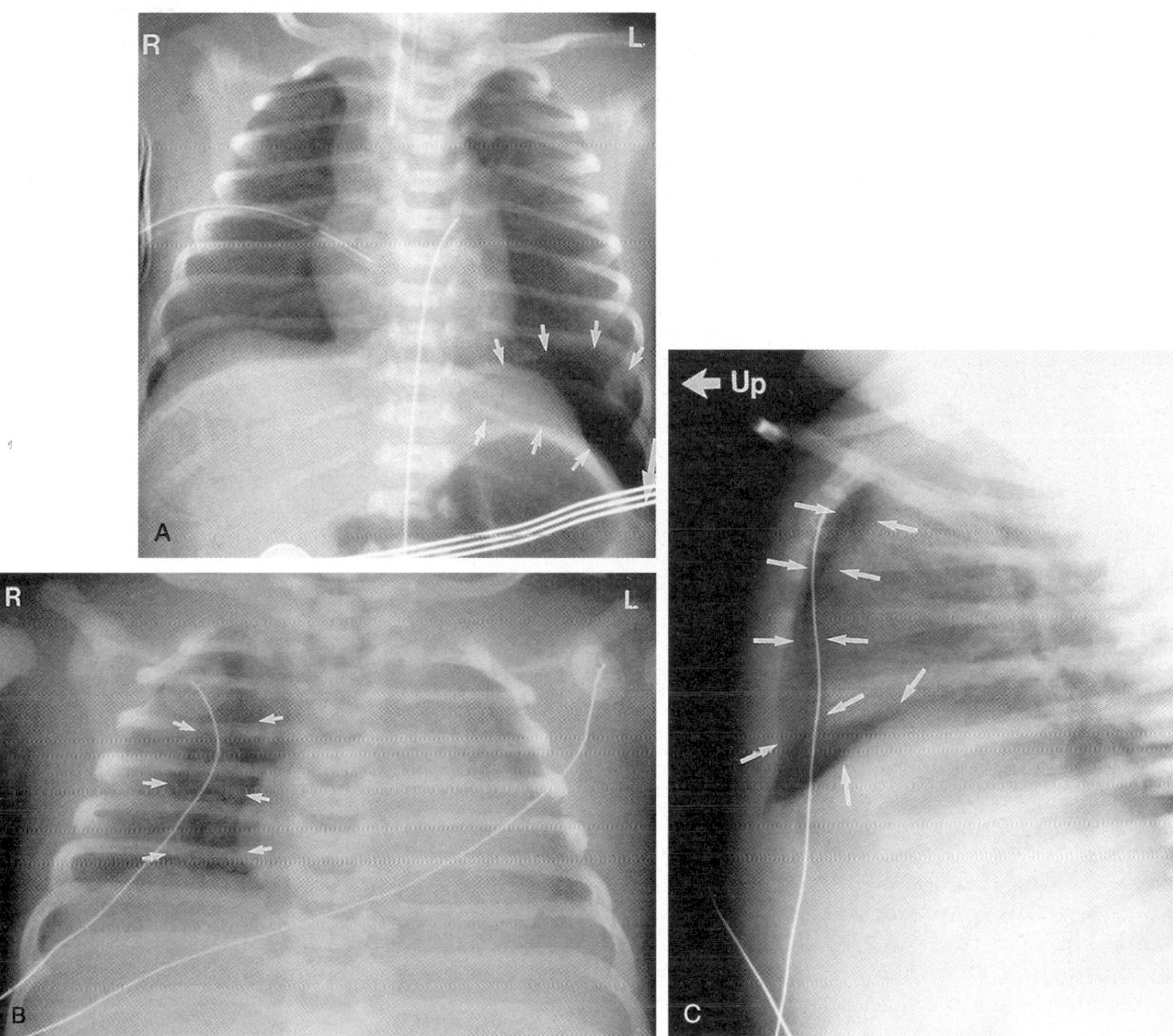

FIGURE 9-16 ■ Pneumothorax on supine chest x-ray *A,* In this infant, a right chest tube has already been placed because a pneumothorax is present. However, a lucency at the left lung base *(small arrows)* represents a loculated pneumothorax. Note, in addition, a deep sulcus sign *(large arrow). B,* An anteroposterior (AP) view of the chest in another infant demonstrates a lucency or dark area overlying the medial aspect of the right lung and outlining the right cardiac border. This represents an anterior medial right pneumothorax. *C,* A lateral view of the chest with this patient supine is the best way to see an anterior pneumothorax. It will be seen as a dark collection of air in the retrosternal region and in the anterior costophrenic angle *(arrows).*

Asthma

Asthma is one of the most common pulmonary disorders in children. Reversible airway obstruction can range from mild to life threatening. Asthma and wheezing (easy inspiration and difficult expiration) should be differentiated from stridor (difficult inspiration and easier expiration). The latter indicates an upper airway obstruction. The initial workup of asthma includes history, physical examination, and pulmonary function tests (particularly forced expiratory volume in 1 sec [FEV_1]). In young children, it is important to exclude inhaled foreign bodies, cystic fibrosis, enlarged lymph

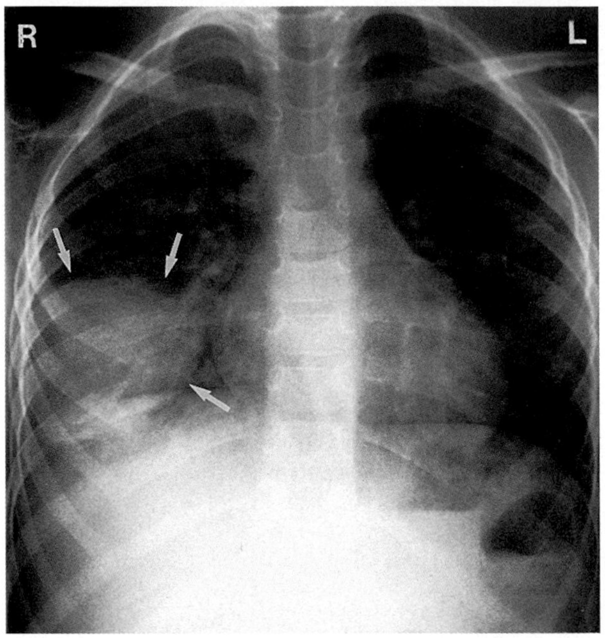

FIGURE 9-17 ■ Round pneumonia. A posteroanterior (PA) view of the chest demonstrates a rounded density in the right lower lobe *(arrows)*. Usually this will progress to a standard lobar consolidation of a typical pneumonia.

nodes, or neoplasms obstructing the bronchi. For patients with known asthma and a simple attack, a chest x-ray is not indicated. If there is suspicion of a complicating factor (fever or pneumonia) or a poor response to therapy, a chest x-ray is indicated.

Cystic Fibrosis

Cystic fibrosis is caused by a dysfunction of the exocrine glands producing thick mucus that accumulates in the lungs, causing bronchitis and recurrent pneumonias. It is an autosomal recessive disorder and is the most common lethal genetic disease affecting whites. Pulmonary findings are present in essentially all cases by the time a child is age 10 years or older. The most obvious finding is hyperinflation. Essentially, the chest x-ray looks like that of an adult with chronic obstructive pulmonary disease (COPD), with an increased AP diameter and flattening of the hemidiaphragms. In addition, the lungs generally appear "dirty." Peribronchial thickening and bronchiectasis are found with many pulmonary markings at the lung bases (Fig. 9-18). These are not lobar or segmental infiltrates.

Children with cystic fibrosis also are prone to a wide variety of gastrointestinal problems, including meconium ileus, meconium peritonitis, rectal prolapse, volvulus, intussusception, pancreatitis, jaundice, and growth failure or vitamin deficiencies. You should suspect cystic fibrosis in any child with recurrent respiratory or gastrointestinal symptoms.

PEDIATRIC ABDOMINAL IMAGING

Congenital diaphragmatic hernia has already been mentioned, but you should be aware of a number of other congenital abnormalities of the bowel in neonates

Esophageal Fistula

Tracheoesophageal fistula (TEF) may be suspected in an infant who has had polyhydramnios. This is usually clinically apparent, because of excessive salivation; as soon as an attempt is made to feed the child, aspiration, coughing, and choking occur. Ninety-five percent of patients with a TEF will have a blind-ending esophagus. The diagnosis is usually made by passing a small, soft feeding tube down the esophagus to the blind end and taking a lateral x-ray. If necessary, air can be injected to help visualization. Instillation of barium or other contrast material is rarely, if ever, indicated. In those few patients with an "H-type" fistula and a patent esophagus, it may take months to arrive at the diagnosis, but the disorder should be suspected in a child with recurrent pneumonias or chronic cough. You should remember that 40% of patients with TEF have associated cardiac and other gastrointestinal anomalies. The VATER syndrome describes the association among *v*ertebral anomalies (hemivertebra), *a*nal atresia, (*t*racheo-*e*sophageal fistula), and *r*adial limb dysplasia.

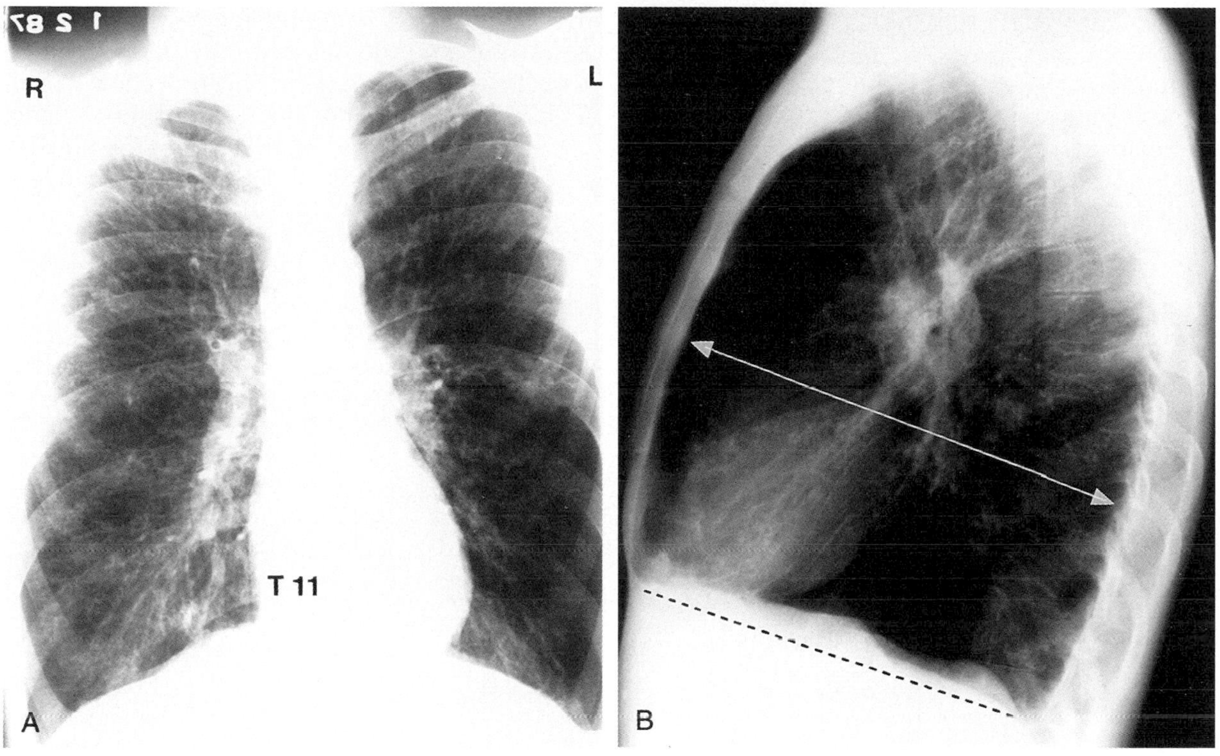

FIGURE 9-18 ■ Cystic fibrosis. *A,* The posteroanterior (PA) view of the chest in this young teenager demonstrates marked hyperinflation, with the hemidiaphragms being flattened and pushed down to the level of the posterior eleventh ribs. Diffuse bronchial thickening throughout both lungs is shown. *B,* The lateral view of the chest shows an increase in anteroposterior (AP) diameter and flattening of the hemidiaphragms. These findings in an adult would normally be associated with chronic obstructive pulmonary disease, but in a teenager or child, they are almost certainly due to cystic fibrosis.

Acute Gastroenteritis

The usual clinical presentation is acute onset of diarrhea, vomiting, or both. Dehydration is the major complication. Acute gastroenteritis is usually due to viruses (Rotavirus or Norwalk agent). In extremely ill patients, a stool culture or toxin assay is indicated. If the patient has abdominal pain or distention, the differential diagnosis includes appendicitis, intussusception, or bowel obstruction. In these circumstances, a plain and upright film of the abdomen or a CT scan may be helpful. These are discussed in more detail in Chapter 6. For simple gastroenteritis, no imaging studies are indicated.

Bowel Obstruction

Air should normally be seen in the abdomen of the neonate in the following temporal progression: in the stomach 2 hours after birth, in the small bowel at 6 hours, and in the rectum by 24 hours. Hypertrophic pyloric stenosis is the second most common gastrointestinal (GI) condition requiring surgery in the first 2 months of life. Pyloric stenosis is more common in male infants and should be suspected if a maternal or sibling history of the condition exists. The typical clinical symptom is nonbilious vomiting during the second to fourth week of life. A palpable olive-shaped mass may be found to the right of the umbilicus. A plain x-ray of the abdomen will show a stomach that is dilated to more than 7 cm, and peristaltic waves can sometimes be seen, giving the stomach a caterpillar appearance. The diagnosis is confirmed by using abdominal ultrasound to visualize the thickened pyloric muscle. The pyloric muscle should not be more than 4 mm in thickness (mucosa to outside wall) or greater than 18 mm in length (Fig. 9-19).

Duodenal atresias, midgut volvulus, and pyloric stenosis are apparent because they produce obstruction and vomiting. Under these circumstances, consult the radiologist as to what imaging procedure would be best. The approximate level of obstruction in the bowel is typically determined on the plain film by seeing how far bowel gas has progressed through the GI tract. If gas is seen only in the stomach or the stomach and duodenum (the "double-bubble" sign), a proximal obstruction is likely. Duodenal atresia or midgut volvulus should be suspected in a

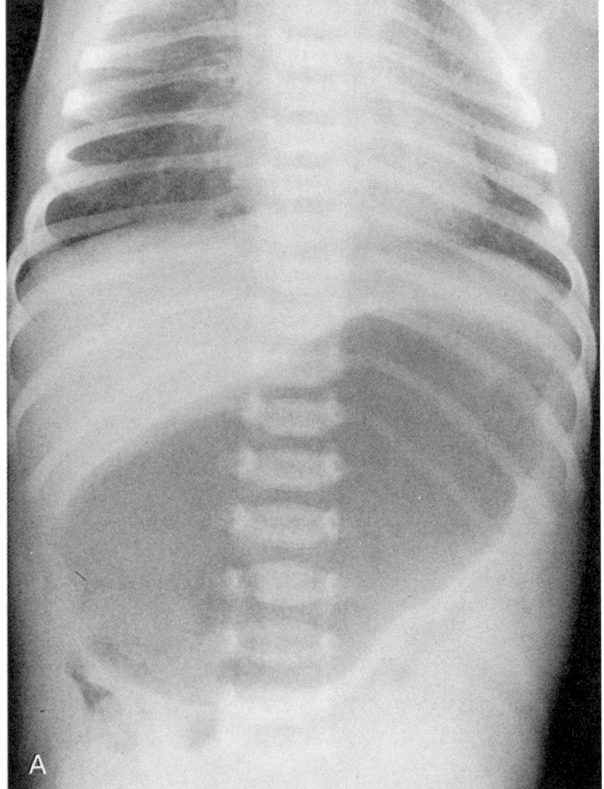

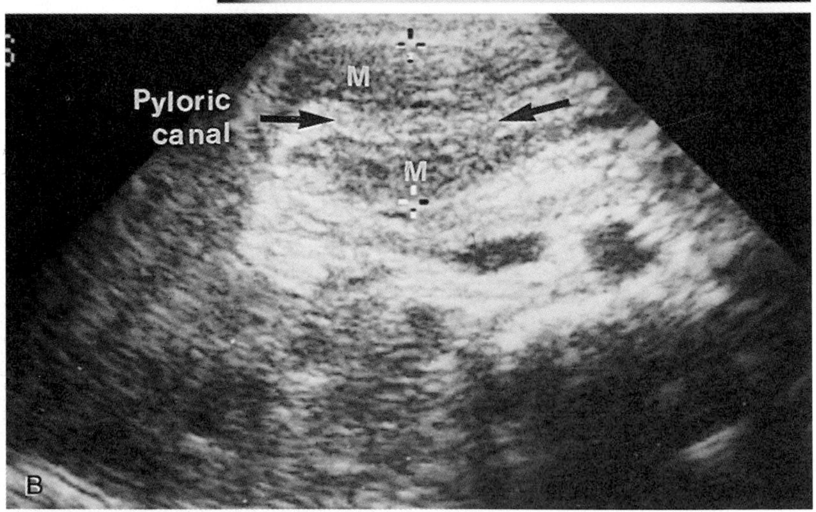

FIGURE 9-19 ■ **Pyloric stenosis.** *A,* A KUB (kidneys, ureters, bladder) image of the abdomen shows a markedly dilated, gas-filled stomach. *B,* A transverse ultrasound study of the upper abdomen shows the thickened pyloric muscle (M) on both sides of the pyloric canal.

birth with polyhydramnios and an infant who has bile-stained vomiting. Duodenal atresia is the most common cause of the double-bubble sign, with annular pancreas being the next most common. Duodenal bands, webs, and midgut volvulus are less frequent. Duodenal atresia has been associated with Down syndrome. Midgut volvulus, although less common, is important to consider, because a high mortality rate occurs without intervention. A midgut volvulus occurs when the small bowel and proximal colon rotate about the axis of the superior mesenteric artery; this can cause arterial compromise and gangrene.

If air is seen beyond the duodenum but not into the distal small bowel or colon, you should think of midlevel lesions. Atresias can occur in the jejunum and ileum. With any of these entities, even with x-ray contrast studies, it is not possible to tell with certainty either the site of or the length of the atresia or even to differentiate an atresia from a midgut volvulus. As a result, most pediatric surgeons are content with the plain x-ray findings before proceeding to surgery. Occasionally some will request a barium enema to look for a microcolon before surgery.

If gas is seen throughout most of the abdomen of a neonate but not in the region of the rectum, a distal small bowel or colon obstruction should be suspected. This may be the result of either a meconium ileus or Hirschsprung's disease. A note of caution should be entered here relative to the appearance of bowel gas in a neonate or very young child. Gas in the small bowel and colon look exactly the same, and you should not allow yourself to think that you can tell the difference. Rather, differential diagnoses are made on the basis of whether gas is seen in the proximal or distal "bowel."

Meconium ileus is seen in 50% of patients with cystic fibrosis. On an enema performed with water-soluble contrast, the colon is seen to be very small (microcolon), because it was unused during fetal life (Fig. 9-20). Hirschsprung's disease is due to the absence of neural cells in the distal segment of the colon; these children are seen in the first 6 weeks of life with obstruction or constipation. This disorder should be suspected in any infant who fails to pass meconium in the first 24 hours of life. In about 75% of patients, the abnormal segment is restricted to

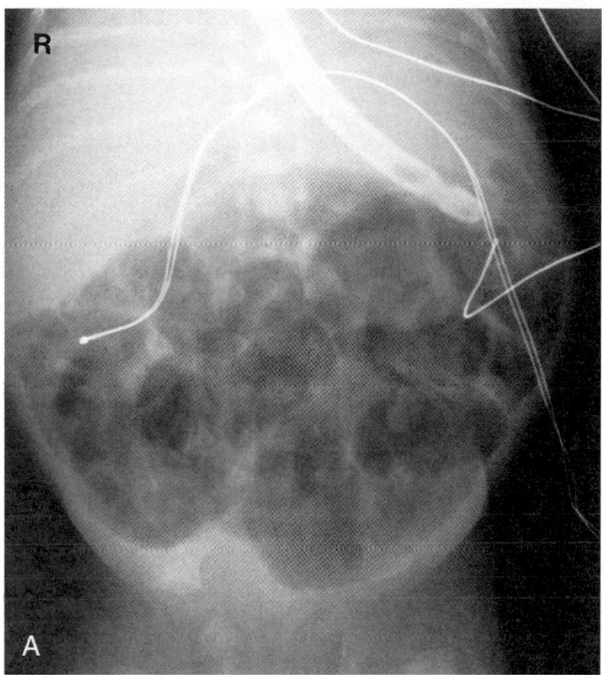

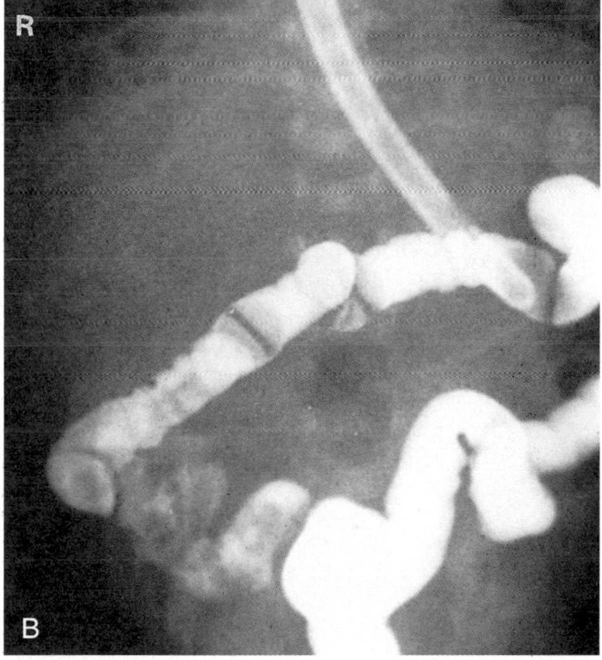

FIGURE 9-20 ■ Meconium ileus. *A,* An anteroposterior (AP) view of the abdomen demonstrates dilated bowel. In a child of this age, it is not possible to differentiate the colon from the small bowel. However, no gas is seen within the rectum. B, A Gastrografin enema has been performed, and the colon is noted to be very small (a microcolon). Intraluminal defects are seen in the colon at the level of the ileocecal valve, because usually obstruction at this level results from the thick tenacious meconium adhering to small bowel.

the rectosigmoid colon. On a barium enema, a narrowed segment may be identified (Fig. 9-21).

Intussusception is invagination of a segment of bowel into more distal bowel and usually occurs with ileum telescoping into colon. Forty percent of patients are initially seen between ages 3 months and 18 months, most with pain and vomiting. A lesser number have an associated abdominal mass or rectal bleeding. Intussusception is rarely seen in neonates. Clinically the children have an acute onset of colicky pain, and they may cry, draw up their knees, and vomit. Sometimes a sausage-shaped mass can be felt in the upper abdomen. Radiographically, plain x-rays are often normal. If the intussusception has occurred within 24 hours before the patient is seen, a radiologist has a good chance of reducing it with a water-soluble contrast enema. Currently, however, most radiologists prefer to reduce intussusception simply by using air (Fig. 9-22). If this fails, surgery is necessary. Reduction by a radiologist should not be attempted if clinical signs of peritonitis or shock are found. Other relatively common lesions to bear in mind when it looks as though there is a proximal bowel obstruction in a child aged 6 to 30 months are an incarcerated inguinal hernia and appendicitis.

Necrotizing Enterocolitis

Necrotizing enterocolitis is the most common GI emergency in premature infants. It usually develops within the first week after birth but can be seen up to 2 months after birth. Clinical signs are abdominal tenderness, rectal bleeding, and a septic shock–like appearance. The earliest radiographic sign is air within the wall of the bowel

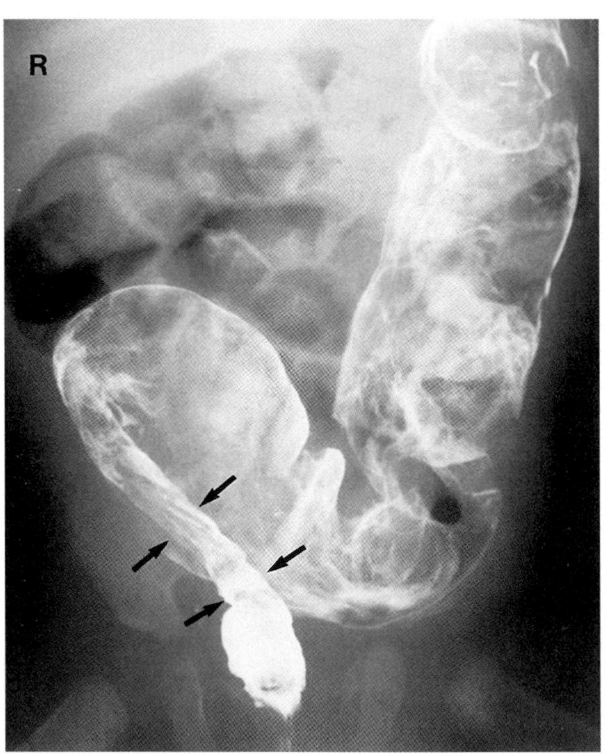

FIGURE 9-21 ■ Hirschsprung's disease. This abnormality is due to an absence of myenteric plexus cells in the distal colon. A barium enema demonstrates a narrowed segment in the rectum and a markedly dilated sigmoid and descending colon.

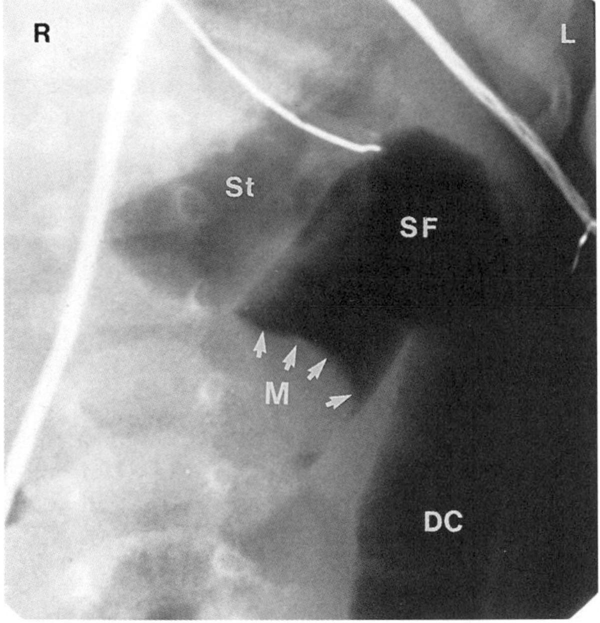

FIGURE 9-22 ■ Intussusception. This 3-year-old had colicky abdominal pain and rectal bleeding. Invagination of a segment of bowel into more distal bowel can be seen. Ileocolic and ileoileocolic intussusceptions represent 90% of occurrences. Here, a film has been obtained while the radiologist is reducing the intussusception with air. Air is seen in the distal colon (DC) and the splenic flexure (SF), and the mass (M) representing the leading portion of the intussuscepted segment is clearly identified.

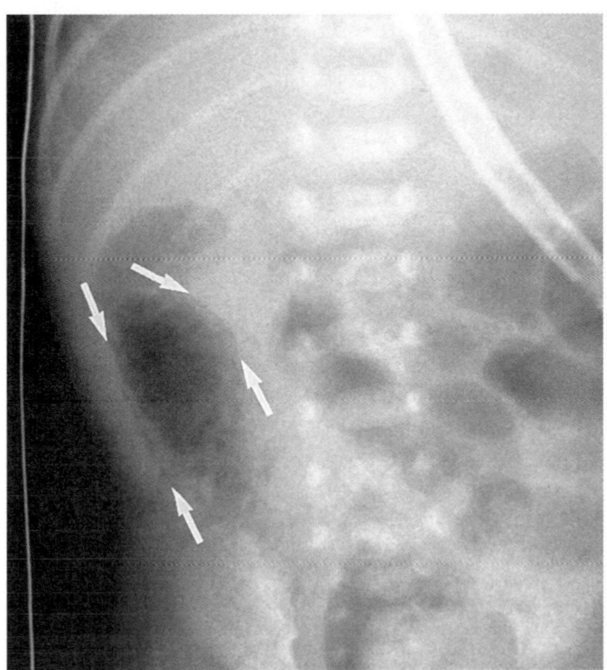

FIGURE 9-23 ■ **Necrotizing enterocolitis.** This represents the most common gastrointestinal emergency in premature infants. A plain x-ray of the abdomen of this 5-day-old infant shows abnormal collections of air within the bowel wall *(arrows).*

(pneumatosis) or a bubbly appearance of the bowel. Another early finding is small bowel dilatation due to an adynamic ileus (Fig. 9-23). Common complications and indications for surgery include free air within the peritoneal cavity, which indicates a bowel perforation. Gas in the portal vein also may be identified. In contrast with adults, in whom this condition generally portends a fatal outcome, the outcome in children with portal venous air is not so bad.

On a supine view, if a large amount of free air is noted within the peritoneal cavity, the air will outline the falciform ligament of the liver (the "football sign") (Fig. 9-24). This is a fairly subtle sign; a large amount of air may be present in the peritoneal cavity, and, on a supine film, you may easily overlook it. For this reason, a left lateral decubitus view, which will show air over the lateral margin of the liver, is often recommended.

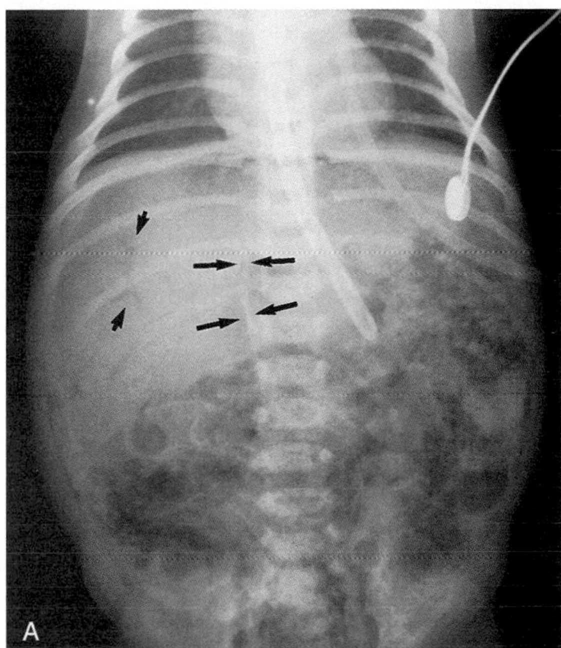

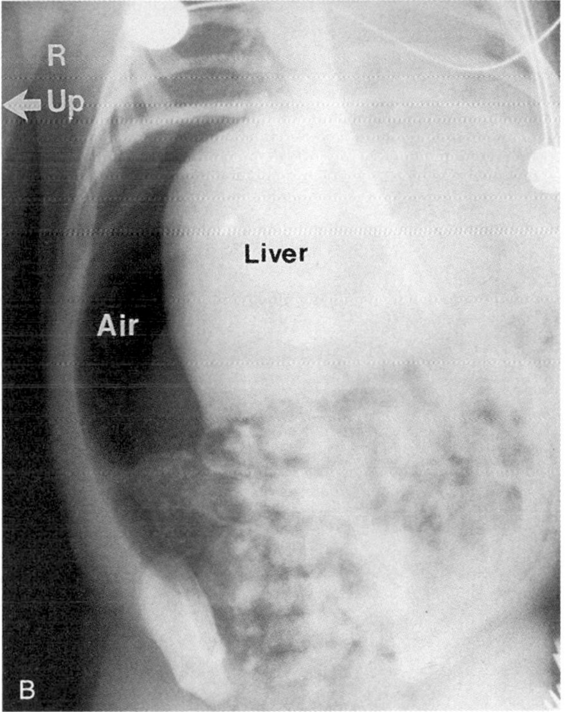

FIGURE 9-24 ■ **Complications of necrotizing enterocolitis.** A, A supine abdominal x-ray of the abdomen demonstrates diffuse mottled air throughout the bowel wall and shows air within the portal venous system *(short arrows)* as well. The falciform ligament is outlined by free air *(long arrows)* anteriorly in the peritoneal cavity. To the uninitiated, the amount of free air is difficult to appreciate. *B,* A left lateral decubitus view obtained in the same patient immediately afterward demonstrates a very large amount of free air overlying the surface of the liver.

Meckel's Diverticulum

Meckel's diverticulum is a vestigial remnant of the omphalomesenteric duct, and it may contain gastric mucosa. Clinical signs are painless rectal bleeding and, occasionally, intestinal obstruction. Meckel's diverticulum follows what is known as the rule of twos. It occurs in 2% of the population; it usually is first seen before age 2 years; and the diverticulum is usually located in the ileum within 2 feet of the ileocecal valve. If gastric mucosa is present in the diverticulum, ulceration and hemorrhage may result. In patients with rectal bleeding before age 2 years, Meckel's diverticulum should be considered. The imaging study of choice is a nuclear medicine scan done with technetium pertechnetate. This concentrates in the normal and ectopic gastric mucosa and allows identification of Meckel's diverticulum (Fig. 9-25).

Neonatal Jaundice

In some very young infants (2 to 3 weeks old), jaundice may develop. The usual diagnostic dilemma is whether the infant has neonatal hepatitis or biliary atresia. The imaging test of choice is a nuclear medicine hepatobiliary scan. This involves giving a small amount of radioactive tracer that is concentrated by the liver and then excreted via the biliary system. If any excretion into the small bowel is detected on the images, biliary atresia is excluded. Occasionally, in patients with severe hepatitis, follow-up images are needed at 24 hours after injection, to be certain of the diagnosis.

Adbominal Masses

Abdominal masses in children are usually initially worked up by clinical examination and

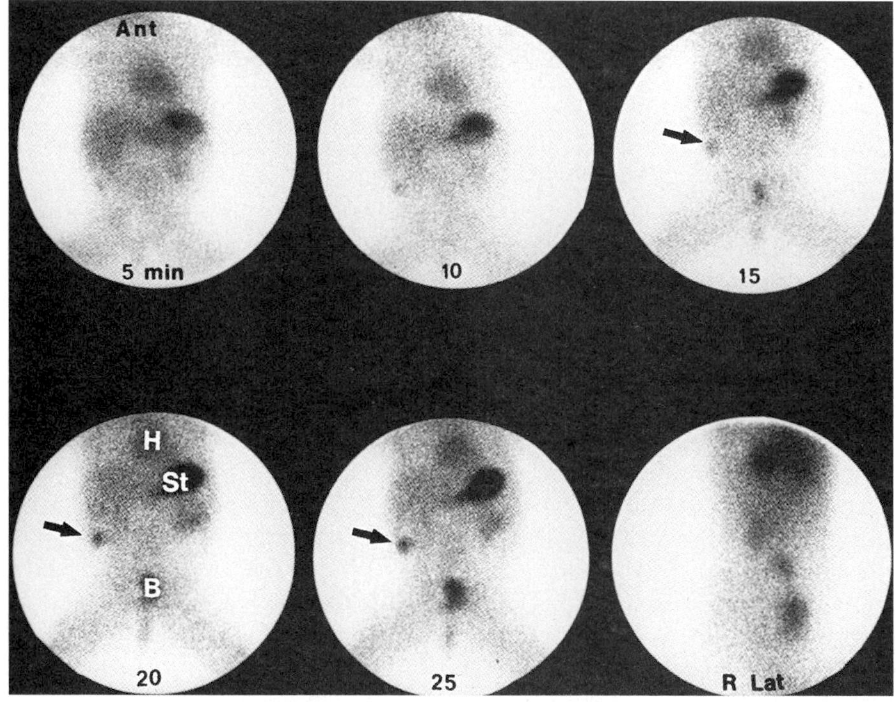

FIGURE 9-25 ■ Meckel's diverticulum. In this 2-year-old child with unexplained rectal bleeding, a nuclear medicine study was performed using radioactive material that concentrates in gastric mucosa (technetium-99m pertechnetate). Sequential 5-min images of the abdomen are obtained. On the 20-min image, the heart (H), stomach (St), and bladder (B) are clearly seen as well as an ectopic focus of activity *(arrow)* representing a Meckel's diverticulum.

a plain x-ray of the abdomen. The differential diagnosis of an abdominal mass varies with the child's age. A mass in the abdomen of a child of any age most likely arises from the kidneys. In a neonate, 55% of masses are renal in origin (hydronephrosis or multicystic dysplastic kidney), and the remainder are usually gastrointestinal duplications, cysts, and hemangioendotheliomas of the liver.

If a mass appears to be in the flank in an older infant or child, Wilms' tumor, neuroblastoma, and hydronephrosis account for about 80% of the lesions. Other possibilities include abscesses, cysts, and hepatoblastomas. Neuroblastomas have calcification approximately 90% of the time (Fig. 9-26) and are usually seen in patients younger than 2 years. They appear as masses external to the kidney and tend to displace the kidney rather than deform it. Because neuroblastomas arise from neural tissue, they also are relatively common in the region of the adrenal glands, along the sympathetic chain, and in the posterior mediastinum (Fig. 9-27). Wilms' tumor begins within the kidney, and on an intravenous pyelogram, it will be seen as a mass within the kidney, deforming the normal collecting system (Fig. 9-28). Wilms' tumors are bilateral 10% of the time and are rarely calcified. The average age of presentation is 2 years to 3 years, which is older than the usual age for neuroblastomas.

Rectal Bleeding

Rectal bleeding in children should be classified as dark or bright red and painless or painful. Dark red blood usually indicates upper GI origin, and the differential diagnosis includes foreign body, varices, peptic ulcer, and bowel duplication. Painful dark or bright rectal bleeding is associated with volvulus, mesenteric thrombosis, and Meckel's diverticulum.

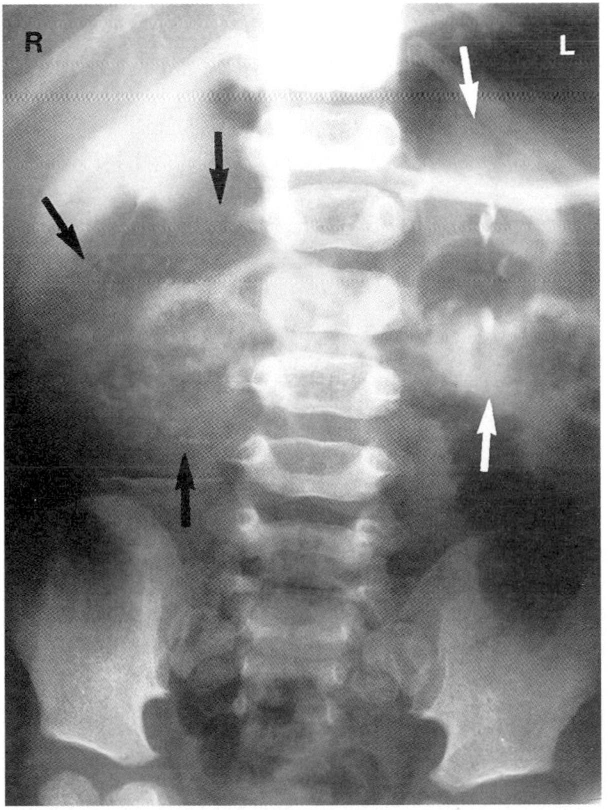

FIGURE 9-26 ■ **Retroperitoneal neuroblastoma.** On this intravenous pyelogram, the left kidney appears to be functioning well *(white arrows)*. On the right, no functional kidney is identified, but the multiple scattered tiny amorphous calcifications are often seen with this tumor.

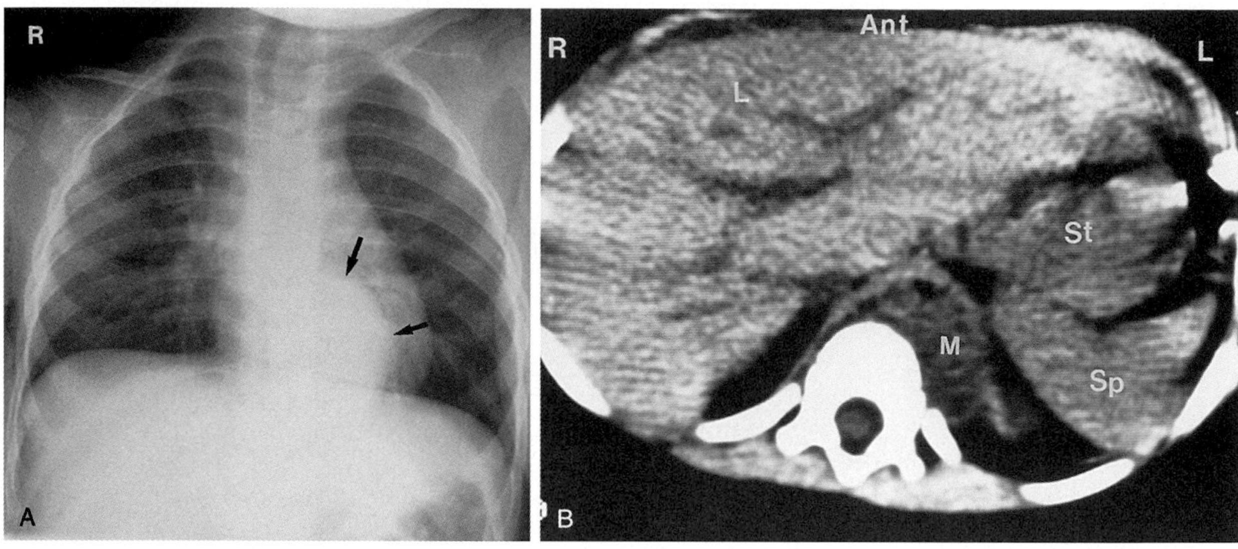

FIGURE 9-27 ■ Posterior mediastinal neuroblastoma. *A,* A posteroanterior (PA) view of the chest demonstrates a rounded retrocardiac mass *(arrows)*. *B,* On a transverse computed tomography scan, the liver (L), spleen (Sp), and stomach (St) are seen, with a mass (M) in the left paraspinous region.

Bright red painless bleeding may be due to a polyp, neoplasm, colitis, or sigmoid intussusception. Painful bright red bleeding is most commonly due to an anal fissure, hemorrhoids, or rectal prolapse; for these, no imaging studies are usually needed. Rectal bleeding in young children can also be due to an allergy to formula.

The workup of any rectal bleeding should begin with a rectal examination. If an obvious cause is not identified and particularly if associated pain, vomiting, guarding, rebound, or abdominal distention is present, a surgical consultation should be obtained. The imaging workup depends on which of the causes is thought to be most likely, although either endoscopy or a plain x-ray of the abdomen with an air or barium enema is often obtained.

Urinary Abnormalities

Two relatively common urinary problems in children are hydronephrosis and ureterovesicular reflux. The most common cause of hydronephrosis in a child is an obstruction at the junction of the lower portion of the renal pelvis and the upper ureter (UPJ). The entity is bilateral in 20% of cases. The initial imaging test of choice is an intravenous pyelogram. Although the dilated collecting system can be visualized with ultrasound, usually not enough anatomic detail of the ureter is found, and no information about renal function is provided. Postoperative follow-up functional studies in these children are usually done with a nuclear medicine furosemide (Lasix) renogram, because the radiation dose is lower with no risk of a contrast reaction. If only information about the degree of dilatation of the collecting system is desired, ultrasound is the test of choice.

Ureterovesicular reflux is due to maldevelopment of the flap valve that is created as the ureter crosses obliquely through the bladder wall. Less commonly, it can be due to ectopic insertion of a ureter when ureteral duplication is found or to a ureterocele. On a contrast study, any visible reflux of urine from the bladder into a ureter is abnormal. If severe, it is surgically repaired because of the increased risk of infection. The most common imaging method is a cystogram. A catheter is placed, contrast is put into the bladder, and the radiol-

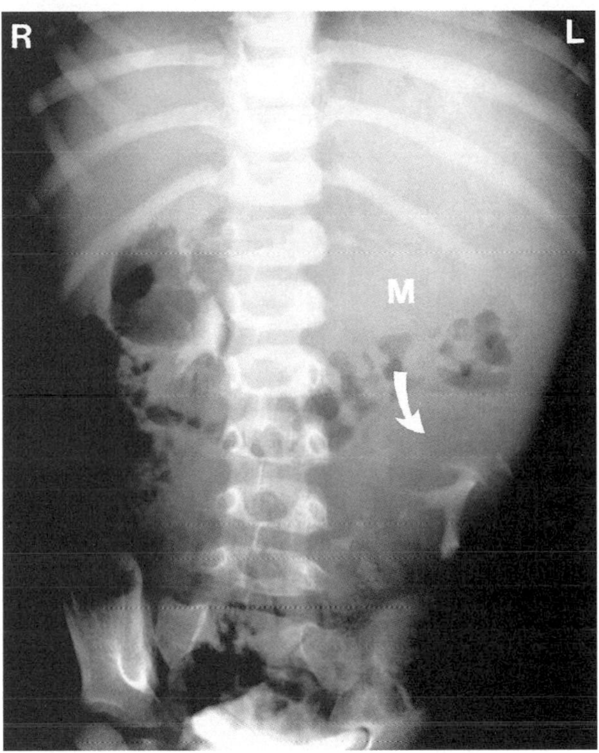

FIGURE 9-28 ■ **Wilms' tumor.** On this intravenous pyelogram, the collecting system of the right kidney is identified along the lateral border of L1, L2, and L3. The collecting system of the left kidney (*arrow*) has been displaced inferiorly by a mass (M), and the collecting system has been distorted, suggesting that the mass is intrarenal in origin. This is a common way of differentiating an intraparenchymal Wilms' tumor from an extrarenal neuroblastoma.

ogist looks for contrast in the ureters. This involves a relatively high radiation dose to the child's gonads, but the anatomic resolution is good. If repeated evaluations of reflux are necessary, a nuclear medicine cystogram can provide good quantitative information with a much lower dose.

Multicystic dysplastic kidney is a unilateral process resulting from a severe UPJ obstruction in utero. As a result, no functional renal parenchyma is present, and the kidney is represented by a large number of noncommunicating cysts. Calcification may be present, with absent or only very small renal vessels. A retrograde pyelogram shows a blind-ending ureter. Surgery is not immediately necessary. Another congenital condition is called multilocular cystic nephroma, which has large cystic areas. Calcifications in this entity are rare.

Neonatal or infantile polycystic disease is not initially seen with a dominant abdominal mass. Each has ectasia of renal tubules, but no obvious cysts are visible by imaging methods. Ultrasound is the test of choice in the neonatal form; most tubules are ectatic, and death usually occurs in months or years. Little associated hepatic fibrosis develops. In the infantile form, about 20% of the tubules are ectatic, and symptoms do not appear for 3 to 6 months. Moderate hepatic fibrosis is seen. In the juvenile form, fewer tubules are ectatic, and symptoms appear at age 1 to 5 years. The liver fibrosis is severe in this form, and death results from portal hypertension.

Suggested Textbooks on the Topic

Kuhn JP, Slovis T, Haller J: Caffey's Pediatric Diagnostic Imaging, 10th ed. Philadelphia, WB Saunders, 2003.

Swischuk L: Emergency Imaging of the Acutely Ill or Injured Child, 5th ed. Philadelphia, Lippincott Williams & Wilkins, 2003.

Appendix

TABLE A-1 ■ **Typical Price Range of Some Imaging Procedures***

Diagnostic Radiology	
Chest	$30–130
Abdomen	25–115
Pelvis	24–140
Hand	25–100
Ankle	25–100
Barium enema	120–450
Intravenous pyelogram	80–310
Mammogram (bilateral)	72–160
Computed Tomography	
Brain without contrast	195–950
Chest without contrast	250–900
Abdomen and pelvis with contrast	560–1980
Magnetic Resonance	
Brain with contrast	500–1900
Lumbar spine	470–1550
Knee	420–800
Nuclear Medicine	
Bone	110–420
Myocardial perfusion with wall motion	330–800
Ultrasound	
Fetal	115–400
Right upper quadrant	100–350

*Price includes hospital and physician charges. The lower end of the range is the fee paid by Medicare, and the upper end is the total fee charged (as compared with paid). Many contracted imaging services offer 20% to 40% discounts on charged fees. Considerable additional charges for contrast agents or radiopharmaceuticals can be hundreds of dollars per procedure.

TABLE A-2 ■ **Radiation Doses from Various Examinations**

Examination	Effective Dose* mSv (mrem)	Gonadal Dose mSv (mrem)
Routine X-rays		
Extremities	0.01 (1)	< 0.01 (<1)
Skull	0.22 (22)	< 0.01 (<1)
Chest (2 views)	0.1 (10)	0.01 (1)
KUB (abdomen 1 view)	0.6 (60)	1/2 (100/220)†
Lumbar spine	1.3 (130)	2.2/7.2 (220/720)
Pelvis or hips	0.5 (50)	2.1/6.0 (210/600)
Barium enema	4.1 (410)	1.75/9.00(175/900)
CT scans		
Head or body	1.1 (110)	—
Nuclear Medicine Scans		
Bone	4.4 (440)	3.2/4.4 (320/440)
Lung	1.5 (150)	2.3/0.3 (230/30)
Cardiac (thallium)	7.0 (700)	19.0/5.6 (1900/560)
Hepatobiliary	3.7 (370)	0.2/0.5 (20/50)
Ultrasound or Magnetic Resonance Imaging	None	None

*The effective dose from natural background radiation in the United States is 3 mSv (300 mrem) per year.
†Refers to male/female. Gonadal dose in the female approximates dose to the fetus in a pregnant female.

Index

Note: Page numbers followed by the letter f refer to figures and those followed by t refer to tables.